Nursing Research

Principles and Methods

SIXTH EDITION

Nursing Research

Principles and Methods

DENISE F. POLIT, Ph.D.
President
Humanalysis, Inc.
Saratoga Springs, New York

BERNADETTE P. HUNGLER, R.N., Ph.D.
Associate Professor, Retired
Boston College School of Nursing
Chestnut Hill, Massachusetts

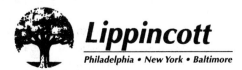

Lippincott
Philadelphia • New York • Baltimore

Acquisitions Editor: Margaret Zuccarini
Sponsoring Editor: Sara Lauber
Senior Project Editor: Erika Kors
Senior Production Manager: Helen Ewan
Senior Production Coordinator: Michael Carcel
Assistant Art Director: Kathy Kelley-Luedtke

6th Edition

9 8 7 6 5 4 3

Library of Congress Cataloging in Publications Data

Polit, Denise.
   Nursing research: principles and methods/Denise F. Polit, Bernadette P. Hungler. —6th ed.
      p. cm.
   Includes bibliographical references and index.
   ISBN 0-7817-1562-8 (alk. paper)
   1. Nursing—Research—Methodology. I. Hungler, Bernadette P.
  II. Title.
      [DNLM: 1. Nursing Research—methods. WY 20.5P769n 1999]
   RT81.5.P64 1999
610.73'072—dc21
DNLM/DLC
for Library of Congress   98-39678
                                                                    CIP

Care has been taken to confirm the accuracy of the information presented and to describe generally accepted practices. However, the authors, editors, and publisher are not responsible for errors or omissions or for any consequences from application of the information in this book and make no warranty, express or implied, with respect to the contents of the publication.

The authors, editors and publisher have exerted every effort to ensure that drug selection and dosage set forth in this text are in accordance with current recommendations and practice at the time of publication. However, in view of ongoing research, changes in government regulations, and the constant flow of information relating to drug therapy and drug reactions, the reader is urged to check the package insert for each drug for any change in indications and dosage and for added warnings and precautions. This is particularly important when the recommended agent is a new or infrequently employed drug.

Some drugs and medical devices presented in this publication have Food and Drug Administration (FDA) clearance for limited use in restricted research settings. It is the responsibility of the health care provider to ascertain the FDA status of each drug or device planned for use in their clinical practice.

To James

whose energy and intellect are an inspiration,
and whose love and support made this edition possible

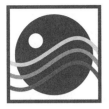

PREFACE

This sixth edition of *Nursing Research: Principles and Methods* presents extensive changes to this award-winning textbook. This edition retains all of the features that have made this textbook popular in the past, while introducing innovations that we think will make it more useful to a broader audience of those who are learning how to do research, as well as to the growing number of nurses who are learning to appraise research reports critically. The uses to which the first five editions have been put suggest that we have reached both producers and consumers of nursing research.

NEW TO THIS EDITION

- **Balanced presentation of qualitative and quantitative research methods.** For the first time, this textbook discusses the methods associated with naturalistic inquiries (qualitative studies) in a manner roughly parallel to the description of methods more typically used in traditional scientific research (quantitative studies). The text compares and contrasts qualitative and quantitative studies with regard to each aspect of a study—from the posing of a question to the analysis and interpretation of research information. This treatment represents an important innovation that is unprecedented in nursing research textbooks and that acknowledges the growing importance of qualitative studies in nursing.

- **A new chapter on qualitative research design and approaches.** This chapter (Chapter 10) discusses major approaches to qualitative inquiry, and design features associated with different qualitative traditions, such as ethnography, phenomenology, and grounded theory.

- **Expanded discussion of multimethod research.** The increasing number of qualitative inquiries has been accompanied by a growing interest in mixed method research that involves both qualitative and quantitative approaches in a single study. This edition offers greater coverage of design options for such investigations.

ORGANIZATION OF THE TEXT

The content of this edition is organized into six main parts.

- **Part I—Introduction to Nursing Research** serves as the overall introduction to fundamental concepts in nursing research. Chapter 1 summarizes the history and future of nursing research, discusses the philosophical underpinnings of qualitative research versus quantitative research, and describes the major purposes of nursing research. Chapter 2 presents an overview of the steps in the research process for both qualitative and quantitative studies and defines some key research terms. Chapter 3 focuses on the development of research questions and the formulation of research hypotheses.

- **Part II—Contexts for Nursing Research** further sets the stage for learning about the research process by discussing several types of contexts for nursing research: the context of prior knowledge through literature reviews (Chapter 4); conceptual and theoretical contexts (Chapter 5); and the ethical context of research with human beings (Chapter 6).
- **Part III—Designs for Nursing Research** presents material relating to the design of nursing research studies. Chapter 7 describes some fundamental principles of research design. Chapter 8 goes on to discuss many specific aspects of research design for quantitative studies, while Chapter 9 describes mechanisms of research control for quantitative studies. Chapter 10 is devoted to research designs for qualitative studies, and Chapter 11 discusses mixed method research designs in which methods for qualitative and quantitative inquiry are blended. Chapter 12 presents various designs and strategies for selecting samples of study participants.
- **Part IV—Measurement and Data Collection** deals with the collection of research data. Chapter 13 discusses the design of a data collection plan, and the subsequent three chapters present materials on specific data collection methods such as self-reports (Chapter 14), observation (Chapter 15), and biophysiologic and other methods (Chapter 16). Chapter 17 discusses the concept and measurement, as well as methods of assessing data quality.
- **Part V—The Analysis of Research Data** discusses methods of analyzing qualitative and quantitative data. Chapters 18, 19, and 20 present an overview of univariate, inferential, and multivariate statistical analyses, respectively. Chapter 21 describes the development of an overall data analytic strategy for quantitative

studies. Chapter 22 discusses methods of doing qualitative analyses. Chapter 23 describes the use of computers in analyzing research data.
- **Part VI—Communication in the Research Process** focuses on communication in research: writing about research (Chapter 24), critiquing written reports (Chapter 25), using the results of published studies in nursing practice (Chapter 26), and preparing research proposals (Chapter 27).

KEY FEATURES

Many of the features successfully used in previous editions have been retained in this sixth edition. Among the basic principles that helped to shape this and earlier editions of this book are (1) an unswerving conviction that the development of research skills is critical to the nursing profession; (2) a fundamental belief that research is an intellectually and professionally rewarding enterprise; and (3) a conviction that learning about research methods need be neither intimidating nor dull. Consistent with these principles, we have tried to present the fundamentals of research methods in a way that both facilitates understanding and stimulates curiosity and interest. Key features of our approach include the following:

- **Research Examples.** Each chapter concludes with one or two actual research examples (usually one quantitative and one qualitative study) designed to highlight critical points made in the chapter and to sharpen the reader's critical thinking skills. In addition, many real and fictitious research examples are used to illustrate key points in the text. The use of relevant examples is crucial to the development of both an understanding of and an interest in the research process. We also hope that the inclusion of many research ideas will stimulate students' thinking about a research project.

- **Clear, "user friendly" style.** Our writing style is designed to be easily digestible and nonintimidating. Concepts are introduced carefully and systematically, difficult ideas are presented clearly and from several vantage points, and readers are assumed to have no prior exposure to technical terms.
- **Specific practical tips on doing research.** The textbook is filled with practical guidance on how to translate the abstract notions of research methods into realistic strategies for conducting research. Nearly every chapter concludes with a series of "tips" for applying the chapter's lessons to real-life situations. The development of these suggestions stems from our belief that there is often a large gap between what gets taught in a research methods textbook and what a researcher needs to know in conducting a study. Beyond these features in each chapter, there are three "how to" chapters that are designed to promote a smoother transition to actual research situations—how to design a research study, how to develop a data collection plan, and how to develop a data analysis plan.
- **Aids to student learning.** Several features are used to enhance and reinforce learning and to help focus the student's attention on specific areas of text content, including the following: detailed but succinct summaries at the end of each chapter; tables and figures that provide examples and graphic materials in support of the text discussion; study suggestions at the end of each chapter; and lists of suggested methodologic and substantive readings at the end of each chapter.

TEACHING-LEARNING PACKAGE

Nursing Research: Principles and Methods (6th edition) has an ancillary package designed with both students and instructors in mind.

- **The Study Guide** augments the textbook and provides the student with exercises that correspond to each text chapter. The Study Guide also includes two actual research reports.
- **The Instructor's Manual and Testbank** includes a chapter that corresponds to every chapter in the textbook. Each chapter contains a statement of intent, student objectives, new terms in the chapter, comments on selected research examples in the textbook, answers to certain Study Guide exercises, and test questions and answers.

We hope that the content and organization of this book continues to meet the needs of a broad spectrum of nursing students and nurse researchers.

Denise F. Polit, Ph.D.
Bernadette P. Hungler, R.N., Ph.D.

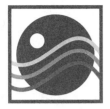

ACKNOWLEDGMENTS

This sixth edition, like the previous five editions, depended on the contribution of many individuals. We are deeply appreciative of those who made all six editions possible. In addition to all those who assisted us with the earlier editions, the following individuals deserve special mention.

Many faculty and students who used the text during the past 15 years have made invaluable suggestions for its improvement, and to all of you we are very grateful. In particular, we would like to acknowledge the continuing feedback from the nursing students and faculty at Boston College. Wanda Anderson and Marilyn Grant made important contributions to Chapter 5. Several of the examples used in the text and in the accompanying Study Guide were developed from ideas provided by Sarah Cimino, Ellen Mahoney, and Toni Hayes.

We also extend our warmest thanks to those who helped to turn the manuscript into a finished product. Sheila Singleton deserves special mention for her ongoing support in this and in earlier editions. The staff at Lippincott-Raven has been of tremendous assistance in the support they have given us over the years. We are indebted to Margaret Zuccarini, Sara Lauber, Erika Kors, Jody DeMatteo, and all the others behind the scenes for their fine contributions.

Finally, we thank our friends and family, who provided ongoing support and encouragement throughout this enterprise.

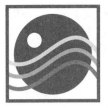

CONTENTS

CHAPTER 27

Writing a Research Proposal   671

Nursing Research
Principles and Methods

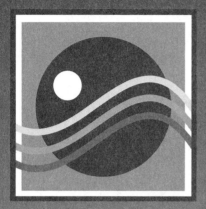

PART I

The Scientific
Research Process

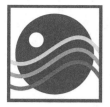

CHAPTER **1**

Introduction to Nursing Research

Nursing research involves a systematic search for and validation of knowledge about issues of importance to the nursing profession. Nursing research has experienced remarkable growth in the past three decades, providing nurses with an increasingly sound base of knowledge from which to practice. Yet many health care questions remain to be answered by nurse researchers—and many answers remain to be utilized by practicing nurses.

The purpose of this book is to acquaint members of the nursing profession with the fundamentals of research methods. This introductory chapter presents an overview of several important nursing research issues.

NURSING RESEARCH IN PERSPECTIVE

A consensus has emerged among nursing leaders that nurses at all levels should develop research skills. In this section, we discuss the rationale for this view.

The Importance of Research in Nursing

The ultimate goal of any profession is to provide its clientele with maximally effective and efficient services. A profession seeking to improve the practice of its members and to enhance its professional stature strives for the continual development of a relevant body of knowledge. Nursing research represents a critically important tool for the nursing profession to acquire such knowledge.

Professionalism. Nurses increasingly recognize the need to extend the base of nursing knowledge as part of professional responsibility and endorse research investigations as a way to achieve this objective. Moreover, nurses are committed to the evolution of a fairly distinct body of knowledge that separates nursing from other professions. Nursing is only one of several professions involved in the delivery of health care. Information from nursing investigations helps to define better the unique role that nursing plays.

Accountability. During the 1970s, nursing leaders pointed out that the quality of nursing care cannot be improved until information-based accountability becomes as much a part of nursing's tradition as humanitarianism. Nurses who incorporate research evidence into their clinical decisions are being professionally accountable to their clients and are also helping nursing to achieve its own professional identity.

3

Social Relevance of Nursing. Nurses today are being asked more than ever before to document their role in the delivery of health services. People are recognizing health care as a right rather than a privilege and, with spiraling costs, are asking various groups of health professionals how their services contribute to the total delivery of health care. This increased interest in examining health care practices makes it essential for nurses to evaluate the efficacy of their practices and to modify or abandon those practices shown to have no effect on client health.

Research and Decision Making in Nursing Practice. Many nurses use the Standards of Clinical Nursing Practice established by the American Nurses' Association (1991) both as their method of clinical practice and to evaluate the quality of their nursing care. The process requires nurses to engage in many decision-making activities. What will be assessed? What nursing diagnoses result from the assessment? What plan of care is most likely to produce the desired outcomes? What nursing interventions are necessary? How will the results be evaluated in terms of their effectiveness? Research conducted by nurses can potentially play a pivotal role at each phase of the nursing process by helping nurses to make more informed decisions.

The Consumer–Producer Continuum of Nursing Research

Nurses and nursing students have assumed a variety of roles in relation to disciplined research, forming a continuum that reflects their degree of active participation in the conduct of research. At one end of the continuum are those nurses whose involvement in research is indirect or passive. **Consumers** of nursing research read reports of studies, typically to keep up to date on information that may be relevant to their practice or to develop new skills. Nurses are increasingly expected to maintain, at a minimum, this level of involvement with research.

At the other end of the continuum are the **producers** of nursing research: nurses who actively participate in the design and conduct of research studies. At one time, most nurse researchers were academicians who taught in schools of nursing, but nurses in practice settings are increasingly doing their own research.

Between these two extremes lie a variety of research-related activities in which nurses engage as a way of enriching their professional lives and contributing to their clients. These activities include the following:

- Participating in a **journal club** in a practice setting, which involves regular meetings among nurses to discuss and critique research articles
- Attending professional conferences that present research findings
- Evaluating completed research for its possible utilization in the practice setting
- Discussing the implications and relevance of research findings with clients
- Assisting in the collection of research information (e.g., distributing questionnaires to patients or observing and recording patients' behaviors)
- Reviewing proposed methods for gathering research information with respect to their feasibility in a clinical setting
- Collaborating in the development of an idea for a research project
- Participating on an institutional committee whose mission is to review the ethical aspects of proposed research before it is undertaken
- Incorporating research findings into nursing practice or nursing education

In all these activities, nurses who have some research skills are in a better position to make a contribution to the nursing profession and to the base of nursing knowledge. Because of this fact, almost all accredited baccalaureate nursing programs include research content as a requirement for nursing students.

HISTORICAL EVOLUTION OF NURSING RESEARCH

Most people would agree that research in nursing began with Florence Nightingale. Her landmark publication, *Notes on Nursing* (1859), describes her early research interest in environmental factors that promote physical and emotional well-being. Nightingale's most widely known research contribution involved her data collection and analysis relating to factors affecting soldier mortality and morbidity during the Crimean War. Based on her skillful analyses and presentations, she was successful in effecting some changes in nursing care—and, more generally, in public health. During several years after Nightingale's work, however, little was added to the nursing literature concerning nursing research.

The Early Years

The pattern that nursing research followed subsequent to Florence Nightingale was closely aligned to the problems confronting nursing. For example, most of the studies conducted between 1900 and 1940 concerned nursing education. In 1923, one group, the Committee for the Study of Nursing Education, studied on a national level the educational preparation of nurse teachers, administrators, and public health nurses and the clinical experiences of nursing students. The committee issued what has become known as the Goldmark Report, which identified many inadequacies in the educational backgrounds of the groups studied and concluded that advanced educational preparation was essential. Partly as a result of that study, hospitals began employing registered nurses to give nursing care that freed student nurses from heavy service demands. As more nurses received university-based education, studies concerning students—their differential characteristics, problems, and satisfactions—became more numerous.

During the 1940s, studies concerning nursing education continued, spurred on by the unprecedented demand for nursing personnel that resulted from World War II. For example, Brown (1948) reassessed nursing education in her study initiated at the request of the National Nursing Council for War Service. The findings from the study, like those of the Goldmark Report, revealed numerous inadequacies in nursing education. Brown recommended that the education of nurses occur in collegiate settings. Many subsequent research investigations concerning the functions performed by nurses, nurses' roles and attitudes, hospital environments, and nurse–patient interactions stemmed from the Brown report.

A number of forces combined during the 1950s to put nursing research on a rapidly accelerating upswing that is still being experienced today. An increase in the number of nurses with advanced educational degrees, the establishment of a nursing research center at the Walter Reed Army Institute of Research, an increase in the availability of funds from the government and private foundations, and the inception of the American Nurses' Foundation—which is devoted exclusively to the promotion of nursing research—were major forces that provided impetus to the research movement in nursing during this period.

Until the 1950s, nurse researchers had few outlets for reporting their studies to the nursing community. The *American Journal of Nursing*, first published in 1900, began on a limited basis to publish some studies in the 1930s. The increasing number of research studies being conducted during the 1950s, however, created the need for a journal in which the findings from these studies could be published; thus, *Nursing Research* came into being in 1952.

Nursing research took a twist in the 1950s not experienced by research in other professions, at least not to the same extent as in nursing. Nurses studied themselves: Who is the nurse? What does the nurse do? Why do individuals choose to enter nursing? What are the characteristics of the ideal nurse? How do other groups perceive the nurse?

Nursing Research in the 1960s

The 1960s was the period during which terms such as *conceptual framework, conceptual model, nursing process,* and *theoretical base of nursing practice* began to appear in nursing literature and to influence views about the role of theory in nursing research. Funding continued to be available both for the educational preparation of nurses and for nursing research projects.

Nursing leaders increasingly expressed concern about the lack of research in nursing practice. Several professional nursing organizations established priorities for research investigations during this period. The Western Interstate Council for Higher Education in Nursing developed content for graduate education in the clinical areas of community health, maternal–child, medical–surgical, and psychiatric nursing and conducted workshops for faculty on the application of research knowledge.

Another important development in this decade was the establishment of a nursing archive by the Mugar Library at Boston University in the late 1960s. One purpose of the archive is to foster nursing research. Also, the *International Journal of Nursing Studies* was first published in 1963.

Nursing Research in the 1970s

By the 1970s, the growing number of nurses conducting research studies and the discussions of theoretical and contextual issues surrounding nursing research created the need for additional sources of communication. Three additional journals that focus on nursing research—*Advances in Nursing Science, Research in Nursing & Health,* and the *Western Journal of Nursing Research*—were established in that decade.

In the 1970s, there was also a change in emphasis in nursing research from areas such as teaching, administration, curriculum, recruitment, and nurses themselves to the improvement of client care—signifying a growing awareness by nurses of the need for a scientific base from which to practice. Nursing leaders strongly endorsed this direction for nursing studies. Lindeman (1975), for example, conducted a study to ascertain the views of nursing leaders concerning the focus of nursing studies. Clinical problems were identified as the highest priorities for nursing research.

Research skills among nurses continued to improve in the 1970s. The cadre of nurses with earned doctorates steadily increased, especially during the later part of the 1970s. The availability of both predoctoral and postdoctoral research fellowships facilitated advanced preparation in research skills.

Nursing Research in the 1980s

The 1980s brought nursing research to a new level of development. An increase in the number of qualified nurse researchers, the widespread availability of computers for the collection and analysis of information, and an ever-growing recognition that research is an integral part of professional nursing led nursing leaders to raise new issues and concerns. Increasing attention was given to the types of questions being asked, the methods of collecting and analyzing that would maximize what could be learned, the linking of research to theory, and the utilization of research findings in practice.

Several events provided impetus for nursing research. Of particular importance was the establishment in 1986 of the National Center for Nursing Research (NCNR) at the National Institutes of Health by congressional mandate. The purpose of NCNR was to promote—and financially support—research training and research projects relating to patient care. Additionally, the Center for Research for Nursing was created in 1983 by the American Nurses'

Association. The Center's mission is to develop and coordinate a research program to serve as the source of national data for the profession.

Several nursing groups developed priorities for nursing research during the 1980s. For example, in 1985, the American Nurses' Association Cabinet on Nursing Research established priorities that helped focus research more precisely on aspects of nursing practice. Finally, several new research-related journals were established in the late 1980s: *Applied Nursing Research*, *Scholarly Inquiry for Nursing Practice*, and *Nursing Science Quarterly*. The journal *Applied Nursing Research* is notable for its intended audience: It includes research reports on studies of special relevance to practicing nurses.

The 1990s and the Future of Nursing Research

After a long crusade by nursing organizations, nursing research was strengthened and given more national visibility when NCNR was promoted to full institute status within the National Institutes of Health: in 1993, the **National Institute of Nursing Research** (NINR) was born. The birth of NINR helps put nursing research more into the mainstream of research activities enjoyed by other health disciplines. Funding for nursing research is also growing. In 1986, the NCNR had a budget of $16.2 million, whereas in fiscal year 1996, the budget for NINR was about $55 million.

Two more research journals were inaugurated during the 1990s—*Clinical Nursing Research* and *Qualitative Health Research*. These journals emerged in response to the growth in clinically oriented and in-depth research among nurses.

During the 1990s, some of the research undertaken by nurses is being guided by priorities established by prominent nurse researchers, who were brought together by NCNR for two Conferences on Research Priorities (CORP). The priorities established by CORP #1, for research through 1994, were as follows: low birthweight, HIV infection, long-term care, symptom management, nursing informatics, health promotion, and technology dependence. In 1993, CORP #2 established the following as research emphases for a portion of NINR's funding from 1995 through 1999:

- *Community-based nursing models*: To examine community-based nursing strategies designed to promote health and reduce risks of disease and disabilities from chronic conditions, particularly among rural, underserved, and minority populations
- *Nursing interventions in HIV and AIDS*: To evaluate the effectiveness of biobehavioral nursing interventions to foster health-promoting behaviors in individuals at risk for HIV and AIDS, and to ameliorate the effects of illness in those already infected
- *Cognitive impairment*: To develop and test biobehavioral and environmental approaches to remedy cognitive impairment, and to examine prevention strategies that target those at risk
- *Chronic illness*: To test interventions that increase individual and family adaptation to chronic illness
- *Immunocompetence*: To identify behavioral factors and test interventions that promote immunocompetence

The future promises to be challenging and exciting for nurse researchers, who are continuing to strengthen the knowledge base for nursing practice. Studies are more likely to be directed toward the practice of nursing than they were in the past. In addition to identifying and pursuing high-priority research areas, there is a growing interest in building a firmer knowledge base by repeating studies, using the procedures used in previous research but with different clients, in different clinical settings, and at different times. Another trend is the growing interest in **outcomes research**—research designed to assess and document the effectiveness of health care service. There is also an increasing emphasis on developing mechanisms for utilizing the results of nursing research in actual practice, and this emphasis is likely to become stronger in the years ahead.

SOURCES OF KNOWLEDGE FOR NURSING

Nursing research is designed to yield important knowledge about phenomena of interest to nurses and their clients. Knowledge of relevance to nurses has many roots. Think for a moment about some facts you have learned relating to the practice of nursing. For example, as nursing students, we learn facts such as "washing hands between patients reduces the spread of bacteria" and "the output of fluids for a patient should be comparable in amount to the intake of fluids per day." What is the source of this and other similar information? Some of the facts we learn are derived from systematic research, but some are not. A brief discussion of some alternative sources of knowledge shows how research-based information is different.

Tradition

Many questions are answered and problems solved on the basis of inherited customs or tradition. Within our culture, certain "truths" are accepted as given. For example, as citizens of the United States, most of us accept, without demanding proof, that democracy is the highest form of government. This type of knowledge often is so much a part of our heritage that few of us seek verification. The discipline of nursing, like other disciplines, also has its store of information passed on to us by tradition or custom. For example, one of the tasks traditionally performed by nurses is the change-of-shift report for each and every patient, whether or not the patient's condition has changed. The question of whether it might

be more productive or effective under certain circumstances to make a report for only those patients whose conditions have changed has not been seriously addressed.

Tradition offers some advantages as a source of knowledge. It is efficient in the sense that each individual is not required to begin anew in an attempt to understand the world or certain aspects of it. Tradition or custom also facilitates communication by providing a common foundation of accepted truth. Nevertheless, tradition poses some problems for human inquiry. Many traditions have never been evaluated for their validity. Indeed, by their nature, traditions may interfere with the ability to perceive alternatives. Walker's (1967) research on ritualistic practices in nursing suggests that some traditional nursing practices, such as the routine taking of a patient's temperature, pulse, and respirations, may be dysfunctional. The Walker study illustrates the potential value of critical appraisal of custom and tradition before accepting them as truth.

Authority

In our complex society, there are authorities—people with specialized expertise—in every field. We are constantly faced with making decisions about matters with which we have had no direct experience; therefore, it seems natural to place our trust in the judgment of people who are authoritative on an issue by virtue of specialized training or experience. As a source of understanding, however, authority has shortcomings. Authorities are not infallible, particularly if their expertise is based primarily on personal experience; yet, like tradition, their knowledge often goes unchallenged. Although nursing practice would flounder if every piece of advice from nursing educators were challenged by students, nursing education would be incomplete if students never had occasion to pose such questions as: How does the authority (the instructor) *know?* What evidence is there that what I am learning is true?

Experience and Trial and Error

Our own experiences represent a familiar and functional source of knowledge. The ability to generalize, to recognize regularities, and to make predictions based on observations is an important characteristic of the human mind. Despite the obvious utility of experience, it has limitations as a basis of understanding. First, each individual's experience may be too restricted to develop generalizations. A nurse may notice, for example, that two or three cardiac patients follow similar postoperative sleep patterns. This observation may lead to some interesting discoveries with implications for nursing interventions, but does the one nurse's observation and experience justify widespread changes in nursing care? A second limitation of experience as a source of knowledge lies in the fact that the same objective event is generally experienced or perceived differently by two individuals. Whose experience constitutes truth?

Closely related to experience is the method of trial and error. In this approach, alternatives are tried successively until we find one that answers our questions or solves our problems. Probably, we have all used the trial-and-error method at some time in our lives, including in our professional work. For example, many patients dislike the taste of potassium chloride solution. Nurses try to disguise the taste of the medication in various ways until one method meets with the approval of the patient. Trial and error may offer a practical means of securing knowledge, but it is fallible and inefficient. This method is haphazard and unsystematic, and the knowledge obtained is often unrecorded and, hence, inaccessible to subsequent problem solvers.

Logical Reasoning

The solutions to many of our perplexing problems are developed by means of logical thought processes. Logical reasoning as a method of knowing combines experience, our intellectual faculties, and formal systems of thought. **Inductive reasoning** is the process of developing generalizations from specific observations. For example, a nurse may observe the anxious behavior of (specific) hospitalized children and conclude that (in general) children's separation from their parents is stressful. **Deductive reasoning** is the process of developing specific predictions from general principles. For example, if we assume that separation anxiety does occur in hospitalized children (in general), then we might predict that the (specific) children in Fairview Hospital whose parents do not room-in would manifest symptoms of stress.

Both systems of reasoning are useful as a means of understanding and organizing phenomena, and both play a role in nursing research. Neither system of thought, however, is without limitations when used alone as a basis of knowledge. The quality of knowledge arrived at through inductive reasoning depends highly on *which* specific examples are used as the basis for generalization. The reasoning process itself offers no mechanism for evaluating whether the examples are really typical and has no built-in checks for self-correction. Deductive reasoning is not itself a source of new information; it is, rather, an approach to illuminating relationships as one proceeds from the general (an assumed truth) to the specific. Deductive logic depends, furthermore, on the truth of the generalizations (called **premises**) to arrive at valid conclusions.

Disciplined Research

Research conducted within a disciplined format is the most sophisticated method of acquiring knowledge that humans have developed. Research combines important features of induction and deduction, together with several other characteristics, to create systems of obtaining knowledge that, although fallible, tend to be more reliable than tradition, authority, experience, or inductive or deductive reasoning alone.

Some of the knowledge that has been incorporated into the nursing profession has been borrowed from research in other disciplines, such as psychology, medicine, anthropology, health care administration, and education. Borrowing involves the use of knowledge and information from other disciplines to influence nursing practice. Nurses throughout the world, however, have come to recognize the need to create a distinct base of knowledge for the nursing profession, and nursing research has become the most widely accepted way to achieve this objective. As we discuss next, disciplined research in nursing is richly diverse with regard to the questions asked and the methods used.

PARADIGMS FOR NURSING RESEARCH

A **paradigm** is a world view, a general perspective on the complexities of the real world. Paradigms for human inquiry are often characterized in terms of the ways in which they respond to basic philosophical questions:

- *Ontologic*: What is the nature of reality?
- *Epistemologic*: What is the relationship between the inquirer and that being studied?
- *Axiologic*: What is the role of values in the inquiry?
- *Methodologic*: How should the inquirer obtain knowledge?

Disciplined inquiry in the field of nursing is being conducted mainly within two broad paradigms, both of which have legitimacy for nursing research.* This section describes the

two alternative paradigms and broadly outlines their associated methodologies.

The Positivist Paradigm

The traditional scientific approach to conducting research has its underpinnings in the philosophical paradigm known as **positivism**. Positivism is rooted in 19th century thought, guided by such philosophers as Comte, Mill, Newton, and Locke. Positivism is a reflection of a broader cultural phenomenon that, in the humanities, is referred to as **modernism,** which emphasizes the rational and the scientific. Although strict positivist thinking—sometimes referred to as **logical positivism**—has been challenged and undermined, a modified positivist position remains a dominant force in scientific research.

The fundamental ontologic assumption of positivists is that there is a reality *out there* that can be studied and known (an **assumption** refers to a basic principle that is believed to be true without proof or verification). Adherents of the scientific approach assume that nature is basically ordered and regular and that an objective reality exists independent of human observation. In other words, the world is assumed not to be merely a creation of the human mind. The related assumption of **determinism** refers to the belief that phenomena are not haphazard or random events but rather have antecedent causes. If a person has a cerebrovascular accident, the scientist assumes that there must be one or more reasons that can be potentially identified and understood. Much of the activity in which a scientific researcher within a positivist paradigm is engaged is directed at understanding the underlying causes of natural phenomena.

Because of their fundamental belief in an objective reality, positivists seek to be as objective as possible in their pursuit of knowledge. Positivists attempt to hold their personal beliefs and biases in check insofar as possible during their research to avoid contaminating

---

*Other inquiry paradigms exist, including several that collectively have been labeled **critical theory** or **critical inquiry** (e.g., feminism, neo-Marxism). It is beyond the scope of this book to discuss these other paradigms.

the phenomena under investigation. The positivists' scientific approach involves the use of orderly, disciplined procedures that are designed to test the researchers's ideas about the nature of the phenomena being studied and the relationships among them.

The methods associated with positivism and the scientific approach are discussed in a subsequent section.

The Naturalistic Paradigm

The **naturalistic** paradigm (which is sometimes referred to as the **phenomenologic** or **constructivist** paradigm) began as a countermovement to positivism with writers such as Weber and Kant. Just as positivism reflects the cultural phenomenon of modernism that burgeoned in the wake of the industrial revolution, natu-

ralism is an outgrowth of the pervasive cultural transformation that is usually referred to as **postmodernism**. Postmodern thinking emphasizes the value of **deconstruction**—that is, of taking apart old ideas and structures—and **reconstruction**—that is, putting ideas and structures together in new ways. The naturalistic paradigm represents a major alternative system for conducting disciplined inquiry in the field of nursing. Table 1-1 compares the major assumptions of the positivist and naturalistic paradigms.

For the naturalistic inquirer, reality is not a fixed entity but rather is a construction of the individuals participating in the research; reality exists within a context, and many constructions are possible. Naturalists thus take the position of relativism: if there are always multiple interpretations of reality that exist in

TABLE 1-1 Major Assumptions of the Positivist and Naturalistic Paradigms

ASSUMPTION	POSITIVIST PARADIGM	NATURALISTIC PARADIGM
Ontologic (What is the nature of reality?)	Reality exists; there is a real world driven by natural causes.	Reality is multiple and subjective, mentally constructed by individuals.
Epistemologic (How is the inquirer related to those being researched?)	Inquirer is independent from those being researched; the findings are not influenced by the researcher.	The inquirer interacts with those being researched; findings are the creation of the interactive process.
Axiologic (What is the role of values in the inquiry?)	Values and biases are to be held in check; objectivity is sought.	Subjectivity and values are inevitable and desirable.
Methodologic (How is knowledge obtained?)	Deductive processes Emphasis on discrete, specific concepts Verification of researcher's hunches Fixed design Tight controls over context Emphasis on measured, quantitative information; statistical analysis Seeks generalizations	Inductive processes Emphasis on entirety of some phenomenon, holistic Emerging interpretations grounded in participants' experiences Flexible design Context bound Emphasis on narrative information; qualitative analysis Seeks patterns

people's minds, then there is no process by which the ultimate truth or falsity of the constructions can be determined.

Epistemologically, the naturalistic paradigm assumes that knowledge is maximized when the distance between the inquirer and the participants in the study is minimized. The voices and interpretations of those under study are key to understanding the phenomenon of interest, and subjective interactions are the primary way to access them. The findings from a naturalistic inquiry are the product of the interaction between the inquirer and the participants. The methodologies associated with the two paradigms are discussed next.

Paradigms and Methods: Quantitative and Qualitative Research

The two alternative perspectives on the nature of reality have strong implications for the methods of knowledge acquisition. The methodologic distinction typically focuses on differences between **quantitative research,** which is most closely allied with the positivist tradition, and **qualitative research,** which is most often associated with naturalistic inquiry—although positivists sometimes engage in qualitative studies, and naturalistic researchers sometimes collect quantitative information. This section provides an overview of the methods associated with the two alternative paradigms. Note that this discussion accentuates the differences in methods as a heuristic device; in reality, there is often greater blurring—and richness—of methods than this introductory discussion implies.

THE SCIENTIFIC METHOD AND QUANTITATIVE RESEARCH

The traditional, positivist **scientific approach** to inquiry refers to a general set of orderly, disciplined procedures used to acquire information. The traditional scientist uses deductive reasoning to generate hunches that are tested in the real world. In **scientific research**—the application of the scientific approach to the study of a question of interest—the researcher moves in an orderly and systematic fashion from the definition of a problem and the selection of concepts on which to focus, through the design of the study and collection of information, to the solution of the problem. By **systematic,** we mean that the scientific investigator progresses logically through a series of steps, according to a prespecified plan of action.

The scientific researcher uses, to the extent possible, mechanisms designed to control the study. **Control** involves imposing conditions on the research situation so that biases are minimized and precision and validity are maximized. The problems that are of interest to nurse researchers—for example, obesity, compliance with a regimen, or perceptions of pain—are highly complicated phenomena, often representing the effects of various forces. In trying to isolate relationships between phenomena, the researcher using a scientific approach attempts to control factors that are not under direct investigation. For example, if a scientist is interested in exploring the relationship between diet and heart disease, steps are usually taken to control other potential contributors to coronary disorders, such as stress and cigarette smoking, as well as additional factors that might be relevant, such as a person's age and gender. The mechanisms of scientific control are discussed at length in this book.

In addressing research questions, the scientist gathers **empirical evidence**—evidence that is rooted in objective reality and gathered directly or indirectly through the human senses. The requirement to use empirical evidence as the basis for knowledge means that the findings of a scientific investigation are to be grounded in reality rather than in the personal beliefs or hunches of the researcher. Empirical evidence, then, consists of observations made known through sight, hearing, taste, touch, or smell. Observations of the presence or absence of skin inflammation, the heart rate of a patient, or the weight of a newborn infant are all examples of empirical observations.

Evidence for a scientific study is gathered according to a specified plan, using formal instruments to collect the needed information. Usually (but not always) the information gathered in a scientific study is **quantitative**—that is, numeric information that results from some type of formal measurement and that is analyzed with statistical procedures.

An important goal of a scientific study is to understand phenomena, not in isolated circumstances alone, but in a broad, general sense. For example, the scientific researcher is typically not as interested in understanding why Ann Jones has cervical cancer as in understanding what general factors lead to this form of carcinoma in Ann and in others. (Of course, a health practitioner would want to take advantage of the general knowledge obtained in the course of scientific research in an effort to assist a particular individual.) The desire to go beyond the specifics of the situation is an important feature of the scientific approach. In fact, the degree to which research findings can be generalized to individuals other than those who participated in the study (referred to as the **generalizability** of the research) is a widely used criterion for assessing the quality of a traditional research study.

The scientific approach—sometimes referred to as the **biomedical model**—has enjoyed considerable stature as a method of inquiry, and it has been used productively by nurse researchers studying a wide range of nursing problems. This is not to say, however, that scientific research can solve all nursing problems or that the scientific method has been without criticism. One important limitation is that the scientific method cannot be used to answer moral or ethical questions. Many of our most persistent and intriguing questions about the human experience fall into this area (e.g., Should euthanasia be practiced? Should abortion be legal?). Given the many moral issues that are linked to medicine and health care, it is inevitable that the nursing process will never rely exclusively on scientific information.

The scientific approach also must contend with problems of measurement. To study a phenomenon, the scientist attempts to measure it. For example, if the phenomenon of interest is patient morale, a researcher might want to assess if a patient's morale is high or low, or higher under certain conditions than under others. Although there are reasonably accurate measures of physiologic phenomena, such as blood pressure, body temperature, and cardiac activity, comparably accurate measures of such psychological phenomena as patient morale, pain, or self-image have not been developed.

A final issue is that nursing research tends to focus on human beings, who are inherently complex and diverse. The scientific method typically focuses on a relatively small portion of the human experience (e.g., weight gain, depression, chemical dependency) in a single study. Complexities tend to be controlled and, insofar as possible, eliminated in scientific studies rather than studied directly, and this narrowness of focus can sometimes obscure insights.

NATURALISTIC METHODS AND QUALITATIVE RESEARCH

Naturalistic methods of inquiry attempt to deal with the issue of human complexity by exploring it directly. Researchers in the naturalistic tradition emphasize the inherent complexity of humans, the ability of humans to shape and create their own experiences, and the idea that truth is a composite of realities. Consequently, naturalistic investigations place a heavy emphasis on understanding the human experience as it is lived, generally through the careful collection and analysis of narrative, subjective—that is, **qualitative**—materials.

Researchers who reject the traditional scientific approach believe that a major limitation of the classical model is that it is **reductionist**—that is, it reduces human experience to only the few concepts under investigation, and those concepts are defined in advance by the researcher rather than emerging from the experiences of those under study. Naturalistic researchers tend to emphasize the dynamic, holistic, and individual aspects of the human experience and attempt to capture those aspects in their entirety, within the context of those who are experiencing them.

Flexible, evolving procedures are used to capitalize on findings that emerge in the course of the study. Naturalistic inquiry always takes place in the **field** (i.e., in naturalistic settings), often over an extended period of time. The collection of information and its analysis typically progress concurrently in naturalistic research—as the researcher sifts through the existing information, insights are gained, new questions emerge, and further evidence is sought to amplify or confirm the insights. Through an inductive process, the researcher integrates the evidence to develop a theory or framework that helps explain the processes under observation.

Naturalistic studies result in rich, in-depth information that has the potential to elucidate the multiple dimensions of a complicated phenomenon. The findings from in-depth qualitative research are rarely superficial, but there are nevertheless several limitations of the approach. Human beings are used directly as the instrument through which information is gathered, and humans are an extremely intelligent and sensitive—but fallible—tool. The subjectivity that enriches the analytic insights in the hands of a skillful researcher can lead to trivial "findings" among less competent inquirers.

A further potential limitation is that the subjective nature of the inquiry may give rise to questions about the idiosyncratic nature of the conclusions. Would two naturalistic researchers studying the same phenomenon in the same setting arrive at the same results? It is difficult to know, and the situation is further complicated by the fact that most naturalistic studies involve a relatively small group of people under study. Questions about the generalizability of the findings from naturalistic inquiries can sometimes loom large.

Multiple Paradigms and Nursing Research

Paradigms should be viewed as lenses that help us to sharpen our focus on a phenomenon of interest—not as blinders that limit our intellectual curiosity. The emergence of alternative paradigms for the study of nursing problems is, in our view, a healthy and desirable trend in the pursuit of new knowledge. Although a researcher's world view may be paradigmatic, knowledge itself is not. The knowledge base in nursing would be slim, indeed, if there were not a rich array of approaches and methods available within the two paradigms—methods that are often complementary in their strengths and limitations. We believe that intellectual pluralism should be encouraged and fostered.

Thus far, we have emphasized the differences between the two paradigms and their associated methods so that their distinctions would be easy to understand. Subsequent chapters of this book will further elaborate on differences in jargon, methods, and research products. It is equally important, however, to note that the alternative paradigms have many features in common, only some of which will be mentioned here:

- *Ultimate goals.* The ultimate aim of disciplined inquiry, regardless of the underlying paradigm, is to gain understanding about the world in which we live. Both quantitative and qualitative researchers seek to capture the true state of affairs with regard to an aspect of the world in which they are interested, and both groups can make significant—and mutually beneficial—contributions.
- *External evidence.* Although the word *empiricism* has come to be allied with the scientific approach, it is nevertheless the case that researchers in both traditions gather and analyze external evidence that is collected through their senses. That is, neither qualitative nor quantitative researchers are armchair analysts, relying exclusively on

their own beliefs and views of the world for their conclusions. Information is gathered from others in a deliberate fashion.

- *Reliance on human cooperation.* Because evidence for nursing research comes primarily from human participants, the need for human cooperation is inevitable. To understand people's characteristics and experiences, researchers must persuade them to participate in the investigation *and* to act and speak candidly. For certain topics, the need for candor and cooperation is a challenging requirement—for researchers in either tradition.
- *Ethical constraints.* Research with human beings is guided by ethical principles that sometimes interfere with the researcher's ultimate goal. For example, if a researcher's aim is to test a potentially beneficial intervention, is it ethical to withhold the treatment from some people to see what happens? As discussed later in the book (see Chapter 6), ethical dilemmas often confront researchers, regardless of their paradigmatic orientation.
- *Fallibility of disciplined research.* Although disciplined nursing research in both paradigms is often of high quality, a general caveat holds true: virtually every research study contains some flaw. Every research question can be addressed in an almost infinite number of ways, and inevitably there are tradeoffs. In most situations, there are financial constraints that lead to less-than-ideal research design decisions. Even when tremendous resources are devoted to an investigation, there are bound to be some shortcomings. This does not mean that small, simple studies have no value. It means that no single study can ever definitively answer a research question. Each completed study adds to a body of accumulated knowledge. If the same question is posed by several researchers, each of whom obtains the same or similar results, increased confidence can be placed in the answer to the question. It is precisely be-

cause of the fallibility of any single study that it is important to understand the tradeoffs and decisions that investigators make when evaluating the adequacy of those decisions.

In summary, despite important philosophical and methodologic differences, researchers using the traditional scientific approach and more naturalistic methods share some overall goals and are faced with many similar constraints and challenges. In our view, the selection of an appropriate method depends to some degree on the researcher's personal taste and philosophy, but it also depends in large part on the nature of the research question, a topic we discuss at length in the next section. If a researcher asks what the effects of surgery are on circadian rhythms (biologic cycles), the researcher really needs to express the effects through the careful quantitative measurement of various bodily characteristics subject to rhythmic variation. On the other hand, if a researcher inquires about the process by which parents learn to cope with the death of a child, the researcher may be hard pressed to quantify such a process. Personal world views of the researchers help to shape the types of question they ask.

In reading about the alternative paradigms for nursing research, you likely were more attracted to one of the two paradigms—the paradigm that corresponds most closely to your view of the world and of reality. It is important, however, to learn about and respect both approaches to disciplined inquiry and to recognize their respective strengths and limitations. In this textbook, we attempt to provide a solid overview of the methods associated with both qualitative and quantitative research. We readily admit that more pages are devoted to the traditional scientific approach and quantitative research than to naturalistic methods and qualitative research. Our rationale for this imbalance is threefold:

1. The methods associated with scientific research inherently are more deliberate and clearly defined. The fluidity that

is the hallmark of naturalistic inquiry means that there are fewer "rules" that have to be understood to comprehend or design a study.

2. The language of naturalistic inquiry is more conversational, and thus there is less technical terminology and jargon than in the case of the scientific approach. Qualitative analysis, for example, is inherently easier to understand (but not necessarily easier to do) than statistical analysis.

3. Most studies in nursing research continue to be quantitative.

Both qualitative and quantitative approaches have strengths and limitations, which are identified throughout this book. It is precisely because the strengths of one approach complement the limitations of the other that both are essential to the further development of nursing knowledge.

THE PURPOSES OF NURSING RESEARCH

The general purpose of nursing research is to answer questions or solve problems of relevance to the nursing profession. Research purposes in nursing can be further described in several ways.

Specific Aims of Quantitative and Qualitative Research

Various types of questions are addressed by nurse researchers, and certain types are more amenable to qualitative than to quantitative inquiry, and vice versa. This section examines some of the specific aims of qualitative and quantitative research in nursing.

IDENTIFICATION

Qualitative researchers often conduct a study to examine phenomena about which little is known. In some cases, so little is known that

the phenomenon has yet to be clearly identified or named or has been inadequately defined or conceptualized. The in-depth, probing nature of qualitative research is well suited to the task of answering such questions as, "What is this phenomenon?" and "What is its name?" (Table 1-2). An example of a qualitative nursing study that involved questions of identification is Cohen's (1995) study of parents' uncertainty with regard to chronic, life-threatening illnesses of their children. In her analysis, Cohen identified the concept of *triggers* that heighten parents' awareness of uncertainty and also identified seven types of triggers.

In quantitative research, by contrast, the researcher begins with a phenomenon that has been previously studied or defined—sometimes in a qualitative study. Thus, in quantitative research, identification typically precedes the inquiry.

DESCRIPTION

The main objective of many nursing research studies is the description and elucidation of phenomena relating to the nursing profession. The researcher who conducts a descriptive investigation observes, counts, describes, and classifies. Phenomena that nurse researchers have been interested in describing are varied. They include topics such as stress and coping in patients, pain management, adaptation processes, health beliefs, rehabilitation success, and time patterns of temperature readings.

Description can be a major purpose for both qualitative and quantitative researchers. Quantitative description involves the prevalence, incidence, size, and measurable attributes of a phenomenon. Table 1-2 summarizes some of the descriptive questions posed by quantitative researchers. As an example, Seifert, Frye, Belknap, and Anderson (1995) did a study to determine the characteristics of nurses' medication administration through enteral feeding catheters. These investigators wanted to describe

TABLE 1-2	**Research Purposes and Research Questions**	

PURPOSE	TYPES OF QUESTIONS: QUANTITATIVE RESEARCH	TYPES OF QUESTIONS: QUALITATIVE RESEARCH
Identification		What is the phenomenon? What is its name?
Description	How prevalent is the phenomenon? How often does the phenomenon occur? What are the characteristics of the phenomenon?	What are the dimensions of the phenomenon? What variations exist? What is important about the phenomenon?
Exploration	What factors are related to the phenomenon? What are the antecedents of the phenomenon?	What is the full nature of the phenomenon? What is really going on here? What is the process by which the phenomenon evolves or is experienced?
Explanation	What are the measurable associations between phenomena? What factors caused the phenomenon? Does the theory explain the phenomenon?	How does the phenomenon work? Why does the phenomenon exist? What is the meaning of the phenomenon? How did the phenomenon occur?
Prediction and control	What will happen if we alter a phenomenon or introduce an intervention? If phenomenon X occurs, will phenomenon Y follow? How can we make the phenomenon happen or alter its nature or prevalence? Can the occurrence of the phenomenon be controlled?	

such things as the *percentage* of patients receiving medications through feeding catheters and the *average number* of feeding catheter obstructions.

Qualitative researchers use in-depth methods to describe the dimensions, variations, and importance of phenomena. For example, Dellasega and Mastrian (1995) conducted a qualitative study designed to identify and describe specific stressors experienced by family members during and after making the decision to place an elder in a long-term skilled care facility. In-depth interviews with seven individuals led to a description of the decision-making process.

EXPLORATION

Like descriptive research, exploratory research begins with some phenomenon of interest; but rather than simply observing and describing the phenomenon, exploratory research is aimed at investigating the full nature of the phenomenon, the manner in which it is manifested, and the other factors with which it is related. For example, a descriptive quantitative study of patients' preoperative stress might seek to document the degree of stress patients experience before surgery and the percentage of patients who actually experience it. An exploratory study might ask the following: What factors are related to a patient's stress level? Is a patient's stress related to behaviors of the nursing staff? Does a patient's behavior change in relation to the level of stress experienced? For example, Picot (1995) conducted an exploratory quantitative study of African American caregivers who provided care to an elderly demented or confused relative. Her study was designed to explore the relationship between the caregivers' coping and such factors as perceived caregiving demands, rewards, and costs.

Exploratory studies are undertaken when a new area or topic is being investigated, and qualitative methods are especially useful for exploring the full nature of a little-understood phenomenon. Exploratory qualitative research is designed to shed light on the various ways in which a phenomenon is manifested and on underlying processes. As an example, Jablonski (1994) explored the full dimensionality of the process and experience of being mechanically ventilated, based on in-depth interviews with 12 patients.

EXPLANATION

The goals of explanatory research are to understand the underpinnings of specific natural phenomena and to explain systematic relationships among phenomena. Explanatory research is often linked to **theories**, which represent a method of deriving, organizing, and integrating ideas about the manner in which phenomena are interrelated. Whereas descriptive research provides new information and exploratory research provides promising insights, explanatory research attempts to offer understanding of the underlying causes or full nature of a phenomenon.

In quantitative research, theories are used deductively as the basis for generating explanations that are then tested empirically. That

is, based on some previously developed theory or body of evidence, the researcher makes specific explanatory predictions that, if upheld by the data, add further credibility to the theory. For example, Bull, Maruyama, and Luo (1995) tested a complex statistical model of factors influencing family caregivers' responses and health outcomes after an elder's discharge from the hospital for acute episodes of chronic illness.

In qualitative studies, the researcher often searches for explanations about how or why a phenomenon exists or what a phenomenon means as a basis for *developing* a theory that is grounded in rich, in-depth, experiential evidence. For example, Redfern-Vance and Hutchinson (1995), using qualitative data, generated a theory designed to illuminate the social psychological processes of women who begin to change their behavior after repeatedly contracting sexually transmitted diseases.

PREDICTION AND CONTROL

With our current level of knowledge, technology, and theoretical progress, there are numerous problems that defy absolute comprehension and explanation. Yet it is frequently possible to make predictions and to control phenomena based on findings from research, even in the absence of complete understanding. For example, research has shown that the incidence of Down syndrome in infants increases with the age of the mother. We can predict that a woman aged 40 years is at higher risk of bearing a child with Down syndrome than is a woman aged 25 years. We can partially control the outcome by educating women about the risks and offering amniocentesis to women over age 35 years. Note, however, that the ability to predict and control in this example does not depend on an explanation of *why* older women are at a higher risk of having an abnormal child.

In many nursing and health-related studies—typically, quantitative ones—prediction and control are key objectives. Studies that are designed to test the efficacy of a nursing intervention are ultimately concerned with controlling patient outcomes or with affecting the costs of care. For example, Gebauer, Kwo, Haynes, and Wewers (1998) investigated the impact of a nurse-managed smoking cessation intervention for pregnant women. Many other nursing studies are designed to identify predictive factors in relation to patient outcomes. For instance, the main purpose of a study by Hendrich, Nyhuis, Kippenbrock, and Soja (1995) was to identify factors that could be used to predict the risk of experiencing a hospital fall.

Basic and Applied Research

Sometimes, the purpose of scientific inquiry is classified according to the direct practical utility of the information gained. **Basic research** is undertaken to accumulate information or to formulate or refine a theory. Basic research is not designed to solve immediate problems but rather to extend the base of knowledge in a discipline for the sake of knowledge and understanding. For example, a researcher may perform an in-depth, qualitative study of the normal process of grieving.

Applied research is focused on finding a solution to an immediate problem. Applied research has as its final goal the systematic planning of induced change in a troublesome situation. For example, a study of the effectiveness of a nursing intervention to ease the grieving process would be considered applied research. We need basic research for the discovery of general principles of human behavior and biophysiologic processes, but applied research tells us how these principles can be put to use to solve problems in the practice of nursing. Qualitative and quantitative researchers engage in both basic and applied research, but in qualitative studies, there is somewhat more emphasis on basic knowledge than on specific problem-solving information.

In nursing, as in medicine, the feedback process between basic and applied research

appears to operate more freely than in the case of other disciplines. The findings from applied research almost immediately pose questions for basic research, whereas the results of basic research often suggest clinical applications to a practical problem.

RESEARCH EXAMPLES

Throughout this book, we present brief descriptions of actual studies recently conducted by nurse researchers. (In the accompanying *Study Guide* we offer descriptions of *fictitious* studies, for students to critique.) The descriptions focus on aspects of the study emphasized in the chapter. In most cases, a review of the actual report in the nursing journal would enhance the assessment process and would provide a useful supplementary assignment.

Research Example of a Quantitative Study

Hauber, Rice, Howell, and Carmon (1998) were interested in better understanding the relationship between anger and blood pressure readings in children. The researchers noted that a number of studies have examined the association of anger and blood pressure readings in adults, but that there is less information about the association for children. The investigators gathered information from a sample of 230 third-graders. Anger was measured in three ways: (1) as a transient emotional condition—state anger; (2) as a more enduring personality characteristic—trait anger; and (3) as one of three patterns of anger expression—anger-out/open anger expression, anger suppression, and anger reflection and control. These measures of anger were obtained in a classroom setting, and blood pressure readings (BPRs) were subsequently taken.

The findings indicated that BPRs were not related to the measures of trait anger or state anger. However, the researchers found that as anger suppression increased, diastolic BPR decreased. And, as anger reflection and control increased, both systolic and diastolic BPR decreased. The investigators concluded that blood pressure readings need to be taken in all children as part of their well-child examinations and that "strategies to manage anger may also need to be considered" (p. 10).

Research Example of a Qualitative Study

Walcott-McQuigg, Sullivan, Dan, and Logan (1995) conducted a study to explore the factors influencing weight control behavior among college-educated African American women. The researchers noted that African American women have consistently been found to be more overweight than European American women, and so they sought to identify potential cultural, social, and psychological factors influencing their weight control behavior. Face-to-face, in-depth interviews were conducted with 36 African American women in their homes. The interviews explored personal weight control behavior among the study participants, factors such as emotions and beliefs that influenced the participants' behavior, and opinions about African American women's weight control behavior in general. The interviews suggested six factors that influenced the women's individual weight control practices: emotions/feelings, beliefs, life events, self-control, discipline, and commitment. Factors related to the African American culture were also identified by the women, such as eating and cooking patterns and cultural values relating to food, health, and body image. The authors concluded that, "recognition of psychosocial determinants of weight control behavior may enable health professionals to design unique interventions relevant to African American women" (p. 502).

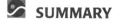 **SUMMARY**

Nursing research involves a systematic search for knowledge relating to the nursing profession. Nurses engage in research for a number of reasons. Research has an important role to play in helping nursing establish a solid knowledge base for its practice. Additionally, the systematic accrual of nursing information facilitates a better definition of the parameters of nursing and helps to document the unique contribution nursing makes to health care. There is a growing consensus that knowledge of nursing research is needed to enhance the professional practice of all nurses—including both **consumers of research** (who read and evaluate studies) and **producers of research** (who design and undertake research studies). Nurses may assume a variety of additional research-related roles in the course of their practices.

Nursing research began with Florence Nightingale and gained slow acceptance until the 1950s, when it accelerated rapidly. Since the 1970s, the emphasis in nursing research has been on clinical practice. Nurses are increasingly studying problems such as health promotion, prevention of illness, the efficacy of nursing interventions, and the needs of special health-risk groups. The establishment of the **National Institute of Nursing Research** at the National Institutes of Health in 1993 attests to the growth and current importance of nursing research.

Nursing research begins with questions about nursing phenomena or with a problem to be solved. Disciplined research stands in contrast to several other sources of knowledge and understanding, such as tradition, voices of authority, personal experience, trial and error, and logical reasoning.

Disciplined inquiry in nursing is being conducted within two broad **paradigms**—world views with underlying **assumptions** about the nature of reality. One paradigm is known as **positivism**. Positivists assume that there is an objective reality that is not dependent on human observation for its existence and that natural phenomena are basically regular and orderly. The related assumption of **determinism** refers to the belief that events are not haphazard but rather the result of prior causes. The naturalistic paradigm, by contrast, assumes that reality is not a fixed entity but is rather a construction of human minds—and thus "truth" is a composite of multiple constructions of reality. Each of these paradigms, with its associated assumptions, have implications for the methods of acquiring knowledge.

The positivist paradigm is associated with the traditional **scientific approach**, which is a systematic, disciplined, and controlled process often aimed at identifying underlying causes of phenomena. Scientists base their findings on **empirical evidence**, which is evidence that is rooted in objective reality and collected by way of the human senses or their extensions. The scientific approach strives for **generalizability** and for the development of explanations or theories about the relationships among phenomena. The scientific approach often involves the collection and analysis of numeric information—that is, it often involves **quantitative research**. Although the scientific approach offers a number of distinct advantages as a system of inquiry, it is not without its share of shortcomings, including its narrow focus on a small range of human experience and the difficulty of quantitatively measuring complex phenomena.

Researchers within the naturalistic paradigm place a heavy emphasis on understanding the human experience as it is lived, generally by the collection and analysis of subjective, narrative materials through flexible procedures that evolve in the **field**; consequently, this paradigm usually involves **qualitative research**. Research in both paradigms can contribute to the further development of nursing knowledge.

Research can be categorized in terms of its aims or objectives. Identification, description, exploration, explanation, prediction, and control of natural phenomena represent the most common goals of a research investigation. Within each broad aim, qualitative and quantitative researchers pose different types of questions. Research can also be described in terms of the direct, practical utility that it sets out to achieve. **Basic research** is designed to extend the base of information for the sake of knowledge. **Applied research** focuses on discovering solutions to immediate problems.

STUDY ACTIVITIES

Chapter 1 of the *Study Guide to Accompany Nursing Research: Principles and Methods, 6th ed.*, offers suggested questions for reinforcing concepts presented in this chapter. Additionally, the following study questions can be addressed:

1. What are some of the current changes occurring in the health care delivery system, and how could these changes influence nursing research?
2. Consider one or two nursing "facts" that you possess, and then trace the facts back to some source. Is the basis for your knowledge tradition, authority, experience, or scientific research?
3. Explain the ways in which scientific knowledge differs from knowledge based on tradition, authority, trial and error, and logical reasoning.
4. How does the assumption of scientific determinism conflict with or coincide with superstitious thinking? Take, as an example, the superstition associated with four-leaf clovers or a rabbit's foot.
5. How does the ability to predict phenomena offer the possibility of their control?
6. Below are a few research problems. For each problem, specify whether you think it is essentially a basic or applied research question. Justify your response.
   a. Is the stress level of patients related to the level of information they possess about their medical status?
   b. Do students who get higher grades in nursing school become more effective nurses than students with lower grades?
   c. Does the early discharge of maternity patients lead to later problems with breastfeeding?

d. Can the incidence of decubitus ulcers be affected by a certain massaging technique?

e. Is individual contraceptive counseling more effective than group-based instruction in minimizing unwanted pregnancies?

⧉ SUGGESTED READINGS

Methodologic and Theoretical References

American Nurses' Association. (1991). *Standards of clinical nursing practice.* Kansas City, MO: ANA.

American Nurses' Association Cabinet on Nursing Research. (1985). *Directions for nursing research: Toward the twenty-first century.* Kansas City, MO: American Nurses' Association.

Brown, E. L. (1948). *Nursing for the future.* New York: Russell Sage.

D'Antonio, P. (1997). Toward a history of research in nursing. *Nursing Research, 46,* 105–110.

Guba, E. G. (Ed.). (1990). *The paradigm dialog.* Newbury Park, CA: Sage.

Kuhn, T. S. (1970). *The structure of scientific revolutions* (2nd ed.). Chicago: University of Chicago Press.

Lincoln, Y. S., & Guba, E. G. (1985). *Naturalistic inquiry.* Beverly Hills: Sage.

Lindeman, C. A. (1975). Delphi survey of priorities in clinical nursing research. *Nursing Research, 24,* 434–441.

Nightingale, F. (1859). *Notes on nursing: What it is, and what it is not.* Philadelphia: J. B. Lippincott.

Oiler, C. (1982). The phenomenological approach in nursing research. *Nursing Research, 31,* 178–181.

O'Sullivan, P. S., & Goodman, P. A. (1990). Involving practicing nurses in research. *Applied Nursing Research, 3,* 169–173.

Schlotfeldt, R. M. (1992). Why promote clinical nursing scholarship? *Clinical Nursing Research, 1,* 5–8.

Walker, V. H. (1967). *Nursing and ritualistic practice.* New York: Macmillan.

Substantive References

Bull, M. J., Maruyama, G., & Luo, D. (1995). Testing a model for posthospital transition of family caregivers for elderly persons. *Nursing Research, 44,* 132–138.

Cohen, M. H. (1995). The triggers of heightened parental uncertainty in chronic, life-threatening childhood illness. *Qualitative Health Research, 5,* 63–77.

Dellasega, C., & Mastrian, K. (1995). The process and consequences of institutionalizing an elder. *Western Journal of Nursing Research, 17,* 123–140.

Gebauer, C., Kwo, C. Y., Haynes, E. F., & Wewers, M. E. (1998). A nurse-managed smoking cessation intervention during pregnancy. *Journal of Obstetric, Gynecologic, and Neonatal Nursing, 27,* 47–53.

Hauber, R. P., Rice, M. H., Howell, C. C., & Carmon, M. (1998). Anger and blood pressure readings in children. *Applied Nursing Research, 11,* 2–11.

Hendrich, A., Nyhuis, A., Kippenbrock, T., & Soja, M. E. (1995). Hospital falls: Development of a predictive model for clinical practice. *Applied Nursing Research, 8,* 129–139.

Jablonski, R. S. (1994). The experience of being mechanically ventilated. *Qualitative Health Research, 4,* 186–207.

Picot, S. J. (1995). Rewards, costs, and coping of African American caregivers. *Nursing Research, 44,* 147–152.

Redfern-Vance, N., & Hutchinson, S. A. (1995). The process of developing personal sovereignty in women who repeatedly acquire sexually transmitted diseases. *Qualitative Health Research, 5,* 222–236.

Seifert, C. F., Frye, J. L., Belknap, D. C., & Anderson, D. C. (1995). A nursing survey to determine the characteristics of medication administration through enteral feeding catheters. *Clinical Nursing Research, 4,* 290–305.

Walcott-McQuigg, J. A., Sullivan, J., Dan, A., & Logan, B. (1995). Psychosocial factors influencing weight control behavior of African American women. *Western Journal of Nursing Research, 17,* 502–520.

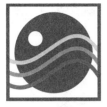

CHAPTER **2**

Overview of the Research Process

![] BASIC RESEARCH TERMINOLOGY

Research, like nursing or any other discipline, has its own language and terminology—its own jargon. Some terms are used by both qualitative and quantitative researchers (although in some cases, the connotations differ), whereas others are used predominantly in connection with one or the other approach. New terms are introduced throughout this textbook. However, we devote a large part of this chapter to some fundamental terms and concepts whose meaning should be mastered so that more complex ideas can be grasped. The purpose of this chapter is to make the rest of this book more manageable by familiarizing readers with the basics of research terminology and with the progression of steps that are undertaken in a research project.

The Study

Before turning to a discussion of the terms that are the building blocks of qualitative and quantitative research, let us consider a few basic terms that are used in research circles. Regardless of the methods used, when researchers address a problem or answer a question, it is usu-

ally said that they are doing a **study**, but the endeavor may also be referred to as an **investigation** or a **research project**.

Research studies with humans involve two sets of people: those who are doing the research and those who are providing information. In a quantitative study, the people who are being studied are sometimes referred to as the **subjects** or the **study participants**, as shown in Table 2-1. (Subjects who provide information to the researchers by answering questions directly—e.g., by filling out a questionnaire—may be called **respondents.**) The term subjects implies that people are *acted upon* by the researchers; however, in a qualitative study, the individuals cooperating in the study play an active rather than a passive role and are therefore usually referred to as **informants** or study participants.

The person who undertakes the research is called the **researcher** or **investigator** (or sometimes—more often in quantitative studies—the **scientist**). A study may be undertaken by a group of people working together rather than by a single researcher. For example, a team of nurse researchers and clinical nurses might collaborate on addressing a problem of clinical relevance. When a study is undertaken by a research team, the main person directing the

TABLE 2-1 Key Terms Used in Quantitative and Qualitative Research		
CONCEPT	**QUANTITATIVE TERM**	**QUALITATIVE TERM**
Person contributing information	Subject Study participant Respondent	— Study participant Informant
Person undertaking the study	Researcher Investigator Scientist	Researcher Investigator —
That which is being investigated	— Concepts Constructs Variables	Phenomena, topics Concepts — —
System of organizing concepts	Theory, theoretical framework Conceptual framework, conceptual model	Theory —
Information gathered	Data (numeric values)	Data (narrative descriptions)
Connections between concepts	Relationships (cause-and-effect, functional)	Patterns of association

investigation is referred to as the **project director** or **principal investigator**. Two or three researchers collaborating equally are sometimes called **co-investigators**.

Phenomena, Concepts, and Constructs

Conceptualization refers to the process of developing and refining abstract ideas. Research is almost always concerned with abstract rather than tangible phenomena. For example, the terms *good health, pain, emotional disturbance, patient care*, and *grieving* are all abstractions that are formulated by generalizing about particular manifestations of human behavior and characteristics. These abstractions are often referred to as **concepts**. (In qualitative studies, researchers often use the term **phenomena** or **topics**).

The term **construct** is also encountered frequently in the research literature, especially with regard to quantitative studies. Like a concept, a construct refers to an abstraction or mental representation inferred from situations, events, or behaviors. Kerlinger (1986) distinguishes concepts from constructs by noting that constructs are abstractions that are deliberately and systematically invented (or constructed) by researchers for a specific purpose. For example, *self-care* in Orem's model of health maintenance may be considered a construct. In practice, the terms construct and concept are often used interchangeably, although by convention, a construct often refers to a slightly more complex abstraction than a concept.

Theories and Conceptual Models

A **theory** is a systematic, abstract explanation of some aspect of reality. Concepts are the building blocks of theories. In a theory, concepts are knitted together into a coherent system in an effort to explain the way in which our world and the people in it function. Theories play a role in both qualitative and quantitative research.

In a quantitative study, the researcher often starts with a theory or a **conceptual model** (the distinction is discussed in Chapter 5). On the basis of an existing theory, the researcher makes predictions about how phenomena will behave in the real world *if the theory is true*. In other words, the researcher uses deductive reasoning to develop from the general theory some specific predictions that can be tested empirically. The results of the research are used to reject, modify, or lend credence to the theory.

In qualitative research, the investigators use the information gathered from the participants inductively as the basis for developing a theory. The participants' input is the starting point from which the researcher begins to conceptualize, seeking to explain patterns, commonalities, and relationships emerging from the researcher–participant interactions. The goal is to arrive at a theory that explains phenomena *as they occur*, not as they are preconceived. Inductively generated theories from a qualitative study are sometimes subjected to more controlled confirmation through quantitative research.

Variables

Within the context of a quantitative research investigation, concepts are usually referred to as **variables**. A variable, as the name implies, is something that varies. Weight, blood pressure readings, preoperative anxiety levels, and body temperature are all variables; that is, each of these properties varies or differs from one person to another. To the quantitative researcher, nearly all aspects of human beings and their environment are considered variables. For example, if everyone had black hair and weighed 125 pounds, hair color and weight would not be variables. If it rained continuously and the temperature were a constant 70°F, weather would not be a variable, it would be a **constant**. But it is precisely because people and conditions *do* vary that most research is conducted. The bulk of all quantitative research activity is aimed at trying to understand how or why things vary and to learn how differences in one variable are related to differences in another. For example, lung cancer research is concerned with the variable of lung cancer. It is a variable because not everybody has the disease. Researchers have studied what variables might be linked to lung cancer and have discovered that cigarette smoking appears to be related. Again, smoking is a variable because not everyone smokes. A variable, then, is any quality of a person, group, or situation that varies or takes on different values—typically, numeric values.

CONTINUOUS, DISCRETE, AND CATEGORICAL VARIABLES

Sometimes, a variable can take on a wide range of different values. A human being's age, for instance, can take on values from zero to more than 100—and the values are not necessarily whole numbers. Such variables are sometimes referred to as **continuous variables** because their values can be represented on a continuum. At least in theory, a continuous variable can assume an infinite number of values between two points. For example, consider the variable *weight*, which is a continuous variable. Between 1 and 2 pounds, there is an unlimited number of values: 1.005, 1.7, 1.3333, and so on.

By contrast, a **discrete variable** is one that has a finite number of values between any two points, representing discrete quantities. For example, if people were asked how many children they had, they might answer 0, 1, 2, 3, or more. The value for number of children is discrete, because a number such as 1.5 is not a meaningful value. Between the values 1 and 3, the only possible value is 2.

Other variables take on a small range of values that do not inherently represent a quantity.

The variable gender, for example, has only two values (male and female). Variables of this type, which take on only a handful of discrete values, are referred to as **categorical variables**. Other examples of categorical variables include marital status (married, single, divorced, widowed, other) and blood type (A, B, AB, and O). When categorical variables take on only two values, they are sometimes referred to as **dichotomous variables**. Some examples of categorical variables that are dichotomous are pregnant/not pregnant, HIV positive/HIV negative, and alive/dead.

ACTIVE VERSUS ATTRIBUTE VARIABLES

Variables are often existing characteristics of the research subjects, such as age, health beliefs, weight, or grip strength. Variables such as these are sometimes called **attribute variables**. In many research situations, however, the investigator creates or designs a variable. For example, if a researcher is interested in testing the effectiveness of ice chips as opposed to effervescent ginger ale in refreshing the mouth after vomiting, some individuals would be given ice chips and others would receive ginger ale. For the purpose of this study, the type of mouth care is a variable because different individuals receive ice chips or ginger ale. Kerlinger (1986) refers to these variables that the researcher creates or designs as **active** variables.

DEPENDENT VERSUS INDEPENDENT VARIABLES

An important distinction can be made between two types of variables in a research study, and this distinction needs to be mastered before proceeding to later chapters. It is the distinction between the independent variable and the dependent variable. Many research studies are aimed at unraveling and understanding the causes underlying phenomena. Does a nursing intervention *cause* more rapid recovery? Does smoking *cause* lung cancer? The presumed **cause** is referred to as the **independent variable**, and the presumed effect is referred to as the **dependent variable**.

Variability in the dependent variable is presumed to *depend* on variability in the independent variable. For example, the researcher investigates the extent to which lung cancer (the dependent variable) depends on smoking behavior (the independent variable). Or, an investigator may be concerned with the extent to which patients' perception of pain (the dependent variable) depends on different types of nursing approaches (the independent variable).

The terms independent variable and dependent variable are frequently used to indicate direction of influence rather than a causal connection. For example, let us say that a researcher is studying nurses' attitudes toward abortion and finds that older nurses hold less favorable opinions about abortion than younger nurses. The researcher might be unwilling to infer that the nurses' attitudes were *caused* by their age. Yet the direction of influence clearly runs from age to attitudes. That is, it would make little sense to suggest that the attitudes caused or influenced age. Even though in this example the researcher does not infer a causal relationship between age and attitudes, it is appropriate to conceptualize attitudes toward abortion as the dependent variable and age as the independent variable.

The dependent variable usually is the variable that the researcher is interested in understanding, explaining, or predicting. In lung cancer research, it is the carcinoma that is of real interest to the research scientist, not smoking behavior per se. In studies of the effectiveness of therapeutic treatments for alcoholics, it is the drinking behavior of the subjects that is the dependent variable. Although a great deal of time, effort, and resources may be devoted to designing new therapies (the independent variable), they are of interest primarily as they relate to improvements in drinking behavior and overall functioning of alcoholics.

Many of the dependent variables that are studied by researchers have a multiplicity of causes or antecedents. If we were interested in studying the factors that influence people's weight, for example, we might consider their height, physical activity, and eating habits as the independent variables. Just as a study may examine more than one independent variable, two or more dependent variables may be of interest to the researcher. For example, an investigator may be concerned with comparing the effectiveness of two methods of nursing care delivery (primary versus functional) for children with cystic fibrosis. Several dependent variables could be designated as measures of treatment effectiveness, such as length of stay in the hospital, number of recurrent respiratory infections, dyspnea on exertion, and so forth. In short, it is common to design studies with multiple independent and dependent variables.

It is important to understand that variables are not inherently dependent or independent. A variable that is dependent in one study could be an independent variable in another study. For example, a researcher may find that the religious background of a nurse (the independent variable) has an effect on the nurse's attitude toward death and dying (the dependent variable). Another study, however, may analyze the extent to which nurses' attitudes toward death and dying (the independent variables) affect their job performance (the dependent variable). To illustrate this point with another example, consider a study that examines the relationship between contraceptive counseling (the independent variable) and unplanned pregnancies (the dependent variable). Yet another research project could study the effect of unplanned pregnancies (the independent variable) on the incidence of child abuse (the dependent variable). In short, the designation of a variable as independent or dependent is a function of the role the variable plays in a particular investigation. Table 2-2 presents

TABLE 2-2 Examples of Independent and Dependent Variables in Quantitative Nursing Studies

RESEARCH QUESTION	INDEPENDENT VARIABLE	DEPENDENT VARIABLES
What is the effect of alternative nondieting interventions on eating restraint and body dissatisfaction among obese women? (Ciliska, 1998)	Alternative interventions	Eating restraint, body dissatisfaction
Is abuse during childhood related to women's victimization throughout adulthood? (Draucker, 1997)	Childhood abuse	Adult victimization
What is the effect of regular, active exercise during the last trimester of pregnancy on maternal weight gain and infant birthweight? (Horns, Ratcliffe, Leggett, & Swanson, 1996)	Amount of exercise	Maternal weight gain, infant birthweight
What is the effect of pain on facial and cry behavior, heart rate, and palmar sweating in infants 0 to 12 months of age? (Fuller & Conner, 1995)	Pain level	Facial and cry behavior, heart rate, palmar sweating

some examples of research questions posed by nurse researchers and specifies the dependent and independent variables.

Some researchers use the term **criterion variable** or **criterion measure** rather than dependent variable. In studies that analyze the consequences of a treatment, therapy, or some other type of intervention, it is usually necessary to establish criteria against which the success of the intervention can be assessed—hence, the origin of the expression criterion variable. Others use the term **outcome variable**—the variable capturing the outcome of interest—in lieu of dependent variable. The term dependent variable, however, is broader and more general in its implications and applicability. Therefore, we use the term dependent variable more frequently than criterion or outcome variable, although in many situations, the terms are equivalent and interchangeable.

HETEROGENEITY

A term that is frequently used in connection with variables is heterogeneity. When an attribute is extremely varied in the group under investigation, the group is said to be **heterogeneous** with respect to that variable. If, on the other hand, the amount of variability is limited, the group is described as relatively **homogeneous**. For example, with respect to the variable height, a group of 2-year-old children is likely to be more homogeneous than a group of 18-year-old adolescents. The degree of **variability** or **heterogeneity** of a group of subjects has implications for the design of a study.

OPERATIONAL DEFINITIONS OF VARIABLES

In a quantitative study, the researcher usually clarifies and defines the variables under investigation at the outset. To be useful, the definition must specify how the variable will be observed and measured in the actual research situation. Such a definition has a special name. An **operational definition** of a concept is a specification of the operations that

the researcher must perform to collect the required information.

Variables differ considerably in the facility with which they can be operationalized. The variable weight, for example, is easy to define and measure. We may use the following as our definition of weight: the heaviness or lightness of an object in terms of pounds. Note that this definition designates that weight will be determined according to one measuring system (pounds) rather than another (kilograms). The operational definition might specify that the subjects' weight will be measured to the nearest pound using a spring scale with subjects fully undressed after 10 hours of fasting. This operational definition clearly indicates both to the investigator and to the consumer what is meant by the variable weight.

Unfortunately, many of the variables of interest in nursing research are not operationalized as easily and directly as is weight. There are multiple methods of measuring most variables, and the researcher must choose the method that best captures the variables as he or she conceptualizes them. For example, patient well-being may be defined in terms of both physiologic and psychological functioning. If the researcher chooses to emphasize the physiologic aspects of patient well-being, the operational definition may involve a measure such as heart rate, white blood cell count, blood pressure, or vital capacity. If, on the other hand, well-being is conceptualized for the purposes of research as primarily a psychological phenomenon, the operational definition will need to identify the method by which emotional well-being will be assessed, such as the responses of the patient to certain questions or the behaviors of the patient as observed by the researcher.

Some readers of a research report may not agree with the way that the investigator has conceptualized and operationalized the variables. Nevertheless, precision in defining the terms has the advantage of communicating exactly what the terms mean. If the researcher is reluctant to be explicit, it will be difficult for others to gauge the full meaning and implications of the research findings. Table 2-3 presents some operational definitions from several quantitative nursing research studies.

Qualitative researchers generally do not define the concepts in which they are interested in operational terms before gathering information. This is because of their desire to have the meaning of concepts defined by those being studied. Nevertheless, in summarizing the results of a study, all researchers should be careful in describing the conceptual and methodologic bases of key research concepts.

Data

The **data** (singular, datum) of a research study are the pieces of information obtained in the course of the investigation. In a quantitative study, the researcher identifies the variables of interest, develops operational definitions of those variables, and then collects the relevant data from the research subjects. The variables, because they vary, take on different values. The actual values of the study variables constitute the data for a research project.

In quantitative studies, the researcher collects primarily **quantitative data**—that is, information that is in numeric form. For example, suppose we were conducting a quantitative study in which the variable of primary inter-

est was *depression*. In such a study, we would try to measure how depressed different study participants were. For example, we might ask the question, "Thinking about the past week, how depressed would you say you have been on a scale from 0 to 10, where 0 means 'not at all' and 10 means 'the most possible'?" Box 2-1 presents some quantitative data from three fictitious respondents. The subjects have provided a number corresponding to their degree of depression—9 for subject 1 (a high level of depression), 0 for subject 2 (no depression), and 4 for subject 3 (very mild depression). The numeric values for all subjects in the study, collectively, would comprise the data on depression.

In qualitative studies, the researcher collects primarily **qualitative data,** which are usually narrative descriptions. Narrative information can be obtained by having conversations with the participants, by making detailed notes about how participants behave in naturalistic settings, or by obtaining narrative records from participants, such as diaries. As an example, suppose we were studying depression qualitatively. Box 2-2 presents some qualitative data from three study participants responding conversationally to the question, "Tell me about how you've been feeling lately—have you felt sad or depressed at all, or have you generally been in good spirits?" Here, the data consist of fairly rich and detailed

TABLE 2-3 Examples of Operational Definitions from Quantitative Nursing Studies	
CONCEPT	**OPERATIONAL DEFINITION**
Energy intake in Buffalo rats	Grams of pulverized rat chow eaten after 6 hours of feeding (McCarthy, 1997)
Weight cycling	Body weight gain and loss greater than 10 pounds within the past 2 years (Popkess-Vawter, Wendel, Schmoll, & O'Connell, 1998)
Postoperative pain in abdominal surgical patients	Sensory component of pain: patient's score on the Sensation of Pain Scale (a 10-point scale) and amount of narcotic intake 24 hours after ambulation (Good, 1995)

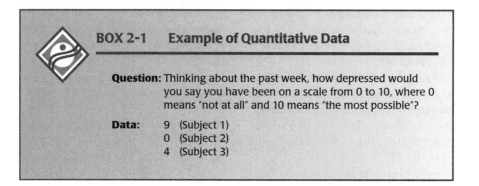

BOX 2-1   Example of Quantitative Data

Question: Thinking about the past week, how depressed would you say you have been on a scale from 0 to 10, where 0 means "not at all" and 10 means "the most possible"?

Data: 9   (Subject 1)
0   (Subject 2)
4   (Subject 3)

narrative descriptions of each participant's emotional state.

In both qualitative and quantitative research, the collection and analysis of the research data are typically the most time-consuming aspects of a study. The analysis of qualitative data is a particularly labor-intensive process.

Relationships

Researchers are rarely interested in a single isolated concept or phenomenon, except in some descriptive studies. As an example of a descriptive study, a researcher might do research primarily to determine the percentage of high school students who have ever used drugs. In this example, there is only one variable or concept: never used drugs versus ever used drugs. Usually, however, researchers study phenomena in relation to other phenomena—that is, they explore or test **relationships**. Generally speaking, a relationship is a bond or a connection between phenomena; for example, researchers repeatedly have found that there is a relationship between cigarette smoking and lung cancer. Both qualitative and quantitative studies examine relationships among phenomena.

In a quantitative study, the researcher is primarily interested in the relationship between the independent variable and the dependent

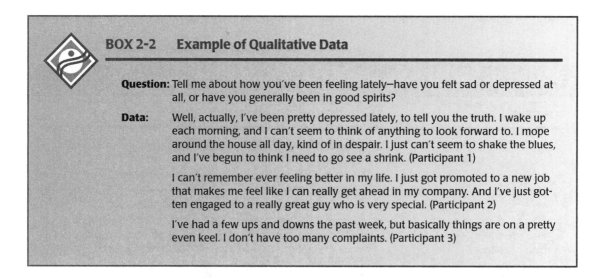

BOX 2-2   Example of Qualitative Data

Question: Tell me about how you've been feeling lately—have you felt sad or depressed at all, or have you generally been in good spirits?

Data: Well, actually, I've been pretty depressed lately, to tell you the truth. I wake up each morning, and I can't seem to think of anything to look forward to. I mope around the house all day, kind of in despair. I just can't seem to shake the blues, and I've begun to think I need to go see a shrink. (Participant 1)

I can't remember ever feeling better in my life. I just got promoted to a new job that makes me feel like I can really get ahead in my company. And I've just gotten engaged to a really great guy who is very special. (Participant 2)

I've had a few ups and downs the past week, but basically things are on a pretty even keel. I don't have too many complaints. (Participant 3)

variable. The research question asks whether variation in the dependent variable is systematically related to variation in the independent variable. Relationships are usually expressed in quantitative terms, such as *more than*, *less than*, and so on. For example, let us consider as a possible dependent variable a person's body weight. What variables are related to (associated with) a person's weight? Some possibilities include height, metabolism, caloric intake, and exercise. For each of these four independent variables, we can make a tentative relational statement:

Height: Taller people will weigh more than shorter people.

Metabolism: The lower a person's metabolic rate, the more he or she will weigh.

Caloric intake: People with higher caloric intake will be heavier than those with lower caloric intake.

Exercise: The greater the amount of exercise, the lower will be the person's weight.

Each of these statements expresses a hypothesized relationship between weight (the dependent variable) and a measurable independent variable. The terms more than and lower than imply that as we observe a change in one variable, we are likely to observe a corresponding change in the other. If Nate is taller than Tom, we would expect (in the absence of any other information) that Nate is also heavier than Tom.

Quantitative studies are often conducted to determine whether relationships exist among variables, as suggested by the following research questions: Is there a relationship between the frequency of turning patients and the incidence and severity of decubitus? Is prematurity related to the incidence of nosocomial viral infections? Most quantitative research is conducted to determine whether relationships do or do not exist among variables and often to *quantify* how strong the relationship is.

Quantitative variables can be related to one another in different ways. One type of relationship is referred to as a **cause-and-effect** (or **causal**) **relationship**. Within the positivist paradigm, natural phenomena are assumed not to be random or haphazard; if phenomena have antecedent factors or causes, they are presumably discoverable. For instance, in our example about a person's weight, we might speculate that there is a causal relationship between caloric intake and weight: eating more calories causes weight gain. As an example of an actual quantitative study that was concerned with causal relationships, Anderson, Lane, and Chang (1995) studied the effect of deep-water tub baths on heat loss in healthy newborns 2 to 3 hours after their birth.

Not all relationships between variables can be interpreted as cause-and-effect relationships. There is a relationship, for example, between a person' pulmonary artery and tympanic temperatures: people with high readings on one tend to have high readings on the other. We cannot say, however, that pulmonary artery temperature *caused* tympanic temperature, nor that tympanic temperature *caused* pulmonary artery temperature, despite the relationship that exists between the two variables. This type of relationship is sometimes referred to as a **functional relationship** (or an **associative relationship**) rather than as a causal relationship. As an example, Evans, Dick, and Clark (1995) studied the relationship between maternal sleep during the week before labor and labor outcomes (e.g., length of time in labor, type of delivery).

Qualitative researchers are not concerned with quantifying relationships, nor with testing and confirming causal relationships. Rather, qualitative researchers seek patterns of association as a way of illuminating the underlying meaning and dimensionality of phenomena of interest. Patterns of interconnected themes and processes are identified as a means of understanding the whole. For example, King, Collins, and Liken (1995) studied the values of caregivers of patients with dementing disease in relation to their patterns of using community services.

Research Control

Research control plays a critical role in quantitative research. It is a topic to which considerable attention is paid in this book. Chapter 9, in particular, discusses methods of achieving control in quantitative research. The concept is so important, however, that some basic ideas about control are presented here.

Essentially, **research control** is concerned with holding constant the possible influences on the dependent variable under investigation so that the true relationship between the independent and dependent variables can be understood. In other words, research control attempts to eliminate any contaminating factors that might otherwise obscure the relationship between the variables that are really of interest. A detailed example should clarify this point.

Let us suppose that a researcher is interested in studying whether teenage women are at higher risk of having low-birthweight infants than are older mothers *because of their age*. In other words, the researcher wants to test whether there is something about the physiologic development of women that causes differences in the birthweight of their babies. Existing studies have shown that, in fact, teenagers have a higher rate of low-birthweight babies than women in their 20s. The question for this researcher, however, is whether age itself causes this difference or whether there are other mechanisms that can account for or influence the relationship between maternal age and infant birthweight. The researcher in this example would want to design the study in such a way that these other factors are controlled. But what are the other factors? To answer this, the researcher must ask the following critical question:

> *What variables could affect the dependent variable under study while at the same time be related to the independent variable?*

In the current study, the dependent variable is infant birthweight, and the independent variable is maternal age. Two variables are prime candidates for concern as contaminating factors (although there are several other possibilities): the nutritional habits of the mother and the amount of prenatal care received. Teenagers tend to be less careful than older women about their eating patterns during pregnancy and are also less likely to obtain adequate prenatal care. Both nutrition and the amount of care could, in turn, affect the baby's birthweight. Thus, if these two factors are not controlled, then any observed relationship between the mother's age and her baby's weight at birth could be caused by the mother's age itself, her diet, or her prenatal care. It would be impossible to know what the underlying cause really is.

These three possible explanations are shown schematically as follows:

1. Mother's age → infant birthweight
2. Mother's age → prenatal care → infant birthweight
3. Mother's age → nutrition → infant birthweight

The arrows here symbolize a causal mechanism or an influence. In examples 2 and 3, the effect of maternal age on infant birthweight is mediated by prenatal care and nutrition, respectively; for this reason, these variables are usually referred to as **mediating variables**. The researcher's task is to design a study in such a way that the true explanation is made clear. Both nutrition and prenatal care must be controlled if the researcher's goal is to learn if explanation 1 is valid.

How can the researcher impose such control? There are a number of ways, as discussed in Chapter 9, but the general principle underlying each alternative is the same: the competing influences—often referred to as the **extraneous variables** of the study—must be held constant. The extraneous variables to be controlled must somehow be handled in such a way that they are not related to the independent or dependent variable. Again, an example should help make this point more clear. Let us say we want to compare the birthweights of infants born to two groups of women: those aged 15 to 19 years and those aged 25 to 29 years. We must then design a study in such a way that the nutritional and prenatal health care practices of the two groups are comparable, even though, in general, the two groups are not comparable in these respects. Table 2-4 illustrates how we might deliberately select subjects for the study in such a way that both older and younger mothers had similar eating habits and amounts of prenatal attention. By building this comparability into the two groups of mothers, we have held nutrition and prenatal care constant. If the babies' birthweights in the two groups differ (as they, in fact, did in Table 2-4), then we might be able to infer that age (and not diet or prenatal care) influenced the birthweights of the infants. If the two groups do not differ, however, then we might be left to tentatively conclude that it is not the mother's age per se that causes young women to have a higher percentage of low-birthweight babies, but rather some other variable or set of variables, such as nutrition or prenatal care. (Note that although we have designated prenatal care and nutrition as the extraneous variables in this particular study, they are not at all extraneous to a full understanding of factors influencing infant birthweight; in other studies, nutritional practices and frequency of prenatal care might well be the independent variables.)

By exercising research control in this example, we have taken a step toward explaining the relationship between variables. The world is extremely complex, and many variables are interrelated in complicated ways. When studying a particular problem within the positivist paradigm, it is difficult to examine this complexity directly; the researcher must generally be content to analyze a couple of relationships at a time and put the pieces together like a jigsaw puzzle. That is why even modest studies can make contributions to knowledge. The extent of the contribution, however, is often directly related to how well a researcher is able to control contaminating influences.

In the present example, we identified three variables that could affect a baby's birthweight, but dozens of others could have been suggested, such as maternal stress, mothers' use of drugs or alcohol during pregnancy, sonogram testing, and so on. Researchers need to isolate the independent and dependent variables in which they are interested and then pinpoint from the dozens of possible candidates those extraneous variables that need to be controlled.

It is often impossible to control all the variables that affect the dependent variable, and not necessary to do so. It is essential to control a variable only if it is simultaneously related to both the dependent and independent variables. Figure 2-1 illustrates this notion. In this figure, each circle represents the variability associated with a particular variable. The large circle in the center represents the dependent variable, infant birthweight. Overlapping circles indicate

TABLE 2-4 Fictitious Example of Controlling Two Variables in a Research Study				
AGE OF MOTHER (YEARS)	RATING OF NUTRITIONAL PRACTICES	NUMBER OF PRENATAL VISITS	INFANT BIRTHWEIGHT
15–19	33% Good	33% 1–3 visits	20% $\leq$2500 g
	33% Fair	33% 4–6 visits	80% >2500 g
	33% Poor	33% >6 visits	
25–29	33% Good	33% 1–3 visits	9% $\leq$2500 g
	33% Fair	33% 4–6 visits	91% >2500 g
	33% Poor	33% >6 visits	

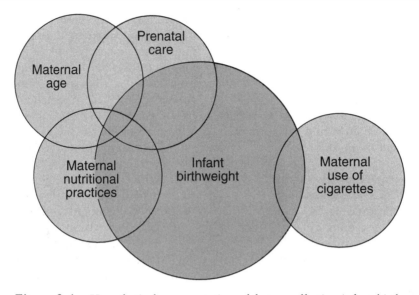

Figure 2-1. Hypothetical representation of factors affecting infant birth-weight.

the degree to which the variables are related to each other. In this hypothetical example, four variables are shown as being related to infant birthweight: the mother's age, the amount of prenatal care she receives, her nutritional practices, and her smoking practices during pregnancy. The first three variables are also related to each other; this is shown by the fact that these three circles overlap not only with infant birthweight but also with each other. That is, younger mothers tend to have different patterns of prenatal care and nutrition than older mothers. The mother's prenatal use of cigarettes, however, is unrelated to these three variables. In other words, women who smoke during their pregnancies (according to this hypothetical representation) are as likely to be young as old, to eat properly as not, and to get adequate prenatal care as not. If this representation is accurate, then it would not be essential to control smoking in a study of the effect of maternal age on infant birthweight. If this scheme is incorrect—if teenage mothers smoke more or less than older mothers—then the mother's smoking

practices ideally should be controlled because maternal smoking is related to birthweight.

Figure 2-1 does not represent infant birthweight as being totally determined by the four other variables. The darkened area of the birthweight circle designates unexplained variability in infant birthweight. That is, other circles or determinants of birthweight are needed for us to understand fully what causes babies to be born weighing different amounts. Genetic characteristics, events occurring during the pregnancy, and medical treatments administered to the pregnant woman are examples of other factors that contribute to an infant's weight at birth. Dozens, and perhaps hundreds, of circles would need to be sketched onto Figure 2-1 for us to understand fully the complex interrelationships between infant birthweight and other phenomena. In designing a study, we might be interested in the effect of only one variable (such as maternal age) on the dependent variable. This is perfectly respectable—indeed, often necessary. However, researchers conducting a quantitative study should attempt to control those variables that overlap with both the independent and dependent variables to understand fully the relationship between the main variables of interest. In Figure 2-1, if there are other variables that belong in the darkened area that are also related to maternal age, then those extraneous variables ideally should be controlled because uncontrolled extraneous variables can lead to erroneous or misleading conclusions.

Research rooted in the naturalistic paradigm is rarely concerned with the issue of control. With their emphasis on a holistic perspective and the individuality of human experience, qualitative researchers typically adhere to the view that to impose controls on a research setting is to remove irrevocably some of the meaning of reality.

MAJOR STEPS IN A QUANTITATIVE STUDY

One of the first decisions a researcher makes before embarking on a study involves the selection of a paradigm to guide the inquiry. As discussed in the previous chapter, the researcher generally works within a paradigm that is consistent with his or her world view, and that gives rise to the type of questions that excite the researcher's curiosity. The maturity of the concept of interest also may lead to one or the other paradigm: when little is known about a topic, a qualitative approach is often more fruitful than a quantitative one. After the appropriate paradigm is identified, the progression of activities differs for the qualitative and quantitative researcher.

In a quantitative study, a researcher moves from the beginning point of a study (the posing of a question) to the end point (the obtaining of an answer) in a logical sequence of predetermined steps that is similar across studies. In some studies, the steps overlap, whereas in others, certain steps are unnecessary. Still, there is a general flow of activities that is typical of a quantitative study. This section describes that flow, and the next section describes how qualitative studies differ.

Phase 1: The Conceptual Phase

The early steps in a quantitative research project typically involve activities that have a strong conceptual or intellectual element. These activities include thinking, reading, conceptualizing, reconceptualizing, theorizing, and reviewing ideas with colleagues or advisers. During this phase, the researcher calls on such skills as creativity, deductive reasoning, insight, and a firm grounding in previous research on the topic of interest.

STEP 1: FORMULATING AND DELIMITING THE PROBLEM

The first step is to develop a research problem and **research questions**. Good research depends to a great degree on good questions. Without a significant, interesting problem, the most carefully and skillfully designed research project is of little value.

Quantitative researchers generally proceed from the selection of broad topic areas of interest to the development of specific questions that are amenable to empirical inquiry. In developing a research question to be studied, nurse researchers must consider its substantive dimensions (Is this research question of theoretical or clinical significance?); its methodologic dimensions (How can this question best be studied?); its practical dimensions (Are adequate resources available to conduct a study?); and its ethical dimensions (Can this question be studied in a manner consistent with guidelines for the protection of subjects?).

STEP 2: REVIEWING THE RELATED LITERATURE

Quantitative research is typically conducted within the context of previous knowledge. To build on existing theory or research, the quantitative researcher strives to understand what is already known about a research problem. A thorough **literature review** provides a foundation upon which to base new knowledge and generally is conducted well before any data are collected in a quantitative study.

A familiarization with previous studies can also be useful in suggesting research topics or in identifying aspects of a problem about which more research is needed. Thus, a literature review sometimes precedes the delineation of the problem.

STEP 3: DEFINING THE THEORETICAL FRAMEWORK

Theory is the ultimate aim of science in that it transcends the specifics of a particular time, place, and group of people and aims to identify regularities in the relationships among variables. When quantitative research is performed within the context of a theoretical framework—that is, when previous theory is used as a basis for generating predictions that can be tested through empirical research—it is more likely that its findings will have broad significance and utility.

STEP 4: FORMULATING HYPOTHESES

A **hypothesis** is a statement of the researcher's expectations about relationships between the variables under investigation. A hypothesis, in other words, is a prediction of expected outcomes; it states the relationships that the researcher expects to find as a result of the study.

The research question identifies the concepts under investigation and asks how the concepts might be related; a hypothesis is the predicted answer. For example, the initial research question might be phrased as follows: Is preeclamptic toxemia in pregnant women associated with stress factors present during pregnancy? This might be translated into the following hypothesis or prediction: Pregnant women with a higher incidence of emotionally disturbing or stressful events during pregnancy will be more likely

than women with a lower incidence of stress to experience preeclamptic toxemia. Most quantitative studies are designed to test a priori hypotheses through statistical analysis.

Phase 2: The Design and Planning Phase

In the second major phase of a quantitative research project, the investigator makes a number of decisions about the methods to be used to address the research question and carefully plans for the actual collection of data. Sometimes, the nature of the question dictates the methods to be used, but more often than not, the researcher has considerable flexibility to be creative and must make many decisions. These methodologic decisions generally have crucial implications for the validity and credibility of the study findings. If the methods used to collect and analyze the research data are seriously flawed, then little confidence can be put in the conclusions. Much of this book is designed to acquaint readers with a range of methodologic options and to give them skills to evaluate their appropriateness for various research problems.

STEP 5: SELECTING A RESEARCH DESIGN

The **research design** is the overall plan for obtaining answers to the questions being studied and for handling some of the difficulties encountered during the research process. The design normally specifies which of the various types of research approach will be adopted and how the researcher plans to implement scientific controls to enhance the interpretability of the results. In quantitative studies, research designs tend to be highly structured and to include tight controls designed to eliminate the effects of contaminating influences.

For studies using traditional scientific methods, a wide variety of research designs are available. A basic distinction is the difference between **experimental research** (in which the researcher actively introduces some form of intervention) and **nonexperimental research** (in which the researcher collects data without trying to make any changes or introduce any treatments). For example, if a researcher gave bran flakes to one group of subjects and prune juice to another to evaluate which method facilitated elimination more effectively, then the study would involve an **intervention** (because the researcher intervened in the normal course of things) and would be considered experimental. If the researcher compared elimination patterns of two groups of people whose regular eating patterns differed—for example, some normally took foods that stimulated bowel elimination and others did not—then the study would not involve an intervention and would be considered nonexperimental. Experimental designs generally offer the possibility of greater control over extraneous variables than nonexperimental designs.

STEP 6: IDENTIFYING THE POPULATION TO BE STUDIED

The term **population** refers to the aggregate or totality of all the objects, subjects, or members that conform to a set of specifications. In quantitative studies, the researcher identifies the population to be studied during the planning phase. For example, a researcher might specify nurses (RNs) and residence in the United States as the attributes of interest; the study population would then consist of all licensed RNs who reside in the United States. We could in a similar fashion define a population consisting of *all* children under 10 years of age with muscular dystrophy in the state of California, or *all* the change-of-shift reports for the year 1998 in Massachusetts General Hospital.

The requirement of defining a population for a research project arises from the need to specify the group to which the results of a study can be applied. Before selecting actual subjects, the quantitative researcher needs to know what characteristics the study participants should possess.

STEP 7: SPECIFYING METHODS TO MEASURE THE RESEARCH VARIABLES

To address a quantitative research problem, the researcher must develop a method to observe or measure the research variables as accurately as possible. In most situations, the quantitative researcher begins by carefully defining the research variables to clarify exactly what each one means. Then the researcher needs to select or design an appropriate method of operationalizing the variables, that is, of collecting the data. A variety of quantitative data collection approaches exist. **Biophysiologic measurements** often play an important role in nursing research. Another popular form is **self-reports**, wherein subjects are asked about their feelings, behaviors, attitudes, and personal traits. Another technique is through **observation**, wherein the researcher collects data by observing people's behavior and recording relevant aspects of it.

Data collection methods vary in the structure imposed on the research subjects. Quantitative approaches tend to be fairly structured and controlled and generally involve the use of a formal instrument that obtains exactly the same information from every subject. The task of measuring research variables and developing a **data collection plan** is a complex and challenging process that permits a great deal of creativity and choice. Before finalizing the data collection plan, the researcher must carefully evaluate whether the chosen approach is likely to capture the concepts under study accurately.

STEP 8: DESIGNING THE SAMPLING PLAN

Research studies as a rule use as subjects only a small fraction of the population, referred to as a **sample**. The advantage of using a sample is that it is more practical and less costly than collecting data from the population. The risk is that the selected sample might not adequately reflect the behaviors, traits, symptoms, or beliefs of the population.

Various methods of obtaining a sample are available to the quantitative researcher. These methods vary in cost, effort, and level of skills required, but their adequacy is assessed by the same criterion: the **representativeness** of the selected sample. That is, the quality of the sample for quantitative studies is a function of how typical, or representative, the sample is of the population with respect to the variables of concern in the study. Sophisticated sampling procedures can produce samples that have a high likelihood of being representative. The most sophisticated sampling methods are referred to as **probability sampling**, which uses random procedures for the selection of the sample. In a probability sample, every member of the population has an equal probability of being included in the sample. With **nonprobability sampling**, by contrast, there is no way of ensuring that each member of the population could be selected; consequently, the risk of a **biased** (unrepresentative) sample is greater. The design of a **sampling plan** includes the selection of a sampling method, the specification of the sample size, and the selection of procedures for recruiting the subjects.

STEP 9: FINALIZING AND REVIEWING THE RESEARCH PLAN

Normally, researchers have their research plan reviewed by several individuals or groups before proceeding with the actual implementation of the plan. When a researcher is seeking financial support for the conduct of a study, the research plan is generally presented as a formal proposal to a funding source. Even when proposed projects are considered to be of sufficiently high quality for funding, the reviewers generally offer suggestions for improving the study design. Students conducting a study as part of a course or degree requirement must also have their plans reviewed by faculty advisers. Even under other circumstances, however, the researcher is well advised to have individuals external to the project check the preliminary plans. An experienced researcher

with a fresh perspective on a research problem can often be invaluable in identifying pitfalls and shortcomings that otherwise might not have been recognized. Finally, before proceeding with a study, researchers often need to have their research plan approved by special committees to ensure that the plan does not violate ethical principles.

STEP 10: CONDUCTING THE PILOT STUDY AND MAKING REVISIONS

Often, the principal focus of a pilot study is assessment of the adequacy of the data collection plan. The researcher may need to know, for example, if technical equipment is functioning properly. If questionnaires are used, it is important to know whether respondents understand the questions and directions or if they find certain questions objectionable in some way; this is generally referred to as **pretesting** the questionnaire.

A pilot study should be carried out with as much care as the major study so that any detected weaknesses will be truly representative of inadequacies inherent in the major study. Subjects for a pilot study should possess the same characteristics as individuals who will compose the main sample. That is, pilot subjects should be chosen from the same population as subjects for the major study. It is often useful to question the individuals who participate in a pilot study concerning their reactions to and overall impressions of the project.

When the data from the test run have been collected and scrutinized, the researcher should make the revisions and refinements that, in her or his judgment, would eliminate or reduce problems encountered during the pilot study. If extensive revisions are required, it may prove advisable to have a second trial run that incorporates those revisions.

Phase 3: The Empirical Phase

The empirical portion of a quantitative study involves the collection of **research data and the** preparation of those data for analysis. In many studies, the empirical phase is the most time-consuming part of the investigation, although the amount of time spent collecting data varies considerably from one study to the next. If data are collected by distributing a written questionnaire to intact groups, this task may be accomplished in a day or so. More often, however, the data collection requires several weeks, or even months, of work.

STEP 11: COLLECTING THE DATA

The actual collection of data in a quantitative study often proceeds according to a preestablished plan. The researcher's plan typically specifies procedures for the actual collection of data (e.g., where and when the data will be gathered); for describing the study to participants; for obtaining their consent; and, if necessary, for training the individuals who will be involved in the collection of the research data.

A considerable amount of both clerical and administrative work is required in the data collection task. The investigators typically must be sure, for example, that enough materials are available to complete the study; that participants are informed of the time and place that their presence may be required; that research personnel (such as interviewers) are conscientious in keeping their appointments; that schedules do not conflict; and that a suitable system of maintaining confidentiality of information has been implemented.

STEP 12: PREPARING THE DATA FOR ANALYSIS

After the data are collected, a few preliminary activities must be performed before the actual analysis of the data can begin. For instance, it is normally necessary to look through questionnaires to determine if they are usable. Sometimes, such forms are left almost entirely blank or contain other indications of misinterpretation or noncompliance. Another step that should be taken at this point is to assign iden-

tification numbers to the responses or observations of different subjects, if this was not done previously.

Frequently, a step known as coding is required. **Coding** refers to the process of translating verbal data into categories or numeric form. For example, patients' responses to a question about the quality of nursing care they received during hospitalization might be coded into positive reactions, negative reactions, neutral reactions, and mixed reactions. Another preliminary step that is generally necessary is transferring research information from written documents onto computer files so that the data can be analyzed by computer.

Phase 4: The Analytic Phase

The quantitative data gathered in the empirical phase are not reported to the consumers of research in raw form. They are subjected to various types of analysis and interpretation, which occurs in the fourth major phase of a project.

STEP 13: ANALYZING THE DATA

The data themselves do not provide us with answers to our research questions. Ordinarily, the amount of data collected in a study is rather extensive and, therefore, needs to be processed and analyzed in some orderly, coherent fashion so that relationships can be discerned. Quantitative information is generally analyzed through statistical procedures. **Statistical analyses** cover a broad range of techniques, from some simple procedures to complex and sophisticated methods. The underlying logic of statistical tests, however, is relatively easy to grasp, and computers and pocket calculators have eliminated the need to get bogged down with detailed arithmetic operations.

STEP 14: INTERPRETING THE RESULTS

Before the results of a study can be communicated effectively, they must be organized and interpreted in some systematic fashion. **Interpretation** refers to the process of making sense of the results and of examining the implications of the findings within a broader context. The process of interpretation begins with an attempt to explain the findings, within the context of the theoretical framework, prior knowledge in the area, and the limitations of the study.

If the research hypotheses have been supported, an explanation of the results is usually straightforward because the findings fit into a previously conceived argument. If the hypotheses are not supported, then the investigator must develop some possible explanations. Is the underlying conceptualization wrong or perhaps inappropriate for the research problem? Or do the findings reflect problems with the research methods rather than the theory (e.g., was the measuring tool inappropriate)? To provide sound explanations for obtained findings, then, the researcher not only must be familiar with the literature on a topic and with the conceptual underpinnings of the problem but also must be able to understand the methodologic weaknesses of the study. A researcher should be in a position to evaluate critically the decisions that he or she made in designing the study and to recommend alternatives to others interested in the same research problem.

Phase 5: The Dissemination Phase

The previous (analytic) phase brings the researcher full circle: it provides the answers to the questions posed in the first phase of the project. However, the researcher's job is not complete until the results of the study are disseminated.

STEP 15: COMMUNICATING THE FINDINGS

The results of a research investigation are of little utility if they are not communicated to others. Even the most compelling hypothesis, the most careful and thorough study, and the most dramatic results are of no value to the nursing community if they are unknown. An-

other—and often final—task of a research project, therefore, is the preparation of a **research report** that can be shared with others.

The research report can take various forms: term papers, dissertations, journal articles, papers for presentation at professional conferences, books, and so on. **Journal articles**—that is, short reports appearing in such professional journals as *Nursing Research*—are generally the most useful because such reports are available to a broad audience. Nurse researchers have many journals available for publishing their research reports.

STEP 16: UTILIZING THE FINDINGS

Many interesting studies have been conducted by nurses without having any effect on nursing practice or nursing education. Ideally, the concluding step of a high-quality study is to plan for its utilization in the real world. Although nurse researchers may not themselves be in a position to implement a plan for utilizing research findings, they can contribute to the process by including in their research reports recommendations regarding how the results of the study could be incorporated into the practice of nursing and by disseminating their findings to practicing nurses.

Organization of a Quantitative Research Project

The steps described in the preceding section represent an idealized conception of what researchers do. The research process rarely follows a neatly prescribed pattern of sequential procedures. Developments in one step, for example, may require alterations in a previously completed activity. Nevertheless, for the quantitative researcher, careful organization is very important.

Almost all research projects are conducted under some time pressure. Students in research courses may have end-of-term deadlines; government-sponsored research involves funds granted for a specified time. Those who may not have such formal time constraints—such as graduate students working on dissertations—normally have their own goals for project completion. Setting up a timetable in advance may be an important step toward meeting such goals. This means that it is useful to make projections about what tasks should be completed by what point in time. Having deadlines for tasks—even tentative ones—helps to impose some structure and delimits tasks that might otherwise continue indefinitely, such as the selection of a problem and review of the literature.

Unfortunately, it is not possible to give even approximate figures for the relative percentage of time that should be spent on each task in a quantitative study. Some projects require many months to develop and pilot test the measuring instruments, whereas other studies use previously existing instruments. The write-up of the study may take many months or only a few days. Clearly, however, not all of the steps will be equally time-consuming. It would make little sense to simply divide the time available by the total number of tasks.

Let us suppose that during a 12-month period we were studying the following problem: Does the presence of fathers in the delivery room affect the mothers' perception of pain? Figure 2-2 presents a hypothetical schedule for the research tasks to be completed. (The selection of the problem is not included because the research topic has already been identified.) Note that many activities overlap and that some tasks are projected to involve little time in terms of time elapsed on the calendar.

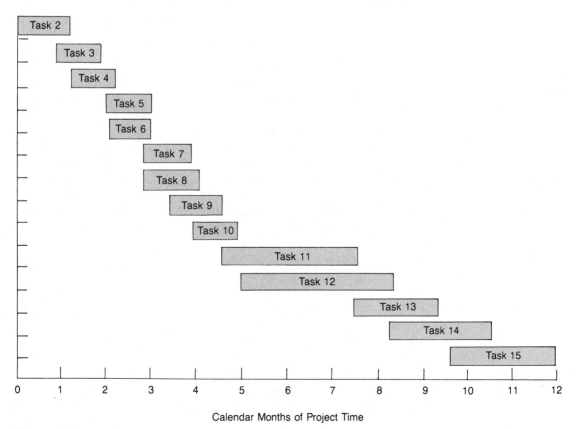

Figure 2-2. Breakdown of project tasks by time allotted.

In developing a schedule of this sort, a number of considerations should be kept in mind, including the level of knowledge and competence of the researcher. Resources available to the researcher, in the form of research funds and personnel, will greatly influence the time estimates. It is also important to consider the practical aspects of performing the study, which were not all enumerated in the preceding section. Obtaining supplies, securing the necessary permissions, having forms or instruments approved by granting agencies or supervisors, and holding meetings are all time-consuming, but often necessary, activities.

Individuals differ in the kinds of tasks that are appealing to them. Some people greatly enjoy the preliminary phase, which has a strong intellectual component, whereas others are more eager to collect the data, a task that is often more interpersonal in nature. The researcher should attempt, however, to allocate a reasonable amount of time to do justice to each activity.

ACTIVITIES IN A QUALITATIVE STUDY

As we have just seen, quantitative research involves a fairly linear progression of tasks—the researcher lays out in advance the steps to be taken to maximize the integrity of the study and then follows those steps as faithfully as possible. In a qualitative study, by contrast, the progression is closer to a circle than to a straight line—the qualitative researcher is continually examining and interpreting data and making decisions about how to proceed based on what has already been discovered.

Because the qualitative researcher has a flexible approach to the collection and analysis of data, it is impossible to define the flow of activities precisely—the flow varies from one study to another, and researchers themselves do not know ahead of time exactly how the study will proceed. However, the following sections attempt to give you a feel for how a qualitative

study is conducted by describing some major activities and indicating how and when they might be performed.

Conceptualizing and Planning a Qualitative Study

Like quantitative researchers, qualitative researchers generally begin with a broad topic area to be studied. However, qualitative researchers are usually interested in an aspect of a topic that is poorly understood and about which little is known. Therefore, they do not develop hypotheses or pose highly refined research questions before going into the field. The general topic area may be narrowed and clarified on the basis of self-reflection and discussion with colleagues (or clients), but usually the researcher proceeds with a fairly broad research question that allows the focus to be sharpened and delineated more clearly once the study is under way. Initially, the qualitative researcher places few boundaries or delimitations on the research question.

There are conflicting ideas among qualitative researchers regarding the performance of a literature review at the outset of the study. At one extreme are those who believe that the researcher should not consult the literature at all before collecting data. The concern is that prior studies might exert an undue influence on the researcher's conceptualization of the phenomena under study. According to this view, the phenomena should be elucidated based on the participants' viewpoints rather than on any prior information. Others feel that the researcher should conduct at least a cursory upfront literature review to obtain some possible guidance (including guidance in identifying the kinds of biases that have emerged in studying the topic). In any event, qualitative researchers typically find a relatively small body of relevant previous work because of the nature of the questions they ask.

During the planning phase, the qualitative researcher must also identify a **site** for the data collection. Before entering the field, the researcher must select a site that is consistent with the topic under study. For example, if the topic is the health care beliefs of the urban poor, an inner-city neighborhood with a high percentage of low-income residents must be identified. The researcher may have to identify further the types of **setting** within the site where data collection will occur—for example, in homes, clinics, work places, and so on. In many cases, the researcher needs to make preliminary contacts with key actors in the selected site to ensure cooperation and access to informants; that is, the researcher needs to **gain entrée** into the site or settings within it.

As indicated in the prior section, quantitative researchers do not begin to collect any data until the research design has been finalized. In a qualitative study, by contrast, the research design is often referred to as an **emergent design**—a design that emerges during the course of data collection. However, before going into the field, the researcher must have some sense of how much time is available for field work and must also arrange for and test any equipment that might be needed. For example, most qualitative studies involve audiotaping (in some cases videotaping) interviews with informants.

Conducting the Qualitative Study

In a qualitative study, the activities of sampling, data collection, data analysis, and interpretation take place in an iterative fashion. The qualitative researcher begins by talking with or observing a few people who have first-hand experience with the phenomenon under study. The discussions and observations are loosely structured, allowing for a full range of beliefs, feelings, and behaviors to be expressed. Analysis and interpretation are ongoing, concurrent activities used to guide the kinds of people to sample next and the types of questions to ask or observations to make. The actual process of data analysis involves clustering together related types of narrative information into a coherent scheme. The analysis of qualitative data is an intensive, time-consuming activity.

As analysis and interpretation progress, the researcher begins to identify themes and categories, which are used to build a descriptive theory of the phenomenon. The kinds of data obtained and the people selected as participants tend to become increasingly focused and purposeful as a theory emerges. Theory development and verification shape the sampling process—as the theory develops, the researcher seeks participants who can confirm and enrich the theoretical understandings, as well as participants who can potentially challenge them and lead to further theoretical development.

A quantitative researcher decides in advance how many subjects to include in the study, but a qualitative researcher's sampling decisions are guided by the data themselves. **Many qualitative researchers use the principle of saturation,** which occurs when themes and categories in the data become repetitive and redundant, such that no new information can be gleaned by further data collection.

In a quantitative study, the researcher seeks to collect high-quality data by selecting methods in advance and by measuring instruments that were previously demonstrated to be accurate and rigorous. The qualitative researcher, by contrast, must take steps to demonstrate the trustworthiness of the data while in the field. The central feature of these efforts is to confirm that the findings accurately reflect the experiences and viewpoints of the participants, rather than the perceptions of the researcher. One confirmatory activity, for example, involves going back to participants and sharing preliminary interpretations with them so that they can evaluate whether the researcher's thematic analysis is consistent with their experiences.

Disseminating Qualitative Findings

Qualitative nursing researchers also strive to share their findings with other nurses and other health care specialists. Qualitative research reports are increasingly being published in the nursing literature. Qualitative findings, because of their depth and richness, also lend themselves more readily to book-length manuscripts than do quantitative findings. Regardless of the researcher's position about when a literature review should be conducted, qualitative researchers usually include a summary of prior research in their reports as a means of providing context for the study.

Quantitative reports almost never contain any **raw data**—data exactly in the form they were collected, which are numeric values. Qualitative reports, by contrast, are generally filled with rich verbatim passages directly from the participants. The excerpts are used in an evidentiary fashion to support or illustrate the researcher's interpretations and theoretical formulations.

Like quantitative researchers, qualitative nurse researchers want to see their findings utilized by other nurses. Qualitative findings often are used as the basis for the formulation of hypotheses that are tested by quantitative researchers. Qualitative findings are also used in the development of assessment tools for both research and clinical purposes. Most important, qualitative studies help to shape nurses' perceptions of a problem or situation and their conceptualizations of potential solutions.

RESEARCH EXAMPLES

This section presents brief overviews of a quantitative and a qualitative study. Our overview deals primarily with the key concepts of the studies. You may wish to consult the full research report in thinking about the differences between qualitative and quantitative studies.

Research Example of a Quantitative Study

Brandt, Andrews, and Kvale (1998) initiated a study to explore whether there was a relation-ship between the quality of mother-infant interactions during the early postpartum period and breastfeeding outcome at 6 weeks postpartum. To be eligible for the study, women had to be in the third trimester of their pregnancies and had to express a desire to breastfeed their infants for at least 8 weeks. A sample of 42 pregnant Latina women were recruited into the study.

The quality of mother-infant interactions was measured shortly after birth (between 28 and 90 hours postpartum) in the homes of the study participants, using a tool called the Nursing Child Assessment Feeding Scale (NCAFS). The NCAFS consists of six subscales, each of which lists a series of caregiver and/or infant behaviors that a nurse observer looks for during a routine feeding. For example, one of the subscales measures the degree to which the mother fosters the child's social-emotional growth. Scores from the six subscales are summed for a total score that can range from 1 to 76, with higher scores reflecting higher quality interactions. Breastfeeding outcome (breastfeeding one or more times a day versus not breastfeeding at all) was assessed 6 weeks later.

The findings indicated that women who continued to breastfeed at 6 weeks postpartum had significantly higher scores on the NCAFS scale than women who had weaned by 6 weeks. The researchers concluded that for mothers and newborns evidencing early difficulties in attachment, assistive interventions and careful follow-up would be beneficial.

Research Example of a Qualitative Study

Langner (1993) conducted an in-depth study of the process of caring for an elderly relative. Her focus was on the process by which the family member copes with the day-to-day caregiving experience, the dilemmas to which it gives rise, and the coping strategies used to deal with the dilemmas.

Twenty-three primary caregivers of an elderly relative participated in the study. Each participant was interviewed on three separate occasions over a 4-month period, beginning shortly after the older relative was discharged from the hospital. All interviews, which yielded narrative, conversational data, were tape recorded and transcribed. Questions for the interviewing evolved from the ongoing analysis of data. Three major strategies for managing the caregiving process emerged from the analysis. One theme, establishing and maintaining a routine, is exemplified by the following excerpt:

> We have a regular schedule now. I get up at 5:30 every morning, and I'm at work between 8:30 and 9:00. I do his sponge bath, breakfast, get all the medicines ready and put them in little cups for the day. There is a fair amount of planning that you do. I wasn't organized at first . . . . But now we have a regular schedule, and we follow that schedule every day as much as we can. I feel like I've got things under better control these days (p. 586).

Langner concluded that the strategies used by family caregivers were instrumental in helping them to manage the caregiving passage because they fostered feelings of control and satisfaction.

SUMMARY

A research **study** (or **investigation** or **research project**) is undertaken by one or more **researchers** (or **investigators** or **scientists**). The people who provide information to the researchers are referred to as **subjects, study participants,** or **respondents** in quantitative research or as study participants or **informants** in qualitative research.

Researchers investigate **phenomena, concepts,** and **constructs,** which are abstractions or mental representations inferred from behavior or events. Concepts are the building blocks of **theories,** which are systematic explanations of some aspect of the real world. In quantitative studies, the concepts under investigation are referred to as **variables.** A variable is a characteristic or quality that varies from one person or object to another. The blood type, grip strength, and hair color of a person are variables. These variables, which are inherent characteristics of a person that the researcher measures or observes, are referred to as **attribute variables.** When a researcher actively creates a variable, as when a special **intervention** or treatment is introduced, the variable may be referred to as an **active variable.** Variables that can take on an infinite range of values along a specified continuum are referred to as **continuous variables** (e.g., height and weight). A **discrete variable,** by contrast, is one that has a finite number of values between two points (e.g., number of children). Variables that have distinct categories that do not represent a quantity are **categorical variables** (e.g., gender and blood type).

An important distinction for quantitative researchers is differentiation between the dependent and independent variables of a study. The **dependent variable** is the behavior, characteristic, or outcome that the researcher is interested in understanding, explaining, predicting, or affecting. The dependent variable (or **criterion variable, outcome variable**) is the presumed consequence or effect of the independent variable. The **independent variable** is the presumed cause of, antecedent to, or influence on the dependent variable. Groups that are highly varied with respect to some attribute are described as **heterogeneous;** groups with limited **variability** are described as **homogeneous.** In an actual quantitative study, the variables are generally clarified and defined in such a way that they are amenable to observation or measurement. The **operational definition** of a concept is the specification of the procedures and tools required to make the needed measurements.

The term **data** is used to designate the information that is collected during the course of a study. Data may take the form of narrative information (**qualitative data**) or numeric values (**quantitative data**). Researchers usually are not interested in studying concepts in isolation but rather in learning about the **relationship** between two or more concepts simultaneously. A relationship refers to a bond or connection (or pattern of association) between two phenomena. Quantitative researchers focus on the relationship between the independent variables and dependent variables.

In a quantitative study, the steps involved in the conduct of an investigation are fairly standard, and the researcher progresses in a fairly linear fashion from posing a research question to answering it. The conceptual phase involves (1) defining the problem to be studied and the **research question** to be addressed; (2) doing a **literature review**; (3) developing a **theoretical framework**; and (4) formulating **hypotheses** to be tested. The design and planning phase include (5) selecting a **research design**; (6) specifying the **population**; (7) specifying the methods to measure the research variables; (8) selecting a **sample**; (9) finalizing the research plan; and (10) conducting a **pilot study** and making revisions. The empirical phase involves (11) collecting the data and (12) preparing the data for analysis. The analytic phase includes (13) analyzing the data through **statistical analysis** and (14) interpreting the results. The dissemination phase involves (15) communicating the findings and (16) promoting their utilization. The conduct of quantitative studies requires careful planning and organization. The preparation of a timetable with expected deadlines for task completion is generally recommended.

The flow of activities in a qualitative study is more flexible and less linear than in a quantitative one. The qualitative researcher begins with a broad question regarding the phenomenon of interest, often focusing on a little-studied aspect. The focus is less likely to be sharpened by reviewing the literature than by the actual process of data collection and analysis. In the early phase, the researcher selects a **site** and then seeks to **gain entrée** into it and into the specific **settings** in which data collection will occur. The research design is typically an **emergent design** that takes shape

in the field. Once in the field, the researcher selects informants, collects data, and then analyzes and interprets them in an iterative fashion. Early analysis leads to refinements in sampling and data collection, until **saturation** (redundancy of information) is achieved. The qualitative researcher concludes by writing a research report.

STUDY ACTIVITIES

Chapter 2 of the *Study Guide to Accompany Nursing Research: Principles and Methods, 6th ed.*, offers various exercises for reinforcing concepts presented in this chapter. Additionally, the following study questions can be addressed:

1. Suggest ways of operationally defining the following concepts: nursing competency, patients' time to first voiding after surgery, aggressive behavior, patients' level of pain, home health hazards, postsurgical recovery, and body image.

2. Name five continuous, five discrete, and five categorical variables; identify which, if any, are dichotomous.

3. Identify which of the following variables could be active variables and which are attribute variables (some may be both): height, degree of fatigue, cooperativeness, noise level on hospital units, length of stay in hospital, educational attainment, self-esteem, nurses' job satisfaction.

4. In the following research problems, identify the independent and dependent variables:
   a. How do nurses and physicians differ in the ways they view the extended role concept for nurses?
   b. Does problem-oriented recording lead to more effective patient care than other recording methods?

c. Do elderly patients have lower pain thresholds than younger patients?

d. How are the sleeping patterns of infants affected by different forms of stimulation?

e. Can home visits by nurses to released psychiatric patients reduce readmission rates?

✎ SUGGESTED READINGS

Methodologic References

Kerlinger, F. N. (1986). *Foundations of behavioral research* (3rd ed.). New York: Holt, Rinehart & Winston.

Morse, J. M., & Field, P. A. (1995). *Qualitative research methods for health professionals* (2nd ed.). Thousand Oaks, CA: Sage Publications.

Substantive References

Anderson, G. C., Lane, A. E., & Chang, H. P. (1995). Axillary temperature in transitional newborn infants before and after tub bath. *Applied Nursing Research, 8,* 123–128.

Brandt, K. A., Andrews, C. M., & Kvale, J. (1998). Mother-infant interaction and breast-feeding outcome 6 weeks after birth. *Journal of Obstetric, Gynecologic, and Neonatal Nursing, 27,* 169–174.

Ciliska, D. (1998). Evaluation of two nondieting interventions for obese women. *Western Journal of Nursing Research, 20,* 119–135.

Draucker, C. B. (1997). Early family life and victimization in the lives of women. *Research in Nursing & Health, 20,* 399–412.

Evans, M. L., Dick, M. J., & Clark, A. S. (1995). Sleep during the week before labor: Relationships to labor outcomes. *Clinical Nursing Research, 4,* 238–252.

Fuller, B. F., & Conner, D. A. (1995). The effect of pain on infant behaviors. *Clinical Nursing Research, 4,* 253–273.

Good, M. (1995). A comparison of the effects of jaw relaxation and music on postoperative pain. *Nursing Research, 44,* 52–57.

Horns, P. N., Ratcliffe, L. P., Leggett, J. C., & Swanson, M. S. (1996). Pregnancy outcomes among active and sedentary primiparous women. *Journal of Obstetric, Gynecologic, and Neonatal Nursing, 25,* 49–54.

King, S., Collins, C., & Liken, M. (1995). Values and the use of community services. *Qualitative Health Research, 5,* 332–347.

Langner, S. R. (1993). Ways of managing the experience of caregiving to elderly relatives. *Western Journal of Nursing Research, 15,* 582–594.

McCarthy, D. O. (1997). Short-term regulation of energy intake in hypophagic tumor-bearing rats. *Research in Nursing & Health, 20,* 425–429.

Popkess-Vawter, S., Wendel, S., Schmoll, S., & O'Connell, K. (1998). Overeating, reversal theory, and weight cycling. *Western Journal of Nursing Research, 20,* 67–83.

CHAPTER 3

Research Problems, Research Questions, and Hypotheses

OVERVIEW OF RESEARCH PROBLEMS

A research study begins as a problem that a researcher would like to solve or as a question (or set of questions) that a researcher would like to answer. The question or problem often evolves from a broad topic area, and researchers usually find it necessary to devote some time to delimiting and explicating the problem. Quantitative researchers, in particular, are apt at an early stage to formulate a refined and specific research question or hypothesis that guides the development of a research design and the plan for the collection and analysis of data. This chapter discusses the formulation and evaluation of research questions and hypotheses. We begin by clarifying some related terms.

Basic Terminology

At the most general level, a researcher is interested in a **topic,** which is sometimes referred to as the **focus** of the research. Examples of research topics are adolescent smoking, patient compliance, coping with disability, and pain

management. Within each of these broad topic areas are many potential research problems.

A **research problem** is a situation involving an enigmatic, perplexing, or troubling condition. Both qualitative and quantitative researchers identify a research problem within a broad topic area of interest. The purpose of disciplined research is to "solve" the problem—or to contribute to its solution—by accumulating sufficient information to lead to understanding or explaining it. A **problem statement** articulates the problem to be addressed.

A **research question** is a statement of the specific query the researcher wants to answer to address the research problem. The research questions guide the types of data to be collected in the study. If a researcher makes a specific prediction regarding the answers to the research questions, he or she poses a **hypothesis** that is tested empirically.

Other related terms are sometimes used in research reports. For example, many reports include a **statement of purpose** (or purpose statement), which is the researcher's summary of the overall goal of a study. A researcher might also identify several specific **research aims** or **objectives**—the specific accomplishments the researcher hopes to achieve by conducting the study. The objectives include obtaining answers to the research questions or testing the research hypotheses but may also encompass some broader aims (e.g., developing recommendations for changes to nursing practice based on the study results).

These various terms are not always consistently defined in research methods textbooks, and differences between the terms are often subtle. Table 3-1 illustrates the interrelationships among them as we have defined them.

Research Problems and Paradigms

Although there is some overlap in the type of research problems that can be addressed within the context of the two major paradigms, there are certain problems that are better suited for studies using qualitative versus quantitative methods. Quantitative studies usually involve concepts that are fairly well developed, about which there is an existing body of literature, and for which reliable methods of measurement have been developed. Generally, a quantitative researcher is likely to pursue a research problem that has been previously studied but has yielded results that need verification, clarification, or extension. For example, a quantitative study might be undertaken to determine if postpartum depression is higher among women who are employed 6 months after delivery than among those who stay home with their babies. There are relatively accurate mea-

---

TABLE 3-1   Example of Terms Relating to Research Problems

TERM	EXAMPLE
Topic or focus	Side effects in chemotherapy patients
Research problem	Nausea and vomiting are common side effects among chemotherapy patients, and interventions to date have been only moderately successful in reducing these effects. New interventions that can reduce or prevent these side effects need to be identified.
Statement of purpose	The purpose of the study is to test an intervention to reduce chemotherapy-induced side effects—specifically, to compare the effectiveness of patient-controlled and nurse-administered antiemetic therapy for controlling nausea and vomiting in chemotherapy patients.
Research question	What is the relative effectiveness of patient-controlled antiemetic therapy versus nurse-controlled antiemetic therapy in chemotherapy patients with regard to (a) medication consumption and (b) control of nausea and vomiting?
Hypotheses	1. Subjects receiving antiemetic therapy by a patient-controlled pump will report less nausea than subjects receiving the therapy by nurse administration. 2. Subjects receiving antiemetic therapy by a patient-controlled pump will vomit less than subjects receiving the therapy by nurse administration. 3. Subjects receiving antiemetic therapy by a patient-controlled pump will consume less medication than subjects receiving the therapy by nurse administration.
Aims or objectives	This study seeks to accomplish the following objectives: (1) to develop and implement two alternative procedures for administering antiemetic therapy for patients receiving moderate emetogenic chemotherapy (patient controlled versus nurse controlled); (2) to test three hypotheses concerning the relative effectiveness of the alternative procedures on medication consumption and control of side effects; and (3) to use the findings to develop recommendations for possible changes to therapeutic procedures.

sures of depression that would yield quantitative information about the level of depression in a sample of employed and nonemployed postpartum women.

Qualitative studies are often undertaken because some aspect of a concept is poorly understood and the researcher wants to develop a rich, comprehensive, and context-bound understanding of a phenomenon. In the example of postpartum depression, a qualitative study would not be well suited to comparing levels of depression among the two groups of women, but it would be ideal for fully exploring the underlying mechanisms that lead to postpartum depression in both groups.

SOURCES OF RESEARCH PROBLEMS

Students are sometimes puzzled about the origins of research problems. Where do ideas for research problems come from? How does a researcher select a topic area and develop research questions? In this section, we suggest some sources for identifying a research problem or topic. The five most common sources are experience, the nursing literature, social issues, theories, and ideas from others.

Experience

The nurse's everyday experience provides a rich supply of problems for investigation. Whether you are a student nurse, practicing nurse, nurse educator, or nursing administrator, there are sure to be occurrences or situations that you have found puzzling or problematic. You may be well along the way to developing a research idea if you have ever asked the following kinds of questions: Why are things done this way? What information would help to solve this problem? What would happen if . . . ? What is the process by which this situation arose? For the beginning researcher in particular, experience is often the most compelling source for topics. Immediate problems that are in need of

solution or that excite the curiosity are relevant and interesting and, thus, may generate more enthusiasm than abstract and distant problems inferred from a theory.

An important ingredient for a successful research project is the investigator's curiosity. As you are performing your nursing functions, you are bound to find a wealth of research ideas if you are curious about why things are the way they are or about how things could be improved if something were to change.

Nursing Literature

Ideas for research projects often come from reading the nursing literature. The beginning nurse researcher can profit from regularly reading nursing journals, especially ones that report the results of nursing studies, such as *Nursing Research, Applied Nursing Research,* or the *Western Journal of Nursing Research.* Many nursing specialty journals (e.g., *Heart & Lung*) also publish research studies. Reading published reports may help neophyte researchers to find a problem amenable to investigation and may also help to familiarize them with the wording of research problems and the actual conduct of research studies.

Published research reports may suggest problem areas indirectly by stimulating the reader's imagination or interest in a topic and directly by specifying further areas in need of investigation. For example, Friedman (1997) studied the sources of social support among older women with heart failure. She concluded that "future study of older women's support sources beginning earlier in the illness experience and assessing change at frequent intervals over a longer time period would allow the process of support acquisition, factors affecting change in support and support sources, and the impact on psychological well-being to be examined more fully" (p. 326).

Inconsistencies in the findings reported in nursing literature often generate ideas for research studies. For example, there are inconsistencies regarding which irrigation fluid (e.g., water, cranberry juice, or cola) is most effective in maintaining the patency of patients' feeding tubes. Such discrepancies could lead to the design of a study to resolve the matter.

A researcher may also wonder whether a study similar to one reported in a journal article would yield comparable results if applied in a different setting or with a different population. **Replications** are needed to establish the validity and generalizability of previous findings.

In summary, a familiarity with existing research or with problematic and controversial nursing issues that have yet to be understood and investigated systematically is an important route to developing a research topic. The student who is actively seeking a problem to study, such as the student required to do an empirical thesis, will find it useful to read widely in areas of interest. In Chapter 4, we deal more extensively with the procedures of doing a research literature review.

Social Issues

Sometimes, topics are suggested by more global contemporary social or political issues of relevance to the health care community. For example, the feminist movement has raised questions about such topics as gender equity, sexual harassment, and domestic violence. The civil rights movement has led to research on minority health problems, access to health care, and other relevant topics. Thus, an idea for a study may stem from a familiarity with social concerns or controversial social problems.

Theory

The fourth major source of research problems (primarily among quantitative researchers) lies in the theoretical systems and conceptual schemes that have been developed in nursing and other related disciplines. To be useful in nursing practice, theories must be tested through research for their applicability to the hospital unit, the emergency room, the classroom, and other nursing environments.

If a researcher decides to base a research project on an existing theory, deductions from the theory must be developed. Essentially, the researcher must ask the following questions: If this theory is correct, what kind of behavior would I expect to find in certain situations or under certain conditions? What kind of evidence would support this theory? This process would eventually result in a specific problem that could be subjected to systematic investigation.

Let us look at an example of how a problem can be derived from a conceptual system. Levine (1973) postulated a conceptual framework for nursing that concerns conservation. She explains nursing as conserving the patient's energy, structural integrity, personal integrity, and social integrity. From this theory, the researcher could formulate specific predictions about expected findings. For example, it might be hypothesized that primary nursing is more effective in conserving the patient's energy and social integrity than is team nursing. By developing measures of energy expenditure and social integration, this hypothesis could be tested scientifically.

Ideas From External Sources

External sources can sometimes provide the impetus for a research idea. In some cases, a research topic may be given as a direct suggestion. For example, a faculty member may give students a list of topics from which to choose or may actually assign a specific topic to be studied. Entities that sponsor funded research, such as the federal government, often identify broad or specific topics on which research proposals are encouraged. For example, in recent years, government agencies have requested a variety of AIDS-related research projects. For beginning students, it is often useful to have some guiding suggestions on the development of a research problem. Even when a research area is suggested, however, it is better for the researcher to identify the aspect of the problem that is of greatest interest because curiosity is a critical ingredient in successful research.

Research ideas sometimes represent a response to priorities that are established within the nursing profession, examples of which were discussed in Chapter 1. Priorities for nursing research have been established by many nursing specialty practices. Priority lists can often serve as a useful starting point for exploring research topics.

Often, ideas for studies emerge as a result of a brainstorming session. By discussing possible research topics with peers, advisers, or researchers with advanced skills, ideas often become clarified and sharpened or enriched and more fully developed. Professional conferences often provide an excellent opportunity for such discussions.

⬥ DEVELOPMENT AND REFINEMENT OF RESEARCH PROBLEMS

Unless a research problem is developed on the basis of theory or an explicit suggestion from an external source, the actual procedures for developing a research topic are difficult to describe. The process is rarely a smooth and orderly one; there are likely to be many false starts, several inspirations, and several setbacks in the initial efforts to develop a research problem statement. The few suggestions offered here are not intended to imply that there are techniques for making this first step easy but rather to encourage the beginning researcher to persevere in the absence of instant success.

Selecting a Topic

The development of a research problem is essentially a creative process that depends on imagination, insight, and ingenuity. In the early stages, when research ideas are being generated, it is wise not to be critical of them immediately. It is much better to begin by just relaxing and jotting down general areas of interest as they come to mind. At this point, it matters little if the terms used to remind you of your ideas are abstract or concrete, broad or specific, technical or colloquial—the important point is to put some ideas on paper. Examples of some broad topics that may come to mind include communication with patients, anxiety in hospitalized children, pain among cancer patients, postpartum depression, and postoperative loss of orientation.

After this first step, the ideas can be sorted in terms of interest, knowledge about the topics, and the perceived promise that the topics hold for a research project. When the most fruitful idea has been selected, the rest of the list should not be discarded; it may be necessary to return to it.

Narrowing the Topic

Once you have identified one or more general topics of interest, you will need to begin asking questions that will lead to a researchable problem. Some examples of question stems that may help you focus your inquiry include the following:

- What is going on with . . . ?
- What can be done to solve . . . ?
- What causes . . . ?
- What is the extent of . . . ?
- Why do . . . ?
- When do . . . ?
- What influences . . . ?
- How intense are . . . ?
- What conditions prevail before . . . ?
- What characteristics are associated with . . . ?
- What are the consequences of . . . ?
- What is the relationship between . . . ?
- How effective is . . . ?
- What differences exist between . . . ?
- What factors contribute to . . . ?

Here again, early criticism of ideas is often counterproductive in this basically creative endeavor. Try not to jump to the conclusion that an idea sounds trivial or uninspired without giving it more careful consideration or without exploring it with fellow students, colleagues, or advisers. It is best not to worry at this point whether another researcher has already done a similar study. Totally original and unique problems are rare, despite the almost infinite range of possible topics. At the same time, no two studies are ever identical, so that every study has the potential of making some contribution to knowledge.

Beginning researchers often develop problems that are too broad in scope or too complex and unwieldy for their level of methodologic expertise. The transformation of the general topic into a workable problem is typically accomplished in a number of uneven steps, involving a series of successive approximations. Each step should result in progress toward the goals of narrowing the scope of the problem and sharpening and defining the concepts.

As the researcher moves from a general topic of interest to more specific researchable problems, it is likely that more than one potential problem area will emerge. Let us consider the following example. Suppose you were working on a medical unit and observed that some patients always complained about having to wait for pain medication when certain nurses were assigned to them and, yet, these same patients offered no complaints when other nurses were assigned to them. You wonder why this phenomenon occurs. The general problem area is discrepancy in complaints from patients regarding pain medications administered by different nurses. You might ask the following: What accounts for this discrepancy? How can I improve the situation? Such questions are not actual research questions because they are too broad and vague. They may, however, lead you to ask other questions, such as the following: How do the two groups of nurses differ? What characteristics are unique to each group of nurses? What characteristics do the group of complaining patients share? At this point, you

may observe that the cultural background of the patients and nurses appears to be a relevant factor. This may direct you to a review of the literature for studies concerning ethnic subcultures in relation to nursing interventions, or it may provoke you to discuss the observations with peers. The result of these efforts may be several researchable questions, such as the following:

- What is the essence of patient complaints among patients of different ethnic backgrounds?
- How do complaints by patients of different ethnic backgrounds get expressed by patients and perceived by nurses?
- How do the interactions between nurses and patients differ among nurses and patients with the same or dissimilar ethnic backgrounds?
- Is the ethnic background of nurses related to the frequency with which they dispense pain medication?
- Is the ethnic background of patients related to the frequency and intensity of their complaints of having to wait for pain medication?
- Does the number of patient complaints increase when the patients are of dissimilar ethnic backgrounds as opposed to when they are of the same ethnic background as the nurse?
- Do nurses' dispensing behaviors change as a function of the similarity between their own ethnic background and that of the patients?

All these questions stem from the same general problem, yet each would be studied in a different manner—for example, some suggest a qualitative approach and others suggest a quantitative one. A quantitative researcher, for instance, might become curious about nurses' dispensing behaviors, based on some interesting evidence in the literature regarding ethnic differences. Both ethnicity and nurses' dispensing behaviors are variables that can be measured in a straightforward and reliable manner.

A qualitative researcher who noticed differences in patient complaints would likely be more interested in understanding the *essence* of the complaints, the patients' *experience* of frustration, the *process* by which the problem got resolved, or the full *nature* of the nurse–patient interactions regarding the dispensing of medications. These are aspects of the research problem that would be difficult to measure quantitatively.

Researchers choose the final problem to be studied based on several factors, including its inherent interest to them and its compatibility with a paradigm of preference. In addition, tentative problems usually vary in their feasibility and worth. It is at this point that a critical evaluation of ideas is appropriate.

Evaluating Research Problems

No rules have been established for making a final selection of a research problem. Some criteria, however, should be kept in mind in the decision-making process. The four most important considerations are the significance, researchability, and feasibility of the problem and its interest to the researcher.

SIGNIFICANCE OF THE PROBLEM

A crucial factor in selecting a problem to be studied is its significance to nursing. New information regarding the research problem should have the potential of contributing to the body of knowledge in nursing in a meaningful way. The researcher should pose the following kinds of questions: Is the problem an important one? Will patients, nurses, or the broader health care community or society benefit by the knowledge that will be produced? Will the results lead to practical applications? Will the results have theoretical relevance? Will the findings challenge (or lend support to) untested assumptions? Will the study help to formulate or alter nursing practices or policies? If the answer to all these questions is no, then the problem should be abandoned.

RESEARCHABILITY OF THE PROBLEM

Not all problems are amenable to study through scientific investigation. Problems or questions of a moral or ethical nature, although provocative, are incapable of being researched. An example of such a problem is whether nurses should join unions. The answer to a question about unionization is ultimately based on a person's values. There are no right or wrong answers, only points of view. The problem is more suitable to a debate than to systematic research. To be sure, it is possible to ask related questions that could be researched. For instance, each of the following questions could be investigated in a research project:

- What are nurses' attitudes toward unionization?
- Do younger nurses hold more favorable opinions of unions than older nurses?
- Does a person's role (nurse versus nursing administrator versus hospital administrator) affect his or her perceptions of the consequences of unions on the delivery of health care?
- Is opposition to unionization for nurses based primarily on perceived outcomes to patients and clients or on outcomes to the nursing profession?

The findings from these hypothetical projects would have no bearing, of course, on whether nurses *should* join unions, but the information could be useful in developing a comprehensive understanding of the issues and in facilitating decision making.

In a quantitative study, researchable problems are ones that involve variables capable of being precisely defined and measured. For example, suppose the researcher was trying to determine what effect early discharge had on the well-being of patients. Well-being is too broad and fuzzy a concept to measure as it is stated. The researcher would have to sharpen the concept so that it could be observed and measured. That is, the researcher would have to establish criteria against which the patients' progress toward well-being could be assessed.

When a new area of inquiry is being pursued, however, it may be impossible to define the concepts of interest in precise terms. In such cases, it may be appropriate to address the problem using in-depth qualitative research. The problem may then be stated in fairly broad terms to permit full exploration of the concept of interest.

FEASIBILITY OF ADDRESSING THE PROBLEM

A problem that is both significant and researchable may still be inappropriate if a study addressing it is not feasible. The issue of feasibility encompasses a variety of considerations. Not all of the following factors are relevant for every potential problem, but most of them should be kept in mind in making a final decision.

Time and Timing. Most studies have deadlines or at least informal goals for their completion. Therefore, the problem must be one that can be adequately studied within the time allotted. This means that the scope of the problem should be sufficiently restricted that enough time will be available for the various steps and activities reviewed in Chapter 2. It is usually wise to be generous in allocating time to the various tasks because research activities often require more time to accomplish than one anticipates. Qualitative studies are often especially time-consuming. A related consideration is the timing of the project. Some of the research steps—especially data collection—may be more readily performed at certain times of the day, week, or year than at other times. For example, if the problem focused on patients with peptic ulcers, the research might be more easily conducted in the fall and spring because of the increase in the number of patients with peptic ulcers during these seasons than in the summer or winter months. When the timing requirements of the tasks do not match the periods available for their performance, the feasibility of the project may be jeopardized.

Availability of Study Participants. In any study involving humans, the researcher needs to consider whether individuals with the desired characteristics will be available and willing to cooperate. Securing people's cooperation may in some cases be easy (e.g., getting nursing students to complete a questionnaire in a classroom), but other situations may pose more difficulties for the researcher. Some people may not have the time, others may have no interest in participating in a study that has little personal benefit, and others may not feel well enough to participate. Fortunately, people usually *are* willing to cooperate with a researcher if the demands on their time and comfort are minimal. If the research is time-consuming, additional effort and the payment of a monetary incentive may be necessary to obtain a sufficiently large sample of study participants. An additional problem may be that of identifying and locating people with the needed characteristics. For example, if we were interested in studying the coping strategies of individuals who had lost a family member through suicide, we would have to develop a plan for identifying prospective participants.

Cooperation of Others. Often, it is insufficient to obtain the cooperation of prospective study participants alone. If the study participants are children, mentally incompetent people, or senile individuals, it is almost always necessary to secure the permission of parents or guardians. In institutional settings, such as hospitals, clinics, public schools, or industrial firms, access to clients, members, personnel, or records usually requires administrative approval. Many health care facilities require that any project be presented to a panel of reviewers for approval before permitting the study to be conducted. In many qualitative studies, a critical requirement is gaining entrée into an appropriate community or institutional setting from key **gatekeepers**.

Facilities and Equipment. All studies have some resource requirements, although in some cases, the needs may be modest. It is prudent to consider what facilities and equipment will be needed and whether they will be available before embarking on a project so that disappointments and frustration can be prevented. The following is a partial list of considerations that fall into this category:

- Will space be required, and can it be obtained?
- Will telephones, office equipment, or other supplies be required?
- If technical equipment and apparatus are needed, can they be secured, and are they functioning properly? Will audio-taping or videotaping equipment be required, and is it of sufficient sensitivity for the research conditions? Will laboratory facilities be required, and are they available?
- Are duplicating or printing services available, and are they reliable?
- Will transportation needs pose any difficulties?
- Will a computer be required for the collection or analysis of the data, and are computing facilities easily obtainable?

Money. Monetary requirements for research projects vary widely, ranging from $10 to $20 for small student projects to hundreds of thousands of dollars for large-scale, federally sponsored research. The investigator on a limited budget should think carefully about projected expenses before making the final selection of a problem. Some major categories of research-related expenditures are the following:

- Literature costs—index cards, books and journals, reproduction of articles, and computerized literature search service charges
- Personnel costs—payments to individuals hired to help with the data collection (e.g., doing interviews, coding, data entry, transcribing, word processing)
- Study participant costs—payment to participants as an incentive for their cooperation or to offset their own expenses (e.g., transportation or baby-sitting costs)
- Supplies—paper, envelopes, computer disks, audiotapes, and so forth
- Printing costs—payment to printers for printing forms, questionnaires, participant recruitment notices, and so on
- Equipment—laboratory apparatus, audio or video recorders, calculators, and the like
- Computer-related expenses
- Laboratory fees for the analysis of bio-physiologic data
- Other service charges, such as the costs of duplicating materials
- Transportation costs
- Postage and shipping costs

Experience of the Researcher. The problem should be chosen from a field about which the investigator has some prior knowledge or experience. The researcher will have a difficult time in adequately developing a study on a topic that is totally new and unfamiliar. In addition to substantive knowledge, the issue of technical expertise should not be overlooked. A beginning researcher usually has limited methodologic skills and so should avoid research problems that might require the development of sophisticated measuring instruments or that involve complex data analyses.

Ethical Considerations. A research problem may not be feasible because the investigation of the problem would pose unfair or unethical demands on the participants. The ethical responsibilities of researchers should not be taken lightly. People engaged in research activities should be thoroughly knowledgeable about the rights of human or animal subjects. An overview of major ethical considerations concerning human study participants is presented in Chapter 6 and should be reviewed when considering the feasibility of a prospective project.

INTEREST TO THE RESEARCHER

If the tentative problem passes the tests of researchability, significance, and feasibility, there is still one more criterion for its selection: the researcher's own interest in the problem. Genuine interest in and curiosity about the chosen research problem are important prerequisites to a successful study. A great deal of time and energy are expended in any research investigation, and interest and enthusiasm ebb and flow throughout the time required for completion of the project. The problem selected should extend the researcher's personal knowledge as well as the base of knowledge for others.

Personal interest in a research problem is least likely to be high when the topic has been suggested or assigned to the researcher by others. Beginning research students often seek out suggestions and may be grateful for assistance in selecting a topic area; often, such assistance can be helpful in getting started. Nevertheless, it is rarely wise to be talked into a research topic toward which you are not personally inclined. If you do not find a problem attractive or stimulating during the beginning phases of a study—when the opportunity for creativity and intellectual reasoning is at its highest—then you are bound to regret your choice later in the project.

COMMUNICATING THE RESEARCH PROBLEM

It is clear that a study cannot progress without the choice of a problem; it is less clear, but nonetheless true, that the problem and the research questions should be carefully stated in written form before proceeding with the design of the study or with field work. Putting one's ideas in writing is often sufficient to illuminate ambiguities and uncertainties. This section discusses the wording of problem statements, statements of purpose, and research questions, and the following major section discusses hypotheses.

Problem Statements

Problematic situations for nurses or their clients are at the heart of a nursing research investigation. A problem statement is an expression of the dilemma or disturbing situation that needs investigation for the purposes of providing understanding and direction. A problem statement identifies the nature of the problem that is being addressed in the study and, typically, its context and significance.

Generally, the problem statement should be broad enough to include central concerns, but it also needs to be narrow enough in scope to serve as a guide to study design. Here is an example of a problem statement from a quantitative study:

> Hazardous noise is an important occupational health problem because it leads to hearing loss and may lead to increased stress and other deleterious physiologic effects.* . . . More than 30 million workers are exposed to hazardous noise on the job. . . Use of hearing protection devices, specifically ear plugs and/ or ear muffs, is known to reduce noise exposure and prevent noise-induced hearing loss. . . . There are, however, relatively few investigators who have examined factors related to the low use of hearing protection by workers. (Lusk, Ronis, & Hogan, 1997)

In this example, the general topic is hazardous on-the-job noise, but the investigators narrowed the scope of their inquiry to factors affecting the low use of hearing protection by workers. This problem statement asserted the nature of the health problem and indicated its breadth (30 million workers). This problem statement also provided a rationale and justification for conducting a new study: the dearth of existing studies on the topic.

---

*Citations to studies that support the researchers' assertions have been omitted from this excerpt.

The problem statement for a qualitative study similarly expresses the nature of the problem, its context, and its significance, as in the following example:

> Women are at high risk for the development of coronary artery disease (CAD). . . . In response to hormonal changes after menopause, a shift in the ratio between protective high density lipoproteins and hazardous low density lipoproteins occurs. This shift is associated with a dramatic increase in the incidence of CAD with postmenopausal women. . . . Although considerable research has focused on the experiences of CAD in men, little has been done to investigate the experience of women. . . . Therefore, this study focused on the experiences of postmenopausal women after diagnosis with CAD. (LaCharity, 1997)

As in the previous example, the researchers have clearly articulated the nature of the problem and the justification for conducting a new study. Problem statements generally appear early in a research report and are often interwoven with a review of the literature, which provides context by documenting knowledge gaps.

Statements of Purpose

Many researchers first articulate their goals formally as a broad statement of purpose, worded in the declarative form. The statement captures—usually in one or two sentences—the essence of the study. The purpose statement establishes the general direction of the inquiry and provides a synopsis of its overall goal. The words *purpose* or *goal* usually appear in a purpose statement (e.g., The purpose of this study was. . . , or, The goal of this study was . . .), but sometimes the words *intent*, *aim*, or *objective* are used instead.

In a quantitative study, a statement of purpose should identify the key study variables and their possible interrelationships as well as the nature of the population of interest, as in the following example: The purpose of this research was to investigate the effect of renal transplant patients' dependency level on their rate of recovery. This statement indicates the population of interest (renal transplant patients), the independent variable (the patients' dependency level), and the dependent variable (rate of recovery).

In qualitative studies, the statement of purpose indicates the nature of the inquiry, the key concept or phenomenon under investigation, and the nature of the group, community, or setting under study, as in the following example: The purpose of this study is to describe the decision-making process of adult children with regard to the placement of elderly parents in nursing homes. This statement indicates that the central phenomenon of interest is the decision-making process relating to nursing home placement, and the group under study is adult children with parents in need of care.

The statement of purpose communicates more than just the nature of the problem. Through the researcher's selection of verbs, a statement of purpose suggests the manner in which the researcher seeks to solve the problem or the state of knowledge on the topic. That is, a study whose purpose is to *explore* or *describe* some phenomenon is likely to be an investigation of a little-researched topic; such a study often involves a qualitative approach. A statement of purpose for a qualitative study may also imply a flexible design through the use of verbs such as *understand*, *discover*, and *develop*. By contrast, a purpose statement indicating that the purpose is to *test* the effectiveness of some intervention or to *compare* two alternative nursing strategies suggests a study with a better established knowledge base, using a quantitative approach and perhaps a design with tight scientific controls. Note that the researcher's choice of verbs in a statement of purpose should connote a certain degree of objectivity. A statement of purpose indicating that the intent of the study was to *prove*, *demonstrate*, or *show* something suggests a bias on the part of the researcher. Some examples of

TABLE 3-2	Examples of Statements of Purpose From the Nursing Research Literature		
STATEMENT OF PURPOSE		**KEY CONCEPTS OR VARIABLES***	**POPULATION OR STUDY GROUP**
Quantitative Studies			
The purpose of this study is to examine patient characteristics that predict referral to outpatient cardiac rehabilitation following hospitalization for myocardial infarction (MI) or coronary artery bypass surgery (CABG). (Burns, Camaione, Froman, & Clark, 1998)		Patient characteristics (IV) Referal to outpatient cardiac rehabilitation (DV)	MI and CABG patients
The purpose of this study was to determine whether the use of perinatal discussion groups for expectant fathers with an emphasis on teaching coping skills would positively influence spousal relations. (Diemer, 1997)		Discussion group intervention (IV) Spousal relations (DV)	Expectant fathers
Qualitative Studies			
The purpose of this study was to describe reported patterns of violence of homeless battered women and their experiences in search for shelter. (Clarke, Pendry, & Kim, 1997)		Patterns of violence, experience in shelter search	Homeless battered women
The purpose of this study was to explore the experience of prolonged bed rest from the perspective of women with high-risk pregnancies. (Gupton, Heaman, & Ashcroft, 1997)		Prolonged bed rest experience	Women with high-risk pregnancies

*IV, independent variable; DV, dependent variable.

well-worded statements of purpose from quantitative and qualitative nursing research studies are presented in Table 3-2.

Research Questions

Research questions are, in some cases, direct rewordings of statements of purpose, phrased interrogatively rather than declaratively, as in the following examples:

- What is the relationship between the dependency level of renal transplant recipients and their rate of recovery?
- What is the process by which adult children make decisions regarding the placement of their elderly parents in nursing homes?

The question form has the advantage of simplicity and directness. Questions invite an answer and help to focus the researcher's and the reader's attention on the kinds of data that would have to be collected to provide that answer. Some research reports thus omit a statement of purpose and state only the research question.

Other researchers use a set of research questions to clarify or lend greater specificity to the purpose statement. For example, the statement of purpose might be the following: The purpose of this research was to study the effects of infertility on the psychosocial functioning of married couples. Some specific research questions stemming from this overall purpose might be as follows:

- What percentage of husbands and wives in infertile couples suffer from depression?
- Do husbands in infertile couples differ from wives with respect to their levels of depression?
- What are the coping strategies used by husbands and wives to deal with their infertility?

In a quantitative study, research questions identify the key variables (most often, the independent and dependent variables), the relationships among them if a relationship is being studied, and the population under study. If a set of questions is used to elaborate upon a broad statement of purpose, the research question would delineate, in fairly specific terms, the measurable research variables (e.g., level of depression).

In qualitative studies, the research questions often evolve and change over the course of the study. At the outset, the research question is fairly broad, giving the researcher the flexibility to explore the phenomenon in depth, to narrow (or even redirect) the focus of the inquiry in the field, and to evolve in more than one direction. The qualitative researcher ideally begins with a question that provides a general starting point but does not prohibit discovery. Thus, at the beginning, the qualitative research question may be little

more than a broad query regarding the study focus (e.g., Why do some patients complain about waiting for pain medications?). As the researcher collects and analyzes data, the research question becomes progressively more focused (e.g., What is the essence of patient complaints, and how are these complaints expressed by patients of different ethnic backgrounds?). In a research report, only the final research question is usually presented.

Some examples of research questions from quantitative and qualitative nursing studies are presented in Table 3-3.

RESEARCH HYPOTHESES

What Is a Research Hypothesis?

In quantitative studies, researchers often present a statement of purpose and then one or more hypotheses. A hypothesis is a tentative prediction or explanation of the relationship between two or more variables; a hypothesis thus translates a research question into a precise prediction of expected outcomes. In a qualitative study, the researcher does not begin with a hypothesis, in part because there is generally too little known about the topic to justify a hypothesis and in part because qualitative researchers want their inquiry to be guided by participants' viewpoints rather than by their own. Thus, our discussion here focuses on hypotheses used to guide the inquiry in quantitative research.

Research questions, as we have seen, are usually queries about how phenomena are related and interact. Hypotheses, on the other hand, are proposed solutions or answers to these research queries. For instance, the research question might ask: Does room temperature affect the optimal placement time of rectal temperature measurements in adults? As a tentative solution to this problem, the researcher might predict the following: Cooler

TABLE 3-3 Examples of Research Questions From the Nursing Research Literature	
RESEARCH QUESTION	**VARIABLES OR CONCEPT**
Quantitative Studies	
How do children's preoperative focus of attention on the stress of surgery relate to their preoperative coping? (LaMontagne, Johnson, Hepworth, & Johnson, 1997)	Children's focus of attention (IV) Preoperative coping (DV)
What is the relationship between anger frequency, intensity, and suppression and blood pressure among women? (Thomas, 1997)	Anger frequency, intensity, and suppression (IV) Blood pressure (DV)
Qualitative Studies	
How do recently graduated nurses describe nursing care provided to culturally diverse clients in hospital settings? (Kirkham, 1998)	Perceptions of nursing care provided to culturally diverse clients
Among those responsible for selecting a nursing home for an elderly family member or friend, why and how does the decision to institutionalize get made? (McAuley, Travis, & Safewright, 1997)	Decision making regarding institutionalization of elders

IV, independent variable; DV, dependent variable.

room temperatures require longer placement times for rectal temperature measurements in adults than warmer room temperatures.

Hypotheses sometimes follow directly from a theoretical framework. The scientist reasons from theories to hypotheses and tests those hypotheses in the real world. The validity of a theory is never examined directly. Rather, it is through hypotheses that the worth of a theory can be evaluated. Let us take as an example the general theory of reinforcement. This theory maintains that behavior or activity that is positively reinforced (rewarded) tends to be learned or repeated. Because nurses play an important teaching and guiding role in hospitals or clinical settings, there are many opportunities for this general theory to be incor-

porated into the context of nursing practice. The theory itself is too abstract to be put to an empirical test. Nevertheless, if the theory is valid, then it should be possible to make predictions (hypotheses) about certain kinds of behavior in hospitals. For example, the following hypotheses have been deduced from reinforcement theory: (1) Elderly patients who are praised (reinforced) by nursing personnel for self-feeding require less assistance in feeding than patients who are not praised; and (2) Pediatric patients who are given a reward (e.g., a balloon or permission to watch television) when they cooperate during nursing procedures tend to be more compliant during those procedures than nonrewarded peers. Both of these propositions can be put to a test in the real world. If the hypotheses are confirmed, the theory is supported, and we can place more confidence in it.

Not all hypotheses are derived from theory. Even in the absence of a theoretical underpinning, well-conceived hypotheses can offer direction and suggest explanations in a quantitative study. Perhaps an example will clarify this point. Suppose we hypothesized that nurses who have received a baccalaureate education are more likely to experience stress in their first nursing job than are nurses with a diploma-school education. We could justify our speculation on the grounds of a theory (e.g., role conflict theory, cognitive dissonance theory), on the basis of earlier studies, as a result of personal observations, or on the basis of some combination of these.

> The development of predictions in and of itself forces the researcher to think logically, to exercise critical judgment, and to tie together earlier research findings.

Now let us suppose the above hypothesis is not confirmed by the evidence collected; that is, we find that baccalaureate and diploma nurses demonstrate an equal amount of stress in their first nursing assignment.

> The failure of data to support a prediction forces the investigator to analyze the theory or previous research critically, to review the limitations of the study's methods carefully, and to explore alternative explanations for the findings.

The use of hypotheses in quantitative studies tends to induce critical thinking and, hence, to facilitate understanding and interpretation of the data.

To illustrate further the utility of hypotheses, suppose we conducted the investigation guided only by the research question, Is there a relationship between a nurse's basic preparation and the degree of stress experienced on the first job? The investigator without a hy-

pothesis is, apparently, prepared to accept any results. The problem is that it is almost always possible to explain something superficially after the fact, no matter what the findings are. Hypotheses guard against superficiality and minimize the possibility that spurious results will be misconstrued.

Characteristics of Workable Hypotheses

An essential characteristic of a workable research hypothesis is that it states the relationship between two or more measurable variables. The variables that are related to one another through the hypothesis are the independent variable (the presumed cause or antecedent) and the dependent variable (the presumed effect or phenomenon of primary interest).

One of the most common flaws of the predictions of beginning researchers is their failure to make a relational statement. The following prediction is not an acceptable research hypothesis: Pregnant women who receive prenatal instruction by a nurse regarding the postpartum experience are not likely to experience postpartum depression. This statement expresses no anticipated relationship; in fact, there is only one variable (postpartum depression), and a relationship by definition requires at least two variables. This prediction, however, can be altered to make it a suitable hypothesis with an independent variable and dependent variable: Pregnant women who receive prenatal instruction are less likely to experience postpartum depression than pregnant women with no prenatal instruction. Here, the dependent variable is the women's depression, and the independent variable is their receipt versus nonreceipt of prenatal instruction.

The relational aspect of the prediction is embodied in the phrase *less than*. If a hypothesis lacks a phrase such as more than, less than, greater than, different from, related to, associated with, or something similar, it is not amenable to testing in a quantitative study. As an example of why this is so, consider the original prediction: Pregnant women who receive prenatal instruction are not likely to experience postpartum depression. How would we know whether this hypothesis was supported—what absolute standard could be used to decide whether to accept or reject the hypothesis? To illustrate the problem more concretely, suppose we asked a group of mothers who have been given instructional sessions on the postpartum experience the following question 1 month after delivery: On the whole, how depressed have you been since you gave birth? Would you say (1) extremely depressed, (2) moderately depressed, (3) somewhat depressed, or (4) not at all depressed?

Based on this question, how could we compare the actual outcome with the predicted outcome? Would *all* the women questioned have to say they were not at all depressed? Would the prediction be supported if 51% of the women said they were not at all depressed *or* only somewhat depressed? There is no adequate way of testing the accuracy of the prediction. A test is simple, however, if we modify the prediction, as suggested above, to the following: Pregnant women who receive prenatal instruction are less likely to experience postpartum depression than those with no prenatal instruction. We could simply ask two groups of women with different prenatal instruction experiences to respond to the question and then compare the responses of the two groups. The absolute degree of depression of either group would not be at issue.

Hypotheses, ideally, should be based on sound, justifiable rationales. The most defensible hypotheses follow from previous research findings or are deduced from a theory. When a relatively new area is being investigated, the researcher may have to turn to logical reasoning or personal experience to justify the predictions. There are, however, few problems for which research evidence is totally lacking.

A good hypothesis should be consistent with an existing body of research findings. This requirement in some cases may be difficult to satisfy because it is not uncommon to find conflicting results on some topics in the research literature. Obviously, when the findings from previous research are inconsistent, it is impossible for the hypothesis to be consistent with all the findings. The researcher must then make a decision, and a good solid basis for such a decision is the critical evaluation of the methods used in earlier studies. The investigator should attempt to understand *why* conflicting results occurred through an examination of the research approach.

Derivation of Hypotheses

Many students ask the question, How do I go about the task of developing hypotheses? There are no formal rules for deriving hypotheses, but two basic processes—induction and deduction—constitute the intellectual machinery involved in deriving hypotheses.

An **inductive hypothesis** is a generalization based on observed relationships. The researcher observes certain patterns, trends, or associations among phenomena and then uses these observations as a basis for a tentative explanation or prediction. Related literature should be examined to learn what is already known on a topic, but an important source of ideas for inductive hypotheses is the researcher's own experiences, combined with intuition and critical analysis. For example, a nurse might notice that presurgical patients who ask a lot of questions relating to pain or who express many pain-related apprehensions have a more difficult time in learning appropriate postoperative procedures. The nurse could then formulate a hypothesis that could be tested through more rigorous scientific procedures. The following hypothesis might be derived: Patients who are stressed by fears of pain will have more difficulty in deep breathing and coughing after their surgery than patients who are not stressed.

The other mechanism for deriving hypotheses is through deduction. Theories of how phenomena behave and interrelate cannot be tested directly. Through deductive reasoning, a researcher can develop scientific expectations or hypotheses based on general theoretical principles. Inductive hypotheses begin with specific observations and move toward generalizations; **deductive hypotheses** have as a starting point theories that are applied to particular situations.

Although a full explication of deductive logic is beyond the scope of this book, the following syllogism illustrates the reasoning process involved:

- All human beings have red and white blood cells.
- John Doe is a human being.
- Therefore, John Doe has red and white blood cells.

In this simple example, the hypothesis is that John Doe does, in fact, have red and white blood cells, a deduction that could be verified.

If a nurse researcher is familiar with a theory relating to phenomena of interest, the theory can serve as a valuable point of departure for the development of hypotheses. The researcher must ask the question: If this theory is correct or valid, what will the logical consequences be in terms of a situation that interests me? In other words, the researcher deduces that if the general theory is true, specific outcomes or consequences can be expected. The specific predictions derived from general principles must then be subjected to further testing through the collection of empirical data. If these data are in fact congruent with hypothesized outcomes, then the theory is strengthened.

The advancement of nursing research depends on both inductive and deductive hypotheses. Ideally, a cyclical process is set in motion

wherein the researcher makes observations, formulates hypotheses inductively, makes systematic and controlled observations, develops theoretical systems, deduces hypotheses, seeks new systematic observations, rethinks the hypotheses or theories, modifies them inductively, and so forth. The scientific researcher needs to be an organizer of concepts (think inductively), a logician (think deductively), and, above all, a critic and a skeptic of resulting formulations.

Testing the Hypothesis

The testing of hypotheses constitutes the heart of most empirical investigations that are quantitative. It must again be emphasized, however, that neither theories nor hypotheses are ever proved in an ultimate sense through hypothesis testing. It is inappropriate to say that the data proved the validity of the hypothesis or that the conclusions proved the worthiness of the theory. Such statements are inappropriate not only because they are incongruent with the limitations of research methods but also because they are inconsistent with the fundamentally skeptical attitudes of scientists. Scientists are basically doubters and skeptics, who are constantly seeking objective, replicable evidence as a basis for understanding natural phenomena. Findings are always considered tentative. Certainly, if the same results are produced repeatedly in a large number of investigations, then greater confidence can be placed in the conclusions. Hypotheses, then, come to be accepted or believed with mounting evidence, but ultimate proof is rarely possible; nor, for that matter, is ultimate falsification of a hypothesis possible.

Let us look more closely at why this is so. Suppose we hypothesize that there is a relationship between height and weight. We predict that, on the average, tall people weigh more than short people. We would then take a sample of people, obtain height and weight measurements, and analyze the data. Now suppose we happened by chance to choose a sample that consisted of short, fat people, and tall, thin people. Our results might then indicate that there is no relationship between an individual's height and weight. Would we then be justified in stating that this study proved that height and weight in humans are unrelated?

A second example illustrates the converse principle. Suppose we hypothesize that taller people are better nurses than shorter people. This hypothesis is used here only to illustrate a point because, in reality, one might suspect that there is no relationship between height and a nurse's job performance. Now suppose that, by chance again, we hit on a sample of nurses in which the taller nurses happened to receive better job evaluations by their supervisors than the shorter nurses. Could we conclude definitively that height is related to a nurse's performance? These two examples illustrate the difficulty of using observations from a sample to generalize to the broader group (the population) from which the sample has been taken. Other problems, such as the accuracy of our measures, the validity of underlying assumptions, the reasonableness of our logical deductions, and rapid changes in technologies and in society, prohibit us from concluding with finality that our hypotheses are proved.

Wording the Research Hypothesis

A workable hypothesis states a relationship between two (or more) variables and is capable of empirical testing. In this section, we look at how the hypothesis should be stated and provide examples of various kinds of hypotheses.

A good hypothesis is worded in simple, clear, and concise language and provides a definition of the variables in concrete, operational terms. These two requirements may be in conflict if the operational definition needs extensive explanation, in which case the variables should be operationally defined separately. The hypothesis should, however, be specific enough so that the reader understands

what the variables are and whom the researcher will be studying.

SIMPLE VERSUS COMPLEX HYPOTHESES

For the purpose of this book, we define **a simple hypothesis** as a hypothesis that expresses an expected relationship between *one* independent and *one* dependent variable. A **complex hypothesis** refers to a prediction of a relationship between two (or more) independent variables and/or two (or more) dependent variables. Sometimes, complex hypotheses are referred to as **multivariate hypotheses** because they involve multiple variables.

We give some concrete examples of both types of hypotheses, but let us first explain the differences in abstract terms. Simple hypotheses state a relationship between a single independent variable, which we will call X, and a single dependent variable, which we will label Y. Our Y variable is the predicted effect, outcome, or consequence of our X variable, which is the presumed cause, antecedent, or precondition. The nature of this relationship is presented in Figure 3-1A. In this figure, the hatched area of the circles, representing variables X and Y, can be taken to signify the strength of the relationship between these two variables. If there were a one-to-one correspondence between variables X and Y, the two circles would completely overlap, and the entire area would be hatched. If the variables were totally unrelated, the circles would not converge or overlap at all.

In the real world, most phenomena are the result not of one variable but of a complex network of many variables. A person's weight, for example, is affected simultaneously by such factors as the person's height, diet, bone structure, activity level, and metabolism. If the dependent variable—Y in Figure 3-1A—were weight, and the independent variable—X—were a person's caloric intake, we would not be able to explain or understand individual variation in weight completely. For example, knowing that Matt Jones' daily caloric intake averaged 2500 calo-

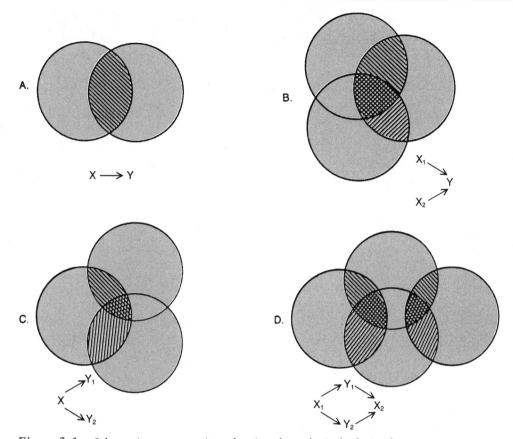

Figure 3-1. Schematic representation of various hypothetical relationships.

ries would not allow us a precise prediction of his weight. Knowledge of other factors, such as Matt Jones' exercise habits, would improve the accuracy with which his weight could be predicted.

Figure 3-1*B* presents a schematic representation of the simultaneous effect of two independent variables on a single dependent variable. The complex hypothesis would state the nature of the relationship between Y on the one hand and X_1 and X_2 on the other. To pursue the example above, the hypothesis might be: Taller people (X_1) and people with higher caloric intake (X_2) will weigh more (Y) than shorter people and people with lower caloric intake. As the figure shows, a larger proportion of the area of Y is hatched when there are

two independent variables than when there is only one. This means that caloric intake *and* height do a better job in helping us understand variations in weight (Y) than caloric intake alone. Complex hypotheses thus have the advantage of allowing researchers to capture some of the complexity of the real world. It is not always possible to design a study with complex hypotheses. A number of practical considerations, including the researcher's technical skills, resources, and time, may render the testing of complex hypotheses impossible or inadvisable. An important goal of research, however, is to explain the dependent variable as thoroughly as possible, and two or more independent variables are typically more successful than one alone.

TABLE 3-4   Examples of Simple and Complex Hypotheses

HYPOTHESES	INDEPENDENT VARIABLE	DEPENDENT VARIABLE	SIMPLE OR COMPLEX
Older patients are at higher risk of experiencing a fall than younger patients.	Age of patients	Falling behavior	Simple
Infants born to heroin-addicted mothers have lower birthweights than infants with nonaddicted mothers.	Addiction versus nonaddiction of mother	Birthweight of infant	Simple
Structured *pre*operative support is more effective in reducing surgical patients' perceptions of pain and requests for analgesics than structured *post*operative support.	Timing of nursing intervention	Patients' pain perceptions; requests for analgesics	Complex
Positive health practices are favorably affected by high self-esteem and greater amounts of social support.	Self-esteem; social support	Health practices	Complex

Just as a phenomenon can be understood as resulting from more than one independent variable, so a single independent variable can have an effect on, or can be antecedent to, more than one phenomenon. Figure 3-1C illustrates this type of relationship. A number of studies have found, for example, that cigarette smoking (the independent variable, X), can lead to both lung cancer (Y_1) and coronary disorders (Y_2). This type of complex hypothesis is common in studies that try to assess the impact of a nursing intervention on a variety of criterion measures of patient well-being. Finally, a more complex type of hypothesis,* which links two or more independent variables to two or more dependent variables, is shown in Figure 3-1D. An example might be a hypothesis that smoking *and* the consumption of alcohol during pregnancy might lead to

lower birthweights *and* lower Apgar scores in infants.

Table 3-4 presents four specific examples of simple and complex hypotheses. Most of these hypotheses would need further elaboration in terms of the specification of operational definitions, but each of these hypotheses is potentially testable, and each delineates a predicted relationship.

Although researchers typically adopt a certain style in the phrasing of hypotheses, some degree of flexibility is allowed. The same hypothesis can generally be stated in a variety of ways as long as the researcher specifies (or implies) the relationship that will be tested. For example, the first hypothesis from Table 3-4 can be acceptably reworded in the following ways:

1. Older patients are more at risk of experiencing a fall than younger patients.
2. There is a relationship between the age of a patient and the risk of falling.

---

*A special kind of complex hypothesis, known as the *interaction hypothesis,* is described in Chapter 8.

3. The older the patient, the greater the risk that she or he will fall.
4. Older patients differ from younger ones with respect to their risk of falling.
5. Younger patients tend to be less at risk of a fall than older patients.
6. The risk of falling increases with the age of the patient.

Other variations are also possible. The important point to remember is that the hypothesis should specify the independent and dependent variables and the anticipated relationship between them.

DIRECTIONAL VERSUS NONDIRECTIONAL HYPOTHESES

Sometimes, hypotheses are described as being either directional or nondirectional. A **directional hypothesis** is one that specifies the expected direction of the relationship between variables. That is, the researcher predicts not only the existence of a relationship but also the nature of the relationship. In the six versions of the same hypothesis given above, versions 1, 3, 5, and 6 are directional because there is an explicit expectation that older patients are at greater risk of falling than younger ones.

A **nondirectional hypothesis**, by contrast, does not stipulate the direction of the relationship. Such a hypothesis predicts that two or more variables are related but makes no projections concerning the exact nature of the association. Versions 2 and 4 in the example illustrate the wording of nondirectional hypotheses. These hypotheses state the prediction that a patient's age and the risk of falling are related; they do not stipulate, however, whether the researcher thinks that older patients or younger ones are at greater risk.

Deductive hypotheses derived from theory are almost always directional because theories attempt to explain phenomena and, hence, provide a rationale for expecting variables to behave in certain ways. Existing studies also support

ply, typically, a basis for directional hypotheses. When there is no theory or related research, when the findings of related studies are contradictory, or when the researcher's own experience results in ambivalent expectations, the investigator may use nondirectional hypotheses. Some people argue, in fact, that nondirectional hypotheses are generally preferable because they connote a degree of impartiality or objectivity. Directional hypotheses, it is said, carry the implication that the researcher is intellectually committed to a certain outcome, and such a commitment might lead to bias. This argument fails to recognize that researchers typically *do* have hunches about the outcomes, whether they state those expectations explicitly or not. Directional hypotheses have three distinct advantages: (1) they demonstrate that the researcher has thought critically and carefully about the phenomena under investigation, (2) they make clear to the readers of a research report the expectations that guided the research, and (3) they may permit a more sensitive statistical test of the hypothesis. This last point, which refers to whether the researcher chooses a one-tailed or two-tailed statistical test, is a fine point that is discussed in Chapter 19.

RESEARCH VERSUS STATISTICAL HYPOTHESES

Hypotheses are sometimes classified as being either research hypotheses or statistical hypotheses. **Research hypotheses** (also referred to as substantive, declarative, or scientific hypotheses) are statements of expected relationships between variables. All the hypotheses in Table 3-4 are research hypotheses. Such hypotheses indicate what the researcher expects to find as a result of conducting the study.

The logic of statistical inference operates on principles that are somewhat confusing to many beginning students. This logic requires that hypotheses be expressed such that *no* relationship is expected. **Statistical or null hypotheses** state that there is no relationship between the independent and dependent variables. The null form of hypothesis 2 in Table 3-4 would be as follows: Infants born to heroin-addicted mothers have birthweights comparable to those of infants born to nonaddicted mothers. The null hypothesis might be compared with the assumption of innocence of an accused criminal in our system of justice: the variables are assumed to be "innocent" of any relationship until they can be shown "guilty" through appropriate statistical procedures. The null hypothesis represents the formal statement of this assumption of innocence.

TIPS ON DEVELOPING RESEARCH PROBLEMS, RESEARCH QUESTIONS, AND HYPOTHESES

For those of you who are planning to conduct a study, we offer a few tips on developing research problems, research questions, and hypotheses:

- As noted earlier in this chapter, your personal experiences as a nurse or nursing student are a provocative source of ideas for research topics. Here are some hints on how to proceed:
  - Watch for recurring problems and see if you can discern a pattern in situations that lead to the problem.
    Example: Why do many patients complain of being tired after being transferred from a coronary care unit to a progressive care unit?
  - Think about aspects of your work that are irksome, frustrating, or do not result in the intended outcome—then try to identify factors contributing to the problem that could be changed.
    Example: Why is supper-time so frustrating in a nursing home?
  - Critically examine some of the decisions you make in the performance of your functions. Are these decisions based on tradition, or are they based on systematic

evidence that supports their efficacy? Many practices in nursing that have become custom might be challenged.
    Example: What would happen if visiting hours in the intensive care unit were changed from 10 minutes every hour to the regularly scheduled hours existing in the rest of the hospital?

- As an alternative to identifying problematic situations, identify aspects of nursing that you most enjoy or in which you have the greatest interest. For example, think about what course work has been most interesting to you, what rotation you most enjoyed, or what part of your job you like the best. Then do some reading in the research literature on this general area to see if a topic suggests itself.

- In a pinch, do not hesitate to replicate a study that is reported in the research literature. Replications provide a valuable learning experience and have the potential to make meaningful contributions because they can corroborate (or challenge) earlier findings.

- If you develop a statement of purpose, be careful in your choice of verbs because the verb communicates information about the nature of your research design and possibly about your level of expertise. Among the verb choices are the following: describe, explore, examine, investigate, address, understand, compare, evaluate, test, assess, explain, and predict.

- In wording your research questions or statement of purpose, it may be useful to look at published research reports for models. However, you may find that some reports fail to state unambiguously the study purpose or specific research questions. Thus, in some studies, you may have to infer the full nature of the research problem from several sources, such as the title of the report. In other reports, the purpose or questions are clearly stated but may be difficult to locate. Researchers most often state their purpose or questions at the end of the introductory section of the report.

- Although most quantitative research studies *do* test hypotheses, only a minority of research reports formally state up front what those hypotheses are. In designing a quantitative study of your own, do not be afraid to make a prediction, that is, to state a hypothesis. Being wrong (or having insufficient evidence to demonstrate that you are right) is part of the learning process.
- If you formulate hypotheses, avoid stating them in null form. When statistical tests are performed, the underlying null hypothesis is usually assumed without being explicitly stated.

RESEARCH EXAMPLES

Table 3-5 presents hypotheses that have appeared in nursing research reports and that illustrate the proper wording of research hypotheses in areas of interest to nurse researchers. The remainder of this section describes the methods in which the research problem and research questions were communicated in two nursing studies, one quantitative and one qualitative.

TABLE 3-5 Examples of Hypotheses from the Nursing Research Literature	
HYPOTHESIS	**VARIABLES***
Perceived social support is positively related to psychosocial adjustment to breast cancer. (Budin, 1998)	Perceived social support (IV); psychosocial adjustment to breast cancer (DV)
Attendance at an outpatient pulmonary rehabilitation (OPR) program will have positive effects on self-efficacy and exercise endurance among patients with chronic obstructive pulmonary disease. (Sherer & Schmieder, 1997)	Attendance in OPR program (IV); self-efficacy, exercise endurance (DVs)
The stronger a nurse's expectation for a physician to collaborate or compromise, the stronger the nurse's intention to collaborate in specific patient care conflict situations with the physician (Keenan, Cooke, & Hillis, 1998)	Nurses' expectation for physician collaboration (IV); nurses' intention to collaborate (DV)
The availability of adequate self-care resources is directly related to the emotional well-being of caregivers of cognitively impaired adults. (Irvin & Acton, 1996)	Availability of self-care resources (IV); emotional well-being of caregivers (DV)
Endotracheal suctioning using room-temperature normal saline will result in a greater decline in PaO_2 and heart rate alterations than body-temperature normal saline. (Gunderson & Stoeckle, 1995)	Temperature of saline (IV); arterial blood gases, heart rate (DVs)

*IV, independent variable; DV, dependent variable.

Research Example
of a Quantitative Study

Landis and Whitney (1997) were interested in studying the effects of sleep deprivation on wound healing. The problem that the investigators identified was described early in the research report as follows: "Questions regarding the possible effects of sleep loss on tissue repair and mechanisms by which sleep loss might negatively affect wound healing have been raised, but no investigators have systematically evaluated the impact of sleep loss on tissue repair at cellular and subcellular levels" (p. 259).

The investigators' statement of purpose appeared near the end of their introductory section. It was phrased as follows: "The purpose of this study was to determine the effects of 72 hours of sleep loss on cellular markers of the proliferative and early collagen biosynthesis phases of wound healing" (p. 261).

The investigators also had specific hypotheses: "We hypothesized that if sleep loss impaired wound healing, there would be a reduced number of fibroblasts and other cells, and lower levels of DNA, protein, and hydroxyproline in ePTFE tissue samples from rats after sleep loss compared to controls" (p. 261).

The researchers tested their hypotheses by comparing six sleep-deprived rats with six control rats, all of whom had miniature wounds from inserted tubing, in terms of various physiologic outcome variables. They concluded that the study provided no evidence that sleep deprivation impairs cellular and biochemical indicators of tissue repair.

Research Example
of a Qualitative Study

Artinian (1995) focused on the topic of the helping relationship, a central concept in the practice of nursing. She noted that the helping relationship has various forms, ranging from the minimal involvement of neutrality to the intense involvement of a "special relationship." Artinian was especially interested in studying involvement at the intense end of the spectrum in the context of caring for cancer patients. She noted that existing research had not provided a systematic examination of the *process* of developing special relationships. Her statement of purpose, which was located in the first paragraph of her report, was stated as follows: "The purpose of this study was to explore and describe the process of how nurses form special relationships with cancer patients" (p. 292).

Artinian elaborated upon her statement of purpose by posing four specific research questions (p. 293):

1. Under what conditions do special nurse–patient relationships form?
2. What are the activities that characterize a special relationship? How are these different from the activities of other relationships?
3. What strategies do nurses use to foster or limit special relationships?
4. What are the consequences of special relationships?

To address these questions, Artinian conducted in-depth interviews with 32 oncology nurses who had worked for more than 6 months on cancer units.

SUMMARY

A **research problem** is a perplexing or enigmatic situation that a researcher wants to address through disciplined inquiry. The **problem statement** articulates the nature, context, and significance of a problem to be studied. The most common sources of ideas for nursing research problems are experience, relevant literature, social issues, theory, and external sources, such as peers and advisers. The researcher usually begins a research project by identifying a broad **topic** or **focus** of interest. After a topic has been tentatively selected, the researcher must begin the task of narrowing the scope of the problem and identifying questions that are consistent with a paradigm of choice.

A number of criteria should be considered in assessing the value of a research problem. First, the problem should be significant—answers to the research question should contribute to nursing practice or nursing theory in a meaningful way. Second, the problem should be researchable; questions of a moral or ethical nature are inappropriate. Third, a problem may have to be abandoned if the investigation is not feasible. Feasibility involves the issues of time, cooperation of study participants and other people, availability of facilities and equipment, experience of the researcher, and ethical considerations.

Researchers communicate their research aims in research reports as problem statements, statements of purpose, research questions, and/or hypotheses. A **statement of purpose** is a summary of the overall goal of the study. In both qualitative and quantitative studies, the purpose statement identifies the key concepts (variables) and the study group or population. The purpose statement usually communicates, through the researcher's selection of verbs, the status of knowledge on the topic and the overall approach to the problem. A **research question** states the specific query the researcher wants to answer to address the research problem.

Quantitative studies may also present one or more hypotheses. A **hypothesis** is a statement of predicted relationships between two or more variables. A workable hypothesis states the anticipated association between the independent and dependent variables. A hypothesis that predicts a result for only one variable is essentially untestable because there is typically no criterion for assessing absolute, as opposed to relative, outcomes. A good hypothesis also should be justifiable; it should be consistent with existing theory or knowledge (or with the researcher's own experiences) and with logical reasoning.

Hypotheses can be classified according to various characteristics. **Simple hypotheses** express a predicted relationship between one in-

dependent variable and one dependent variable, whereas **complex hypotheses** state an anticipated relationship between two or more independent variables and two or more dependent variables. A **directional hypothesis** specifies the expected direction or nature of a hypothesized relationship. **Nondirectional hypotheses** denote a relationship but do not stipulate the precise form that the relationship will take. Another distinction is between research and statistical hypotheses. **Research hypotheses** predict the existence of relationships; **statistical** or **null hypotheses** express the absence of any relationship. After hypotheses are developed and refined in a quantitative study, they are subjected to an empirical test through the collection, analysis, and interpretation of data. Hypotheses are never proved or disproved in an ultimate sense—they are accepted or rejected, supported or not supported by the data. Through replication of studies, hypotheses and theories can gain increasing acceptance, but scientists, who are essentially skeptics, avoid the use of the word *proof*.

STUDY ACTIVITIES

Chapter 3 of the *Study Guide to Accompany Nursing Research: Principles and Methods, 6th ed.*, offers various exercises and study suggestions for reinforcing the concepts presented in this chapter. Additionally, the following study questions can be addressed:

1. Think of a frustrating experience you have had as a nursing student or as a practicing nurse. Identify the problem area. Ask yourself a series of questions until you have one that you think is researchable. Evaluate the problem in terms of the criteria of a researchable problem discussed in this chapter.

2. Examine the following five problem statements. Are they researchable problems as stated? Why or why not? If a problem statement is not researchable, modify it in

such a way that the problem could be studied scientifically.

   a. What are the factors affecting the attrition rate of nursing students?

   b. What is the relationship between atmospheric humidity and heart rate in humans?

   c. Should nurses be responsible for inserting nasogastric tubes?

   d. How effective are walk-in clinics?

   e. What is the best approach for conducting patient interviews?

3. Examine a recent issue of a nursing research journal. Find an article that does not present a formal, well-articulated problem statement. Write a problem statement for that study in both declarative and interrogative form.

4. Below are five hypotheses. For each hypothesis, give a possible problem statement from which the hypothesis might have been developed.

   a. Absenteeism is higher among nurses in intensive care units than among nurses in other wards.

   b. Patients who are not told their diagnoses report more subjective feelings of stress than do patients who are told their diagnosis.

   c. Patients receiving intravenous therapy report greater nighttime sleep pattern disturbances than patients not receiving intravenous therapy.

   d. Patients with roommates call for a nurse less often than patients without roommates.

   e. Women who have participated in Lamaze classes request pain medication during labor less often than women who have not taken these classes.

5. For each of the five hypotheses in suggestion 4, do the following: (a) indicate whether the hypothesis is simple or complex and directional or nondirectional; (b) state the independent and dependent variables; and (c) state the hypotheses in null form.

SUGGESTED READINGS

Methodologic References

Kerlinger, F. N. (1986). *Foundations of behavioral research*. (3rd ed.). New York: Holt, Rinehart and Winston.

Kirk-Smith, M. (1996). Clinical evaluation: Deciding what questions to ask. *Nursing Times, 92,* 8–14.

Martin, P. A. (1994). The utility of the research problem statement. *Applied Nursing Research, 7,* 47–49.

Moody, L., Vera, H., Blanks, C., & Visscher, M. (1989). Developing questions of substance for nursing science. *Western Journal of Nursing Research, 11,* 393–404.

Substantive References

Artinian, B. M. (1995). Risking involvement with cancer patients. *Western Journal of Nursing Research, 17,* 292–304.

Budin, W. C. (1998). Psychosocial adjustment to breast cancer in unmarried women. *Research in Nursing & Health, 21,* 155–166.

Burns, K. J., Camaione, D. N., Froman, R. D., & Clark, B. A. (1998). Predictors of referral to cardiac rehabilitation and cardiac exercise. *Clinical Nursing Research, 7,* 147–163.

Clarke, P. N., Pendry, N. C., & Kim, Y. S. (1997). Patterns of violence in homeless women. *Western Journal of Nursing Research, 19,* 490–500.

Diemer, G. A. (1997). Expectant fathers: Influence of perinatal education on stress, coping, and spousal relations. *Research in Nursing & Health, 20,* 281–293.

Friedman, M. M. (1997). Social support sources among older women with heart failure. *Research in Nursing & Health, 20,* 319–328.

Gunderson, L. P., & Stoeckle, M. L. (1995). Endotracheal suctioning of the newborn piglet. *Western Journal of Nursing Research, 17,* 20–31.

Gupton, A., Heaman, M., & Ashcroft, T. (1997). Bed rest from the perspective of high-risk pregnant women. *Journal of Obstetric, Gynecologic, and Neonatal Nursing, 26,* 423–432.

Irvin, B. L., & Acton, G. J. (1996). Stress mediation in caregivers of cognitively impaired adults: Theoretical model testing. *Nursing Research, 45,* 160–166.

Keenan, G. M., Cooke, R., & Hillis, S. L. (1998). Norms and nurse management of conflicts: Keys to understanding nurse-physician collaboration. *Research in Nursing & Health, 21,* 59–72.

Kirkham, S. R. (1998). Nurses' descriptions of caring for culturally diverse clients. *Clinical Nursing Research, 7,* 125–146.

LaCharity, L. A. (1997). The experiences of postmenopausal women with coronary artery disease. *Western Journal of Nursing Research, 19,* 583–607.

LaMontagne, L. L., Johnson, J. E., Hepworth, J. T., & Johnson, B. D. (1997). Attention, coping, and activity in children undergoing orthopaedic surgery. *Research in Nursing & Health, 20,* 487–494.

Landis, C. A., & Whitney, J. D. (1997). Effects of 72 hours sleep deprivation on would healing in the rat. *Research in Nursing & Health, 20,* 259–267.

Lusk, S. L., Ronis, D. L., & Hogan, M. M. (1997). Test of the Health Promotion Model as a causal model of construction workers' use of hearing protection. *Research in Nursing & Health, 20,* 183–194.

McAuley, W. J., Travis, S. S., & Safewright, M. P. (1997). Personal accounts of the nursing home search and selection process. *Qualitative Health Research, 7,* 236–254.

Scherer, Y. K., & Schmeider, L. E. (1997). The effect of a pulmonary rehabilitation program on self-efficacy, perception of dyspnea, and physical endurance. *Heart & Lung, 26,* 15–22.

Thomas, S. P. (1997). Women's anger: Relationship of suppression to blood pressure. *Nursing Research, 46,* 324–330.

Other Reference Cited

Levine, M. E. (1973). *Introduction to clinical nursing* (2nd ed.). Philadelphia: F. A. Davis.

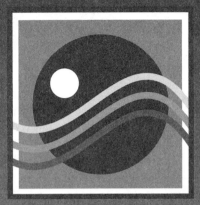 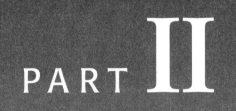

Contexts
for Nursing Research

CHAPTER **4**

The Knowledge Context: Literature Reviews

Researchers almost never conduct a study in an intellectual vacuum; their studies are usually undertaken within the context of an existing knowledge base. Researchers often undertake a **literature review** to familiarize themselves with that knowledge base—although, as noted in Chapter 2, some qualitative researchers deliberately avoid an in-depth literature search before entering the field to circumvent having their inquiries constrained or biased by prior thought on the topic.

The term literature review is used in two ways by the research community. The first refers to the activities involved in identifying and searching for information on a topic and developing an understanding of the state of knowledge on that topic. A researcher may thus say that he or she is "doing a literature review" before conducting a study. The term is also used to designate a written summary of the state of the art on a research problem. Both the search and the write-up are important in the research process.

This chapter discusses several aspects of a literature review: first, the functions that a literature review can play in a research project; second, the kinds of material covered in a lit-

erature review; third, suggestions concerning where to find appropriate references and how to record the information once it is located; fourth, tips on how to read research reports; and finally, the organization and presentation of a written literature review.

PURPOSES OF A LITERATURE REVIEW

Literature reviews can serve a number of important functions in the research process. By examining some of their specific functions, we hope to clarify their value.

Source for Research Ideas

Familiarizing oneself with practical or theoretical issues relating to a problem area often helps the researcher to generate ideas or focus on a research topic. A review of the literature may, in some cases, precede the identification of a topic. Readings in areas of general interest can be extremely useful in alerting the researcher to unresolved research problems or to new applications suitable for a project. When a general topic has already been selected, readings on that topic help to bring the problem into sharper focus and aid in the formulation of appropriate research questions.

Orientation to What Is Already Known

One of the major functions of a research literature review is to ascertain what is already known in relation to a problem of interest. Acquaintance with the current state of knowledge enables those engaged in doing research to avoid unintentional duplication of a study and to focus on aspects of the problem about which there is relatively little knowledge. Of course, there are situations in which a deliberate decision to replicate a study is made, but here too, the researcher needs to be familiar with existing research to make that type of decision.

Nurses who are not researchers also are often interested in learning about the current state of knowledge with regard to a particular issue, as a means of improving their practice or identifying potential solutions to problems. For example, a nurse may be interested in learning about nursing strategies for reducing pain during neonatal circumcision. In such a situation, the nurse would need to turn to the research literature to find out about recent developments. Nurses' abilities to utilize research findings in their practice effectively depends on their capacity to evaluate the research literature.

Provision of a Conceptual Context

For both qualitative and quantitative researchers, a literature review is important for developing a broad conceptual context into which a research problem will fit. When a study is linked with other research, the findings can be better understood within the existing base of knowledge. The accumulation of research-based knowledge is analogous to the fitting together of a jigsaw puzzle. Your piece of the puzzle, small though it may be, may help to join together other parts of the puzzle.

The review also serves the essential function of providing you, as a researcher, with a perspective on the problem necessary for interpreting the results of your study. The comparison of the results of a study with earlier findings is often a good point of departure for suggesting new research either to resolve conflicts or to extend the base of knowledge.

Finally, a written review included in a research report is useful to the nursing community in that it communicates the context within which the study was conducted.

Information on the Research Approach

An important role of the literature review, particularly for students engaged in their first research project, is to suggest ways of going about the business of conducting a study on a topic of interest. In other words, the review can be useful in pointing out the research strategies and specific procedures, measuring instruments, and statistical analyses that might be productive in pursuing the research problem. The research literature can also suggest the extraneous variables that should be controlled.

Research reports differ considerably in the amount of detail they include concerning specific methodologic procedures, but it is not unusual for a report to provide complete documentation of the investigator's methods, including a description of the measuring instruments used. When the actual instrument is not published with the report, it is almost always possible to obtain a copy by writing to the author.

SCOPE OF A LITERATURE SEARCH

Most readers are undoubtedly familiar with locating library documents and organizing them. However, a review of research literature differs in a number of respects from other kinds of term papers or summaries that students are called on to prepare. In this section, the type of information that should be sought in conducting a research review is examined, and other issues relating to the breadth and depth of the review are considered.

Types of Information to Seek

Written materials vary considerably in their quality, their intended audience, and the kind of information they contain. The researcher performing a review of the literature ordinarily comes in contact with a wide range of documents and, thus, has to be selective in deciding what to read or what to include in a written review. How are such decisions to be made? There is, unfortunately, no easy answer to this question, but we can offer a number of suggestions that may prove useful.

The first step in selecting appropriate materials is to make sure that you have been thorough in tracking down most of the relevant references. The next main section of this chapter addresses the issue of locating good source materials.

The type of information included in academic or other nonfictional documents can be classified roughly into five categories: (1) research findings, facts, and statistics; (2) theory or interpretation; (3) methods and procedures; (4) opinions, beliefs, or points of view; and (5) anecdotes, clinical reports, or narrations of incidents and situations. Table 4-1 summarizes the functions that each type of information normally serves in a literature review. A brief description of the utility of the various kinds of information follows.

1. *Research findings.* This category of information represents the results of research investigations; it clearly constitutes one of the most important types of information for a research review. Research findings provide information on what is already known on a topic, based on prior empirical investigations. As Table 4-1 indicates, published studies can also inspire new research ideas and can help in the development of the conceptualization and design of new research. Normally, research findings are available in a variety of sources, including books, encyclopedias, conference proceedings, and, especially, scholarly journals such as *Nursing Research.* Depending on the topic, it may be useful to review research findings in the nursing literature as well as in the literature of related disciplines, such as sociology, psychology, medicine, or physiology. Because research reports are often difficult for beginning students to understand, a section of this chapter is devoted to suggestions on reading published research studies.

TABLE 4-1	Summary of the Uses of Various Types of Information for Research Reviews			
	REVIEW FUNCTION			
TYPE OF INFORMATION	Source of Research Ideas	Information on What Is Known	Conceptual Context	Research Approach
Research	X	X	X	X
Theoretical explications	X		X	
Methodology				X
Opinions and viewpoints	X		X	
Clinical reports and anecdotes	X		X	

2. *Theory*. The second type of information deals with broader, more conceptual issues of relevance to the topic of interest. Descriptions of theory are useful in providing a conceptual context for a research problem but may also be useful in suggesting a research topic. Sometimes, a theory is briefly summarized in research reports and journal articles. However, a full description of a theory is more likely to be found in books.

3. *Methodology*. The third type of information that should be sought in a literature review concerns the methods of conducting a study on the topic of interest. That is, in reviewing the literature, the researcher should pay attention not only to what has been found but also to *how* it was found. What approaches have other researchers used? How have they measured their variables or conceptualized the phenomena in which they were interested? What procedures did they use to analyze their data? Although modifications of existing approaches, designs, or instruments may be necessary, it is usually possible to find techniques that can serve as a foundation for research activities. Research reports concerning similar problems are especially useful.

4. *Opinions and viewpoints*. The general and specialty nursing literature contains numerous papers and articles that focus on an author's opinions or attitudes concerning a topic of interest. Such articles are inherently subjective, presenting the suggestions and points of view of the authors. Opinion articles are often an important source of ideas and contextual information for studies that focus on controversial or emerging issues in nursing.

5. *Case reports, clinical descriptions, and anecdotes*. Descriptions of clinical situations or special problems appear frequently in nursing, medical, and health-related literature. These articles relate the experiences and clinical impressions of the authors or describe the condition and treatment of one or two patients. For instance, Comport (1997) presented a case report of a pregnant patient with severe aortic stenosis. The report included a description of the multidisciplinary plan of clinical care of the patient.

Case reports, anecdotes, and opinion articles may serve to broaden the researcher's understanding of a problem, particularly if the researcher is relatively unfamiliar with the underlying issues. Such sources may also illustrate a point, demonstrate a need for rigorous research, or ignite a researcher's curiosity. However, they have limited utility in literature reviews for research studies because of their subjective or idiosyncratic nature. Beginning researchers should avoid the temptation of relying heavily on such sources in their review of the literature, particularly if they are preparing a written review. This is not to say that such materials are uninteresting or unimportant, but they are generally inappropriate in summarizing knowledge and theories concerning a research question.

Depth and Breadth of Literature Coverage

Beginning students are often troubled by the question of how limited or broad their literature search should be. Once again, there is no convenient formula giving a precise number of references to be tracked down. The extensiveness of the literature review depends on a number of factors. For written reviews, one determinant is the nature of the document being prepared. Doctoral dissertations often include a thorough and extensive review that covers materials that are directly and indirectly related to the problem area. Reports in research journals, on the other hand, tend to have a brief literature review covering only highly pertinent findings from other studies. Another factor to consider is the researcher's own level of knowledge and expertise. Inexperienced researchers who are relatively unfamiliar with a topic may have to cover more materials than more experienced researchers to feel secure about their level of understanding.

The breadth of a literature review depends to a great extent on how well researched the topic is. If there have been 20 published studies on a specific problem, it would be difficult for the researcher to come to conclusions about the current state of knowledge on a topic without reading all 20 reports. However, it is not necessarily true that the literature task is more easily accomplished if the topic has not been heavily researched. Literature reviews on new topics or little-researched problems may need to involve reviews of a broad spectrum of peripherally related studies to develop a meaningful context.

Students embarking on their first research review should strive for relevancy and quality rather than quantity in selecting references for a written review of the literature. A common misconception is that the quality of the review depends on the number of references included. A small review covering pertinent studies and organized in a coherent fashion is of more value than a rambling presentation of questionably relevant information.

With respect to the depth of coverage in a written review, the most important criterion is, once again, relevancy. Research that is highly related to the problem or theory usually merits fairly detailed coverage. Studies that are only indirectly related can often be summarized in a sentence or two.

Primary and Secondary Sources

References can be categorized as being either primary or secondary sources. Although this distinction probably is familiar to most readers, it is sufficiently important to merit a comment here. A **primary source,** from the point of view of the research literature, is the description of an investigation written by the person who conducted it. For example, most of the articles appearing in research journals, such as

Nursing Research, Research in Nursing & Health, and the *Western Journal of Nursing Research*, are original research reports and are, therefore, primary sources. A **secondary source** is a description of a study or studies prepared by someone other than the original researcher. Review articles that summarize the literature on a topic are secondary sources. When you have completed and written up a review of the literature on a topic, your document will be considered a secondary reference. If you go on to collect new data on the same topic, however, your description of the research problem, methods, and results of the study will be a primary source reference for others doing a literature review.

Primary and secondary sources play important, but different, roles in the literature review task. Secondary sources are useful in providing bibliographic information on relevant primary sources. However, secondary descriptions of studies should not be considered substitutes for the primary sources. Secondary sources typically fail to provide sufficient detail about research studies. An even more serious limitation of secondary sources is that it is rarely possible to achieve complete objectivity in summarizing and reviewing written materials. We must accept our own values and biases as one filter through which information passes—although we should certainly make every effort to control such biases. However, we should not have to accept as a second filter the biases of the person who prepared a summary of research studies. Literature reviews should rely on primary sources whenever possible.

LOCATING RELEVANT LITERATURE FOR A RESEARCH REVIEW

The ability to identify and locate articles and books on a research topic is an important skill. However, it is a skill that requires adaptability—rapid technologic changes such as the expanding use of the Internet are making manual methods of finding information from print resources in many subject areas obsolete, and more sophisticated methods of searching the literature are being introduced continuously. Because the changes are ongoing and the risk of our presenting outdated information is high, we present only a brief glimpse of currently available resources for locating research literature. We urge you either to consult with librarians at your institution or to search the Internet for more updated information, using the Internet addresses we provide here and their linkages.

Electronic Literature Searches

Most college and university libraries now offer students the capability of performing their own searches of **electronic databases**—that is, huge bibliographic files that can be accessed by computer. Although electronic literature retrieval has been available since the 1970s, it was initially necessary to have the search performed by a librarian, usually at considerable cost. The expanding development of **end-user systems** has made it possible for those without specialized computer expertise to conduct their own electronic searches on a terminal or personal computer in a library—or even in their own homes, dorm rooms, or offices.

Access to the various databases is made possible through various sources and methods. Several competing commercial vendors offer electronic information retrieval services for numerous bibliographic databases. Currently, the most widely used service providers (and their websites and e-mail addresses) are the following:

- *Aries Knowledge Finder.* Website: http://www.ariessys.com; e-mail: WebMaster@ariessys.com
- *Ovid.* Website: http://www.ovid.com; e-mail: webmaster@ovid.com
- *PaperChase.* Website: http://www.paper-chase.com; e-mail: pch@bidmc.harvard.edu
- *SilverPlatter.* Website: http://www.silver-platter.com; e-mail:editor@silverplatter.com

All of these services are designed to provide user-friendly retrieval of bibliographic information—they provide menu-driven systems with on-screen support so that retrieval can usually proceed with fairly minimal instruction. However, the services vary with regard to a number of factors, such as number of databases covered, cost, online help, ease of use, special features, methods of access, and mapping capabilities. (**Mapping** is a feature that allows you to search for topics in your own words, rather than needing to enter a term that is exactly the same as a subject heading in the database. The vendor's software translates [maps] the topic you type into the most plausible subject heading.)

Most of the electronic databases of particular interest to the nursing community can be accessed either **online** (i.e., by directly communicating with a host computer over telephone lines or the Internet) or via **CD-ROM** (compact disks that store the bibliographic information). The bibliographic retrieval service providers mentioned earlier usually offer free trial services that allow you to test an online or CD-ROM system before subscribing.

We should also note that the books and other holdings of libraries can almost always be searched electronically using **online catalog systems**. Moreover, through the Internet, the catalog holdings of libraries across the country can be reviewed.

KEY ELECTRONIC DATABASES FOR NURSE RESEARCHERS

The two electronic databases that are most likely to be useful to nurse researchers are CINAHL (**C**umulative **I**ndex to **N**ursing and **A**llied **H**ealth **L**iterature) and MEDLINE® (**Me**dical **Li**terature On-**Li**ne). These two databases are described in some detail in subsequent sections.

In addition to CINAHL and MEDLINE®, the most important bibliographic databases for nurse researchers are as follows:

- AIDSLINE (AIDS Information Online) is a collection of bibliographic citations focusing on research, clinical issues, and health policy issues related to AIDS. The database includes articles from more than 3000 journals published worldwide as well as technical reports, professional meeting abstracts and papers, theses, books, and audiovisual materials.

- Alcohol and Alcohol Problems Science Database (ETOH) contains more than 92,000 bibliographic records of alcohol-related scientific documents from the United States and international sources. The database covers all aspects of alcoholism research, including psychology, psychiatry, physiology, biochemistry, epidemiology, sociology, animal studies, treatment and prevention, and public policy.

- CancerLit is a source of bibliographic information pertaining to all aspects of cancer, including experimental and clinical cancer therapy; chemical, viral, and other cancer-causing agents; mechanisms of carcinogenesis; biochemistry, immunology, and physiology of cancer; and mutagen and growth factor studies. Approximately 200 core journals contribute to this database, with other information drawn from proceedings of meetings, government reports, theses, and monographs.

- EMBASE, the Excerpta Medica database, is a major biomedical and pharmaceutical database indexing more than 3500 international journals in the following fields: drug research, pharmacology, pharmaceutics, toxicology, clinical and experimental medicine, health policy, environmental health, drug dependence and abuse, and biomedical instrumentation; there is selective coverage for nursing. The database currently contains more than 6 million records.

- HealthSTAR contains citations to the published literature on health services, technology, administration, and research. It focuses on both the clinical and nonclinical aspects of health care delivery. The database contains citations and abstracts to journal articles, monographs, technical reports, and government documents from 1975 to the present.

- PsycINFO® covers the professional and academic literature in psychology and related disciplines, including medicine, psychiatry, nursing, sociology, education, pharmacology, physiology, and other areas. This database includes references and abstracts to more than 1300 journals in more than 20 languages and currently contains more than 1 million references. Two subsets of the PsycINFO® database are PsycLIT® and ClinPSYC®. PsycLIT® differs from PsycINFO® in that the former does not index dissertations and reports and covers a shorter year range. ClinPSYC® also omits dissertations and reports and contains references only from the clinically relevant classification codes.

Libraries subscribe to different databases, so these resources are not universally available through your institution. However, all are available through the Internet for a flat monthly or annual rate or an hourly fee. Fees vary by database and service provider but typically range from $10 to $40 per hour of connect time.

THE CINAHL DATABASE

The **CINAHL database** is the most important electronic database for nurses. This database covers references to virtually all English-language and many foreign-language nursing journals as well as to books, book chapters, nursing dissertations, and selected conference proceedings in nursing and allied health fields. Material from more than 950 journals is included in CINAHL, covering fields such as cardiopulmonary technology, emergency services, health education, laboratory technology, medical records, radiologic technology, respiratory therapy, and social sciences.

The CINAHL database covers materials dating from 1982 to the present and contains more than 250,000 records. In addition to bibliographic information (i.e., the author, title, journal, year of publication, volume, and page numbers of a reference), the CINAHL database provides abstracts for more than 300 journals. Supplementary information, such as names of data collection instruments and references cited in the source document, are available for many records in the database. Documents of interest can typically be ordered electronically.

CINAHL can be accessed online or by CD-ROM through Ovid Technology, Silver-Platter Information, Ebsco Publishing, and Aries Systems Corporation (Knowledge Finder). CINAHL also has its own direct online service; information about this option can be obtained over the Internet through the CINAHL website (http://www.cinahl.com).

We will use the CINAHL database to illustrate some of the features of an electronic search. Our example relied on the Ovid Search Software for CD-ROM, but similar features are available through other vendors' software.

Most searches are likely to begin with a **subject search** (i.e., a search for references relating to a specific topic). After selecting the search command from the main menu, you would type in a single word or phrase that captures the essence of the topic, and the computer would then proceed with the search. An important alternative to a subject search is a **textword search** that looks for your topic in text fields of each record, including the title and the abstract.

After you have typed in your topic, the computer will give you feedback on how many "hits" there are in the database—that is, how many matches against your topic. In most cases, the number of hits initially is rather large, and you will want to refine the search to ensure that you retrieve only the most appropriate references. You can limit your search in a number of ways. For example, you can restrict the search to those references for which your topic is the main focus of the document. For most subject headings,

you also can select from a number of subheadings specific to the topic you are searching. You might also want only references published in nursing journals; only those that are for research investigations; only those published in certain years (e.g., after 1990); only those written in English; or only those for dealing with study participants in certain age groups (e.g., adolescents).

To illustrate with a concrete example, suppose we were interested in recent research on treatments for postoperative pain and we began our search by typing in *postoperative pain*. In the CINAHL database, there are 11 subheadings for this topic, three of which (diet therapy, drug therapy, and therapy) relate to treatments. Here is an example of how many hits there were on successive restrictions to the search, using the CINAHL database current to February, 1998:

Search Topic/Restriction	*Hits*
• Postoperative pain	859
• Restrict to main focus	663
• Restrict to drug therapy subheading	339
• Limit to core nursing journals	158
• Limit to research reports	50
• Limit to 1995 through 1998 publications	9

This narrowing of the search—from 859 initial references on postoperative pain to 9 references for recent nursing research reports on drug therapies for postoperative pain—took under 1 minute to perform. Next, we would view the titles of the 9 references on the computer monitor, and we could then display (and print) full bibliographic information for those that appeared especially promising. An example of one of the CINAHL record entries retrieved through this search on postoperative pain treatments is presented in Box 4-1. Each entry shows an accession number that is the unique identifier for each record in the database. Then, the authors and title of the reference are displayed, followed by source information. The source indicates the following:

BOX 4-1   Example of a CINAHL Record Entry

Accession Number
1997029240

Authors
McRae ME. Rourke DA. Imperial-Perez FA. Eisenring CM. Ueda JN.

Institution
UCLA Medical Center, Los Angeles, CA.

Title
Development of a research-based standard for assessment, intervention, and evaluation of pain after neonatal and pediatric cardiac surgery.

Source
Pediatric Nursing. 23(3):263–71, 1997 May–Jun. (32 ref)

Cinahl Subject Headings

Adolescence
Age Factors
Analgesics, Opioid/tu [Therapeutic use]
Analysis of Variance
Child
Child, Preschool
Clinical Assessment Tools
Descriptive Statistics
Extubation/ae [Adverse Effects]
Female
*Heart Surgery/ae [Adverse Effects]
Infant
Infant, Newborn

Male
Pain Measurement/st [Standards]
*Pain Measurement
*Pediatric Nursing
*Postoperative Pain/dt [Drug Therapy]
Postoperative Pain/et [Etiology]
Prospective Studies
Record Review
Reoperation/ae [Adverse Effects]
Retrospective Design
Sedation
T-Tests

Instrumentation
Wong-Baker FACES Pain Rating Scale.

Abstract
This analysis of retrospective and prospective data quantified children (age range 0–18 years, total n = 132) during their stay in a cardiothoracic intensive care unit and examined pain management and sedation practices. Data on both factors that could potentially affect pain and its management, and analgesics/sedatives ordered for and administered to subjects were collected from chart review. In the prospective group, pain intensity was measured twice daily using the Wong-Baker FACES Pain Rating Scale. Repeat cardiac surgical procedure subjects reported significantly more pain than nonrepeat subjects on the first postoperative night. Subjects with sternal incisions reported significantly more pain than subjects with submammary incisions. Not all subjects were premedicated with analgesia for invasive procedures. Significantly greater amounts of analgesia were received by the 0–3 year-old subjects. Large amounts of sedation were used, especially in children under 3 years of age. The results prompted development of a nursing standard to assess and manage pain and sedation in this population. (32 ref)

- Name of the journal (*Pediatric Nursing*)
- Volume (23)
- Issue (3)
- Page numbers (263–271)
- Year and month of publication (1997 May–June)
- Number of cited references (32 ref.)

The printout also shows all the CINAHL subject headings that were coded for this particular entry; any of these headings could have been used in the subject search process to retrieve this reference. Note that the subject headings include both substantive/topical headings (e.g., postoperative pain, sedation) and methodologic headings (e.g., descriptive statistics, prospective studies). Next, when formal, named instruments are used in the study, these are printed under *Instrumentation*. Finally, the abstract for the study is presented.

Based on the abstract, we would then decide whether this reference was pertinent to our inquiry. Once relevant references are identified, the full research reports can be obtained and reviewed. All of the documents referenced in the database can be ordered by mail or facsimile (fax), so it is not necessary for your library to subscribe to the referenced journal. Many of the retrieval service providers (such as Ovid) offer **full text** online services, so that, for certain journals, documents can be browsed directly, linked to other documents, and downloaded.

THE MEDLINE® DATABASE

The MEDLINE® database was developed by the U.S. National Library of Medicine (NLM) and is widely recognized as the premier source for bibliographic coverage of the biomedical literature. MEDLINE® incorporates information from *Index Medicus, International Nursing,* and other sources in the areas of communication disorders, population biology, and reproductive biology. MEDLINE® covers more than 3600 journals and contains more than 8.5 million records.

Because the MEDLINE® database is so large, it is often useful to access a subset of the database rather than the unabridged version that has references dating from 1966 to the present. For example, some subsets of the database cover only references within the previous 5 years. Other subsets include core medical journals, specialty journals, and nursing journals.

The MEDLINE® database can be accessed online or by CD-ROM through Ovid, Aries Knowledge Finder, SilverPlatter, and Paper-Chase, for a fee. This database can also be accessed, however, through the Internet for free. The NLM has produced the Internet Grateful Med, which offers free access not only to MEDLINE® but also to other databases, such as AIDSLINE and HealthSTAR. The website for Internet Grateful Med is http://igm.nlm.nih.gov. The MEDLINE® database can be accessed free of charge through other websites as well, including the following:

- PubMed (http://www.ncbi.nlm.nih.gov/ PubMed)
- Health Gate (http://www.healthgate.com/ HealthGate/MEDLINE/search/shtml)

The advantage of accessing the database through commercial vendors is that they offer superior search capabilities with many special features.

Print Resources

Print-based resources that must be searched manually are rapidly being overshadowed by electronic databases, but their availability should not be ignored—especially because smaller libraries (such as hospital libraries) sometimes rely on these print resources because of cost constraints. Moreover, it is sometimes necessary to refer to printed resources to perform a thorough search that includes early literature on a topic. For example, the CINAHL database does not include references to research reports published before 1982.

Print indexes are books that are used to locate articles in journals and periodicals, books, dissertations, publications of professional organizations, and government documents. Indexes that are particularly useful to nurses are the *International Nursing Index, Cumulative Index to Nursing and Allied Health Literature* (the "red books"), *Nursing Studies Index, Index Medicus,* and *Hospital Literature Index.* Indexes are published periodically throughout the year (e.g., quarterly), with an annual cumulative index. When using a print index, you usually first need to identify the appropriate subject heading.* Subject headings can be located in the index's thesaurus, which lists commonly used terms or **key words.** Once the proper subject heading is determined, you can proceed to the subject section of the index, which lists the actual references.

Abstract journals summarize articles that have appeared in other journals. Abstracting services are generally more useful than indexes because they provide a summary of a study rather than just a title. Two important abstract sources for the nursing literature are *Nursing Abstracts* and *Psychological Abstracts.*

Tips on Locating Research Reports

Locating all relevant information on a research problem is a bit like being a detective. The various electronic and print literature retrieval tools are a tremendous aid, but there inevitably needs to be some digging for, and a lot of sifting and sorting of, the clues to knowledge on a topic. Here are a few suggestions:

- If you are interested in identifying all major research reports on a topic, you need to be flexible and to think broadly about the key words and subject headings that could be related to the topic in which you are interested. For example, if you are interested in anorexia nervosa in adolescents, you might want to look under *anorexia, eating disorders,* and *weight loss,* and perhaps under *appetite, eating behavior, nutrition, bulimia, body weight changes,* and *body image.*

- If the research problem on which your search is focused includes independent and dependent variables, you may need to do separate searches for both. For example, if you were interested in learning about the effect of daily stress on the health beliefs of AIDS patients, you might want to read about the effects of stress (in general) and about people's health beliefs (in general). Moreover, you might also want to learn something generally about AIDS patients and their problems. If you are searching for references electronically, you can also often combine searches, so that the references for two independent searches can be linked (e.g., the search program can identify those references that have both stress and health beliefs as subject headings).

- If you are doing a completely manual search, it is a wise practice to begin the search for relevant references with the most recent issue of the index or abstract journal and then to proceed backward. (Most electronic databases are organized chronologically, with the most recent references appearing at the beginning of a listing.)

- It is rarely possible to identify all relevant studies if you rely on electronic databases exclusively. An excellent method of identifying additional research reports is to find several recently published relevant studies and examine the references at the end. Researchers who are conducting studies on a topic are usually knowledgeable about other research on that topic and refer to major relevant studies as a means of providing a context for their own investigations.

---

*When the researcher is seeking articles published by a particular author, the procedure is to go directly to the author section of the index.

READING RESEARCH REPORTS

Once the researcher has identified potential references, he or she must proceed to locate the actual documents. Academic libraries (i.e., libraries in colleges and universities) are likely to contain many of the journals or books identified in the initial literature search. If a reference cannot be located, it is wise to check with a librarian because most academic libraries have interlibrary loan capabilities that make it possible to obtain a reference from another cooperating library. Additionally, as previously noted, many references can be ordered electronically through a database search provider or even downloaded directly.

For research literature reviews, relevant information will be found mainly in research reports in professional research journals, such as *Nursing Research* or *Western Journal of Nursing Research*. Before discussing how to prepare a written review, we briefly present some suggestions on how to read a research report in a professional journal.

What Are Research Journal Articles?

Research **journal articles** are reports that summarize the highlights of a research investigation. Because journal space is limited, the typical research article is relatively brief—generally only 15 to 25 typewritten double-spaced pages. This means that the researcher must condense a lot of information into a short space.

Research reports are accepted by journals on a competitive basis and are critically reviewed before acceptance for publication. Readers of research journal articles thus have some assurance that the studies have already been scrutinized for their scientific merit. Nevertheless, the publication of an article does not mean that the research findings can be uncritically accepted as true because the validity of the findings depends to a large degree on how the study was conducted; this is why both producers and con-

sumers of research can profit from gaining some knowledge about research methods.

Research reports in journals tend to follow a certain format for the presentation of material and tend to be written in a particular style. The next two sections discuss the content and style of research reports.

Content of Research Reports

Research reports in professional journals typically consist of six major sections: an abstract, an introduction, a method section, a results section, a discussion, and references. These sections are briefly described next to provide some guidelines for what to expect in a research report.

THE ABSTRACT

The **abstract** is a brief description of the study placed at the beginning of the journal article. The abstract answers, in about 100 to 200 words, the following questions: What were the research questions? What methods did the researcher use to address those questions? and What did the researcher discover? Readers can review an abstract to assess whether the entire report should be read. Because researchers know that many people will read only the abstract, they normally strive to communicate only that which is essential for readers to grasp what the study was all about. Box 4-2 presents abstracts from two actual studies—one quantitative and the other qualitative.

THE INTRODUCTION

The purpose of the introductory section of a research report is to acquaint readers with the research problem and with the context within which it was formulated. The introduction often is not specifically labeled "Introduction" but rather follows immediately after the abstract. The introductory section may contain the following elements:

BOX 4-2   Examples of Abstracts From Published Research

Quantitative Study

Little is known about how to assist children with chronic conditions and their families cope with repeated hospitalizations. A two-group, pretest-posttest study was done to determine whether a community-based, stress-point nursing intervention for parents could decrease distress and improve child and family functioning. Fifty participants were randomly assigned to intervention or usual care control groups. The intervention focused on specific, parent-verified child and family issues. Three months after hospitalization, intervention parents had better coping and family functioning than those in the usual care group. Intervention parents' anxiety was initially higher and then lower. There were no child behavior differences between the groups after hospitalization. Intervention children had no developmental regression at 2 weeks and better developmental gains 3 months after discharge than the usual care children. Stress-point intervention for families and their children with chronic conditions improved family coping and functioning, and eliminated hospitalization-induced developmental regression. (Burke, Handley-Derry, Costello, Kauffmann, & Dillon, 1997)

Qualitative Study

Based on in-depth interviews, this article reports how people with disabilities perceive and experience the care given by public health care personnel. A major and disturbing finding is that the informants describe feelings of being violated, transgressed, and infringed upon by the personnel in charge of their care. Because of the way nurses and other health care personnel interact, patients' bodies are often perceived as objects. The article describes some of these feelings, including how the informants construct different body boundaries in order to handle the violation of their body and body zone, and it discusses some features of the health care professions that may cause the informants' feelings of being violated. (Lillestø, 1997)

- *The central phenomena, concepts, or variables under study.* The key topic under investigation is identified.
- *The statement of purpose, research questions, and/or hypotheses to be tested.* The introductory section usually indicates what the researcher set out to accomplish.
- *A review of the related literature.* Current knowledge relating to the study problem is often briefly described so that readers can understand how the study fits in with previous findings and can assess the contribution of the new study.
- *The theoretical framework.* In quantitative studies designed to test a theory, the framework is usually presented in the introduction.
- *The significance of and need for the study.* The introduction to most research reports includes an explanation of why the study is important and how it can contribute to the existing base of knowledge or improve nursing practice.

In summary, the purpose of the introduction is to set the stage for a description of what the researcher did and what the researcher discovered.

THE METHOD SECTION

The purpose of the method section is to communicate to readers what the researcher did to solve the research problem or to answer the research questions. The method section tells readers about major methodologic decisions and often offers rationales for those decisions. For example, a report on a qualitative study often explains why a qualitative approach was considered to be especially appropriate and fruitful.

In a quantitative study, the method section usually describes the following, which may be presented as subsections:

- *The subjects.* Quantitative research reports generally describe the population under study, specifying the criteria by which the researcher decided whether a person would be eligible for the study. The method section also describes the actual research sample, indicating how people were selected or recruited and the number of participants in the sample.
- *The research design.* A description of the study design focuses on the overall research plan, often including the steps the researcher took to minimize biases and to enhance the interpretability of the results by instituting various controls.
- *Instruments and data collection.* An important component of the method section is the discussion of the method or methods used to collect the data. The researcher describes how the critical research variables were operationalized and the specific instruments used to measure the variables. The researcher may also present information concerning the quality of the measuring tools.
- *Study procedures.* The method section usually contains a description of the procedures used during the conduct of the study. For example, if a nursing intervention is being evaluated, then that intervention is fully described. Procedures for data collection are also summarized. The researcher's efforts to protect the rights of human subjects may also be documented in the method section.

In a qualitative report, the researcher discusses many of the same issues as in a quantitative one, although often with different emphases. For example, a qualitative study generally provides much more information about the research setting and the context of the study and less information on sampling. Also, because formal instruments are generally not used to collect data in qualitative studies, there is little discussion about the specific data collection methods, but there may be more information on data collection procedures. Increasingly, reports of qualitative studies are including descriptions of efforts the researcher made to ensure high-quality data. Many qualitative reports also have a subsection on data analysis. Although there are fairly standard ways of analyzing quantitative data, such standardization does not exist for qualitative data, so there is often a need for qualitative researchers to describe briefly their analytic approach.

THE RESULTS SECTION

The results section presents the **research findings**—that is, the results obtained in the analyses of the data. The text summarizes the findings, often accompanied by tables or figures that highlight the most noteworthy results.

Virtually all results sections contain some basic descriptive information, including a description of the study participants (e.g., the average age or the percentages of male and female subjects). In quantitative studies, the researcher provides basic descriptive information for the key variables, using simple statistics. For example, in a study of the effect of prenatal drug exposure on the birth outcomes of infants, the results section might begin by describing the average birthweights and Apgar scores of the infants or the percentage who had a low birthweight (less than 2500 g).

In quantitative studies, the results section typically reports the following additional types of information relating to the statistical analyses performed:

- *The name of any statistical tests used.* A **statistical test** is, simply, a tool for evaluating the believability of the findings. For example, if the percentage of low-birth-weight infants in the sample of drug-exposed infants is computed, how likely is it that the percentage is accurate? If the researcher finds that the average birthweight of drug-exposed infants in the sample is lower than the average birthweight of infants in the sample who were not exposed to drugs, how probable is it that the same would be true for other infants not in the sample? That is, is the relationship between prenatal drug exposure and infant birthweight as observed in the sample *real* and likely to be replicated with a new sample of infants? Statistical tests provide answers to questions such as these. Dozens of statistical tests exist, but they are all based on common principles; readers do not have to know the names of all statistical tests to comprehend the findings.

- *The value of the calculated statistic.* Computers are used almost universally to process research data and compute a value for the particular statistical test used. The value allows the researcher to draw conclusions about the meaning of the results. The actual numeric value of the statistic, however, is not inherently meaningful and need not concern readers of research reports.
- *The significance.* The most important information in the results section is whether the **results** of the statistical tests were significant (not to be confused with important). If a researcher reports that the results are **statistically significant**, it means that, according to the statistical test, the findings are likely to be valid and replicable with a completely new sample of subjects. Research reports also indicate the **level of significance**, which is an index of how probable it is that the findings are reliable. For example, if a report indicates that a finding was significant at the .05 level, this means that only 5 times out of 100 would the obtained result be spurious or haphazard. In other words, 95 times out of 100, similar results would be ob-

tained, and the researcher can therefore have a high degree of confidence that the findings are reliable.

In a qualitative report, the researcher usually organizes the findings according to the major **themes** that emerged directly from the data. The results section of qualitative reports typically has several subsections, the headings of which correspond to the researcher's labels for the themes. For example, Jarrett and Lethbridge (1994) studied women's experiences with waning fertility during midlife and identified the central process as "Looking Forward, Looking Back." Within this overall process were three main themes that were used as headings for the results subsections: Reflecting on Childbearing Years, Doing a Midlife Review, and Anticipating Getting Older. In qualitative studies, excerpts from the actual data are included in the report to support and provide a rich description of the thematic analysis. The results sections of qualitative studies may also present the researcher's emerging theory about the phenomenon under study, although this may also appear in the concluding section of the report.

THE DISCUSSION SECTION

The discussion section of a journal article draws conclusions about the meanings and implications of the study. This section tries to unravel what the results mean and why things turned out the way they did. The discussion in both qualitative and quantitative reports may incorporate the following elements:

- *An interpretation of the results.* The interpretation involves the translation of findings into practical, conceptual, and/or theoretical meaning.
- *Implications.* Researchers may offer suggestions for how their findings could be used to improve nursing, and they may also make recommendations on how best to advance knowledge in the area through further research.

• *Study limitations*. The researcher often is in the best position to discuss study limitations, such as sample deficiencies, design problems, weaknesses in data collection, and so forth. A discussion section that presents these limitations demonstrates to readers that the author was aware of these limitations and probably took them into account in interpreting the findings.

Some researchers, especially those conducting a qualitative study, summarize research literature in their discussion section rather than—or in addition to—the introduction. In such a situation, the researcher uses prior studies as the basis for comparing and contrasting research findings.

THE REFERENCES

Research journal articles conclude with a list of the books, reports, and other journal articles that were referenced in the text of the report. For those interested in pursuing additional reading on a substantive topic, the reference list of a current research study is an excellent place to begin.

The Style of Research Reports

Research reports tell a story. However, the style in which many research journal articles are written—especially reports of quantitative studies—makes it difficult for beginning research consumers to become interested in the story that the researcher is communicating. To unaccustomed audiences, research reports may sound stuffy and pedantic. Four factors—only the first two of which are relevant to qualitative research reports—contribute to this impression:

• *Compactness*. As mentioned previously, journal space is limited, so authors must try to compress many ideas and concepts into the short space available. Some of the interesting, personalized aspects of the investigation often cannot be reported.

• *Jargon*. The authors often use research terms that are assumed to be part of the reader's vocabulary. In most cases, the jargon can be translated into everyday terms, but this is at the expense of efficiency and, in some cases, precision.

• *Objectivity*. The writer of a quantitative research report generally strives to present findings in a manner that suggests neutrality and the absence of personal biases. Quantitative researchers normally take pains to avoid any impression of subjectivity, and thus, research stories are told in a way that makes them sound impersonal. For example, most quantitative research articles are written in the passive voice; that is, personal pronouns are avoided. Use of the passive voice tends to make a report less inviting and lively than use of the active voice, and it tends to give the impression that the researcher did not play an active role in conducting the study. (Qualitative reports, by contrast, are more subjective and personal and are written in a more conversational style.)

• *Statistical information*. Numbers and statistical symbols may intimidate readers who do not have strong mathematic interest or training. Most nursing studies are quantitative, and thus, most research reports summarize the results of statistical analyses. Indeed, nurse researchers have become increasingly sophisticated during the past decade and have begun to use more powerful and complex statistical tools.

A major goal of this textbook is to assist nurses in dealing with these issues.

Tips on Reading Research Reports

As you progress through this textbook, you will acquire skills with which to evaluate various aspects of research reports critically. Some preliminary hints on digesting research reports and dealing with the issues described above follow.

- Grow accustomed to the style of research reports by reading them frequently, even though you may not at this point understand all the technical points. Try to keep the underlying rationale for the style of research reports (as just described) in mind as you are reading.
- We recommend that, at least initially, you read research journal articles rather slowly; it may be useful to first skim the article to get the major points and then read the article more carefully a second time.
- Try not to get bogged down in (or scared away by) the statistical information. Try to grasp the gist of the story without letting symbols and numbers frustrate you.
- Until you become more accustomed to the style and jargon of research journal articles, you may want to translate research articles mentally. You can do this by translating compact paragraphs into looser constructions, by translating jargon into more familiar phrases and terms, by recasting the report into an active voice to get a better sense of the researcher's dynamic role in the research process, and by summarizing the findings with words rather than with numbers. As an example of such a translation, Box 4-3 presents a brief summary of a fictitious study. The top panel is written in the style typically found in research journal articles. The bottom panel presents a translation of the summary that recasts the information into language that is more digestible.
- Although it is certainly important to read research reports with understanding, it is also important to read them critically, especially when you are preparing a written literature review. A critical reading in-

volves an evaluation of the researcher's major conceptual and methodologic decisions. Unfortunately, it is difficult for students to criticize these decisions before they have gained some conceptual and methodologic skills themselves. These skills will be strengthened as you progress through this book, but sometimes, common sense and thoughtful analysis suggest to beginning students flaws in a study. Some of the key questions to ask include the following: Does the way the researcher conceptualized the problem make sense—for example, do the hypotheses seem sensible? Did the researcher conduct a quantitative study when a qualitative one would have been more appropriate? In a quantitative study, were the research variables measured in a reasonable way, or would an alternative method have been better? Additional guidelines for critiquing various aspects of a research report are presented in Chapter 25.

PREPARING A WRITTEN LITERATURE REVIEW

A number of steps are involved in preparing a written review, as summarized in Figure 4-1. As the figure shows, after identifying potential sources, you will need to locate the references and screen them for their relevancy to the topic being reviewed. References that appear appropriate are read and notes taken, and inappropriate references can be discarded. Frequently, one reference will provide citations to many other relevant references, which might send you back to locate additional sources. After all relevant references have been reviewed, you can proceed to organize, analyze, and integrate the body of literature. The written review can then be prepared. This section provides some advice on the last few steps in preparing a written review.

BOX 4-3   Summary of a Fictitious Study and a "Translation"*

Original Version

The potentially negative sequelae of having an abortion on the psychological adjustment of adolescents has not been adequately studied. The present study sought to determine whether alternative pregnancy resolution decisions have different long-term effects on the psychological functioning of young women.

Three groups of low-income pregnant teenagers attending an inner-city clinic were the subjects in this study: those who delivered and kept the baby; those who delivered and relinquished the baby for adoption; and those who had an abortion. There were 25 subjects in each group. The study instruments included a self-administered questionnaire and a battery of psychological tests measuring depression, anxiety, and psychosomatic symptoms. The instruments were administered upon entry into the study (when the subjects first came to the clinic) and then one year after termination of the pregnancy.

The data were analyzed using analysis of variance. The ANOVA tests indicated that the three groups did not differ significantly in terms of depression, anxiety, or psychosomatic symptoms at the initial testing. At the posttest, however, the abortion group had significantly higher scores on the depression scale and were significantly more likely than the two delivery groups to report severe tension headaches. There were no significant differences on any of the dependent variables for the two delivery groups.

The results of this study suggest that young women who elect to have an abortion may experience a number of long-term negative consequences. It would appear that appropriate efforts should be made to follow-up abortion patients to determine their need for suitable treatment.

Translated Version

As researchers, we wondered whether young women who had an abortion had any emotional problems in the long run. It seemed to us that not enough research had been done to know whether any actual psychological harm resulted from an abortion.

We decided to study this question ourselves by comparing the experiences of three types of teenagers who became pregnant—first, girls who delivered and kept their babies; second, those who delivered the babies but have them up for adoption; and third, those who elected to have an abortion. All of the teenagers in the sample were poor, and all were patients at an inner-city clinic. Altogether, we studied 75 girls—25 in each of the three groups. We evaluated the teenagers' emotional state by asking them to fill out a questionnaire and to take several psychological tests. These tests allowed us to assess things like the girls' degree of depression and anxiety and whether they had any complaints of a psychosomatic nature. We asked them to fill out the forms twice: once when they came into the clinic and then again a year after the abortion or the delivery.

We learned that the three groups of teenagers looked pretty much alike in terms of their emotional states when they first filled out the forms. But when we compared how the three groups looked a year later, we found that the teenagers who had abortions were more depressed and were more likely to say they had severe tension headaches than teenagers in the other two groups. The teenagers who kept their babies and those who gave their babies up for adoption looked pretty similar 1 year after their babies were born, at least in terms of depression, anxiety, and psychosomatic complaints.

Thus, it seems that we may be right in having some concerns about the emotional effects of having an abortion. Nurses should be aware of these long-term emotional effects, and it even may be advisable to institute some type of follow-up procedure to find out if these young women need additional help.

---

*The "findings" summarized here are not necessarily accurate.

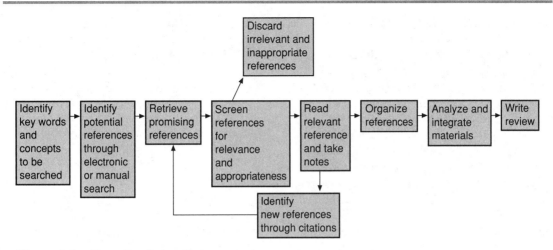

Figure 4-1. Flow of tasks in a literature review.

Abstracting and Recording Notes

Once a document has been determined to be relevant, the entire report should be read carefully and critically, identifying material that is sufficiently important to warrant note taking and observing flaws in the study or gaps in the report. Notes should be taken to remind you of the content of the report and the study's strengths and limitations. The following kinds of information should usually be recorded: the *full* citation for inclusion in your bibliography, the research questions or hypotheses, the theoretical framework, key features of the research methods, and the major findings and conclusions.

Organizing the Review

If the end product of your literature search is to be a written review, a critical task is the organization of the gathered information. Several devices may help in the successful accomplishment of this task. When the literature on a topic is extensive, it is sometimes useful to organize the findings from studies in a summary table. The table could include columns with headings such as Author, Number of Subjects, Type of Design, Method of Measuring

Variables, and Key Findings. Such a table provides a quick overview that allows the reviewer to make sense of a large mass of information. As an example, Tuten and Gueldner (1991), in the introduction to their study of the effectiveness of sodium chloride versus dilute heparin for maintenance of peripheral intermittent intravenous devices, present an excellent table summarizing earlier research.

Most writers find it helpful to work from an outline. If the review is lengthy and complex, it is useful to write out the outline; a mental outline may be sufficient for shorter reviews. The important point is to work out a structure before starting to write so that the presentation has a meaningful and understandable flow. Lack of organization is a common weakness in students' first attempts at writing a literature review.

Some research reviews can be organized in a chronologic fashion by summarizing the history of research on a topic, but this is likely to prove useful only if clear trends over time can be discerned (e.g., early research on factors associated with adolescent pregnancy focused primarily on knowledge of and access to contraception, but recent research has examined more complex social and psychological factors such as poverty, family functioning, and perceived life options). Another approach that can be used if the research is quantitative is to provide an overview of research on the dependent variable, the independent variable, and then the two combined, followed by research on factors that affect the relationship between the two (e.g., the effect of marital status on health if different for men and women). Although the specifics of the organization differ from topic to topic, the overall goal is to structure the review in such a way that the presentation is logical, demonstrates meaningful integration, and leads to a conclusion about what is known and not known about the topic.

Once the main topics and their order of presentation have been determined, a review of the notes is in order. This not only will help you recall materials read earlier but also will lay the groundwork for decisions about where (if at all) a particular reference fits in terms of the outline. If certain references do not seem to fit anywhere, the outline may need to be revised or the reference discarded. Students should avoid the temptation to force a reference into the review if it does not make a contribution. The number of references used in the review is much less important than the relevance of the references, the quality of the summary, and the overall organization.

Content of the Written Literature Review

A written review of the literature should be neither a series of quotes nor a series of abstracts. The central tasks are to organize and summarize the references so they reveal the current state of knowledge on the selected topics and, in the context of a new study, to lay a systematic foundation for the research. The review should point out both consistencies and contradictions in the literature as well as offer possible explanations for the inconsistencies, for example, different conceptualizations or methods.

Studies that are particularly relevant should be described in some detail. However, studies

with comparable findings can often be grouped together and briefly summarized, as in the following fictitious example:

> A number of studies have found that the incidence of phlebitis is directly related to the method of administering intravenous infusions and to certain parameters of materials used in the infusions (Dayton, 1998; Stainback, 1996; Whitman and Coxe, 1997).

It is important to paraphrase, or summarize, a reference source in your own words. The review should demonstrate that thoughtful consideration has been given to the materials. Stringing together quotes from various documents fails to show that previous research and thought on the topic have been assimilated and understood.

Another point to bear in mind is that the review should be as objective as possible. Studies that conflict with personal values should not be omitted from the review. Also, the review should not deliberately ignore a study simply because its findings contradict other studies. Analyze inconsistent results, and evaluate the supporting evidence as objectively as possible.

The literature review should conclude with a summary of the current state of knowledge on the research problem under consideration. The summary not only should point out what has been studied and how adequate the investigations have been but also should make note of any gaps or areas of research inactivity. The summary requires some critical judgment concerning the extensiveness and dependability of information on a topic. If the literature review is conducted as part of a new study, this critical summary should demonstrate the need for the research and should clarify the context within which the hypotheses will be developed.

As you progress through this book, you will become increasingly proficient in critically evaluating the research literature. We hope that you will understand the mechanics of writing a research review once you have completed this chapter, but we do not expect that you will be in a position to write a critical, state-of-the-art review until you have required more research skills.

Style of a Research Review

One of the most common problems for the student researcher preparing a written research review for the first time is adjusting to the style of writing that is used in research reviews. There is a tendency, for example, for students to accept the results of previous research as a fact or as proof that a finding is conclusive or a theory is correct. This tendency is understandable; it is the style of presentation commonly used in many textbooks, opinion articles, and other nonresearch papers. This style stems partly from a desire for clarity and lack of ambiguity for pedantic purposes, but it is also, in part, the result of a common misunderstanding about the degree of conclusiveness that can be achieved through empirical research. No hypothesis or theory can be definitively proved or disproved by empirical testing, and no research question can be definitively answered in a single study.

Every study has some limitations, the severity of which depends to a great extent on the researcher's methodologic decisions. The fact that theories and hypotheses cannot be ultimately proved or disproved does not, of course, mean that we must disregard evidence or challenge every idea we encounter. The problem is partly a semantic one: hypotheses are not *proved*, but they are *supported* by research findings; theories are not *verified* or *confirmed*, but they may be tentatively *accepted* if there is a substantial body of evidence demonstrating their legitimacy. The reviewer must learn to adopt this language of tentativeness in presenting the review of the literature.

A related stylistic problem is the inclination of novice reviewers to intersperse opinions liberally (their own or someone else's) with the findings of research investigations. The review should use statements of opinions sparingly, if at all, and should be explicit about the source

of the opinion. A description of the point of view of a knowledgeable or influential individual may be useful in establishing the need to investigate the problem or in providing a perspective on the topic, but it should occupy a relatively small section of the review. The researcher's own opinions do not belong in a review section, with the exception of an assessment of the quality of existing studies.

The left-hand column of Table 4-2 presents several examples of the kinds of stylistic difficulties we have been discussing in this section. The right-hand column offers some recommendations for rewording the sentences to conform to a more generally acceptable form for a research literature review. Many alternative ways of phrasing these sentences are possible.

RESEARCH EXAMPLES OF RESEARCH LITERATURE REVIEWS

The best way to learn about the style, content, and organization of a research literature review is to read several reviews that appear in the nursing literature. We present two excerpts from reviews here and urge you to read other reviews on a topic of interest to you.

Research Example from a Quantitative Research Report

Holditch-Davis, Barham, O'Hale, and Tucker (1995) conducted a quantitative study to examine the effects of standardized rest periods on the sleep and wake states of preterm infants who are convalescing. The following excerpt represents essentially the entire literature review section of their research report, which appeared in the *Journal of Obstetric, Gynecologic, and Neonatal Nursing*.

One of the most difficult problems for neonatal nurses is modifying the neonatal intensive-care unit environment so that it provides

TABLE 4-2 Examples of Stylistic Difficulties for Research Reviews

INAPPROPRIATE STYLE OR WORDING	RECOMMENDED CHANGE
1. It is known that unmet expectations engender anxiety.	Several experts (Abraham, 1999; Lawrence, 1998) have asserted that unmet expectations engender anxiety.
2. The woman who does not participate in childbirth preparation classes tends to manifest a high degree of stress during labor.	Previous studies have indicated that women who participate in preparation for childbirth classes manifest less stress during labor than those who do not. (Klotz, 1997; Reynolds, 1998; McTygue, 1997)
3. Studies have proved that doctors and nurses do not fully understand the psychobiologic dynamics of recovery from a myocardial infarction.	The studies by Lambalot (1998) and Carter (1997) suggest that doctors and nurses do not fully understand the psychobiologic dynamics of recovery from a myocardial infarction.
4. Attitudes cannot be changed overnight.	Attitudes have been found to be relatively enduring attributes that cannot be changed overnight. (O'Connell, 1997; Valentine, 1999)
5. Responsibility is an intrinsic stressor.	According to Doctor A. Cassard, an authority on stress, responsibility is an intrinsic stressor. (Cassard, 1996, 1998)

Note: All references are fictitious.

appropriate stimulation for the growth and development of preterm infants. Preterm infants are adapted to the uterus, a warm, dark environment that provides kinesthetic stimulation and complex hormonal support. By contrast, the neonatal intensive care unit is a bright and noisy environment with limited diurnal variation, frequent technical procedures, and little positive handling (Duxbury et al., 1984; Gottfried & Gaiter, 1985). Sick infants lack the physiologic reserves to cope with this environment. Critically ill infants become hypoxic in response to such stimulation as noise (Long et al., 1980), technical procedures (Evans, 1991; Peters, 1992), and social touches (Gorski et al., 1983). Even spontaneous changes in sleep-wake states can result in decreased oxygenation (Brazy, 1988; Gabriel et al., 1980).

The intermediate care environment is similar to that of intensive care. Light levels and number of technical procedures are decreased, but preterm infants still experience limited diurnal variation and few social interactions (Blackburn & Barnard, 1985; Gaiter, 1985; Gottfried, 1985). Responses to infant cues are inconsistent. Gottfried (1985) found that nurses responded to fewer than half the cries of premature infants in intermediate or convalescent care. . . .

The sleeping and waking states of preterm infants in particular are affected by the environment. Infants have identifiable sleep-wake states that develop during the preterm period (Curzi-Dascalova et al., 1988; Holditch-Davis, 1990a). Their sleep-wake states are influenced by aspects of the intermediate care environment, such as handling for routine nursing care (Duxbury et al., 1984; Holditch-Davis, 1990b), high levels of light (Moseley et al, 1988), painful procedures (Field & Goldson, 1984; Holditch-Davis & Calhoon,

1989), and interactions between the infants and their parents (Miller & Holditch-Davis, 1992; Minde et al, 1975). However, not all the effects of the intermediate nursery environment are detrimental. For example, interactions with parents appear to decrease arousal and to increase social behaviors (Miller & Holditch-Davis, 1992; Minde et al., 1975). Therefore, determining how the intermediate care nursery (ICN) environment affects sleep-wake states is essential to provide optimal nursing care for preterm infants who are convalescing.

Studies have examined the effects that changes in the ICN have on the sleep-wake states of infants. Gabriel et al. (1981) clustered routine nursing care. Strauch et al. (1993) reduced noise levels for 1 hour on each nursing shift. Fajardo et al. (1990) developed a special nursery with diurnal cycles, reduced noise, demand feedings, and responsive nursing care. Other researchers provided greater day-night differentiation by reducing light and/or noise levels at night (Blackburn & Patteson, 1991; Mann et al., 1986). Modifications of the environment to meet the needs of individual infants also have been examined (Als et al., 1986; Becker et al., 19911). Preterm infants benefitted from these changes, but the nature of the benefits differed between studies. Some of the environmental changes resulted in infants experiencing more sleep and fewer state changes (Fajardo et al., 1990; Gabriel et al., 1981; Strauch et al., 1993); decreased activity levels (Blackburn & Patteson, 1991; Fajardo et al., 1990); or less time on mechanical ventilation and earlier bottle feedings (Als et al., 1986; Becker et al., 1991).

The findings of these studies must be interpreted cautiously because most of the studies have small samples (fewer than 15 per group) (Als et al., 1986; Fajardo et al., 1990; Gabriel et al., 1981; Strauch et al., 1993). Control and experimental groups sometimes were not well matched (Fajardo et al., 1990). Often, experimental groups were studied after control groups (Als et al., 1986; Becker et al., 1991; Gabriel et al., 1981). Yet outcomes for infants studied at later time should be better than those studied at an earlier time, even if a special intervention had no effect, because

neonatal care is constantly improving. These studies all modified multiple aspects of the environment, and it is impossible to determine whether all the modifications were necessary for the beneficial effects.

The purpose of this study was to determine whether modifying a single aspect of the intermediate care environment alters the sleep-wake patterns of preterm infants. (pp. 424–425)

Research Example from a Qualitative Research Report

Brodsky (1995) conducted a qualitative study that explored survivors' perceptions of the psychosocial impact of testicular cancer. Brodsky's introduction, all of which is presented below, contained a brief review that was used to frame the study and highlight the need for in-depth research:

Testicular cancer is the most common malignancy in men aged 15–34 (Ganong & Markovitz, 1987) and incidence rates have risen in the United States in recent decades (Schottenfeld et al., 1980). However, there is still a dearth of information pertaining to the male's experience with testicular cancer and its treatment. This is evident in a review of the literature that reveals only two first-person accounts of men who have had testicular cancer (Fiore, 1979; Moreland, 1982), one survey that focused on the psychological aspects of testicular cancer (Schover & von Eschenbach, 1984), and research that focused on the psychological response of patients cured of advanced cancer (Kennedy et al., 1976).

This lack of information may be due to the fact that in the recent past, few patients ever survived the disease. However, new developments in medical technology have led to increased survival rates. These developments have benefitted patients by keeping them alive, but new problems have been created. These problems pertain to the rehabilitation of patients following treatment. Thus, surviving testicular cancer is a new phenomenon (Donohue et al.,

1978; Einhorn, 1987). As a result of its novelty, we do not yet understand the impact of survival on men's sense of self (Gorzynski & Holland, 1979). We are now at the point where we can begin to explore the nature of the phenomenon. Therefore, the focus of this research was to examine changes in one's sense of self due to the experience of having had testicular cancer. (pp. 78–79)

In the discussion section of Brodsky's report, the findings from the research are compared with those from other studies. Here is an excerpt that helps to provide more context for the new research:

Others who have made observations about the impact of trauma have uncovered similar findings to those of the researcher. In her qualitative study of people and bereavement, Kessler (1987) found that bereavement, much like the experience of testicular cancer, can help many to "appreciate the preciousness of life and discover inner sources of strength."

Similar findings are supported by Kennedy et al. (1976) who concluded "Patients with advanced cancer apparently cured of the disease have a greater appreciation of time, life, people, and interpersonal reactions. . . ."

Data from this study also agree with findings of Gorzynski and Holland (1979) who address psychological adjustments of testicular cancer patients resulting from diagnosis, retroperitoneal lymphadenectomy, and chemotherapy. They suggest that in the diagnostic stage, denial of the seriousness of the disease may lead to delayed treatment and that male physicians delay suggesting an orchiectomy due to their own discomfort and identification with the patient. . . .

Findings also support those of Liss-Levinson (1982) and Farrell (1974). Liss-Levinson recognized males' difficulty with dependency and loss of control. This was verified for almost one half of the respondents in the present study. Farrell (1974) spoke of the men's problems communicating with others on an emotional level. This was reflected in the study by the decision of so few respondents to seek psychiatric assistance in identifying feelings and

communicating them to others. . . . Findings by Schover and von Eschenbach (1984) and Cash et al. (1986) concerning the relationship between body image and psychological well-being were also confirmed. (pp. 93–94)

SUMMARY

The task of reviewing research literature involves the identification, selection, critical analysis, and written description of existing information on the topic of interest. It is usually advisable to undertake a **literature review** on a subject before actually conducting a research project. Such a review can play a number of important roles. First, in the start-up phase of a project, a review of work conducted in an area of general interest can help in the formulation or clarification of a research problem. Second, a scrutiny of previous work acquaints the researcher with what has been done in a field, thereby minimizing the possibility of unintentional duplication. Third, the review provides a conceptual context or framework for the researcher and for the research community, thereby facilitating the accumulation of knowledge. Fourth, the researcher may be in a better position to assess the feasibility of a proposed study by becoming familiar with related work. Finally, the review can be highly useful in providing methodologic suggestions for the actual conduct of the investigation.

The kinds of information available in written documents can be categorized into five broad classes: facts, findings, or results; theory; research procedures or methods; opinions, points of view, or personal commentaries; and clinical case reports, anecdotes, or impressions of a particular event or situation. Another way of categorizing literature is in terms of its being either a primary or secondary source. A **primary source** with respect to the research literature is the original description of a study prepared by the researcher who conducted it; a **secondary source** is a description of the study by a person unconnected with the investigation. Primary sources should be consulted whenever possible in performing the literature review task.

For those preparing a literature review, the first steps are to identify the key concepts and to locate appropriate references. An important bibliographic development to emerge in recent years is the increasing availability of various **electronic databases**, many of which can be accessed through an **online search** or by **CD-ROM**. For nurses, the **CINAHL database** is especially useful. In searching a database, users usually perform a **subject search** for a topic of interest, but other types of search are available. Although electronic information retrieval is now widespread and growing, print resources, such as **print indexes** and **abstract journals**, are also available and are especially useful for locating references published before 1982.

After the researcher has identified and located references, he or she must screen them for relevance and then read them critically. For research reviews, most references are likely to be found in professional journals. Research **journal articles**, which present concise descriptions of research investigations, typically contain six major sections: the **abstract** (a brief summary of the study); the introduction (which explains the study problem and its context; the method section (the strategy the researcher used to address the research problem); the results (the actual **research findings**); the discussion (the interpretation and implications of the findings); and the bibliographic references.

The compactness of research journal articles, the use of technical terms, their impersonal style, and the description of **statistical tests** often make research articles difficult for students to read. Students may need to translate the ideas contained in a research article before trying to digest them.

Skillful note taking and organization can greatly simplify the tasks of analyzing, summarizing, and evaluating literature on a given topic. In preparing a written review, it is important to organize materials in a logical, coherent fashion. The preparation of an outline is recommended, and the development of summary charts often helps in integrating diverse studies. The written review should not be a succession of quotes or abstracts. The role of the reviewer is to point out what has been studied to date, how adequate and dependable those studies are, what gaps there appear to be in the existing body of research, and what contribution a new study would make. The reviewer should present facts and findings in the tentative language that befits scientific inquiry and should remember to identify the sources of opinions, points of view, and generalizations.

STUDY ACTIVITIES

Chapter 4 of the *Study Guide to Accompany Nursing Research: Principles and Methods, 6th ed.*, offers various exercises and study suggestions for reinforcing the concepts presented in this chapter. Additionally, the following study suggestions can be addressed:

1. Read the study by Keeling and her colleagues (1994) entitled, "Postcardiac catheterization time-in-bed study: Enhancing patient comfort through nursing research," *Applied Nursing Research, 7,* 14–17. Write a summary of the problem, methods, findings, and conclusions of the study. Your summary should be capable of serving as notes for a review of the literature.

2. Suppose that you were planning to study counseling practices and programs for rape trauma victims. Make a list of several key words relating to this topic that could be used with indexes or information retrieval systems for identifying previous work.

3. Below are five sentences from literature reviews that require stylistic improvements. Rewrite these sentences to conform to considerations mentioned in the

text. (Feel free to give fictitious references if desired.)

   a. Children are less distressed during immunization when their parents are present.

   b. Young adolescents are unprepared to cope with complex issues of sexual morality.

   c. More structured programs to use part-time nurses are needed.

   d. Intensive care nurses need so much emotional support themselves that they can provide insufficient support to patients.

   e. Most nurses have not been adequately educated to understand and cope with the reality of the dying patient.

4. Suppose you are studying factors relating to the discharge of chronic psychiatric patients. Obtain five bibliographic references for this topic. Compare your references and sources with those of other students.

SUGGESTED READINGS

Methodologic References

American Psychological Association. (1983). *Publication manual* (3rd ed.). Washington, DC: Author.

Cooper, H. M. (1984). *The integrative research review*. Beverly Hills: Sage.

Fox, R. N., & Ventura, M. R. (1984). Efficiency of automated literature search mechanisms. *Nursing Research, 33,* 174–177.

Ganong, L. H. (1987). Integrative reviews of nursing research. *Research in Nursing & Health, 10,* 1–11.

Light, R. J., & Pillemer, D. B. (1984). *Summing up: The science of reviewing research*. Cambridge, MA: Harvard University Press.

Saba, V. K., Oatway, D. M., & Rieder, K. A. (1989). How to use nursing information sources. *Nursing Outlook, 37,* 189–195.

Smith, L. W. (1988). Microcomputer-based bibliographic searching. *Nursing Research, 37,* 125–127.

Turabian, K. L., Grossman, J., & Bennett, A. (1996). *A manual for writers of term papers, theses, and dissertations* (6th ed.). Chicago: University of Chicago Press.

Substantive References

Brodsky, M. S. (1995). Testicular cancer survivors impressions of the impact of the disease on their lives. *Qualitative Health Research, 5,* 78–96.

Burke, S. O., Handley-Derry, M, Costello, E. A., Kauffmann, E., & Dillon, M. C. (1997). Stresspoint intervention for parents of repeatedly hospitalized children with chronic conditions. *Research in Nursing & Health, 20,* 475–485.

Holditch-Davis, D., Barham, L. N., O'Hale, A., & Tucker, B. (1995). Effect of standard rest periods on convalescent preterm infants. *Journal of Obstetric, Gynecologic, and Neonatal Nursing, 24,* 424–432.

Jarrett, M. E., & Lethbridge, D. J. (1994). Looking forward, looking back: Women's experience with waning fertility during midlife. *Qualitative Health Research, 4,* 370–384.

Lillestø, B. (1997). Violation in caring for the physically disabled. *Western Journal of Nursing Research, 19,* 282–296.

Tuten, S. H., & Gueldner, S. H. (1991). Efficacy of sodium chloride versus dilute heparin for maintenance of peripheral intermittent devices. *Applied Nursing Research, 4,* 63–71.

Other Reference Cited

Comport, K. A. (1997). Aortic stenosis in pregnancy: A case report. *Journal of Obstetric, Gynecologic, and Neonatal Nursing, 26,* 67–77.

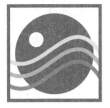

CHAPTER **5**

Conceptual and Theoretical Contexts

Good research generally integrates research findings into an orderly, coherent system. Such integration typically involves linking new research and existing knowledge by performing a thorough review of the prior research on a topic (see Chapter 4) and by identifying or developing an appropriate conceptual framework. These activities are important because they provide a rich context for a research project and because they help the reader to define and delimit the problem to be studied. This chapter discusses theoretical and conceptual contexts for nursing research problems.

THEORIES, MODELS, AND FRAMEWORKS

Many different terms have been used in connection with conceptual contexts for research, including theories, models, frameworks, schemes, and maps. There is considerable overlap in how these terms are used, caused in part by the fact that they are used differently by different writers. We offer some guidance in distinguishing these terms but note that there is often a blur-

ring of these terms in the literature and that our definitions are not universal.

Theories

The term theory is used in many ways. For example, nursing instructors and students frequently use the term to refer to the content covered in classrooms, as opposed to the actual practice of performing nursing activities. The term is sometimes used to refer to someone's hunches or ideas, as in the following statement: My theory is that if you smile at patients and establish rapport with them, they will be more compliant. In both lay and scientific usage, the term **theory** connotes an abstraction or a generalization.

Even within research circles, the term theory is used differently by different authors. Classically, scientists have used theory to refer to an abstract generalization that presents a systematic explanation about how phenomena are interrelated. Thus, the traditional definition requires that a theory embody at least two concepts that are related to one another in a manner that the theory purports to explain.

Others, however, use the term theory less restrictively to refer to a broad characterization of some phenomenon. According to this less restrictive definition, a theory can account for (i.e., thoroughly describe) a single phenomenon. Some authors specifically refer to this type of theory as **descriptive theory**. For example, Fawcett and Downs (1992) define descriptive theories as empirically driven theories that "describe or classify specific dimensions or characteristics of individuals, groups, situations, or events by summarizing commonalities found in discrete observations" (p. 7). Descriptive theory plays an especially important role in qualitative studies. Qualitative researchers often strive to develop a conceptualization of the phenomena under study that is grounded in the actual observations made by the researcher. The uses of theory in qualitative and quantitative studies are described later in this chapter.

As traditionally defined, scientific theories involve a series of propositions regarding the interrelationships among concepts, from which a large number of empirical observations can be deduced. In the writings on scientific theory, one encounters a variety of terms, such as proposition, postulate, premise, axiom, law, principle, and so forth, some of which are used interchangeably and others of which introduce subtleties that are too complex for the beginning researcher. Here, we present a simplified analysis of the components of a theory for the sake of clarity.

COMPONENTS OF A TRADITIONAL THEORY

Theories comprise, first of all, a set of concepts. As we noted in Chapter 2, **concepts** are abstract characteristics of the objects that are being studied. Examples of nursing concepts are adaptation, health, anxiety, nurse–client interaction, and social support. Concepts are the basic ingredients in the formulation of a theory. Second, theories comprise a set of statements or propositions, each of which indicates a relationship among the concepts. Relationships are denoted by such terms as "is associated with," "varies directly with," or "is contingent on." Third, the propositions must form a logically interrelated deductive system. This means that the theory must provide a mechanism for logically arriving at new statements from the original propositions.

Let us consider the following example, which illustrates these three points. Selye (1978) developed a theory of adaptation to stress. This theory postulates that a person's body responds to the nonspecific demands of stress by means of the General Adaptation Syndrome (GAS), which continues until adaptation occurs or death ensues. Stress may be internal or external to the individual and is manifested by the syndrome, which consists of nonspecifically induced changes occurring within the person's body. The GAS consists of three phases—the alarm phase, the phase of adaptation or resistance, and the phase of exhaustion—all of which are reversible if adjustment to stress occurs. A greatly simplified construction of Selye's theory might consist of the following propositions:

1. Humans seek to attain a desired state (e.g., the reduction of stress) by mobilizing the body's general defense mechanisms to overact to maintain life.
2. When the specific defense mechanism is identified by the body for dealing with the sources of stress (such as increased muscular activity), the overactivity of the general mechanisms subsides, and the specific mechanisms overact (such as increasing the oxygen supply in muscular activity).
3. If the specific defense mechanisms are unable to cope with the stress, then the general defense mechanisms reactivate to help the body adjust, or death ensues.
4. During the alarm and exhaustion phases, there is an increase in the production of adrenocortical hormone (ACTH), which subsides during the resistance phase when specific defense mechanisms come into play.

The concepts that form the basis of Selye's theory include stress, the GAS, the body's general defense mechanisms, and the body's specific defense mechanisms. His theory postulates that relationships occur between stress and the body's defense mechanisms, which are activated to cope with the stress. For example, the theory claims that the level of ACTH varies with the stage of the GAS. Selye's propositions readily lend themselves to empirical verification by providing a mechanism for deductive hypothesis generation. We might hypothesize on the basis of Selye's theory that the level of ACTH will be greater before a meal than it is after a meal or that ACTH production is lower during an intravenous infusion than immediately before its inception. On the basis of his theory, we should be able to identify how well the person is coping with the stress by measuring changes in ACTH production. Several nursing studies have been based on Selye's theory of stress and adaptation. For example, Henneman (1989) used Selye's concepts of stress response to evaluate the effect of direct nursing contact on patients. Hardin, Carbaugh, Weinrich, Pesut, and Carbaugh (1992) used Selye's theory to analyze stressors and coping strategies used by adolescents exposed to Hurricane Hugo.

TYPES OF TRADITIONAL THEORIES

Theories differ extensively in their level of generality. So-called **grand theories** or **macrotheories** purport to describe and explain large segments of the environment or of human experience. Some learning theorists, such as Clark Hull, or sociologists, such as Talcott Parsons, have developed highly general theoretical systems that claim to account for broad classes of behavior and social functioning.

Theories that focus on only a piece of reality or human experience and that incorporate a selected number of concepts are sometimes referred to as **middle-range theories**. For example, there are middle-range theories that attempt to explain such phenomena as decision-making behavior, compliance, and infant attachment. This limited scope is consistent with the state of scientific developments in many fields dealing with human behavior.

Theories also vary in their complexity. Here, we refer to the number and intricacy of the concepts involved and the complexity of relationships presumed. Theories in the disciplines dealing with humans often tend to be complex, not only because the subject matter is inherently complex but also because conditional relationships and multiple variables are required at the current level of understanding and conceptualization.

Conceptual Models

Conceptual models, conceptual frameworks, or **conceptual schemes** (we use the terms interchangeably here) represent a less formal attempt at organizing phenomena than theories. As the name implies, conceptual models deal with abstractions (concepts) that are assembled by virtue of their relevance to a common theme. Both conceptual models and theories use concepts as building blocks. What is absent from conceptual models is the deductive system of propositions that assert a relationship between the concepts. Conceptual models provide a conceptual perspective regarding interrelated phenomena but are more loosely structured than theories. A conceptual model broadly presents an understanding of the phenomenon of interest and reflects the assumptions and philosophical views of the model's designer. Conceptual models are not directly testable by researchers in the same way that theories are. However, conceptual models, like theories, can serve as important springboards for the generation of hypotheses to be tested.

Much of the conceptual work that has been done in connection with nursing practice falls into the category we have designated as conceptual models. These models represent world views about the nursing process and the nature of the nurse–patient relationship. A subsequent section of this chapter describes some of the major conceptual models in nursing and illustrates how they have been used in nursing research.

Schematic and Statistical Models

The term **model** is sometimes used to denote a symbolic representation of conceptualizations of phenomena. Within a research context, the models that one is most likely to encounter are mathematic (or statistical) models and schematic models. These models, like conceptual frameworks, are constructed representations of some aspect of our environment. They use abstractions (i.e., concepts) as the building blocks, but they attempt to represent reality with a minimal use of words. A visual or symbolic representation of a theory or conceptual framework often helps to express abstract ideas in a more readily understandable or graphic form than the original conceptualization.

Schematic models are common and are undoubtedly familiar to all readers. A schematic model (also referred to as a **conceptual map**) represents the phenomena of interest figuratively. Concepts and the linkages between them are represented diagrammatically through the use of boxes, arrows, or other symbols. An example of a schematic model is presented in Figure 5-1. This model, known as **Pender's Health Promotion Model**, is described by its developer as "a multivariate paradigm for explaining and predicting the health-promotion component of lifestyle" (Pender, Walker, Sechrist, & Frank-Stromborg, 1990, p. 326). Schematic models of this type can be useful in the research process in clarifying concepts and their associations, in enabling researchers to place a specific problem into an appropriate context, and in revealing areas where further inquiry is needed. Increasingly, nurse researchers are developing such schematic models and testing them using highly sophisticated analytic techniques.

Statistical models are playing a growing role in research endeavors in nursing and re-

lated sciences. These models use symbols to express quantitatively the nature of relationships among variables. Few relationships in the behavioral sciences can be summarized as elegantly as in the mathematic model F = ma (force = mass × acceleration). Because human behavior is so complex and subject to so many influences as yet poorly understood, it is typically possible to model it only in a probabilistic manner. This means that we are not able to develop equations, such as the example of force from mechanics, in which a human behavior can be simply described as the product of two other phenomena. What we can do, however, is describe the probability that a certain behavior or characteristic will exist, given the occurrence of other specified phenomena. This is the function of statistical models. An example of a statistical model is shown below:

$$Y = \beta_1 X_1 + \beta_2 X_2 + \beta_3 X_3 + \beta_4 X_4 + e$$

where Y = nursing effectiveness, as measured by a supervisor's evaluation

X_1 = nursing knowledge, as measured by a standardized test

X_2 = past achievement, as measured by grades in nursing school

X_3 = decision-making skills, as measured by number of nursing diagnoses made

X_4 = empathy, as measured by timing between the patient's request for pain medication and actual administration of pain medication

e = a residual, unexplained factor

$\beta_1, \beta_2, \beta_3,$ and β_4 = weights indicating the importance of $X_1, X_2, X_3,$ and X_4, respectively, in determining nursing effectiveness

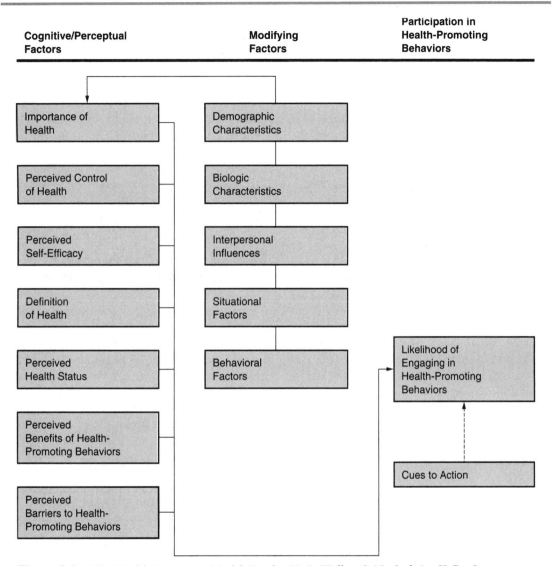

| Cognitive/Perceptual Factors | Modifying Factors | Participation in Health-Promoting Behaviors |

Figure 5-1. The Health Promotion Model (Pender, N. J., Walker, S. N., Sechrist, K. R., & Frank-Stromborg, M. [1990]. Predicting health-promoting lifestyles in the workplace. *Nursing Research, 39,* 331).

Each term in this model is quantified or quantifiable; that is, every symbol can be replaced by a numeric value, such as an individual's score on a standardized test of knowledge (X_1).

What does this equation mean and how does it work? This model constitutes a proposed mechanism for understanding and predicting nursing effectiveness. The model proposes that nurses' on-the-job effectiveness is affected primarily by four factors: the nursing knowledge, past achievement, decision-making skill, and empathy of the nurse. These influences are not presumed to be equally important. The weights (βs) associated with each factor represent a recipe for designating the relative importance of each. If empathy were much more important than past achievement, for example, then the weights might be 2 to 1, respectively (i.e., two parts empathy to one part past achievement). The *e* (or **error term**) at the end of the model represents all those unknown or unmeasurable other attributes that affect one's performance as a nurse. In the quantitative equation, *e* would be set equal to some constant value; it would not vary from one nurse to another because it really constitutes an unknown element in the equation. Once the values of the weights and *e* have been established (through statistical procedures), the model can be used to predict the nursing effectiveness of any nurse for whom we have gathered information on the four *X*s (standardized test scores and so forth). Our prediction of who will make an especially effective nurse will not always be perfectly accurate, in part because of the influence of those unknown factors summarized by *e*. Perfect forecasting is seldom attainable with probabilistic statistical models. However, such a model makes prediction of nursing effectiveness less haphazard than mere guesswork or intuition.

Frameworks

A **framework** is the conceptual underpinnings of a study. Not every study is based on a theory or conceptual model, but every study has a framework. In a study based on a theory, the framework is referred to as the **theoretical framework**; in a study that has its roots in a specified conceptual model, the framework is often called the **conceptual framework** (although the terms conceptual framework and theoretical framework are often used interchangeably).

In many cases, the framework for a study is implicit—that is, not formally acknowledged or described by the researcher. The concepts in which a researcher is interested are by definition abstractions of observable phenomena, and our world view (and views on nursing) shape how those concepts are defined and op-

erationalized. What often happens, however, is that researchers fail to clarify the conceptual underpinnings of their research variables, thereby making it more difficult to integrate research findings. Consider, for example, the concept of *caring*. Caring can be conceptualized as a human trait, a moral ideal, an affect, an interaction, or an intervention (Morse, Solberg, Neander, Bottorff, & Johnson, 1990). A researcher undertaking a study concerned with caring should make clear what **conceptual definition** of caring he or she has adopted—that is, what the framework for the study is.

THE NATURE OF THEORIES AND CONCEPTUAL MODELS

Theories and conceptual models have much in common, including their origin, general nature, purposes, and role in the research process. In this section, we examine some of the general characteristics of conceptual frameworks that provide contexts for nursing research. In this section, we use the term theory in its least restrictive sense.

Origin of Theories and Models

Theories and conceptual models are not discovered by researchers and scientists; they are created and invented by them. The building of a framework depends not only on the observable facts in our environment but also on the originator's ingenuity in pulling those facts together and making sense of them. Thus, theory construction is a creative and intellectual enterprise that can be engaged in by anyone who has imagination, a solid base of knowledge, and the ability to knit together observations and existing knowledge into an intelligible pattern.

Tentative Nature of Theories and Models

Theories and conceptual models can never be proved or confirmed. A theory represents a scientist's best efforts to describe and explain phenomena; today's successful theory may be relegated to tomorrow's intellectual junk yard. This may happen if new evidence or observations discredit or undermine a previously well-accepted framework. It is also possible that a new theoretical system can integrate new observations with the observations on which the old theory was based and result in a more parsimonious explanation of the phenomena in question.

Theories and models that are not congruent with a culture's values and philosophical orientation also may be discredited over time. It is not unusual for a theory to lose supporters because its implications are not in vogue. For example, certain psychoanalytic and structural social theories, which had widespread support for decades, have come to be challenged and revised as a result of the emergence of feminism and changes in society's views about the roles of women. This link between theory and values may surprise those who think of science as being completely objective. It should be remembered, however, that frameworks are deliberately invented by humans; thus, they can never be freed totally from the human perspective, which is amenable to change over time.

Thus, no theory or model, no matter what its subject matter, can ever be considered final and verified. There always remains the possibility that a theory will be modified or discarded. Many theories in the physical sciences have received considerable empirical support, and their well-accepted propositions are often referred to as **laws**, such as Boyle's law of gases. Nevertheless, we have no way of knowing the ultimate accuracy and utility of any theory and should, therefore, treat all theories as tentative. This caveat is nowhere more relevant than in the emerging sciences such as nursing.

Purposes of Theories and Conceptual Models

Theoretical and conceptual frameworks play several interrelated roles in the progress of a sci-ence. Their overall purpose is to make research findings meaningful and generalizable. Theories allow researchers to knit together observations and facts into an orderly scheme. Frameworks are efficient mechanisms for drawing together and summarizing accumulated facts, sometimes from separate and isolated investigations. The linkage of findings into a coherent structure makes the body of accumulated knowledge more accessible and, thus, more useful both to practitioners who seek to implement findings and to researchers who seek to extend the knowledge base.

In addition to summarizing, theories and models can guide the researcher's understanding of not only the *what* of natural phenomena but also the *why* of their occurrence. Theories often provide a basis for predicting the occurrence of phenomena. Prediction, in turn, has implications for the control of those phenomena. A utilitarian framework is one that has potential to bring about desirable changes in people's behavior or the environment.

Theories and conceptual models help to stimulate research and the extension of knowledge by providing both direction and impetus. Many nursing studies have been generated explicitly to examine aspects of a conceptual model of nursing. Thus, frameworks may serve as a springboard for scientific advances.

Relationship Between Theory and Research

The relationship between theory and research is a reciprocal and mutually beneficial one. Theories and models are built inductively from observations, and an excellent source for those observations is prior research and in-depth qualitative studies. Concepts and relationships that are validated empirically through research become the foundation for theory development. The theory, in turn, must be tested by subjecting deductions from it (hypotheses) to further systematic inquiry. Thus, research plays a dual and continuing role in theory building and testing. Theory guides and generates ideas for research; research assesses the worth of the theory and provides a foundation for new theories.

It would be unreasonable to assert that research without a specific theoretical framework cannot make a contribution to knowledge. In nursing research, many facts still need to be accumulated, and purely descriptive inquiries may well form the basis for subsequent theoretical developments. Research that does not test a theory can potentially be linked to a framework at a later time. Although it is not always easy to place one's research problems into a theoretical context, however, it is advantageous for the advancement of nursing science to do so. Some suggestions for linking a study to a conceptual framework are presented later in this chapter.

CONCEPTUAL MODELS USED IN NURSING RESEARCH

Nurse researchers have used both nursing and nonnursing frameworks to provide a conceptual context for their studies. This section briefly summarizes several frameworks that have been found useful by nurse researchers.

Conceptual Models of the Nursing Process

In the past few decades, nurses have formulated a number of conceptual models of nursing practice. These models constitute formal explanations of what the nursing discipline is according to the model developer's point of view. As Fawcett (1989) has noted, four concepts are central to models of nursing:

- Person
- Environment
- Health
- Nursing

The various conceptual models, however, define these concepts differently, link them in diverse ways, and give different emphases to the relationships among them. Moreover, different models emphasize different processes as being central to nursing. For example, Sister Calista Roy's Adaptation Model identifies adaptation of patients as a critical phenomenon (Roy & Andrews, 1991). Rogers (1986), by contrast, emphasizes the centrality of the individual as a unified whole, and her model views nursing as a process in which individuals are aided in achieving maximum well-being within their potential.

The conceptual models were not developed primarily as a base for nursing research. Indeed, these models have thus far had more impact on nursing education, administration, and clinical practice than on nursing research. Nevertheless, nurse researchers are turning increasingly toward these conceptual frameworks for their inspiration and theoretical foundations in formulating research questions and hypotheses. In this section, we briefly examine some of the major conceptual frameworks of nursing and give examples of research that claimed their intellectual roots in these models.

KING'S OPEN SYSTEM MODEL

King's (1981) conceptual model includes three types of dynamic, interacting systems: personal systems (represented by individuals); interpersonal systems (represented by such dyadic interactions as nurse–patient dialogue); and social systems (represented by larger institutions, such as hospitals and families). The social system provides a context in which nurses work. Within King's model, the domain of nursing includes promoting, maintaining, and restoring health. Nursing is viewed as "a process of action, reaction, and interaction whereby nurse and client share information about their perceptions of the nursing situation" (King, 1981, p. 2). King herself conducted a descriptive observational study of nurse–client encounters that yielded a classification of elements in nurse–client interactions. The study provided preliminary support for the proposition that goal attainment was facilitated by accurate nurse–client perceptions, satisfactory communication, and mutual goal setting. Hanna (1993) used King's framework in a study of the effect of a nurse–client transactional intervention on female adolescents' oral contraceptive adherence. Brooks and Thomas (1997) based their study of the perception and judgment of student nurses in clinical decision making on King's model, and the results led the researchers to propose a reconceptualization of King's system.

LEVINE'S CONSERVATION MODEL

Levine's (1973) model focuses on individuals as holistic beings, and the major area of concern for nurses is maintenance of the person's wholeness. The model identifies adaptation as the process by which the integrity or wholeness of individuals is maintained. Levine's model identifies several principles of conservation that aim to facilitate patients' adaptation processes. Through these principles, the model emphasizes the nurse's responsibility to maintain the client's integrity in the threat of assault through illness or environmental influences. Foreman (1989) categorized variables associated with confusion in the elderly according to Levine's conservation principles. Schaefer and Potylycki (1993) based their study of fatigue associated with congestive heart failure on Levine's conservation model.

NEUMAN'S HEALTH CARE SYSTEMS MODEL

Neuman's (1989) model focuses on the person as a complete system, the subparts of which are interrelated physiologic, psychological, sociocultural, spiritual, and developmental factors. In this model, the person maintains balance and harmony between internal and external environments by adjusting to stress and by defending against tension-producing stimuli. Wellness is equated with equilibrium. The primary goal of nursing is to assist in the attainment and maintenance of client system stability. Nursing interventions include activities to strengthen flexible lines of defense, to strengthen resistance to stressors, and to maintain adaptation. Using Neuman's model, Lowry and Anderson (1993) investigated what factors influenced weaning from mechanical ventilation. Ross and Bourbonnais (1985) described the interpersonal, intrapersonal, and extrapersonal stressors identified in the home care of a man after a myocardial infarction. They developed nursing interventions directed toward strengthening the flexible lines of defense and resistance.

OREM'S SELF-CARE MODEL

Orem's (1985) model focuses on each individual's ability to perform self-care, defined as "the practice of activities that individuals initiate and perform on their own behalf in maintaining life, health, and well-being" (p. 35). One's ability to care for oneself is referred to as *self-care* agency, and the ability to care for others is referred to as *dependent-care* agency. In Orem's model, the goal of nursing is to help people meet their own therapeutic self-care demands. Orem identified three types of nursing systems: (1) wholly compensatory, wherein the nurse compensates for the patient's total inability to perform self-care activities; (2) partially compensatory, wherein the nurse compensates for the patient's partial inability to perform these activities; and (3) supportive–educative, wherein the nurse assists the patient in making decisions and acquiring skills and knowledge. Orem's Self-Care Model has generated considerable interest among nurse researchers. For example, Ailinger and Dear (1997) used Orem's self-care theory to study the needs of clients with rheumatoid arthritis. Page and Ricard (1996) conducted a study to describe the self-care requisites of women treated for depression. Aish and Isenberg (1996) explored the effect of nursing care on nutritional self-care among myocardial infarction patients.

PARSE'S THEORY OF HUMAN BECOMING

Rooted firmly in existential phenomenology, Parse's (1992, 1995) theory views a human being as an open system freely able to choose from among a series of options in giving meaning to a situation. Humans and the environment remain independent entities during interchanges, and together they co-create meaning and patterns. The goal of Parse's model in nursing practice is to encourage a client to share his or her thoughts and feelings about the meaning of a situation. The explication of the meaning changes the situation, and new meaning occurs. As new meanings arise, the patterns co-created by client and environment change. Clients may then be guided to plan for change from the known health patterns to new health patterns. Clients are considered and respected as the experts of their own health. The Parse framework is a relatively young one but has already generated several applications in the research literature, particularly among qualitative researchers. For example, Janes, Wells, and Daly (1997) relied on the Parse model in their study of hospitalized elderly patients' experience of being cared for by nurses. Parse herself (1997) studied the lived experience of joy and sorrow among elderly women.

ROGERS'S SCIENCE OF UNITARY HUMAN BEINGS

Rogers's model (1970, 1986) focuses on the individual as a unified whole in constant interaction with the environment. The unitary person is viewed as an energy field that is more than, as well as different from, the sum of the biologic, physical, social, and psychological parts. In Rogers's model, nursing is concerned with the unitary person as a synergistic phenomenon.

Nursing science is devoted to the study of the nature and direction of unitary human development. Nursing practice helps individuals achieve maximum well-being within their potential. Using Rogers's framework, Bernardo (1996) examined parents' reports about their children's behaviors and life events, using injury, illness, and wellness as measures of change. Butcher (1996) sought to enhance understanding of the phenomenon of dispiritedness in later life within the context of Rogers's theory. Sherman (1996) used Rogers's framework to examine relationships among spirituality, perceived social support, death anxiety, and nurses' willingness to care for AIDS patients among a sample of RNs in New York City.

ROY'S ADAPTATION MODEL

In Roy's Adaptation Model (1984, 1991), humans are biopsychosocial adaptive systems who cope with environmental change through the process of adaptation. Within the human system, there are four subsystems: physiologic needs, self-concept, role function, and interdependence. These subsystems constitute adaptive modes that provide mechanisms for coping with environmental stimuli and change. The goal of nursing, according to this model, is to promote patient adaptation during health and illness. Nursing also regulates stimuli affecting adaptation. Nursing interventions generally take the form of increasing, decreasing, modifying, removing, or maintaining internal and external stimuli that affect adaptation. Roy's model has provided a conceptual framework for many nursing studies. Based on Roy's concepts, Bournaki (1997) studied children's age, gender, exposure to past painful experiences, temperament, and fears in relationship to their pain responses to venipuncture. Samarel, Fawcett, and Tulman (1997) tested Roy's model in a study of the effect of support groups on adaptation to early-stage breast cancer. Hamner (1996) tested a proposition of Roy's model that predicted relationships among severity of illness, perceived control, hardiness, anxiety, and length of stay in an intensive care unit.

Other Models Developed by Nurses

In addition to conceptual models that are designed to describe and characterize the entire nursing process, nurses have developed other models and theories that focus on more specific phenomena of interest to nurses. Two important examples are Pender's Health Promotion Model and Mishel's Uncertainty in Illness Theory.

THE HEALTH PROMOTION MODEL

Pender's (1987) Health Promotion Model (HPM) focuses on explaining health-promoting behaviors, using a wellness orientation. According to the model, a schematic model of which is shown in Figure 5–1, *health promotion* is defined as activities directed toward the development of resources that maintain or enhance an individual's well-being. The HPM encompasses two phases: a decision-making phase and an action phase. In the decision-making phase, the model emphasizes seven cognitive/perceptual factors that compose primary motivational mechanisms for acquisition and maintenance of health-promoting behaviors (e.g., perceived barriers to health-promoting behaviors) and five modifying factors that indirectly influence patterns of health behavior (e.g., situational influences). In the action phase, both barriers and cues to action trigger activity in health-promoting behavior. According to the model, people move back and forth in a reciprocal fashion between the two phases. Nurse researchers have applied the HPM to study the factors that differentiate contraceptive use among sexually active adolescent women (Felton, 1996), the use of hearing protection among construction workers (Lusk, Ronis, & Hogan, 1997), and the determinants of exercise and aerobic fitness among outpatients with arthritis (Neuberger, Kasal, Smith, Hassanein, & DeViney, 1994). A more

detailed example of a study using this model is presented at the end of this chapter.

UNCERTAINTY IN ILLNESS THEORY

Mishel's (1988) Uncertainty in Illness Theory focuses on the concept of uncertainty—the inability of a person to determine the meaning of illness-related events. According to this theory, people develop subjective appraisals of meaning to assist them in interpreting the experience of illness and treatment. Uncertainty occurs when people are unable to recognize and categorize stimuli. Uncertainty results in the inability to obtain a clear conception of the situation, but a situation appraised as uncertain will mobilize individuals to use their resources to adapt to the situation. Mishel's conceptualization of uncertainty has been used as a framework for both qualitative and quantitative studies. For example, Baier (1995) conducted an in-depth qualitative study focusing on uncertainty in illness of people with schizophrenia, and Lemaire and Lenz's (1995) quantitative study was designed to identify predictors of uncertainty among menopausal women. Staples and Jeffrey (1997) examined the relationships among quality of life, uncertainty, and hope before bypass surgery among patients and their spouses. Tomlinson, Kirschbaum, Harbaugh, and Anderson (1996) studied the influence of illness severity and family resources on maternal uncertainty during a child's hospitalization for a life-threatening illness.

Other Models Used by Nurse Researchers

Many of the phenomena in which nurse researchers are interested involve concepts that are not unique to nurses, and therefore their studies are sometimes linked to conceptual models that are not models from the nursing profession. Three nonnursing models that have frequently been used in nursing research investigations are the Health Belief Model (HBM), Lazarus and Folkman's Theory of Stress and

Coping, and Ajzen's Theory of Planned Behavior (TPB). These models and examples of nursing studies that were based on them are briefly described next.

THE HEALTH BELIEF MODEL

The HBM has become a popular conceptual framework in nursing, especially in studies focusing on patient compliance and preventive health care practices. The model postulates that health-seeking behavior is influenced by a person's perception of a threat posed by a health problem and the value associated with actions aimed at reducing the threat (Becker, 1978). The major components of the HBM include perceived susceptibility, perceived severity, perceived benefits and costs, motivation, and enabling or modifying factors. Perceived susceptibility refers to a person's perception that a health problem is personally relevant or that a diagnosis of illness is accurate. Even when one recognizes personal susceptibility, action will not occur unless the individual perceives the severity to be high enough to have serious organic or social implications. Perceived benefits refer to the patients' beliefs that a given treatment will cure the illness or help prevent it, and perceived costs refer to the complexity, duration, and accessibility of the treatment. Motivation includes the desire to comply with a treatment and the belief that people should do what is prescribed by health care personnel. Among the modifying factors that have been identified are personality variables, patient satisfaction, and sociodemographic factors. Nurse researchers have used the HBM in connection with studies of early detection of cancer among Chinese women (Hoeman, Ku, & Ohl, 1996), the effects of an age-specific AIDS education program (Rose, 1996), and the effects of a nurse-directed self-management program on dyspnea among patients with chronic obstructive pulmonary disease (Zimmerman, Brown, & Bowman, 1996).

LAZARUS AND FOLKMAN'S THEORY OF STRESS AND COPING

This model (Lazarus, 1966; Folkman & Lazarus, 1988) represents an effort to explain people's methods of dealing with stress, that is, environmental and internal demands that tax or exceed a person's resources and endanger his or her well-being. The model posits that coping strategies are learned, deliberate responses to stressors that are used to adapt to or change the stressors. According to this model, a person's perception of mental and physical health is related to the ways he or she evaluates and copes with the stresses of living. Many nurses have conducted research within the context of this model, including studies of coping among patients with a recurrence of cancer (Mahon & Casperson, 1997), stress among staff nurses resulting from verbal abuse by physicians (Manderino & Berkey, 1997), and problem-focused coping in relation to perceived self-efficacy and social support among HIV-infected mothers (Sharts-Hopko, Regan-Kubinski, Lincoln, & Heverly, 1996).

AJZEN'S THEORY OF PLANNED BEHAVIOR

The Theory of Reasoned Action (TRA) provides a framework for understanding the relationships among a person's attitudes, intentions, and behaviors (Ajzen & Fishbein, 1980). According to the TRA, behavioral intentions are the best predictor of a person's behavior, and behavioral intentions are a function of attitude toward performing the behavior and the subjective norm, which is the person's perception of whether relevant others think the behavior should be performed. The TRA has been used as a framework for nurse researchers in studies of nurses' behaviors regarding the conduct of pain assessment (Nash, Edwards, & Nebauer, 1993) and nurses' intended care behavior with patients who are HIV positive (Laschinger & Goldenberg, 1993).

The Theory of Planned Behavior (TPB; Ajzen, 1988) is an extension of the TRA, which assumed volitional control over behavior. The TPB assumes that behavior is located along a continuum from complete volitional control to no volitional control. Many recent nursing studies have been based on the TPB, including Wambach's (1997) study regarding the prediction of breastfeeding behavior, Hanson's (1997) investigation of cigarette smoking among teenage women, and DiIorio's (1997) research on neuroscience nurses' intentions to care for people with HIV or AIDS.

Theoretical Contexts and Nursing Research

As previously noted, theory and research have reciprocal, beneficial ties. Fawcett (1978) described the relationship between theory and research as a double helix, with theory as the impetus of scientific investigations and with findings from research shaping the development of theory. However, this relationship has not always characterized the progress of nursing science. Many have criticized nurse researchers for producing numerous isolated studies that are not placed in a theoretical context.

This criticism was more justified a decade ago than it is today. Many researchers are developing studies on the basis of conceptual models of nursing. Nursing science is still struggling, however, to integrate accumulated knowledge within theoretical systems. This struggle is reflected, in part, in the number of controversies surrounding the issue of theoretical frameworks in nursing.

One of these controversies concerns whether there should be one single, unified model of nursing or multiple, competing models. Fawcett (1989) has argued against combining different models, noting that "before all nurses follow the same path, the competition of multiple models is needed to determine the superiority of one or more of them" (p. 9). Research

can play a critical role in testing the utility and validity of alternative nursing models.

Another controversy involves the desirability and utility of developing theories unique to nursing. Some commentators argue that theories relating to humans developed in other disciplines, such as physiology, psychology, and sociology (so-called **borrowed theories**), can and should be applied to nursing problems. Others advocate the development of unique nursing theories, claiming that only through such development can knowledge to guide nursing practice be produced.

Until these controversies are resolved, nursing research is likely to continue on its current path of conducting studies within a multidisciplinary and multitheoretical perspective. We are inclined to see the use of multiple frameworks as a healthy and unavoidable part of the development of nursing science.

TESTING, USING, AND DEVELOPING A THEORY OR FRAMEWORK

In a previous section, we described the strong interrelationship between theory and research. The manner in which theory and conceptual frameworks are used by qualitative and quantitative researchers is elaborated on in the following section. In the discussion, the term theory is used in its broadest sense. In other words, the procedures discussed are almost always equally applicable to conceptual frameworks and models and to formal theories.

Qualitative Research and Theory Development

Qualitative researchers often strive to develop a conceptualization of the phenomena under study that is grounded in the actual observations made by the researcher. As we discuss in Chapter 10, these researchers seek to develop what is referred to as a **grounded** theory—an empirically based conceptualization for integrating and making sense of a process or phenomenon.

Theory development in a qualitative study is primarily an inductive process. The qualitative researcher seeks to identify patterns, commonalities, and relationships through the scrutiny of specific instances and events. During the ongoing analysis of data, the qualitative researcher moves from specific pieces of data to abstract generalizations that synthesize and give structure to the observed phenomenon. The goal is to use the data, grounded in reality, to provide a description or an explanation of events as they occur in reality—not as they have been conceptualized in preexisting theories. Most qualitative studies develop theories that can be classified as middle-range theories.

Not all qualitative studies have theory development as a goal. Moreover, some qualitative researchers acknowledge an explicit conceptual model of nursing as a framework for their studies. For example, a number of qualitative nurse researchers acknowledge that the philosophical roots of their studies lie in conceptual models of nursing such as those developed by Parse and Rogers.

Theories in Quantitative Research

Quantitative researchers can link research to theory or models in several ways. The most common approach is to test hypotheses deduced from a previously proposed theory.

TESTING A THEORY

As noted earlier, theories often stimulate new research investigations. For example, a nurse might read several papers relating to Orem's Self-Care Model. As the nurse's reading progresses, the following types of conjectures might arise: "If Orem's Self-Care Model is valid, then one might expect that nursing effectiveness can be enhanced in environments more conducive to self-care (e.g., a birthing room versus a delivery room)" or "Given this conceptual framework, it might be expected that the dependency level of patients (in terms of either their physical or psychologic characteristics) would influence the nature and intensity of effective interventions." These conjectures, derived from a theory or conceptual framework, can serve as a point of departure for testing the adequacy of the theory.

In testing a theory, the researcher deduces implications (as in the preceding examples) and develops research hypotheses. These hypotheses are predictions about the manner in which variables would be related, if the theory were correct and useful. The hypotheses are then subjected to empirical testing through systematic research. A theory is never tested directly. It is the hypotheses deduced from a theory that are subjected to investigations.

Comparisons between the observed outcomes of research and the relationships predicted by the hypotheses are the major focus of the testing process. Through this process, the theory is continually subjected to potential disconfirmation. Repeated failures of research endeavors to disconfirm a theory result in increasing support for and acceptance of a theoretical position. The testing process continues until pieces of evidence cannot be interpreted within the context of the theory but *can* be explained by a new theory that also accounts for all previous findings. From the point of view of theory testing, the goals of a serviceable research project are to devise logically adequate deductions from theory, to develop a research design that reduces the credibility of alternative explanations for observed relationships, and to select methods that assess the theory's validity under maximally heterogeneous situations so that potentially competing theories can be ruled out.

TESTING TWO COMPETING THEORIES

Researchers who directly test two competing theories to explain some phenomenon are in a particularly good position to advance knowledge. Almost all phenomena can be explained in alternative ways, as suggested by the alternative conceptual models of nursing. There are also competing theories for such phenomena as stress, compliance, child development, learning, and grieving. All of these phenomena are of great importance to nursing. Each competing theory for these phenomena suggests alternative approaches to facilitating a positive outcome or minimizing a negative one. It is therefore important to know which explanation has more validity, if we are to design maximally effective nursing interventions.

Typically, researchers have opted to test a single theory in a research investigation. Then, to evaluate the worth of competing theories, they must compare the results of different studies. Such comparisons, however, are often difficult to make because study designs rarely lend themselves to direct comparisons. For example, one study of stress might use a sample of college students, another might use military personnel in a combat situation, and yet another might use terminally ill cancer patients. Each of these studies might use an alternative approach to measuring stress. If the results of these studies support alternative theories of stress to different degrees, it would be difficult to know the extent to which the results reflected differences in the study design rather than differences in the validity of the theories.

The researcher who directly tests two (or more) competing theories, using a single sample of subjects and comparable measures of the key research variables, is in a position to make powerful and meaningful comparisons. Such a study typically requires considerable advance planning and the inclusion of a wider array of measures than would otherwise be the case, but such efforts are to be commended. In recent years, a growing number of nursing investigators have used this approach to generate and refine our knowledge base and to provide promising new leads for further research. For example, Campbell (1989) tested a "grief model" and a "learned helplessness" model to explain women's responses to battering. She found that both theories had some support but that the "learned helplessness" concepts had not been sufficiently operationalized in her study and required further investigation. Yarcheski, Mahon, and Yarcheski (1997) tested two alternative models of positive health practices in adolescents: an explanation that involved future time perspective and another that included the adolescents' perceived health status. The findings suggested that the first model had a better fit with the data than the second model.

FITTING A PROBLEM TO A THEORY

The preceding sections addressed the situation in which a researcher begins with one or more specific theories or conceptual frameworks and uses the theories as the basis for developing hypotheses and a research design. Circumstances sometimes arise in which the problem is formulated before consideration is given to a theoretical framework. Even in such situations, researchers may wish to (or may be required to) devise a theoretical context in an effort to enrich the value and interpretability of their inquiry. Although we recognize that this situation sometimes occurs, we must nevertheless caution that an after-the-fact linkage of theory to a research question is usually considerably less meaningful than the testing of a particular theory of interest. This is especially true for neophyte researchers who may lack a thorough grounding in the theoretical positions of their own or related disciplines.

The search for relevant existing theories can be greatly facilitated by first conceptualizing the nature of the problem on a sufficiently abstract level. For example, take the research question, "Do daily telephone conversations between a psychiatric nurse and a patient for 2 weeks following discharge from the hospital result in lower rates of readmission by short-term psychiatric patients?" This is a relatively concrete research problem but might profitably be viewed as a subproblem for Orem's Self-Care Model, a theory of reinforcement, a theory of social influence, or a theory of crisis resolution. Part of the difficulty in finding a theory is that a single phenomenon of interest can be conceptualized in a number of ways and, depending on the manner chosen, may refer the researcher to conceptual schemes from a wide range of disciplines.

Once the researcher has conceptualized the research problem on an abstract level, the search for a suitable framework can proceed. Textbooks, handbooks, and encyclopedias in the chosen discipline usually are a good starting point for the identification of a framework. These sources usually summarize the status of a theoretical position and document the efforts to confirm and disconfirm it. Journal articles contain more current information but are usually restricted to descriptions of specific studies rather than to broad expositions or evaluations of theories. When a theoretical position has been developed at length or has been supported by extensive empirical observations, entire books may be devoted to its description.

Once a potential conceptual framework has been identified, its utility should be carefully evaluated in terms of its congruity with the problem to be studied and with the researcher's own philosophy and world view. If the framework is judged to be adequate on these grounds, it then becomes the researcher's job to design the study in such a way that it fits the framework.

The task of fitting a problem to a theory should be done with caution. It is true that having a theoretical context enhances the meaningfulness of a research study, but artificially cramming a problem into a theory is not the route to scientific utility. There are many published studies that purport to have a conceptual framework when, in fact, the post hoc nature of the conceptualization is all too evident. If a conceptual framework is really linked to a research problem, then the design of the study, the selection of appropriate data collection strategies, the data analysis, and (especially) the interpretation of the findings *flow* from that conceptualization. We advocate a

balanced and reasoned perspective on this issue: *Researchers should not shirk their intellectual duties by failing to make an attempt to link their problem to broader theoretical concerns, but there is no point in fabricating such a link when it does not exist.*

DEVELOPING A FRAMEWORK IN A QUANTITATIVE STUDY

Many beginning researchers may think of themselves as unqualified to develop a theory or conceptual scheme of their own. But theory development depends much less on one's knowledge of research methods and experience in the conduct of investigations than on one's powers of observation, understanding of a problem, and readings about a substantive issue. There is, therefore, nothing to prevent an imaginative and sensitive person from formulating an original conceptual framework for a study. The conceptual scheme may or may not be a full-fledged formal theory with well-articulated postulates; the scheme should, however, place the issues of the study into some broader perspective.

The basic intellectual process underlying theory development is induction, which refers to the process of reasoning from particular observations and facts to generalizations. The inductive process involves integrating what one has experienced or learned into some concise and general conclusion. For example, if one has observed that Christopher R., Chance S., Alana K., and Sarah T. (all of whom are tonsillectomy patients) have refused to eat their first postoperative meal, one might conclude that loss of appetite characterizes those who have just had a tonsillectomy operation. The observations used in the inductive process need not be personal observations; they may be (and often are in formal theories) the findings and conclusions from other studies. When relationships among variables are arrived at this way, one has the makings of a theory that can be put to a more rigorous scientific test. The first step in theory development, then, is to formulate a generalized scheme of relevant concepts, that is, to perform a conceptual analysis. The product of this step should be a conceptual framework, the worth of which can be assessed through the collection of empirical information.

Let us consider the following simple example. Suppose that we were interested in understanding the factors influencing enrollment in a prenatal education program. We might begin by considering two basic sets of forces: those that promote enrollment and those that hinder it. After reviewing the literature, discussing the problem with colleagues, and developing ideas from our own experiences, we might arrive at a conceptual scheme such as the one presented in Figure 5-2. This framework is undoubtedly incomplete and imperfect, but it does allow us to study a number of research questions *and* to place those problems in perspective. For example, the conceptual scheme suggests that as the availability of social supports declines, the obstacles to participation in a prenatal education program increase. We might then make the following hypothesis: "Single pregnant women are less likely to participate in a prenatal educa-

tion program than married pregnant women," on the assumption that husbands are an important source of social support to women in their pregnancy.

Many nursing studies involve a conceptual framework developed by the researchers. For example, Auvil-Novak (1997) evolved a middle-range theory of chronotherapeutic intervention for postsurgical pain and tested it in three separate chronobiologic studies. Janson-Bjerklie, Ferketich, and Benner (1993) tested their own conceptual model to predict psychosocial and morbidity outcomes in adults with chronic asthma.

TIPS ON FRAMEWORKS IN NURSING STUDIES

Most published nursing studies are not explicitly linked to a conceptual model or theory—despite the widespread acknowledgment that research without theory often undermines the utility of the knowledge gained. In this section, we offer some suggestions on how to strengthen the conceptual basis of nursing studies.

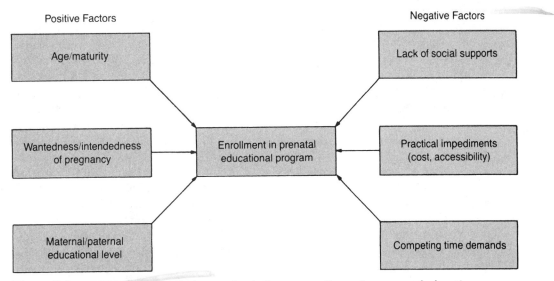

Figure 5-2. Conceptual model—factors that influence enrollment in a prenatal education program.

- Although most nursing studies are not theory driven, virtually all studies have an unacknowledged conceptual basis. Concepts (which become research variables) are by definition abstractions of observable phenomena, and our world view and views on nursing shape how those concepts are defined and operationalized. What often happens, however, is that researchers fail to clarify the conceptual underpinnings of their research variables, thereby making it more difficult to integrate research findings. For example, a researcher undertaking a study concerned with caring should make clear which perspective on caring he or she has adopted. Thus, even if you are not testing a specific theory, it is wise to clarify the conceptual perspective you have on key constructs.

- If you begin with a research problem and are trying to identify a suitable conceptual framework, it is probably wise to confer with others—especially with people who may be familiar with a broad range of theoretical perspectives. By having an open discussion, you are more likely to become aware of your own conceptual perspectives and are thus in a better position to identify an appropriate framework.

- It is often suggested that a theory first be evaluated before it is used as a basis for a research project—an enterprise that may be difficult for beginning researchers. However, some basic evaluative criteria are fairly easy to apply, including the following:

  Is the theory one that has significance—that is, does it address a problem of particular interest to nurses or society?

  Does the theory offer the possibility of explaining or systematically describing some phenomenon?

  Is the theory testable—that is, can the concepts be observed and measured, and can hypotheses be deduced?

For the advanced student, Stevens (1984), Chinn and Jacobs (1994), and Fawcett and Downs (1992) present more extensive and more rigorous criteria for assessing conceptual frameworks in nursing.

- In a qualitative study, evaluation criteria for a theory are somewhat different than in a quantitative study. In qualitative research in which a theory has been developed, the degree of the theory's fit with the data is considered the critical attribute.

- If you begin with a research question and then subsequently identify an appropriate framework, be willing to adapt or augment your original research problem as you gain greater understanding of the framework. The linking of theory and research question often requires an iterative approach.

- If you are basing your study on a specific theory or conceptual framework, be sure to read about the theory from a primary source. It is important to understand fully the conceptual perspective of the theorist. If this perspective is not congruent with your own, it may be that an alternative theory or framework would be more appropriate.

- It may also be useful to read research reports of other studies that were based on the selected framework—even if the research problem is not similar to your own. By reading other studies, you will be better able to judge how much empirical support the theory has received and perhaps how the theory should be adapted.

- Once you have identified an appropriate framework, it is important to strive for maximal congruity between the theory and its components, the research problem and hypotheses, the definition and operationalization of the concepts, and the selection of research design. If you are really testing the utility of the framework, the framework should drive many of your research decisions as well as your interpretation of the findings.

RESEARCH EXAMPLES

Throughout this chapter, we have described studies that used various widely used conceptual and theoretical models. Table 5-1 provides additional examples of nursing studies that used other, less widely used frameworks as their conceptual bases.

This section presents two examples of the linkages between theory and research from the nursing research literature—one from a quantitative study and the other from a qualitative study.

Research Example From a Quantitative Study: Testing the Health Promotion Model

Pender, Walker, Sechrist, and Frank-Stromborg (1990) used the HPM to predict health-promoting lifestyles among employees enrolled in six employer-sponsored health-promotion programs. The researchers noted that when workplace health promotion programs are initially introduced, employee enrollment tends to be high. Over time, however, erratic participation and a high dropout rate tend to characterize many such programs, a situation that concerns both the employers and the health professionals responsible for operating the programs.

Pender and her co-researchers noted that most studies of the determinants of healthy lifestyles have used a prevention-oriented model in which fear of the consequences of illness are

TABLE 5-1 Examples of Additional Theories and Models Used by Nurse Researchers	
RESEARCH QUESTION	**THEORY OR MODEL**
What is the experience of living in a nursing home? (Running, 1997)	Human Caring Theory (Watson)
What are the factors that contribute to mammography use? (Lauver, Nabholz, Scott, & Tak, 1997)	Theory of Care-Seeking Behavior (Triandis)
Do family strengths, sources of motivation, and resources positively affect health promotion processes used in families with preadolescent children? (Ford-Gilbe, 1997)	Developmental Health Model (Allen)
What is the relationship between trait anxiety and patients' evaluation of information they received during hospitalization after myocardial infarction? (Yarcheski, Proctor, & Oriscello, 1998)	Trait-State Anxiety Theory (Spielberger)
Are there any differences in self-efficacy between exercisers and non-exercisers in an elderly population? (Stidwell & Rimmer, 1995)	Self-Efficacy Theory (Bandura)
What are the behaviors of first-born children before and after the birth of a sibling? (Gullicks & Crase, 1993)	Attachment Theory (Bowlby)

viewed as the primary motivation for health-related behavior. In contrast, these researchers used a wellness-oriented framework, the HPM, in their investigation. The model tested by this team of researchers is shown in Figure 5-1. The arrows in this figure denote the hypothesized direction of causal influences. The model includes seven cognitive/perceptual factors that are hypothesized to be influenced by five modifying factors. The cognitive/perceptual factors, which are viewed as directly affecting participation in health-promoting behaviors, are considered to be amenable to change—an important feature of factors proposed as a basis for the design of interventions to promote healthy lifestyles. These seven factors are as follows:

- *Importance of health*—the value placed on health in relation to other personal values
- *Perceived control of health*—the perception of whether health is self-determined, influenced by powerful others, or the result of chance factors
- *Perceived self-efficacy*—the belief that one has the competence and skills to carry out specific actions
- *Definition of health*—the personal meaning of health to each individual
- *Perceived health status*—the self-evaluation of current health as a subjective state
- *Perceived benefits of health-promoting behavior*—the perceived desirability of behavioral outcomes
- *Perceived barriers to health-promoting behaviors*—the perceived hindrances to taking action

Pender and her colleagues tested the utility of the HPM in explaining health-promoting lifestyles among employees who had enrolled in a workplace health-promotion program (thereby suggesting an intent to change their health habits) but who varied greatly in their level of participation in the program. With a sample of nearly 600 subjects, the researchers assessed each of the cognitive/perceptual factors as well as several of the modifying factors. The dependent variable, participation in health-promoting behaviors, was measured by the Health-Promoting Lifestyle Profile, a 48-question scale focusing on such behaviors

as health responsibility, exercise, nutrition, and stress management.

The findings provided some support for the HPM model. In particular, perceptions of control of health, personal efficacy, definition of health, and health status emerged as a constellation of HPM constructs most closely associated with health-promoting lifestyle behaviors among employees enrolled in a work-site health-promotion program. Other hypothesized factors (e.g., valuing health), however, were not significant determinants of a health-promoting lifestyle.

Research Example From a Qualitative Study: Development of a Theory of Caring

As noted earlier in this chapter, many qualitative studies have theory development as an explicit goal. Here, we describe the efforts of a qualitative researcher who developed a middle-range theory of caring on the basis of three separate qualitative inquiries.

Swanson (1991) developed an empirically driven descriptive theory of caring. Using data from three separate qualitative investigations, Swanson inductively derived and then refined a theory of the caring process.

Swanson studied caring in three separate perinatal contexts: as experienced by women who miscarried, as provided by parents and professionals in the newborn intensive care unit, and as recalled by at-risk mothers who had received a long-term public health nursing intervention. Data were gathered through in-depth interviews with study participants and also through observations of care provision. Data from the first study led to the identification and preliminary definition of five caring processes. The outcome of the second study was confirmation of the five processes and refinement of their definitions. In the third study, Swanson confirmed the five processes, redefined one of them, developed subdimensions of each process, and derived a definition of the overall concept of caring: "Caring is a nurturing way of relating to a valued other toward whom one feels a personal sense of commitment and responsibility" (p. 165).

According to Swanson's theory, the five caring processes are as follows:

- Knowing—striving to understand an event as it has meaning in the life of the other
- Being With—being emotionally present to the other
- Doing For—doing for the other as he or she would do for the self if it were at all possible
- Enabling—facilitating the other's passage through life transitions and unfamiliar events
- Maintaining belief—sustaining faith in the other's capacity to get through an event or transition and face a future with meaning

In presenting her theory, Swanson described the five processes, supporting each with rich excerpts from her in-depth interviews. Here is an example of the excerpt illustrating the process of knowing:

> When things weren't right, I could say that things were fine and it was only a matter of time. I mean the nurse would ask certain questions and there would be no way that I could be consistent without telling the truth. And then we would talk, and pretty soon instead of saying it was fine, I would start out with what was really wrong. (p. 163)

Swanson noted that her theory of caring was being used in the development and testing of a caring-based nurse counseling program for women who miscarry. Her theory was also used as a conceptual framework for a qualitative study that examined the interactions of AIDS family caregivers and professional health care providers (Powell-Cope, 1994).

SUMMARY

Theories and conceptual models are the primary means of providing a conceptual context for a study. In its least restrictive definition, a **theory** is a broad and abstract characterization of some phenomenon; this definition encompasses **descriptive theory** that thoroughly describes a phenomenon. As classically defined, a theory is an abstract generalization that systematically explains the relationships among phenomena. The basic components of a theory are concepts; classically defined theories consist of a set of statements about the interrelationships among concepts, arranged in a logically interrelated system that permits new statements to be derived from them. Theories vary in their level of generality and complexity. Some theories attempt to describe large segments of the environment and are called **grand theories** or **macrotheories**, whereas other theories are more restricted in scope. Theories that are more specific to certain phenomena are sometimes referred to as **middle-range theories**.

Conceptual models (also called **conceptual frameworks** or **schemes**) are less fully developed attempts at organizing phenomena than are theories. Concepts are the basic elements of a conceptual scheme, as in theories. In a conceptual framework, however, the concepts are not linked to one another in a logically ordered deductive system. Much of the conceptual work in nursing is more rightfully described as conceptual schemes than as theories. Conceptual frameworks are highly valuable in that they often serve as the springboard for theory development.

The term **model** is often used to denote a symbolic representation of phenomena. Models depict a theory or conceptual scheme through the use of symbols or diagrams. Two types of models frequently used in research are mathematic or **statistical models** and **schematic models** (or **conceptual maps**). Models are useful to scientists because they use a minimal amount of words, which tend to be ambiguous, in representing reality.

A **framework** is the conceptual underpinnings of a study. Not every study is based on a theory or conceptual model, but every study has a framework. In many studies, the framework is implicit and not fully explicated, but ideally, the researcher makes clear what **conceptual definitions** were used for the key concepts under investigation.

The overall objective of theories and frameworks is to make scientific findings meaningful and generalizable. In addition, they help to summarize existing knowledge into coherent systems and stimulate new research by providing both direction and impetus. Theories and conceptual frameworks are created or developed by scientists. Their creation requires imagination on the part of the scientist and congruence with reality and existing knowledge. All theories and frameworks are considered tentative and are never proved.

Nursing research is increasingly drawing on conceptual frameworks and models in its efforts to integrate accumulated knowledge and advance nursing science. Many investigations are based on **borrowed theories** from other disciplines (such as the Health Belief Model), but an increasing number of studies have conceptual models of nursing as their frameworks. Among the major conceptual models of nursing are King's Open Systems Model, Levine's Conservation Model, Neuman's Health Care Systems Model, Orem's Self-Care Model, Parse's Theory of Human Becoming, Rogers's Science of Unitary Human Beings, and Roy's Adaptation Model.

The link between research and theory is a mutually beneficial one. Qualitative studies are often used to develop inductively derived theories. Some qualitative researchers specifically seek to develop **grounded theories,** data-driven explanations to account for phenomena under study. Quantitative studies are more likely to test hypotheses developed on the basis of an existing theory or conceptual model—or to test two competing theories. In other situations, a problem may be developed first and a theory selected to fit the problem. An after-the-fact selection of a theory usually is more problematic and less meaningful than the systematic testing of a particular theory.

STUDY ACTIVITIES

Chapter 5 of the *Study Guide to Accompany Nursing Research: Principles and Methods, 6th ed.,* offers various exercises and study suggestions for reinforcing the concepts presented in this chapter. Additionally, the following study questions can be addressed:

1. Read the following article: Salazar, M. K., & Carter, W. B. (1993). Evaluation of breast self-examination beliefs using a decision model. *Western Journal of Nursing Research, 15,* 403–418. What theoretical basis does the author develop for health conception and health behavior choice? Would you classify the theoretical basis as a theory or as a conceptual framework? Draw a schematic model of the major concepts used in the study.

2. Select one of the nursing conceptual frameworks or models described in this chapter. Formulate a research question and two hypotheses that could be used empirically to test the utility of the conceptual framework or model in nursing practice.

3. Four researchable problems follow. Abstract a generalized issue or issues for each of these problems. Search for an existing theory that might be applicable and appropriate.
   a. What is the relationship between angina pain and alcohol intake?
   b. What effect does rapid weight gain during the second trimester have on the outcome of pregnancy?
   c. Do multiple hospital readmissions affect the achievement level of children?
   d. To what extent do coping mechanisms of individuals differ in health and illness?

4. Read the following article: Kelly-Powell, M. L. (1997). Personalizing choices: Patients' experiences with making treatment decisions. *Research in Nursing &*

Health, 20, 219–227. What evidence does the researcher offer to substantiate that her grounded theory is a good fit with her data?

SUGGESTED READINGS

Theoretical References

Andrews, H. A., & Roy, C. (1986). *Essentials of the Roy Adaptation Model.* Norwalk, CT: Appleton-Century-Crofts.

Ajzen, I. (1988). *Attitudes, personality, and behavior.* Milton-Keynes: Open University Press.

Ajzen, I., & Fishbein, M. (1980). *Understanding attitudes and predicting social behavior.* Englewood Cliffs, NJ: Prentice-Hall.

Batey, M. V. (1977). Conceptualization: Knowledge and logic guiding empirical research. *Nursing Research, 26,* 324–329.

Becker, M. (1978). The Health Belief Model and sick role behavior. *Nursing Digest, 6,* 35–40.

Chinn, P. L., & Jacobs, M. (1994). *Theory and nursing: A systematic approach* (4th ed.). St. Louis: C. V. Mosby.

Craig, S. L. (1980). Theory development and its relevance for nursing. *Journal of Advanced Nursing, 5,* 349–355.

Fawcett, J. (1978). The relationship between theory and research: A double helix. *Advances in Nursing Science, 1,* 49–62.

Fawcett, J. (1994). *Analysis and evaluation of conceptual models of nursing* (3rd ed.). Philadelphia: F. A. Davis.

Fawcett, J., & Downs, F. (1992). *The relationship of theory and research.* (2nd ed.). Philadelphia: F. A. Davis.

Flaskerud, J. H. (1984). Nursing models as conceptual frameworks for research. *Western Journal of Nursing Research, 6,* 153–155.

Flaskerud, J. H., & Halloran, E. J. (1980). Areas of agreement in nursing theory development. *Advances in Nursing Science, 3,* 1–7.

Folkman, S., & Lazarus, R. S. (1988). Coping as a mediator of emotion. *Journal of Personality and Social Psychology, 54,* 466–475.

Hardy, M. E. (1974). Theories: Components, development, evaluation. *Nursing Research, 23,* 100–107.

Hurley, B. A. (1979). Why a theoretical framework in nursing research? *Western Journal of Nursing Research, 1,* 28–41.

King, I. M. (1981). *A theory for nursing: Systems, concepts, and process.* New York: John Wiley and Sons.

Lazarus, R. (1966). *Psychological stress and the coping response.* New York: McGraw-Hill.

Levine, M. E. (1973). *Introduction to clinical nursing* (2nd ed.). Philadelphia: F. A. Davis.

Marriner-Tomey, A. (1993). *Nursing theorists and their work* (3rd ed.). St. Louis: C. V. Mosby.

McFarlane, E. A. (1980). Nursing theory: The comparison of four theoretical proposals (King, Rogers, Roy, Orem). *Journal of Advanced Nursing, 5,* 3–19.

Mishel, M. H. (1988). Uncertainty in illness. *Image—The Journal of Nursing Scholarship, 20,* 225–232.

Morse, J. M., Solberg, S. M., Neander, W. L., Bottorff, J. L., & Johnson, J. L. (1990). Concepts of caring and caring as a concept. *Advances in Nursing Science, 13,* 1–14.

Neuman, B. (1989). *The Neuman systems model* (2nd ed.). Norwalk, CT: Appleton & Lange.

Nicoll, L. H. (1997). *Perspectives on nursing theory* (3rd ed.). Philadelphia: Lippincott-Raven.

Orem, D. E. (1985). *Concepts of practice* (3rd ed.). New York: McGraw-Hill.

Parse, R. R. (1992). Human becoming: Parse's theory. *Nursing Science Quarterly, 5,* 35–42.

Parse, R. R. (1995). *Illuminations: The human becoming theory in practice and research.* New York: NLN Pub. #15–2670.

Pender, N. (1996). *Health promotion in nursing practice* (3rd ed.). Norwalk, CT: Appleton & Lange.

Rogers, M. E. (1970). *An introduction to the theoretical basis of nursing.* Philadelphia: F. A. Davis.

Rogers, M. E. (1986). Science of unitary human beings. In V. Malinski (Ed.), *Explorations on Martha Rogers' science of unitary human beings.* Norwalk, CT: Appleton-Century-Crofts.

Roy, C. (1984). *Introduction to nursing: An adaptation model* (2nd ed.). Englewood Cliffs, NJ: Prentice-Hall.

Roy, C. Sr., & Andrews, H. (1991). *The Roy adaptation model: The definitive statement.* Norwalk, CT: Appleton & Lange.

Sandelowski, M. (1993). Theory unmasked: The uses and guises of theory in qualitative research. *Research in Nursing & Health, 16,* 213–218.

Selye, H. (1978). *The stress of life* (2nd ed.). New York: McGraw-Hill.

Stevens, B. J. (1984). *Nursing theory: Analysis, application, evaluation* (2nd ed.). Boston: Little, Brown.

Substantive References

Ailinger, R. L., & Dear, M. R. (1997). An examination of the self-care needs of clients with rheumatoid arthritis. *Rehabilitation Nursing, 22,* 135–140.

Aish, A. E., & Isenberg, M. (1996). Effects of Orem-based nursing intervention on nutritional self-care of myocardial infarction patients. *International Journal of Nursing Studies, 33,* 259–270.

Auvil-Novak, S. E. (1997). A middle-range theory of chronotherapeutic intervention for postsurgical pain. *Nursing Research, 46,* 66–71.

Baier, M. (1995). Uncertainty in illness for persons with schizophrenia. *Issues in Mental Health Nursing, 16,* 201–212.

Bernardo, M. L. (1996). Parent-reported injury associated behaviors and life events among injured, ill, and well preschool children. *Journal of Pediatric Nursing, 11,* 100–110.

Bournaki, M. (1997). Correlates of pain-related responses to venipunctures in school-aged children. *Nursing Research, 46,* 147–154.

Brooks, E. M., & Thomas, S. (1997). The perception and judgment of senior baccalaureate student nurses in clinical decision making. *Advances in Nursing Science, 19,* 50–69.

Butcher, H. K. (1996). A unitary field pattern portrait of dispiritedness in later life. *Visions: The Journal of Rogerian Nursing Science, 4,* 41–58.

Campbell, J. C. (1989). A test of two explanatory models of women's responses to battering. *Nursing Research, 38,* 18–24.

DiIorio, C. (1997). Neuroscience nurses' intentions to care for persons with HIV/AIDS. *Journal of Neuroscience Nursing, 29,* 50–55.

Felton, G. M. (1996). Female adolescent contraceptive use or nonuse at first and most recent coitus. *Public Health Nursing, 13,* 223–230.

Ford-Gilboe, M. (1997). Family strengths, motivation, and resources as predictors of health promotion behavior in single-parent and two-parent families. *Research in Nursing & Health, 20,* 205–217.

Foreman, M. D. (1989). Confusion in the hospitalized elderly: Incidence, onset, and associated factors. *Research in Nursing & Health, 12,* 21–29.

Gullicks, J. N., & Crase, S. J. (1993). Sibling behavior with a newborn. *Journal of Obstetric, Gynecologic, and Neonatal Nursing, 22,* 438–444.

Hamner, J. B. (1996). Preliminary testing of a proposition from the Roy Adaptation Model. *Image—The Journal of Nursing Scholarship, 28,* 215–220.

Hanna, K. M. (1993). Effect of nurse-client transaction on female adolescents' oral contraceptive adherence. *Image—The Journal of Nursing Scholarship, 25,* 285–290.

Hanson, M. J. S. (1997). The theory of planned behavior applied to cigarette smoking in African-American, Puerto Rican, and non-Hispanic white teenage females. *Nursing Research, 46,* 155–162.

Hardin, S. B., Carbaugh, L., Weinrich, S., Pesut, D., & Carbaugh, C. (1992). Stressors and coping in adolescents exposed to Hurricane Hugo. *Issues in Mental Health Nursing, 13,* 191–205.

Henneman, E. A. (1989). Effect of nursing contact on the stress response of patients being weaned from mechanical ventilation. *Heart & Lung, 18,* 483–489.

Hoeman, S. P., Ku, Y. L., & Ohl, D. R. (1996). Health beliefs and early detection among Chinese women. *Western Journal of Nursing Research, 18,* 518–533.

Janes, N. M., Wells, D. L., & Daly, J. (1997). Elderly patients' experiences with nurses guided by Parse's theory of human becoming. *Clinical Nursing Research, 6,* 205–224.

Janson-Bjerklie, S., Ferketich, S., & Benner, P. (1993). Predicting the outcomes of living with asthma. *Research in Nursing & Health, 16,* 241–250.

Laschinger, H. K. S., & Goldenberg, D. (1993). Attitudes of practicing nurses as predictors of intended care behavior with persons who are HIV positive. *Research in Nursing & Health, 16,* 441–450.

Lauver, D., Nobholz, S., Scott, K., & Tak, Y. (1997). Testing theoretical explanations of mammography use. *Nursing Research, 46,* 32–39.

Lemaire, G. S., & Lenz, E. R. (1995). Perceived uncertainty about menopause in women attending an educational program. *International Journal of Nursing Studies, 32,* 39–48.

Lowry, L. A., & Anderson, B. (1993). Neuman's framework and ventilator dependency. *Nursing Science Quarterly, 6,* 195–200.

Lusk, S. L., Ronis, D. L., & Hogan, M. M. (1997). Test of the Health Promotion Model as a causal model of construction workers' use of hearing protection. *Research in Nursing & Health, 20,* 183–194.

Manderino, M. A., & Berkey, N. (1997). Verbal abuse of staff nurses by physicians. *Journal of Professional Nursing, 13,* 46–55.

Mahon, S. M., & Casperson, D. M. (1997). Exploring the psychosocial meaning of recurrent cancer. *Cancer Nursing, 20,* 178–186.

Nash, R., Edwards, H., & Nebauer, M. (1993). Effect of attitudes, subjective norms, and perceived control on nurses' intention to assess patients' pain. *Journal of Advanced Nursing, 18,* 941–947.

Neuberger, G. B., Kasal, S., Smith, K. V., Hassanein, R., & DeViney, S. (1994). Determinants of exercise and aerobic fitness in outpatients with arthritis. *Nursing Research, 43,* 11–17.

Page, C., & Ricard, N. (1996). Conceptual and theoretical foundations for an instrument designed to identify self-care requisites in women treated for depression. *Canadian Journal of Nursing Research, 28,* 95–112.

Parse, R. R. (1997). Joy-sorrow: A study using the Parse research method. *Nursing Science Quarterly, 10,* 80–87.

Pender, N. J., Walker, S. N., Sechrist, K. R., & Frank-Stromborg, M. (1990). Predicting health-promoting lifestyles in the workplace. *Nursing Research, 39,* 326–332.

Powell-Cope, G. M. (1994). Family caregivers of people with AIDS: Negotiating partnerships with professional health care providers. *Nursing Research, 43,* 324–330.

Rose, M. A. (1996). Effect of an AIDS education program for elder adults. *Journal of Community Health Nursing, 13,* 141–148.

Ross, M. M., & Bourbonnais, F. F. (1985). The Betty Neuman Systems Model in nursing practice: A case study approach. *Journal of Advanced Nursing, 10,* 199–207.

Running, A. (1997). Snapshots of experience: Vignettes from a nursing home. *Journal of Advanced Nursing, 25,* 117–122.

Samarel, N., Fawcett, J., & Tulman, L. (1997). Effect of support groups with coaching on adaptation to early stage breast cancer. *Research in Nursing & Health, 20,* 15–26.

Schaefer, K. M., & Potylycki, M. J. S. (1993). Fatigue associated with congestive heart failure: Use of Levine's Conservational Model. *Journal of Advanced Nursing, 18,* 260–268.

Sharts-Hopko, N. C., Regan-Kubinski, M. J. R., Lincoln, P. S., & Heverly, M. A. (1996). Problem-focused coping in HIV-infected mothers in relation to self-efficacy, uncertainty, social support, and psychological distress. *Image—The Journal of Nursing Scholarship, 28,* 107–111.

Sherman, D. W. (1996). Nurses' willingness to care for AIDS patients and spirituality, social support, and death anxiety. *Image—The Journal of Nursing Scholarship, 28,* 205–213.

Staples, P., & Jeffrey, J. (1997). Quality of life, hope, and uncertainty of cardiac patients and their spouses before coronary artery bypass surgery. *Canadian Journal of Cardiovascular Nursing, 8,* 7–16.

Stidwell, H. F., & Rimmer, J. H. (1995). Measurement of physical self-efficacy in an elderly population. *Clinical Kinesiology, 49,* 58–63.

Swanson, K. M. (1991). Empirical development of a middle range theory of caring. *Nursing Research, 40,* 161–166.

Tomlinson, P. S., Kirschbaum, M., Harbaugh, B., & Anderson, K. H. (1996). The influence of illness severity and family resources on maternal uncertainty during critical pediatric hospitalization. *American Journal of Critical Care, 5,* 140–146.

Wambach, K. A. (1997). Breastfeeding intention and outcome. *Research in Nursing & Health, 20,* 51–59.

Yarcheski, A., Mahon, N. E., & Yarcheski, T. J. (1997). Alternate models of positive health practices in adolescents. *Nursing Research, 46,* 85–92.

Yarcheski, A., Proctor, T. F., & Oriscello, R. G. (1998). Moderators of the relationship between trait anxiety and information received by patients post-myocardial infarction. *Clinical Nursing Research, 7,* 29–46.

Zimmerman, B. W., Brown, S. T., & Bowman, J. M. (1996). A self-management program for chronic obstructive pulmonary disease. *Rehabilitation Nursing, 21,* 253–257.

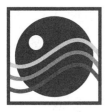

CHAPTER **6**

The Ethical Context of Nursing Research

Nurses continually face ethical issues in their practice; the prolongation of life by artificial means, the institution of tube feedings when patients are unable to sustain oral nourishment, and the testing of new products to monitor care are but a few examples. Situations such as these have led to an increasing number of discussions and debates concerning ethical issues in the delivery of nursing care.

The proliferation of research involving humans has led to similar ethical concerns and debates regarding the protection of the rights of people who participate in nursing research. Ethical concerns are especially prominent in the field of nursing because the line of demarcation between what constitutes the expected practice of nursing and the collection of research information has become less distinct as research by nurses increases. Furthermore, ethics poses particular problems to nurse researchers in some situations because ethical requirements sometimes conflict with methodologic considerations. This chapter discusses the major ethical principles that should be considered in designing research studies.

THE NEED FOR ETHICAL GUIDELINES

When humans are used as study participants in research investigations—as they usually are in nursing research—care must be exercised in ensuring that the rights of those humans are protected. The requirement for ethical conduct may strike you as so self-evident as to require no further comment, but the fact is that ethical considerations have not always been given adequate attention. In this section, we consider some of the reasons that the development of ethical guidelines became imperative.

Historical Background

As modern, civilized humans, we might like to think that systematic violations of moral principles among scientists occurred centuries ago rather than in recent times, but this is not the case. The Nazi medical experiments of the 1930s and 1940s are the most famous example of recent disregard for ethical conduct. The Nazi program of research involved the use of prisoners of war and racial "enemies" in numerous experiments designed to test the limits of human endurance and human reaction to diseases and untested drugs. The studies were unethical not only because they exposed the participants to permanent physical harm and even death but also because the subjects were not given an opportunity to refuse participation.

Some recent examples of ethical transgressions have also occurred in the United States. For instance, between 1932 and 1972, a study known as the Tuskegee Syphilis Study, sponsored by the U.S. Public Health Service, investigated the effects of syphilis among 400 men from a poor black community. Medical treatment was deliberately withheld to study the course of the untreated disease. Another well-known case of unethical research involved the injection of live cancer cells into elderly patients at the Jewish Chronic Disease Hospital in Brooklyn, without the consent of those patients. Even more recently, it was revealed in 1993 that U.S. federal agencies, such as the Atomic Energy Commission, have sponsored radiation experiments since the 1940s on hundreds of people, many of them prisoners or elderly hospital patients. Many other examples of studies with ethical transgressions—often much more subtle than these examples—have emerged to give ethical concerns the high visibility they have today.

Ethical Dilemmas in Conducting Research

Research that violates ethical principles is rarely done specifically to be cruel or immoral, but more typically occurs out of a conviction that knowledge is important and potentially life-saving or beneficial (usually to others) in the long run. There are, unfortunately, research problems in which the rights of participants and the demands of the study are put in direct conflict, resulting in **ethical dilemmas** for the researcher. Here are some examples of situations in which the researcher's need for rigor can be compromised by ethical considerations:

1. *Research question:* How empathic are nurses in their treatment of patients in intensive care units?

   Ethical dilemma: To address this question, the researcher would likely want to observe nurses' behavior while treating patients. Ethical research generally involves explaining the study to participants and obtaining their consent to participate in the study. Yet if the researcher in this example informs the participating nurses that their treatment of patients will be observed, will their behavior be "normal"? If the nurses' behavior is altered because of their awareness of being observed, the entire value of the study could be undermined.

2. *Research question:* What are the feelings and coping mechanisms of parents whose children have a terminal illness?

   Ethical dilemma: To answer this question fully, the researcher may need to probe intrusively into the psychological state of the parents at a highly vulnerable time in their lives; such probing could be painful and even traumatic. Yet knowledge of the parents' coping mechanisms could help to design more effective ways of dealing with parents' grief and anger.

3. *Research question:* Does a new medication prolong life in cancer patients?

   Ethical dilemma: The best way to test the effectiveness of interventions is to administer the intervention to some people but withhold it from others to see if differences between the groups emerge. If the intervention is untested (e.g., a new drug), however, the group receiving the intervention may be exposed to potentially hazardous side effects. On the other hand, the group not receiving the drug may be denied a beneficial treatment.

4. *Research question:* What is the process by which adult children adapt to the day-to-day stresses of caring for a terminally ill parent?

   Ethical dilemma: In a qualitative study, which would be appropriate for this research question, the researcher might become so closely involved with the study participants that they become willing to share "secrets" and privileged information, as they would with a friend. Interviews can become confessions—sometimes of unseemly or even illegal or immoral behavior. In this example, suppose a participant admitted to physically abusing their terminally ill parent—how does the researcher handle that information without undermining a pledge of confidentiality? And, if the researcher divulges the information, how can a pledge of confidentiality be given in good faith to other participants?

As these examples suggest, researchers involved with human participants are sometimes in a bind; they are obligated to advance knowledge, using the best methods available, but they must also adhere to the dictates of ethical rules that have been developed to protect human rights. Another type of dilemma arises from the fact that nurse researchers may be confronted with conflict-of-interest situations, in which their expected behavior as nurses comes into conflict with the expected behavior of researchers (e.g., deviating from a standard research protocol to give needed assistance to a patient). It is precisely because of such conflicts and dilemmas that **codes of**

ethics have been developed to guide the efforts of researchers.

Codes of Ethics

During the past four decades, largely in response to the human rights violations described earlier, various codes of ethics have been developed. One of the first internationally recognized efforts to establish ethical standards is referred to as the **Nuremberg Code,** developed after the Nazi atrocities were made public in the Nuremberg trials. Several other international standards have subsequently been developed, the most notable of which is the **Declaration of Helsinki,** which was adopted in 1964 by the World Medical Assembly and then later revised in 1975.

Most disciplines have established their own code of ethics. The American Nurses' Association (1975) put forth a document entitled *Human Rights Guidelines for Nurses in Clinical and Other Research.* The American Sociological Association published its *Code of Ethics* in 1984. Guidelines for psychologists were published by the American Psychological Association (1982) in *Ethical Principles in the Conduct of Research With Human Participants.* Although there is considerable overlap in the basic principles articulated in these documents, each deals with problems of particular concern to their respective disciplines.

An especially important code of ethics was adopted by the National Commission for the Protection of Human Subjects of Biomedical and Behavioral Research (1978). The commission, established by the National Research Act (Public Law 93–348), issued a report in 1978 that served as the basis for regulations affecting research sponsored by the federal government. The report, sometimes referred to as the *Belmont Report,* also served as a model for many of the guidelines adopted by specific disciplines. The *Belmont Report* articulated three primary ethical principles on which standards of ethical conduct in research are based: beneficence, respect for human dignity, and justice.

THE PRINCIPLE OF BENEFICENCE

One of the most fundamental ethical principles in research is that of **beneficence**, which encompasses the maxim: Above all, do no harm. Most researchers consider that this principle contains multiple dimensions.

Freedom From Harm

Exposing research participants to experiences that result in serious or permanent harm is unacceptable. Research should be conducted only by qualified people, especially if potentially dangerous technical equipment or specialized procedures are used. The researcher must be prepared at any time during the study to terminate the research if there is reason to suspect that continuation would result in injury, disability, undue distress, or death to study participants. When a new medical procedure or drug is being tested, it is almost always advisable to experiment with animals or tissue cultures before proceeding to tests with humans. (Ethical guidelines relating to the treatment of animal subjects should be consulted for research on animals; see, for example, Thomas, Hamm, Perkins, & Raffin, 1988).

Although protecting human beings from physical harm is in many cases straightforward, some psychological consequences of participating in a study may be subtle and thus require closer attention and sensitivity. Sometimes, for example, people are asked questions about their personal views, weaknesses, or fears. Such queries might require individuals to admit to aspects of themselves that they dislike and would perhaps rather forget. The point is not that the researcher should refrain from asking any questions but, rather, that it is nec-essary to think carefully about the nature of the intrusion on people's psyches. Researchers strive to avoid inflicting psychological harm by carefully considering the phrasing of questions, by having **debriefing** sessions that permit participants to ask questions after their participation, and by providing participants with written information on how they may later contact the researchers.

The need for sensitivity on the part of the researcher may be heightened in qualitative studies, which often involve in-depth exploration into highly personal areas. In-depth probing may actually expose deep-seated fears and anxieties that the study participants had previously repressed. Qualitative researchers must thus be especially vigilant in anticipating such problems.

Freedom From Exploitation

Involvement in a research study should not place people at a disadvantage or expose them to situations for which they have not been explicitly prepared. Participants need to be assured that their participation, or the information they might provide to the researcher, will not be used against them in any way. For example, a woman describing her economic circumstances to a researcher should not be exposed to the risk of losing Medicaid benefits; the person reporting drug abuse should not fear exposure to criminal authorities.

The study participant enters into a special relationship with the researcher, and it is critical that this relationship not be exploited in any way. Exploitation may be overt and malicious (e.g., sexual exploitation, use of subjects' identifying information to create a mailing list, and use of donated blood for the development of a commercial product), but it is more likely to be inadvertent. For example, people may agree to participate in a study requiring 30 minutes of their time. The researcher may then decide 1 year later to go back and talk to the participants to follow their progress or circumstances. Unless the researcher had previously explained to the participants that there might be a follow-up study, the researcher might be accused of not adhering to the agreement previously reached and of exploiting the researcher–participant relationship.

Because nurse researchers may have a nurse–patient (in addition to a researcher–participant) relationship, special care may need to be exercised to avoid exploitation of people's vulnerabilities. Researchers should be cognizant of the fact that patients' consent to participate in a study may result from their understanding of the researcher's role as *nurse* not as *researcher*.

In qualitative research, the risk of exploitation may become especially acute because the psychological distance between the investigator and the study participant typically diminishes dramatically as the study progresses. The emergence of a pseudotherapeutic relationship between the researcher and participant is not uncommon, and this imposes additional responsibilities on the researcher—and additional risks that exploitation could inadvertently occur. On the other hand, qualitative researchers are typically in a better position than quantitative researchers to *do good*, rather than just to avoid doing any harm, because of the close relationships they often develop with participants. Munhall (1988) has argued that qualitative nurse researchers have the responsibility of ensuring that the "therapeutic imperative of nursing (advocacy) takes precedent over the research imperative (advancing knowledge) if conflict develops" (p. 151).

Benefits From Research

People agree to participate in research investigations for a number of reasons. They may perceive that there are some direct personal benefits. More often, however, any benefits from the research accrue to society in general or to other individuals. Thus, many individuals may participate in a study out of a desire to be helpful. The researcher should strive insofar as possible to maximize benefits and to communicate candidly the potential risks and benefits to study participants.

The Risk/Benefit Ratio

In deciding to conduct a study, the researcher must carefully assess the risks and benefits that would be incurred. The assessment should weigh the risks and benefits that individual participants might experience, and the assessment should be shared with them so that they can evaluate whether it is in their best interest to participate. Box 6-1 summarizes some of the more salient benefits and costs to which research participants might be exposed. In evaluating the anticipated **risk/benefit ratio**, the researcher might want to consider how comfortable he or she would feel if it were family members participating in the study.

The risk/benefit ratio should also be considered in terms of whether the risks to participants are commensurate with the benefit to society and the nursing profession in terms of the knowledge produced. The general guideline is that the degree of risk to be taken by those participating in the research should never exceed the potential humanitarian benefits of the knowledge to be gained. Thus, the selection of a significant topic that has the potential to improve patient care is the first step in ensuring that research is ethical.

All research involves some risks, but in many cases, the risk is minimal. **Minimal risk,** according to federal guidelines, is defined as anticipated risks that are no greater than those ordinarily encountered in daily life or during the performance of routine physical or psychological tests or procedures. When the risks are not minimal, the researcher must proceed with great caution, taking every step possible to reduce risks and maximize benefits. If the perceived risks and costs to participants outweigh the anticipated benefits of the research,

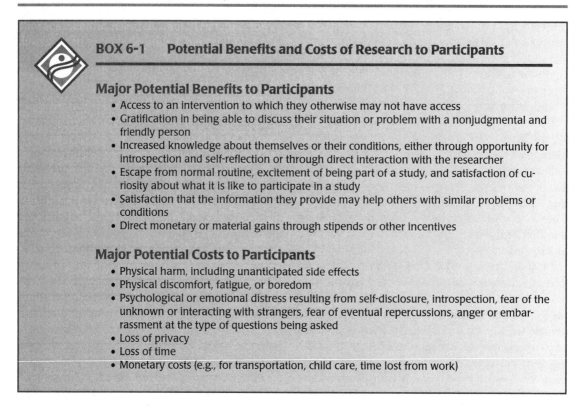

BOX 6-1   Potential Benefits and Costs of Research to Participants

Major Potential Benefits to Participants

- Access to an intervention to which they otherwise may not have access
- Gratification in being able to discuss their situation or problem with a nonjudgmental and friendly person
- Increased knowledge about themselves or their conditions, either through opportunity for introspection and self-reflection or through direct interaction with the researcher
- Escape from normal routine, excitement of being part of a study, and satisfaction of curiosity about what it is like to participate in a study
- Satisfaction that the information they provide may help others with similar problems or conditions
- Direct monetary or material gains through stipends or other incentives

Major Potential Costs to Participants

- Physical harm, including unanticipated side effects
- Physical discomfort, fatigue, or boredom
- Psychological or emotional distress resulting from self-disclosure, introspection, fear of the unknown or interacting with strangers, fear of eventual repercussions, anger or embarrassment at the type of questions being asked
- Loss of privacy
- Loss of time
- Monetary costs (e.g., for transportation, child care, time lost from work)

the research should be either abandoned or redesigned.

In quantitative studies, most of the details of the study are usually spelled out in advance, and therefore a reasonably accurate risk/benefit ratio assessment can be developed. Qualitative studies, however, are often less structured and are likely to evolve as data are gathered, and it may therefore be more difficult to assess all risks at the outset of a study. Qualitative researchers thus must remain sensitive to potential risks throughout the research process.

THE PRINCIPLE OF RESPECT FOR HUMAN DIGNITY

Respect for human dignity is the second ethical principle articulated in the *Belmont Report*. This principle includes the right to self-determination and the right to full disclosure.

The Right to Self-Determination

Humans should be treated as autonomous agents, capable of controlling their own activities and destinies. The principle of **self-determination** means that prospective participants have the right to decide voluntarily whether to participate in a study, without the risk of incurring any penalties or prejudicial treatment. It also means that people have the right to decide at any point to terminate their participation, to refuse to give information, or to ask for clarification about the purpose of the study or specific study procedures.

A person's right to self-determination includes freedom from coercion of any type. **Coercion** involves explicit or implicit threats of penalty from failing to participate in a study or excessive rewards from agreeing to participate. The obligation to honor and protect individuals from coercion may require careful thought when the researcher is in a position of authority, control, or influence over potential participants, as might often be the case in a nurse–patient relationship. The ideal of noncoercion may also need to be considered even when there is not a preestablished relationship. For example, a monetary incentive offered to an economically disadvantaged group—such as the homeless—might be considered mildly coercive; its acceptability might have to be evaluated in terms of the risk/benefit ratio. That is, if risks are high relative to any benefits and the participants are poor, monetary incentives (sometimes referred to as **stipends**) may place undue pressure on prospective participants.

The Right to Full Disclosure

The principle of respect for human dignity encompasses people's right to make informed voluntary decisions about their participation in a study. Such decisions cannot be made without full disclosure. **Full disclosure** means that the researcher has fully described the nature of the study, the participant's right to refuse participation, the researcher's responsibilities, and the likely risks and benefits that would be incurred. The right to self-determination and the right to full disclosure are the two major elements on which informed consent is based. Procedures for obtaining informed consent from study participants are discussed in a later section of this chapter.

Although full disclosure is normally provided to participants before they begin a study, there is often a need for further disclosure at a later point, either in debriefing sessions or in written communications. For example, issues that arise during the course of data collection may need to be clarified, or the participant may want aspects of the study explained once again. Many investigators also offer to send participants summaries of the research findings after the information has been analyzed. In qualitative studies, the consent process may require an ongoing negotiation between the re-

searcher and the participants, as we discuss in a subsequent section.

Issues Relating to the Principle of Respect

Although almost all researchers would, in the abstract, endorse participants' right to self-determination and full disclosure, there are circumstances that make these standards difficult to adhere to in practice. One issue concerns the inability of certain individuals to make well-informed judgments about the costs and benefits associated with participation. Children, for example, may be unable to give truly informed consent. The issue of groups that are vulnerable within a research context is discussed in a subsequent section of this chapter.

Other circumstances occur in which the researcher may feel that the right to full disclosure and self-determination must be violated for the research to yield meaningful information. Researchers concerned with the validity of the study findings are sometimes worried that full disclosure might result in two types of biases: (1) the bias resulting from subjects giving inaccurate information, and (2) the bias resulting from failure to recruit a good sample.

Let us suppose that a researcher is studying the relationship between high school students' substance abuse and their absenteeism from school. That is, the researcher wants to know if students with a high rate of absenteeism are, as a group, more likely to be substance abusers than students with a good attendance record. If the researcher approached potential participants and fully explained the purpose of the study, some students might refuse to participate. The problem is that nonparticipation would be highly selective; one would expect, in fact, that those least likely to volunteer for such a study would be students who are substance abusers—the very group of primary interest in the research. Moreover, by knowing the specific research question, those who do volunteer to participate might be less inclined to give candid responses. The researcher in such a situation might argue that full disclosure would totally undermine his or her ability to conduct the study productively.

Researchers who feel that full disclosure is incompatible with the aims of their research sometimes use two techniques. The first is **covert data collection** or **concealment,** which means the collection of information without the participants' knowledge and, thus, without their consent. This might happen, for example, if a researcher wanted to observe naturalistic behavior in a real-world setting and was concerned that doing so openly would result in changes in the behavior of interest. In such a situation, the researcher might obtain the information through concealed methods, such as by audiotaping or videotaping participants through hidden equipment, observing through a one-way mirror, or observing while pretending to be engaged in other activities. As another example of covert data collection, hospital patients might unwittingly become participants in a study through the researcher's use of existing hospital records. In general, covert data collection may be acceptable as long as the risks are negligible and the participants' right to privacy has not been violated. Covert data collection is least likely to be ethically acceptable if the research is focused on sensitive aspects of people's behavior, such as drug use, sexual conduct, or illegal acts.

The second, and more controversial, technique is the researcher's use of **deception.** Deception can involve either withholding information about the study or providing participants with false information. For example, the researcher studying high school students' use of drugs might describe the research as a study of students' health practices, which is a mild form of misinformation.

The practice of deception is problematic from an ethical standpoint because it interferes with the participants' right to make a truly informed decision regarding the personal costs and benefits of participation. Some people argue that the use of deception is never justified. Others, however, believe that if the study involves minimal risk to subjects and if there are anticipated benefits to the profession and society, then deception may be justified to enhance the validity of the findings. The American Psychological Association's (1982) code of ethics offers the following guideline regarding the use of deception and concealment:

> Methodologic requirements of a study may make the use of concealment or deception necessary. Before conducting such a study, the investigator has a special responsibility to 1) determine whether the use of such techniques is justified by the study's prospective scientific, education, or applied value; 2) determine whether alternative procedures are available that do not use concealment or deception; and 3) ensure that the participants are provided with sufficient explanation as soon as possible. (pp. 35–36)

THE PRINCIPLE OF JUSTICE

The third broad principle articulated in the *Belmont Report* concerns justice. This principle includes the participants' right to fair treatment and their right to privacy.

The Right to Fair Treatment

Study participants have the right to fair and equitable treatment both before, during, and after their participation in the study. Fair treatment includes the following features:

- The fair and nondiscriminatory selection of participants such that any risks and benefits will be equitably shared; participant selection should be based on research requirements and not on the convenience, gullibility, or compromised (or favored) position of certain types of people
- The nonprejudicial treatment of individuals who decline to participate or who withdraw from the study after agreeing to participate
- The honoring of all agreements made between the researcher and the participant,

including adherence to the procedures outlined in advance and the payment of any promised stipends

- Participants' access to research personnel at any point in the study to clarify information
- Participants' access to appropriate professional assistance if there is any physical or psychological damage
- Debriefing, if necessary, to divulge information that was withheld before the study or to clarify issues that arose during the study
- Respectful and courteous treatment at all times

The Right to Privacy

Virtually all research with humans constitutes some type of intrusion into the people's personal lives. Researchers need to ensure that their research is not more intrusive than it needs to be and that the participants' privacy is maintained throughout the study.

Study participants have the right to expect that any information collected during the course of a study will be kept in strictest confidence. This can occur either through anonymity or through other confidentiality procedures. **Anonymity** occurs when even the researcher cannot link a participant with the information for that person. For example, if questionnaires were distributed to a group of nursing home residents and were returned without any identifying information on them, the responses would be considered anonymous. As another example, if a researcher reviewed hospital records from which all identifying information (e.g., name, address, social security number, and so forth) had been expunged, anonymity would again protect the participants' right to privacy. Whenever it is possible to achieve anonymity, the researcher should strive to do so.

In situations in which anonymity is impossible, appropriate **confidentiality procedures** need to be implemented. A promise of confidentiality to participants is a pledge that any

information that the participant provides will not be publicly reported in a manner that identifies the participant or made accessible to parties other than those involved in the research. This means that research information should not be shared with strangers nor with people known to the participants, such as family members, counselors, physicians, and other nurses, unless the researcher has been given explicit permission to share the information.

Researchers can take a number of steps to safeguard the confidentiality of participants, including the following:

- Obtain identifying information (e.g., name, address) from participants only when it is essential to do so.
- Assign an identification (ID) number to each participant and attach the ID number rather than other identifiers to the actual research information.
- Maintain any identifying information and lists of ID numbers with corresponding identifying information in a locked file.
- Restrict access to identifying information to a small number of individuals on a need-to-know basis.
- Enter no identifying information onto computer files.
- Destroy identifying information as quickly as is feasible.
- Have all research personnel who have contact with the research information or identifiers sign pledges of confidentiality.
- Report research information in the aggregate; if information for a specific participant is reported, take steps to disguise the person's identity, such as through the use of a fictitious name together with sparing use of descriptors of the individual.

Qualitative researchers sometimes find that extra precautions are needed to safeguard the privacy of their research participants. Anonymity is almost never possible in qualitative research because the researcher typically is interjected deeply into the lives of those being studied. Moreover, because of the in-depth nature of many qualitative studies, there may be a greater invasion of privacy than is true in quantitative research. Researchers who spend time in the home of a study participant, for example, may have difficulty segregating the public behaviors that the study participant is willing to share from the private behaviors that unfold unwittingly during the course of data collection. A final thorny issue that many qualitative researchers face is adequately disguising study participants in their research reports. Because the number of respondents is typically small and because rich descriptive information is typically obtained, it is sometimes difficult to protect the identities of the participants adequately.

INFORMED CONSENT

Prospective participants who are fully informed about the nature of the research and potential costs and benefits to be incurred are in a position to make thoughtful decisions regarding participation in the study. **Informed consent** means that participants have adequate information regarding the research, are capable of comprehending the information, and have the power of free choice, enabling them to consent to or decline participation in the research voluntarily. This section discusses procedures for obtaining informed consent.

The Content of Informed Consent

Fully informed consent involves the disclosure of the following pieces of information to participants:

1. *Participant status.* Prospective participants should be informed that any data they provide will be used in a study. Patients should be told which health care activities are routine and which are implemented specifically for the purposes of the research.

2. *Study purpose.* The overall purpose of conducting the research should be stated, preferably in lay rather than technical terms. The use to which the research information will be put should also be described.

3. *Type of data.* Prospective participants should be told the type of data that will be collected from them during the course of the study.

4. *Nature of the commitment.* Information regarding the duration of the study should be provided, together with an estimated time commitment at each point of contact.

5. *Sponsorship.* Information on who is sponsoring or funding the study should be mentioned; if the research is a course or degree requirement, this information should be shared.

6. *Participant selection.* The researcher should explain how the prospective participants came to be selected for recruitment into the study; the explanation may also indicate how many people will be participating in the study.

7. *Procedures.* Prospective participants should be given a description of the procedures that will be used to collect the data and of the procedures involved in any special or experimental treatment.

8. *Potential risks or costs.* Prospective participants should be informed of any potential foreseeable risks (physical, psychological, or economic) or costs that might be incurred as a result of participation. The possibility of unforeseeable risks should also be discussed, if appropriate. If injury or damage is possible, treatments that will be made available to participants should be described.

9. *Potential benefits.* Specific benefits to participants, if any, should be described, together with information on possible benefits to others. If participant stipends are to be paid, they should be discussed.

10. *Confidentiality pledge.* Prospective participants should be assured that their privacy will at all times be protected.
11. *Voluntary consent.* The researcher should clearly indicate that participation is strictly voluntary and that failure to comply will not result in any penalties or loss of benefits.
12. *Right to withdraw.* Prospective participants should be informed that even after consenting to cooperate they will have the right to withdraw from the study and to refuse to provide any specific piece of information. Additionally, researchers may, in some cases, need to provide participants with a description of circumstances under which the researcher will terminate their participation or the overall study.
13. *Alternatives.* If appropriate, the researcher should provide information regarding alternative procedures or treatments, if any, that might be advantageous to participants.
14. *Contact information.* The researcher should provide information on whom the participants could contact in the event of further questions, comments, or complaints relating to the research.

In some qualitative studies, especially those requiring repeated contact with the same participants, it is difficult to obtain a meaningful informed consent at the outset. A qualitative researcher does not always know in advance how the study will evolve. For example, because the research design emerges during the data collection and analysis process, the researcher may not know the exact nature of the data to be collected, what the risks and benefits to participants will be, nor how much of a time commitment they will be expected to make. Thus, in a qualitative study, consent is often viewed as an ongoing, transactional process, referred to as **process consent**. In process consent, the researcher continually renegotiates the consent, allowing participants to play a collaborative role in the decision-making process regarding their ongoing participation.

Comprehension of Informed Consent

The information just described is normally presented to prospective participants orally while they are being recruited to participate in a study. As discussed in the next section, researchers often present this information to prospective participants in writing as well. A written form, however, should not take the place of an oral explanation of critical information about the study (unless the study does not involve face-to-face contact with participants). Oral presentations provide opportunities for greater elaboration and for participant questioning. Because informed consent is based on a person's evaluation of the potential costs and benefits of participation, it is important that the critical information be not only communicated but also understood.

Researchers preparing statements for prospective participants should be careful to use simple language, avoiding jargon and technical terms whenever possible. Written statements should be consistent with the participants' reading levels and educational attainment. For participants from a general population (e.g., patients in a hospital), the statement should be written at about the seventh- or eighth-grade reading level.

For studies involving more than minimal risk, researchers need to make special efforts to ensure that prospective participants understand what participation in the research will involve. In some cases, this might involve testing the participants for their comprehension of the informed consent material before deeming them eligible for participation.

Documentation of Informed Consent

Researchers usually document the informed consent process by having participants sign a

consent form. Federal regulations covering studies conducted under the sponsorship of government agencies require written consent, except under two circumstances: (1) when the consent document would be the only record linking the participant and the research information, and participants agree that documentation can be foregone in the interest of protecting their privacy; or (2) when the study involves minimal risk and involves no procedures for which written consent would normally be needed. For example, for studies involving the completion of a questionnaire,

informed consent documentation is normally optional.

The consent form should contain all the information essential to informed consent, as described earlier. An example of a written consent form is presented in Figure 6-1. The prospective participant should have ample time to review the written document before signing it. The document should also be signed by the researcher, and a copy should be retained by both parties.

If the informed consent information is lengthy, government regulations give re-

---

In signing this document, I am giving my consent to be interviewed by an employee of Humanalysis, Inc., a nonprofit research organization based in Saratoga Springs, New York. I understand that I will be part of a research study that will focus on the experiences and needs of mothers of young children in the United States. This study, supported by a grant from the U.S. Department of Health and Human Services, will provide some guidance to people who are trying to help mothers and their children.

I understand that I will be interviewed in my home at a time convenient to me. I will be asked some questions about my experiences as a parent, my feelings about how to raise children, the health and characteristics of my oldest child, and my use of community services. I also understand that the interviewer will ask to have my oldest child present during at least some portion of the interview. The interview will take about $1\frac{1}{2}$ to 2 hours to complete. I also understand that the researcher may contact me for more information in the future.

I understand that I was selected to participate in this study because I was involved in a study of young mothers at the time of my oldest child's birth. At that time, I was recruited into the study, along with about 500 other young mothers, through a hospital or service agency.

This interview was granted freely. I have been informed that the interview is entirely voluntary, and that even after the interview begins I can refuse to answer any specific questions or decide to terminate the interview at any point. I have been told that my answers to questions will not be given to anyone else and no reports of this study will ever identify me in any way. I have also been informed that my participation or nonparticipation or my refusal to answer questions will have no effect on services that I or any member of my family may receive from health or social services providers.

This study will help develop a better understanding of the experiences of young mothers and the services that can be most helpful to them and their children. However, I will receive no direct benefit as a result of participation. As a means of compensating for any fatigue, inconvenience, or monetary costs associated with participating in this study, I have received $25 for granting this interview.

I understand that the results of this research will be given to me if I ask for them and that Dr. Denise Polit is the person to contact if I have any questions about the study or about my rights as a study participant. Dr. Polit can be reached through a collect call at (518) 587-3994.

_____   _____
Date   Respondent's Signature

                                          _____
                                          Interviewer's Signature

Figure 6-1. Sample consent form.

searchers whose studies are funded by federal agencies the option of presenting the full information orally and then summarizing essential information in a **short form**. If a short form is used, however, the oral presentation must be witnessed by a third party, and the signature of the witness must appear on the short consent form. The signature of a third-party witness is also advisable in studies involving more than minimal risk, even when a long and comprehensive consent form is used.

⬛ VULNERABLE SUBJECTS

Adherence to ethical standards such as those discussed thus far is, in most cases, straightforward. However, the rights of special vulnerable groups may need to be protected through additional procedures and heightened sensitivity on the part of the researcher. **Vulnerable subjects** (the term used in federal guidelines) may be incapable of giving fully informed consent (e.g., mentally retarded people) or may be at high risk of unintended side effects because of their circumstances (e.g., pregnant women). Researchers interested in studying high-risk groups should become acquainted with laws and guidelines governing informed consent, risk/benefit ratio assessments, and acceptable procedures for research involving the group of interest. In general, research with vulnerable groups should be undertaken only when the researcher has determined that the risk/benefit ratio is low or when there is no alternative (e.g., studies of childhood development require child participants).

Among the groups that nurse researchers should consider as being especially vulnerable are the following:

- *Children*. Legally and ethically, children do not have the competence to give their informed consent. Generally, the informed consent of children's parents or legal guardians should be obtained. If the child is developmentally mature enough to understand the basic information involved in informed consent (e.g., a 13-year-old), it is advisable to obtain written consent from the child as well, as evidence of respect for the child's right to self-determination.
- *Mentally or emotionally disabled people*. Individuals whose disability makes it impossible for them to weigh the risks and benefits of participation and make an informed decision (e.g., people affected by mental retardation, senility, mental illness, unconsciousness, and so on) also cannot legally or ethically be expected to provide informed consent. In such cases, the researcher should obtain the written consent of each person's legal guardian. However, the researcher should be sensitive to the fact that the legal guardian may not necessarily have the person's best interests in mind. In such cases, informed consent should also be obtained from a person whose primary interest is the person's welfare. As in the case of children, informed consent from prospective participants themselves should be sought to the extent possible in addition to consent from their guardians.
- *Physically disabled people*. For certain physical disabilities, special procedures for obtaining consent may be required. For example, with deaf participants, the entire consent process may need to be in writing. For people who have a physical impairment preventing them from writing or for participants who cannot read and write, alternative procedures for documenting informed consent (such as audiotaping or videotaping the consent proceedings) should be used.
- *The terminally ill*. Terminally ill people who participate in the study can seldom expect to benefit personally from the research, and thus the cost/benefit ratio needs to be carefully assessed. Researchers must also take steps to ensure that if the terminally ill participate in the study, the health care and comfort of these individu-

als are not compromised. Special procedures may be required for obtaining informed consent if they are physically or mentally incapacitated.

- *Institutionalized people.* Nurses often conduct studies using hospitalized or institutionalized people as participants. Special care may be required in recruiting such people because they often depend on health care personnel and may feel pressured into participating or may feel that their treatment would be jeopardized by their failure to cooperate. Inmates of prisons and other correctional facilities, who have lost their autonomy in many spheres of activity, may similarly feel constrained in their ability to give free consent. The government has issued special regulations for the additional protection of prisoners as participants (see Code of Federal Regulations, 1983). Researchers studying institutionalized groups need to emphasize the voluntary nature of participation.

- *Pregnant women.* The government has issued stringent additional requirements governing research with pregnant women (Code of Federal Regulations, 1983). These requirements reflect a desire to safeguard both the pregnant woman, who may be at heightened physical and psychological risk, and the fetus, who cannot give informed consent. The regulations stipulate that a pregnant woman cannot be involved in a study unless the purpose of the research is to meet the health needs of the pregnant woman and risks to her and the fetus are minimized or there is only a minimal risk to the fetus.

EXTERNAL REVIEWS AND THE PROTECTION OF HUMAN RIGHTS

Researchers may not be objective in their assessment of the risk/benefit ratio or in their development of procedures to protect the rights of participants. Biases may arise as a result of the researchers' commitment to an area of knowledge and their desire to conduct a study with as much rigor as possible. Because of the risk of a biased evaluation, the ethical dimensions of a study should normally be subjected to external review.

Most hospitals, universities, and other institutions where research is conducted have established formal committees and protocols for reviewing proposed research plans and procedures before they are implemented. These committees are sometimes called **human subjects committees** or **research advisory panels**. If the institution receives federal funds that help to pay for the costs of research, it is likely that the committee will be called an **Institutional Review Board (IRB)**.

Research involving humans that is sponsored through federal funds (including federally sponsored fellowships) is subject to strict guidelines for evaluating the treatment of study participants. Before undertaking such a study, the researcher must submit research plans to the IRB. The duty of the IRB is to ensure that the proposed plans meet the federal requirements for ethical research. An IRB can approve the proposed plans, require modifications, or disapprove the plans. IRB decisions are usually documented on an approval form, such as the one shown in Figure 6-2. The main requirements governing IRB decisions may be summarized as follows (Code of Federal Regulations, 1983):

- Risks to participants are minimized.
- Risks to participants are reasonable in relation to anticipated benefits, if any, and the importance of the knowledge that may reasonably be expected to result.
- Selection of participants is equitable.
- Informed consent will be sought, as required.
- Informed consent will be appropriately documented.
- Adequate provision is made for monitoring the research to ensure the safety of participants.

REVIEW OF SAFEGUARDS FOR HUMAN SUBJECTS

Proposal/Project Number: Internal _____ Sponsor: _____

Proposal/Project Title: _____

_____

Type of review:

____ Determination of Exemption   ____ Full Board Proposal Review
____ Expedited Review   ____ Ongoing research in certifi-
                                          cation of change

____ Other (Specify): _____

_____

After reviewing the above proposal/project:

Exemption ____ The institutional official has determined that the research is
                   exempt under 45 CFR 46.101 (b) or

Safeguards ____ This Institutional Review Board (or member signing below
                    in the case of expedited review) has determined by unani-
                    mous vote of the members present that:

              ____ Risks to subjects are minimized and are reasonable in rela-
                    tion to anticipated benefits. Selection of subjects is equita-
                    ble, and the privacy of the subjects and confidentiality of the
                    data are adequately protected. Approval is given.

              ____ Approval is given under the following conditions:

              ____ Approval is not given, for the following reasons:

Where applicable, attach summary of controverted issues and their resolution.

_____

Date: _____

Names of Members Present: *Signatures of Members Present:*

_____   _____

_____   _____

_____   _____

_____   _____

_____   _____

Figure 6-2. Sample Institutional Review Board review/approval form.

• Appropriate provisions are made to protect the privacy of participants and the confidentiality of data.

• When vulnerable subjects are involved, appropriate additional safeguards are included to protect their rights and welfare.

Many research projects require a full review by the IRB. For a full review, the IRB convenes meetings at which most IRB members must be present. An IRB must consist of five or more members, at least one of whom is not a researcher (e.g., a member of the clergy or a lawyer may be appropriate). One member of the IRB must also be a person who has no affiliation with the institution and is not a family member of a person affiliated with the institution. The IRB cannot comprise entirely men, women, or members from a single profession. These requirements are designed to safeguard against the possibility of various biases.

For certain kinds of research involving no more than minimal risk to humans, the IRB can use expedited review procedures, which do not require that a meeting be convened. In an **expedited review**, a single IRB member (usually the IRB chairperson or another member designated by the chairperson) carries out the review. Examples of the kinds of research ac-

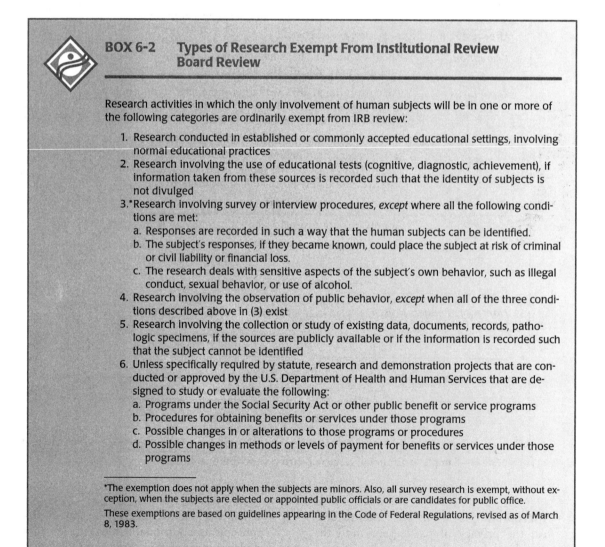

BOX 6-2   Types of Research Exempt From Institutional Review Board Review

Research activities in which the only involvement of human subjects will be in one or more of the following categories are ordinarily exempt from IRB review:

1. Research conducted in established or commonly accepted educational settings, involving normal educational practices
2. Research involving the use of educational tests (cognitive, diagnostic, achievement), if information taken from these sources is recorded such that the identity of subjects is not divulged
3. *Research involving survey or interview procedures, *except* where all the following conditions are met:
   a. Responses are recorded in such a way that the human subjects can be identified.
   b. The subject's responses, if they became known, could place the subject at risk of criminal or civil liability or financial loss.
   c. The research deals with sensitive aspects of the subject's own behavior, such as illegal conduct, sexual behavior, or use of alcohol.
4. Research involving the observation of public behavior, *except* when all of the three conditions described above in (3) exist
5. Research involving the collection or study of existing data, documents, records, pathologic specimens, if the sources are publicly available or if the information is recorded such that the subject cannot be identified
6. Unless specifically required by statute, research and demonstration projects that are conducted or approved by the U.S. Department of Health and Human Services that are designed to study or evaluate the following:
   a. Programs under the Social Security Act or other public benefit or service programs
   b. Procedures for obtaining benefits or services under those programs
   c. Possible changes in or alterations to those programs or procedures
   d. Possible changes in methods or levels of payment for benefits or services under those programs

*The exemption does not apply when the subjects are minors. Also, all survey research is exempt, without exception, when the subjects are elected or appointed public officials or are candidates for public office.

These exemptions are based on guidelines appearing in the Code of Federal Regulations, revised as of March 8, 1983.

tivities that qualify for an expedited IRB review include the following:

- Gathering information from participants 18 years old or older using noninvasive procedures routinely employed in clinical practice (e.g., weighing, testing sensory acuity, electrocardiography, and thermography)
- Collection of blood samples by venipuncture, in amounts not exceeding 450 mL, in an 8-week period, from participants at least 18 years old, in good health, and not pregnant
- Collection of excreta and external secretions, including sweat, uncannulated saliva, placenta removed at delivery, and amniotic fluid at the time of rupture of the membrane before or during delivery
- The study of existing documents, records, pathologic specimens, or diagnostic specimens
- Research on individual behavior or characteristics when the researcher does not man   the participants' behavior and when   udy will not involve stress to the pa   ants

The   egulations also allow certain types of   n to be totally exempt from IRB revie   ese are studies in which there are no apparent risks to human participants. Box 6-2 summarizes the types of research for which investigators can request an exemption from the IRB review process.

TIPS ON ADDRESSING ETHICAL ISSUES IN A RESEARCH STUDY

Not all nurse researchers face ethical dilemmas in their research, but they all must give adequate attention to the protection of the rights of their participants. Below are some suggestions for addressing the ethical aspects of a study.

- Researchers need to give careful thought to ethical requirements during the planning of a research project and to ask themselves continually whether planned safeguards for protecting humans are sufficient. Once the study procedures have been developed, researchers should undertake a self-evaluation of those procedures to determine if they meet ethical requirements. Box 25-17 in Chapter 25 provides some guidelines for such a self-evaluation.
- Not all research is subject to federal guidelines, and so not all studies are reviewed by IRBs or other formal committees. Nevertheless, researchers have a responsibility to ensure that their research plans are ethically acceptable and are thus encouraged to seek an outside opinion regarding the ethical dimensions of a study before it is underway. Advisers may include faculty members, the clergy, representatives from the group that would be asked to participate in the research, or advocates for that group.
- If the research is being conducted within an institution (or if clients are being referred by an institution), it is important to find out early what the institution's requirements are regarding ethical issues. Many clinical agencies have specific protocols and forms for submitting information about the protection of participants. If you are a student with a time constraint for completing a research project, you should consult with the nurse researcher or nursing administration personnel at the agency as quickly as possible to determine the appropriate procedures to follow, the schedule of human subjects committee meetings, and the anticipated date for receiving information regarding the committee's decision.
- There are no firm rules regarding the payment of stipends. In general, stipends are used as incentives to increase the rate of participation in a study; they appear to be especially effective when the group under investigation is known to be difficult

to recruit or when the study is extremely time-consuming or tedious. Stipends range from $1 to hundreds of dollars, but most stipends are in the range of $10 to $25. Federal agencies that sponsor research sometimes do not allow the payment of an outright stipend but will allow for the reimbursement of certain expenses (e.g., for the participants' travel, child care, or lunch money).

 ## RESEARCH EXAMPLES

Because researchers generally attempt to report the results of their research as succinctly as possible, they rarely describe in much detail the efforts they have made to safeguard the rights of their participants. (The absence of any mention of such safeguards does not, of course, imply that no precautions were taken.) Researchers are especially likely to discuss their adherence to ethical guidelines when the study involves more than minimal risk or when the group of people being studied is a vulnerable one. Table 6-1 outlines the procedures used in several studies in which the authors described some of the steps taken to protect human rights. Two research examples that highlight ethical issues are presented below.

Research Example From a Quantitative Study

Holdcraft and Williamson (1991) studied levels of hope among psychiatric and chemically dependent inpatients, noting that hospitalization for these patients might be a time of crisis or despair. Patients in a large general hospital were asked to participate in the study and complete the Miller Hope Scale. Patients in the mental unit were approached within the first 3 days after admission or transfer to the unit. Patients on the chemical dependency unit were told about the study during their transition from the detoxification phase of their treatment. Informed consent was ob-

tained from all study participants. Subjects who agreed to participate completed the questionnaire and returned it in a sealed envelope. The participants were asked to complete the questionnaire a second time to determine if levels of hope changed over the course of their treatment. The participants received the materials and instructions to complete the second questionnaires at discharge. The participants' names were not used on any study materials, except on the consent forms and on a master list of names and code numbers. Consent forms and the list of names were filed in a separate office and destroyed at the completion of the study.

Research Example From a Qualitative Study

Kearney, Murphy, Irwin, and Rosenbaum (1995) conducted a study of how pregnant crack cocaine users perceived their social psychological problems and responded to them. In-depth interviews were conducted with 60 women who reported regular crack cocaine use and who were either pregnant or within 6 months postpartum. Women were solicited through flyers posted in urban neighborhoods and through health and social service agencies.

Interviews with eligible women were conducted in the field setting of the women's choice. Although the pregnancy status of the women was confirmed at the interview by a urine test, drug testing was not performed "in the interest of protection of legally and socially vulnerable participants" (p. 209). The participants were encouraged to participate in the safeguarding of their own privacy: they were invited to use pseudonyms and to decline to provide personal information such as addresses. To prevent an ethical dilemma that might arise because of potential criminal liability of the participants in connection with divulged information on drug use, the researchers obtained a Certificate of Confidentiality from the National Institute of Drug Abuse. The certificate *required* the re-

TABLE 6-1 Examples of Procedures to Protect Study Participants		
PRINCIPLE	**STUDY QUESTION**	**PROCEDURES**
Informed consent Privacy IRB review Risk reduction	How effective is an intervention protocol for increasing safety-seeking behaviors of abused women during pregnancy?	Data collection began after the IRB approved the study. Women were assessed for abuse in a private room, without their male partners present. Study participants completed an informed written consent form. (McFarlane, Parker, Soeken, Silva, & Reel, 1998)
Informed consent Confidentiality Privacy IRB approval	What are the experiences of gay couples when at least one member has been diagnosed with symptomatic HIV infection or AIDS?	Before the initial interview, informed consent was obtained and confidentiality ensured. All interviews were conducted with partners individually (except for one couple who requested a joint interview). IRB approval was obtained. (Powell-Cope, 1995)
Informed consent of minors	What are the behavior patterns of children with Turner syndrome in comparison with those of children with learning disabilities?	Informed consent was obtained from the parents of 8- to 15-year-old children. The children also consented. (Williams, 1994)
Informed consent IRB review Risk reduction Exclusion of vulnerable subjects	What are the effects of different temperature cooling blankets in humans with fever, in terms of time to cool, shivering, and perceived discomfort?	Participants were informed of the study purpose and signed a consent form. Vulnerable subjects (e.g., pregnant women) were excluded. All equipment was carefully tested before the study. IRB approval was secured. (Caruso, Hadley, Shukla, Frame, & Khoury, 1992)

searchers to protect the data from discovery for nonresearch use. The study was reviewed and approved by two IRBs. Informed consent was obtained from each study participant, who was paid a stipend of $40 for cooperating in the study. The researchers were cognizant of the potential for psychological distress: "Due to the emotionally difficult and illicit nature of the interview content, interviewers sought to provide women with maximal control over their disclosures" (p. 209). Interviewers made referrals for drug treatment, health care, and other services to women who requested help.

SUMMARY

Research that involves human beings requires a careful consideration of the procedures to be used to protect their rights. Because research has not always been conducted ethically and because of the genuine **ethical dilemmas** that researchers often face in designing studies that are both ethical and methodologically rigorous, **codes of ethics** have been developed to guide researchers. The three major ethical principles that are incorporated into most guidelines are beneficence, respect for human dignity, and justice.

Beneficence encompasses the maxim: Above all, do no harm. This principle involves the protection of participants from physical and psychological harm, the nonexploitation of participants, and the performance of some good. In deciding to conduct a study, the researcher must carefully weigh the **risk/benefit ratio** of participation to individuals and must also weigh the risks to the participants against the potential benefits to society.

The principle of **respect for human dignity** includes the right to **self-determination**, which means that participants have the freedom to control their own activities, including their voluntary participation in the study. The respect principle also includes the participants' right to full disclosure. **Full disclosure** means that the researcher has fully described to prospective participants the nature of the study and participants' rights. Because full disclosure can lead to potentially misleading and distorted study findings, researchers sometimes feel that this principle can, in certain cases, be violated in the name of good research. When full disclosure poses the risk of biased results, researchers sometimes use **covert data collection** or **concealment**, which means the collection of information without the participants' knowledge or consent. In other research situations, researchers have used **deception** (either withholding information from participants or providing false information) to avoid biases. When deception or concealment is necessary, extra precautions are usually needed to minimize risks and protect the other rights of participants.

The third principle, **justice**, includes the **right to fair treatment** (both in the selection of participants and during the course of the study) and

the **right to privacy**. Privacy of participants can be maintained through **anonymity** (wherein not even the researcher knows the identity of the participants) or through formal **confidentiality procedures**.

Most studies should involve **informed consent** procedures designed to provide prospective participants with sufficient information to make a reasoned decision about the potential costs and benefits of participation. Informed consent normally involves having the participant sign a **consent form**, which documents the participant's voluntary decision to participate after receiving a full explanation of the research. In qualitative studies, consent may need to be renegotiated continually with participants as the study evolves, through **process consent** procedures.

Certain people, sometimes referred to as **vulnerable subjects**, require additional safeguards to protect their rights. These participants may be vulnerable because they are not competent with regard to making an informed decision about participating in a study (e.g., children or mentally retarded people); because their circumstances make them feel that free choice is constrained (e.g., an institutionalized group of participants); or because their circumstances heighten their risk for physical or psychological harm (e.g., pregnant women, the terminally ill).

External review of the ethical aspects of a study is highly recommended and, in many cases, is required by either the agency funding the research or the organization in which the research is being conducted. Most institutions have special review committees for such purposes. Research funded through the federal government is normally reviewed by the **Institutional Review Board (IRB)** of the institution with which the researcher is affiliated. In studies in which risks to participants are minimal, an **expedited review** (review by a single member of the IRB) may be substituted for a full board review; in cases in which there are no anticipated risks, the research may be exempted from review. However, researchers are always advised to consult with at least one external adviser whose perspective allows him or her to evaluate objectively the ethics of a proposed study.

STUDY ACTIVITIES

Chapter 6 of the *Study Guide to Accompany Nursing Research: Principles and Practice, 6th ed.*, offers suggested questions and exercises for reinforcing concepts relating to research ethics. Additionally, the following questions can be addressed:

1. Point out the ethical dilemmas that might emerge in the following studies:
   a. A study of the relationship between sleeping patterns and acting-out behaviors in hospitalized psychiatric patients
   b. A study of the effects of a new drug on human participants
   c. An investigation of an individual's psychological state after an abortion
   d. An investigation of the contraceptive decisions of high school students at a school-based clinic
2. For each of the studies described in question 1, indicate whether you think the study would require a full IRB review or an expedited review, or whether it would be totally exempt from review.
3. For the study described in the research example section (the study by Holdcraft and Williamson, 1991), prepare an informed-consent form that includes required information, as described in the section on informed consent.

SUGGESTED READINGS

References on Research Ethics

American Nurses' Association. (1975). *Human rights guidelines for nurses in clinical and other research*. Kansas City, MO: Author.

American Nurses' Association. (1985). *Code for nurses with interpretive statements*. Kansas City, MO: Author.

American Psychological Association. (1982). *Ethical principles in the conduct of research with human subjects*. Washington, DC: Author.

American Sociological Association. (1984). *Code of ethics*. Washington, DC: Author.

Code of Federal Regulations. (1983). *Protection of human subjects: 45CFR46* (revised as of March 8, 1983). Washington, DC: Department of Health and Human Services.

Cowles, K. V. (1988). Issues in qualitative research on sensitive topics. *Western Journal of Nursing Research, 10,* 163–179.

Damrosch, S. P. (1986). Ensuring anonymity by use of subject-generated identification codes. *Research in Nursing & Health, 9,* 61–63.

Davis, A. J. (1989a). Clinical nurses' ethical decision-making in situations of informed consent. *Advances in Nursing Science, 11,* 63–69.

Davis, A. J. (1989b). Informed consent process in research protocols: Dilemmas for clinical nurses. *Western Journal of Nursing Research, 11,* 448–457.

Munhall, P. L. (1988). Ethical considerations in qualitative research. *Western Journal of Nursing Research, 10,* 150–162.

National Commission for the Protection of Human Subjects of Biomedical and Behavioral Research. (1978). *Belmont report: Ethical principles and guidelines for research involving human subjects*. Washington, DC: U. S. Government Printing Office.

Ramos, M. C. (1989). Some ethical implications of qualitative research. *Research in Nursing & Health, 12,* 57–64.

Rempusheski, V. F. (1991a). Elements, perceptions, and issues of informed consent. *Applied Nursing Research, 4,* 201–204.

Rempusheski, V. F. (1991b). Research data management: Piles into files—locked and secured. *Applied Nursing Research, 4,* 147–149.

Silva, M. C., & Sorrell, J. M. (1984). Factors influencing comprehension of information for informed consent. *International Journal of Nursing Studies, 21,* 233–240.

Thomas, J. A., Hamm, T. E., Perkins, P. L., & Raffin, T. A. (1988). Animal research at Stanford University: Principles, policies, and practices. *New England Journal of Medicine, 318,* 1630–1632.

Thurber, F. W., Deatrick, J. A., & Grey, M. (1992). Children's participation in research: Their right to consent. *Journal of Pediatric Nursing, 7,* 165–170.

Watson, A. B. (1982). Informed consent of special subjects. *Nursing Research, 31,* 43–47.

Substantive References

Caruso, C. C., Hadley, B. J., Shukla, R., Frame, P., & Khoury, J. (1992). Cooling effects and comfort of four cooling blanket temperatures in humans with fever. *Nursing Research, 41,* 68–72.

Holdcraft, C., & Williamson, C. (1991). Assessment of hope in psychiatric and chemically dependent patients. *Applied Nursing Research, 4,* 129–133.

Kearney, M. H., Murphy, S., Irwin, K., & Rosenbaum, M. (1995). Salvaging self: A grounded theory of pregnancy on crack cocaine. *Nursing Research, 44,* 208–213.

McFarlane, J., Parker, B., Soeken, K., Silva, C., & Reel, S. (1998). Safety behaviors of abused women after an intervention during pregnancy. *Journal of Obstetric, Gynecologic, and Neonatal Nursing, 27,* 64–69.

Powell-Cope, G. M. (1995). The experiences of gay couples affected by HIV infection. *Qualitative Health Research, 5,* 36–62.

Williams, J. K. (1994). Behavioral characteristics of children with Turner syndrome and children with learning disabilities. *Western Journal of Nursing Research, 16,* 26–35.

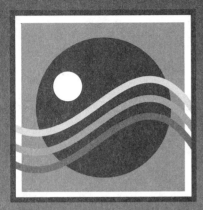

PART **III**

Designs for Nursing Research

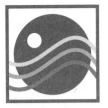

Selecting a Research Design

A researcher's overall plan for obtaining answers to the research questions or for testing the research hypotheses is referred to as the **research design**. The research design spells out the basic strategies that the researcher adopts to develop information that is accurate and interpretable.

The research design incorporates some of the most important methodologic decisions that the researcher makes in conducting a research study. Other aspects of the study—the data collection plan, the sampling plan, and the analysis plan—also involve important decisions, but the research design stipulates the fundamental form that the research will take. For this reason, it is important to have a good understanding of design options when embarking on a research project. The purpose of this chapter is to provide an overview of various research design considerations. Subsequent chapters cover research design issues in greater depth.

ASPECTS OF RESEARCH DESIGN

The researcher's overall plan for addressing the research problem covers multiple aspects of the study's structure. The key factors that are incorporated into a research design are discussed in this section.

Intervention

In some studies, nurse researchers want to test the effects of a specific intervention (e.g., an innovative program to promote breast self-examination or new procedures for monitoring infants in the neonatal intensive care unit). In such studies, called **experimental studies,** the researcher plays an active role by introducing the intervention. In other studies, referred to as **nonexperimental** studies, the researcher observes phenomena as they naturally occur without intervening in any way. The distinction between experimental and nonexperimental designs in quantitative studies is discussed at length in Chapter 8. Qualitative studies are almost always nonexperimental, as we discuss in Chapter 10.

When the study is experimental, the researcher makes decisions about the full nature of the intervention as part of the research design. Among the questions that would be addressed are the following:

- What exactly *is* the intervention? How does it differ from the more usual methods of care?

- What are the procedures to be used with those receiving—and with those *not* receiving—the intervention?
- Who will receive the intervention, and who will not? How will each group be selected or designated?
- What is the dosage or intensity of the intervention?
- Over how long a period will the intervention be administered? When will the treatment begin (e.g., 2 hours after operation)?
- Who will administer the intervention? What are their credentials, and what type of special training or preparation will they receive?
- Will those administering the intervention be fully informed about the nature of the study? Will study participants be fully informed?
- Under what conditions will the intervention be withdrawn or altered?

Comparisons

In most studies, researchers try to develop some type of comparison to provide a context for interpreting their results. In a quantitative study, the researcher typically specifies the nature of the comparisons in advance, whereas in a qualitative study, comparisons may suggest themselves during the course of data collection. Comparisons in research studies can be of various types, the most common of which are as follows:

1. *Comparison between two or more groups.* For example, suppose a researcher wanted to study the emotional consequences of having an abortion. To do this, the researcher might compare the emotional status of women who had an abortion with the status of women from the same health clinic who had an unintended pregnancy but who nevertheless delivered the baby. As another example, a qualitative researcher might study adaptation to menopause among women in different cultural or ethnic groups.

2. *Comparison of a single group at two or more points in time.* For example, the researcher might want to assess patients' levels of stress before and after introducing a new procedure intended to reduce preoperative stress. Or a researcher might want to compare the coping processes of the caregivers of AIDS patients early and later in the caregiving experience.

3. *Comparison of a single group under different circumstances or experiences.* For example, a researcher might compare the heart rates of people undergoing two different types of exercise.

4. *Comparison based on relative rankings.* Researchers addressing questions about relationships among variables are really making comparisons. For example, if the research hypothesis is that there is a relationship between cancer patients' level of pain (the independent variable) and their degree of hopefulness (the dependent variable), the researcher is essentially asking whether patients with high levels of pain feel less hopeful than patients with low levels of pain. Thus, the research question involves a comparison of those with different rankings—high versus low—on both variables.

5. *Comparison with samples from other studies.* Researchers may directly compare their results with results from other studies, sometimes using statistical procedures. This type of comparison typically supplements rather than replaces other types of comparisons. Within quantitative studies, this approach is useful primarily when the measure of the dependent variable is a widely used and accepted measure (e.g., blood pressure measures or scores on a standard measure of depression).

Comparisons are sometimes the central focus of the research, but even when they are not, they provide a context for understanding the findings. In the first example above, in which the researcher was interested in the emotional status of women who had an abortion, the inclusion of a comparison group would allow the researcher to interpret better the findings for the women who had an abortion. If the researcher did not use a comparison group, it would be difficult to know whether the emotional status of the abortion group members was unusual in any way.

In some studies, a natural comparison group suggests itself. For example, if a researcher were testing the effectiveness of a new nursing procedure for a group of nursing home residents, an obvious comparison group would be nursing home residents who were exposed to the standard procedure rather than to the innovation. In other cases, however, the comparison group to be used is less clearcut, and the researcher's decision about a comparison group can have serious consequences for the interpretability of the findings. In the example about the emotional consequences of an abortion, the researcher decided to use women who had delivered a baby as the comparison group. This reflects a comparison focusing on the *outcome* of the pregnancy (i.e., pregnancy termination versus live birth). An alternative comparison group might be women who had a miscarriage. In this case, the comparison focuses not on the outcome (in both groups, the outcome is pregnancy loss) but rather on the *determinant* of the outcome. Thus, in designing a study, the researcher often must be careful to make comparisons that will best illuminate the central issue under investigation. Of course, in some cases, it may be desirable to include two or more types of comparison, but this usually increases the cost of undertaking the study.

Some examples of comparisons incorporated into the design of actual nursing studies are presented in Table 7-1.

Controls for Extraneous Variables

As noted in Chapter 2, the complexity of relationships among human characteristics often makes it difficult to answer research questions unambiguously unless efforts are made to isolate the key research variables and to control other factors extraneous to the research question. Thus, in structured quantitative studies, an important feature of the research design is the specification of steps that will be taken to control extraneous variables. The methods used to enhance research control are discussed in Chapter 9.

In designing a quantitative study, the researcher must make decisions about which extraneous variables to control. If the researcher is using a sophisticated research design or analytic strategy, it may be possible to control for a whole host of extraneous variables, but beginning researchers are more likely to be able to control for only one or two. Familiarity with the research literature often helps to identify especially important variables to control.

Timing of Data Collection

In most studies, data are collected from participants at a single point in time. For example, patients might be asked on a single occasion to discuss their nutritional practices. Some designs, however, call for multiple contacts with participants, either to determine how things have changed over time, to determine the stability of some phenomenon, or to establish a baseline against which the effect of some treatment can later be compared. Thus, in designing a study, the researcher must decide on the number of times data will be collected.

The research design also designates *when*, relative to other events, the data will be collected. For example, the design might call for a sample of pregnant women to be interviewed in the 16th and 30th weeks of gestation, or for blood samples to be drawn after 10 hours of fasting, or for patients to be observed 1 day

TABLE 7-1 Examples of Studies With Various Types of Comparisons	
RESEARCH QUESTION	**NATURE OF THE COMPARISON**
What are the differences in psychosocial adjustment among men on three types of dialysis? (Courts & Boyette, 1998)	Three groups of patients were compared: those on home dialysis, on in-center dialysis, and on peritoneal dialysis.
What is the effect of a self-management program for adults with asthma on compliance with prescribed medications, asthma symptoms, and airway obstruction? (Berg, Dunbar-Jacob, & Sereika, 1997)	Two groups (one in the self-management program and the other not) were compared before and after the intervention.
What is the experience of fatigue and depression before and after low-dose 1-thyroxine supplementation in men and women with minor hyperthyroid disease? (Dzurec, 1997)	One group was compared before and after supplementation; also, men and women were compared.
What are the effects of continuous and intermittent sucking on breathing and sucking during oral feedings in very-low-birthweight infants? (Shiao, 1997)	One group of infants was compared with a nasogastric tube and without it (half the infants got the tube first, the other half got the tube second).
What are the characteristics of women with high versus low levels of anxiety after an abnormal Pap smear result? (Nugent, Tamlyn-Leaman, Isa, Reardon, & Crumley, 1993)	Relative rankings: higher versus lower scores on a measure of anxiety were compared; also, subjects were compared with samples in other studies.

after surgery. The timing should make sense in terms of the overall research objectives.

Research Sites and Settings

The research design must specify the site and setting for the research study. That is, the researcher needs to decide where the data will be collected. As discussed in Chapter 2, the site is the overall location for the research—it could be an overall community (e.g., a Haitian neighborhood in Miami) or an institution within a community (e.g., a hospital in Cleveland). Research sometimes occurs in more than one site because the use of multiple sites can often ensure a larger, more diverse, or more representative sample. For example, in a study of a new nursing inter-

vention, the researchers may wish to implement the intervention in both a public and a private hospital or in both an urban and a rural location.

Settings are the more specific places where data collection will occur. In some cases, the setting and the site are the same, as when the selected site is an institution, and the data are collected exclusively within that setting. When the setting is a larger community, however, the researcher must decide where data should be collected—in homes, on the street, in schools, and so on. Because the nature of the setting can influence the way people behave or feel and how they respond to questions, the selection of an appropriate setting is important. Sometimes, studies take place in **naturalistic settings**, such as in people's homes or places of employment. In-depth qualitative studies are especially likely to be done in natural settings because qualitative researchers are interested in studying the context of participants' experiences. Qualitative researchers sometimes study their participants in multiple settings within the selected site (e.g., in their homes, at clinics, and so on).

At the other extreme, some studies are conducted in highly controlled **laboratory settings**. By laboratory, we do not necessarily mean a setting in which scientific equipment is installed. Here, the term is used in a general sense to refer to a physical location apart from the routine of daily living, which is used by the researcher as the site for the collection of data and where subjects report to participate in the research project.

For nurse researchers, studies are often conducted in quasi-natural settings, such as hospitals, clinics, or other similar facilities. These are settings that are not necessarily natural to the participants (unless the participants are nurses or other health care personnel), but neither are they highly contrived and controlled research laboratories. Nevertheless, it may be important to consider whether the participants are being influenced by being in a setting that may be anxiety-provoking or foreign to their usual experiences.

Table 7-2 describes the settings of several actual nursing studies.

Communication With the Study Participants

In designing the study, the researcher must decide how much information will be provided to the study participants. As discussed in Chapter 6, full disclosure to study partici-

TABLE 7-2 Examples of Studies Conducted in Various Settings	
RESEARCH QUESTION	**SETTINGS**
How effective are directed verbal prompts and positive reinforcement on the level of eating independence of elderly patients with dementia? (Coyne & Hoskins, 1997)	A 60-bed dementia unit of a skilled nursing home facility
What is the experience of being a long-term survivor of AIDS? (Barroso, 1997)	Homes of the informants
What are the self-perceived health concerns among the homeless, and what are the conditions under which they would use health services? (Kinzel, 1991)	Homeless shelters, the streets
What are the risk factors and pregnancy outcomes among pregnant incarcerated women? (Fogel, 1993)	A women's maximum security prison
What are the paths of influence on fifth and eighth graders' self-reported sexual behavior? (Porter, Oakley, Ronis, & Neal, 1996)	Elementary and middle school classrooms
Is nap therapy effective in improving alertness and reducing the frequency of sleep attacks among narcoleptic patients? (Rogers & Aldrich, 1993)	A hospital sleep disorder laboratory

pants before obtaining their consent is highly desirable from an ethical standpoint but may in some cases undermine the value of the research. The researcher should consider the costs and benefits of alternative means of communicating information to study participants. Among the issues that should be addressed are the following:

- How much information about the study aims will be provided to prospective participants while they are being recruited?
- How much information about the study aims will be provided to participants during the informed consent process?
- How will information be provided—orally or in writing?
- Who will provide the information, and what will that person be expected to say in response to additional questions the participants may ask?
- Will there be any debriefing sessions after the data are collected to explain more fully the study purpose or to answer participants' questions?
- Will participants be provided with a written summary of the study results?

Because the nature of the communication with participants can affect participants' cooperation and even the data they provide, these issues should be given careful consideration in designing the research.

OVERVIEW OF RESEARCH DESIGN TYPES

There is no single, easy-to-describe typology of research designs. Research designs vary along a number of dimensions, some of which are related to the factors discussed in the preceding section. Table 7-3 lays out some of the major dimensions of research designs. Many of these dimensions are totally independent of the others. For example, an experimental design can be cross-sectional or longitudinal.

This section describes the major dimensions along which research designs can vary—the major exception being the experimental/nonexperimental dimension, which is covered at length in the next chapter.

Structured Versus Flexible Designs

Research designs vary with regard to how much structure the researcher imposes on the research situation and how much flexibility is allowed in making structural changes once the study is underway. The research designs of most quantitative studies are highly structured and are spelled out in advance of any data collection. In a typical quantitative study, the researcher specifies the nature of any intervention, the nature of the comparisons, the methods to be used to control extraneous variables, the timing of data collection, the study site and setting, and the information to be given to participants—all before a single piece of data is gathered. Once data collection is underway, modifications to the research design are rarely instituted. Indeed, when changes are found to be needed, it is usually the result of a discovery that some aspect of the design did not work. The researcher may then decide to discard all the data gathered before implementing the change—essentially treating the first part of the study as pilot work.

Research design in a qualitative study is more fluid. The qualitative researcher often wants to make deliberate modifications that are sensitive to what is being learned as the data are gathered. For example, interesting types of comparisons may potentially be identified during the collection of data and may drive subsequent data collection decisions. Or the researcher may discover that certain types of settings work better than others for encouraging candor or for observing certain types of natural behavior and may at that point alter the setting for the remaining data collection. The fluidity of the research design in qualita-

TABLE 7-3 Dimensions of Research Designs

DIMENSION	DESIGN	MAJOR FEATURES
Control over independent variable	Experimental	Manipulation of independent variable, control group, randomization
	Quasi-experimental	Manipulation of independent variable, but no randomization or no control group
	Nonexperimental	No manipulation of independent variable
Degree of structure	Structured	Design is specified before data are collected.
	Flexible	Design evolves during the course of data collection.
Type of group comparisons	Between-subjects	Participants in groups being compared are different people.
	Within-subjects	Participants in group being compared are the same people.
Number of data collection points	Cross-sectional	Data are collected at one point in time.
	Longitudinal	Data are collected at multiple points in time over an extended time period.
Occurrence of independent and dependent variables	Retrospective	Study begins with dependent variable and looks backward for cause or influence.
	Prospective	Study begins with independent variable and looks forward for the effect.

tive studies is consistent with their basically exploratory and investigative nature.

Between-Subjects and Within-Subjects Designs

As previously noted, most research designs involve making a comparison. In quantitative research, the hypotheses embody the nature of the comparison to be tested. For example, the hypothesis that the drug tamoxifen reduces the rate of breast cancer in high-risk women could be tested by comparing women who received tamoxifen and those who did not.

Comparisons sometimes involve separate groups of people, as in the above example: those getting the drug tamoxifen are not the same people as those not getting the drug. In another example, if a researcher were interested in comparing the pain tolerance of men and women, the groups being compared would obviously involve different people. This class of design is referred to as **between-subjects designs**.

It is sometimes possible and even desirable to make comparisons for the *same* study participants. For example, a researcher might be interested in studying patients' heart rates before and after a nursing intervention. Another researcher might want to compare lower back pain for patients lying in two different positions. These examples both call for a **within-subjects design**, involving comparisons of the same people under two conditions or at two points in time.

Qualitative studies make both types of comparisons, but they are unlikely to ever refer to their designs in these terms. In quantitative studies, the nature of the comparison has implications for the type of statistical test used.

The Time Dimension

As mentioned earlier, the research design generally specifies when and how often data will be collected in a study. There are four situations in which it might be appropriate to design a study with multiple points of data collection:

1. *Studying time-related processes.* Certain research problems specifically focus on phenomena that evolve over time. Examples include such phenomena as healing, learning, growth, recidivism, and physical development.
2. *Determining time sequences.* It is sometimes important to ascertain the temporal sequencing of phenomena. For example, if it is hypothesized that infertility results in depression, then it would be important to determine that the depression did not precede the fertility problem.
3. *Developing comparisons.* Sometimes, a time dimension is useful for placing findings in a broader context, to determine if changes have occurred over time. For example, a study might be concerned with documenting trends in the smoking behavior of teenagers over a 10-year period. Another example of collecting data over time for comparative purposes is a study in which the intent is to see if changes over time can reasonably be attributed to some intervention.
4. *Enhancing research control.* Some research designs for quantitative studies involve the collection of data at multiple points to enhance the interpretability of the results. For example, when two groups are being compared with regard to the effects of alternative interventions, the collection of data before any intervention occurs allows the researcher to detect—and control—any initial differences between groups.

Because of the importance of the time dimension in designing research, studies are often categorized in terms of how they deal with time. The major distinction is between cross-sectional and longitudinal designs.

CROSS-SECTIONAL DESIGNS

Cross-sectional designs involve the collection of data at one point in time. The phenomena under investigation are captured, as they manifest themselves, during one period of data collection. Cross-sectional studies are especially appropriate for describing the status of phenomena or for describing relationships among phenomena at a fixed point in time. For example, a researcher might be interested in determining whether psychological symptoms in menopausal women are correlated contemporaneously with physiologic symptoms.

Cross-sectional designs are sometimes used for time-related purposes, but the results are often ambiguous. For example, a researcher might test the hypothesis, using cross-sectional data, that a contributor to excessive alcohol consumption is low impulse control, as measured by a psychological test. When both alcohol consumption and impulse control are measured concurrently, however, it is difficult to know which variable influenced the other, if either. Cross-sectional data can most appropriately be used to infer temporal sequencing under two circumstances: (1) when there is evidence or logical reasoning indicating that one variable preceded the other (e.g., in a study of the effects of low birthweight on morbidity in school-aged children, there would be no confusion over whether birthweight, the independent variable, came first); and (2) when there is a strong theoretical framework guiding the analysis.

Cross-sectional studies can also be designed in such a way that processes evolving over time can be inferred, such as when the measurements capture the process at different points in its evolution with different individuals. As an example, suppose we were interested in studying the changes in nursing students' professionalism as they progress through a 4-year baccalaureate program. One way to investigate this issue would be to survey students when they are freshmen and then again every year until they graduate; this would be a longitudinal design. On the other hand, we could use a cross-sectional design by surveying members of the four classes at one point and then comparing the responses of the four groups. If seniors manifested stronger professionalism than freshmen, it might be inferred that nursing students become increasingly socialized professionally by their educational experiences. To make this kind of inference, the researcher must assume that the senior students would have responded as the freshmen responded had they been questioned 3 years earlier or, conversely, that freshmen students would demonstrate increased professionalism if they were surveyed 3 years later. Such a design, which involves a comparison of two different age cohorts, is sometimes referred to as a **cohort comparison design.**

The main advantage of cross-sectional designs in such situations is that they are practical: they are relatively economical and easy to manage. There are, however, a number of problems in inferring changes and trends over time using a cross-sectional design. The overwhelming number of social and technologic changes that characterize our society frequently makes it questionable to assume that differences in the behaviors, attitudes, or characteristics of different age groups are the result of the passage through time rather than the result of cohort or generational differences. In the nursing students example, seniors and freshmen may have different attitudes toward the nursing profession, independent of any experiences during their 4 years of education. In such cross-sectional studies, there are frequently several alternative explanations for the research findings.

LONGITUDINAL DESIGNS

A research project in which data are collected at more than one point in time uses a **longitudinal design.** In this section, we discuss several types of longitudinal studies to present new terminology and to acquaint students with alternative designs.

Trend studies are investigations in which samples from a general population are studied over time with respect to some phenomenon. Different samples are selected at repeated intervals, but the samples are always drawn from the same population. Trend studies permit researchers to examine patterns and rates of change over time and to predict future developments. For example, trend studies have been initiated to analyze the number of students entering nursing programs and to forecast future supplies of nursing personnel.

Cohort studies are a particular kind of trend study in which specific subpopulations are examined over time. The samples are drawn from specific subgroups that are often age-related. For example, the cohort of women born from 1946 to 1950 may be studied at regular intervals with respect to health care utilization. As another example, the cohort of nursing students receiving their bachelor's degree in the 1960s may be periodically surveyed to determine their employment/unemployment patterns.

A sophisticated design known as the **cross-sequential design*** combines the features of cohort studies with a cross-sectional approach. In cross-sequential studies, two or more different age cohorts are studied longitudinally so that both changes over time *and* generational or cohort differences can be detected. For example, a researcher might compare the development

---

*Some researchers refer to this as a **cohort-sequential design,** or as a cohort comparison design with a longitudinal component.

of AIDS awareness over time for both a younger and older cohort of teenagers.

In **panel studies**, the *same* people are used to supply data at two or more points in time. The term **panel** refers to the sample of participants involved in the study. Panel studies typically yield more information than trend studies because the investigator can usually reveal patterns of change and reasons for the changes. Because the same individuals are contacted at two or more points in time, the researcher can identify the individuals who did and did not change and then isolate the characteristics of the subgroups in which changes occurred. As an example, a panel study could be designed to explore over time the antecedent characteristics of people who were later able to quit smoking. Panel studies also allow the researcher to examine how conditions and characteristics at time 1 influence characteristics and conditions at time 2. For example, health outcomes at time 2 could be studied among individuals with different health-related practices at time 1. A panel study is intuitively appealing as an approach to studying change and temporal sequencing but is extremely difficult and expensive to manage. The most serious problem is the loss of participants at different points in the study—a problem that is known as **attrition**. Attrition is a problem for the researcher because those who drop out of the study may differ in important respects from the individuals who continue to participate, resulting in potential biases to the results.

Follow-up studies are similar in design to panel studies. Follow-up investigations are generally undertaken to determine the subsequent development of individuals who have a specified condition or who have received a specified intervention—unlike panel studies, which have samples drawn from a general population. For example, patients who have received a particular nursing intervention or clinical treatment may be followed to ascertain the long-term effects of the treatment. As another example, samples of premature babies may be followed to assess their later perceptual and motor development.

In sum, longitudinal designs are appropriate for studying the dynamics of a variable or phenomenon over time. The number of data collection periods and the time intervals between the data collection points depend on the nature of study. When change or development is rapid, numerous time points at short intervals may be required to document the pattern and make accurate forecasts. By convention, however, the term *longitudinal* implies multiple data collection points over an extended period of time. For example, a study involving the collection of patient data on vital signs postoperatively at 2-hour intervals over a 2-day period would not be described as longitudinal.

Many nursing studies involve a time dimension. Table 7-4 presents a brief description of several nursing studies that have used different research designs to address time-related research questions.

Retrospective Versus Prospective Designs

Many studies are undertaken in an effort to understand the underlying causes of phenomena. In studies that are nonexperimental—that is, in which the researcher does not introduce an intervention—there are two basic types of design that can be used to explore cause-and-effect relationships.

RETROSPECTIVE DESIGNS

Studies with a **retrospective design** are investigations in which some phenomenon existing in the present is linked to other phenomena that occurred in the past, before the study was initiated. That is, the investigator is interested in some presently occurring outcome and attempts to shed light on antecedent factors that have caused it. Many epidemiologic studies are retrospective in nature, and this approach has been used by medical researchers for more than a century. Most of the early cigarette smoking–lung cancer studies were retrospective. In such studies, the researcher would be-

TABLE 7-4	Examples of Studies With a Time Dimension		

RESEARCH QUESTION	DESIGN	SAMPLE
What is the role of age in affecting the psychological well-being of older women with chronic illnesses? (Heidrich, 1996)	Cross-sectional	188 older women, in two age groups: young-old (aged 60–74 years) and old-old (aged 75 years and older)
What are the trends in the academic, achievement, values, and personal attributes of college freshmen aspiring to nursing careers from the 1960s to the 1980s? (Williams, 1988)	Trend study	Samples of 500 college freshmen surveyed in 1966, 1972, 1982, 1983, 1984, and 1985
What are the factors that contribute to turnover, absenteeism, and reduced work schedules in hospital nurses? (Wise, 1993)	Cohort study	A cohort of 404 nurses hired in a 2-year period in five hospitals
What is the utility of the construct "locus of control" in predicting substance use in adolescents? (Bearinger & Blum, 1997)	Cross-sequential	Three waves of data collected at 2-year intervals from 7th, 9th, and 11th grade students
What are the pathways to depressed mood among women in midlife? (Woods & Mitchell, 1997)	Panel study	337 women aged 35–55 years surveyed over a 3-year period
What is the natural evolution of postpartum fatigue among primiparous women? (Troy & Dalgas-Pelish, 1997)	Follow-up study	36 women assessed for fatigue during the first 6 weeks postpartum

gin with a group of lung cancer victims and another group of people without the disease. The researcher would then look for differences between the two groups in antecedent behaviors or conditions, such as smoking habits. In nursing research, as in medical research, retrospective studies are fairly common.

PROSPECTIVE DESIGNS

A study with a nonexperimental **prospective design** starts with presumed causes and then goes forward in time, longitudinally, to the presumed effect. For example, a researcher might want to test the hypothesis that the incidence of rubella during pregnancy is related to

malformations in the offspring. To test this hypothesis prospectively, the investigator would begin with a sample of pregnant women, including some who contracted rubella during their pregnancy and others who did not. The subsequent occurrence of congenital anomalies would be observed, and the researcher would then be in a position to test whether women who contracted the disease during pregnancy were more likely to bear malformed babies than women who did not have rubella when pregnant. Prospective designs are thus the designs used in follow-up studies.

Prospective studies are usually much more costly than retrospective studies. Prospective designs often require large samples, particularly

TABLE 7-5 Examples of Retrospective and Prospective Designs

RESEARCH QUESTION	INDEPENDENT VARIABLE/TIMING OF MEASUREMENT	DEPENDENT VARIABLE/TIMING OF MEASUREMENT
Prospective		
What are the predictors of the development of chronic pain in hospitalized patients? (White, LeFort, Amsel, & Jeans, 1997)	Predictive factors (e.g., length of hospital stay): Time 1	Resolution versus non-resolution of pain: 3 months after Time 1
What are the interdependent contributions of hemodynamics, gas exchange, and pulmonary mechanics to the prediction of weaning outcome in cardiac surgery patients? (Hanneman, 1994)	Cardiopulmonary predictive factors: Time 1, 2 hours after surgery	Ability to be weaned from mechanical ventilation: several hours later
Retrospective		
What is the relationship between the incidence of sexually transmitted disease (STD) among young women and factors such as sexual abuse, sexual precocity, and risk-taking behavior? (Kenney, Reinholtz, & Angelini, 1998)	Antecedent factors (e.g., sexual abuse): Time 1	Incidence of STDs: Time 1
What are the occupational and nonoccupational factors that predict job satisfaction among nurses? (Decker, 1997)	Antecedent factors: Time 1	Job satisfaction: Time 1

if the dependent variable of interest is rare, as in the example of malformed babies and maternal rubella. Another difficulty with prospective studies is that a substantial follow-up period may be necessary before the phenomenon or effect under investigation manifests itself, as is the case in prospective studies of cigarette smoking and lung cancer.

Despite these problems, prospective studies are considerably stronger than retrospective studies. For one thing, any ambiguity concerning the temporal sequence of phenomena is usually resolved in prospective research. In addition, samples are more likely to be representative, and investigators may be in a position

to impose some controls to rule out competing explanations for observed effects.

Some actual research examples of retrospective and prospective designs are presented in Table 7-5.

CHARACTERISTICS OF GOOD DESIGN

In selecting a research design, the researcher should be guided by one overarching consideration: whether the design does the best possible job of providing trustworthy answers to the research questions. In this section, we briefly examine more specific characteristics of good research design.

Appropriateness to the Research Question

The requirement that the research design should be appropriate to the question being asked seems so obvious that it may be overlooked. Generally, a given research problem can be handled adequately with a number of different designs, and the researcher typically has some flexibility in developing a research design. Yet many designs are completely unsuitable for dealing with certain research problems. For example, a loosely structured research design, such as those often used in qualitative studies, might be inappropriate to address the question of whether nonnutritive sucking opportunities among premature infants facilitate early oral feedings. On the other hand, a tightly controlled study may unnecessarily restrict the researcher interested in understanding the processes by which nurses make diagnoses. There are many research questions of interest to nurses for which highly structured designs are unsuitable.

Lack of Bias

A second characteristic of good research design is the absence of bias. **Bias, which** refers to an influence that can distort the results of a study, can operate in a variety of ways, some of which are particularly subtle.

A common source of bias stems from differences among participants in groups that are being compared. When groups are formed on a nonrandom basis, the risk of bias is always present. For example, in a prospective quantitative study of the effect of smoking on lung cancer, an important concern would be that smokers and nonsmokers might differ in ways that have little to do with smoking habits. The problem is that these other differences, rather than smoking, are potentially the "real" cause

of differences in rates of developing lung cancer. Unless these other differences (extraneous variables) are controlled, the resulting biases may make it difficult for the researcher to conclude with confidence that there is a causative link between smoking and lung cancer. Chapter 9 presents a number of techniques that can be used to eliminate or reduce bias in quantitative studies.

In some studies, the researcher's preconceptions might unconsciously bias the objective collection of data. In such a case, the researcher should take steps to minimize this risk. For example, **double-blind** procedures can be used in certain situations. The double-blind technique removes observer biases because neither the participant nor the person collecting the data knows the specific research objectives (nor, if groups are being compared, the group that the participant is in) and thus cannot systematically distort the data or influence participants to respond in a certain way. When this approach is not feasible, other steps can often be taken. For example, in studies in which the data are collected by means of observation, it may be useful to have two or more observers so that at least an estimation of the biases can be made.

Although techniques of research control are often mechanisms for controlling bias, there are situations in which too much control can introduce bias. For example, if the researcher tightly controls the ways in which the key study variables can manifest themselves, it is possible that the true nature of those variables will be obscured. When the key concepts are phenomena that are poorly understood or the dimensions of which have not been clarified, then a design that allows some flexibility is better suited to the study aims.

In qualitative studies, the concept known as triangulation is often used to avoid biases. **Triangulation** refers to the use of multiple referents or methods to draw conclusions about what constitutes the truth and to separate the truth from any biases or other anomalies that may characterize the research data. Triangulation is discussed in greater detail in Chapter 17.

Precision

Quantitative researchers generally try to design a study to achieve the highest possible **precision**, which is achieved through the use of precise measuring tools and through a design that yields control over extraneous variables. Research control actually concerns control over variability in the dependent measures. This concept can best be understood through a specific example.

Suppose we were interested in studying the effect of admission into a nursing home on the level of depression among the elderly. Depression may be the result of various influences; that is, depression varies from one elderly person to another for a variety of reasons. In the present study, we are interested in isolating—as precisely as possible—the portion of the variation in depression that is attributable to nursing home admission. Mechanisms of research control that reduce the variability attributable to extraneous factors can be built into the research design, thereby enhancing precision.

In a quantitative study, the following ratio expresses what the researcher is attempting to assess:

$$\frac{\text{Variation in depression due to nursing home admission}}{\substack{\text{Variation in depression due to other factors} \\ \text{(e.g., age, pain, medical prognosis, social support)}}}$$

This ratio, although greatly simplified here, captures the essence of many statistical procedures. The researcher wants to make the variability in the numerator (the upper half) as large as possible relative to the variability in the denominator (the lower half) to evaluate most clearly the relationship between nursing home admission and levels of depression. The smaller the variability in depression that is due to extraneous variables such as the elderly person's age and prognosis, the easier it will be

for the researcher to detect differences in depression between those who were and those who were not admitted to a nursing home. Designs that enable the researcher to reduce the variability caused by the extraneous variables are said to increase the precision of the research. As a purely hypothetical illustration of why this is so, we will attach some numeric values*: to the ratio, as follows:

$$\frac{\text{Variability due to nursing home admission}}{\text{Variability due to extraneous variables}} = \frac{10}{4}$$

Now, if we can make the bottom number smaller, say by changing it from 4 to 2, then we will have a purer and more precise estimate of the effect of nursing home admission on depression, relative to other influences.

How can a research design help to reduce the variability caused by extraneous variables? Several approaches are discussed in Chapter 9, but we illustrate here with a simple example. The total variability in levels of depression can be conceptualized as having three components:

Total variability in depression = Variability due to nursing home admission + Variability due to age + Variability due to other extraneous variables

This equation can be taken to mean that part of the reason why some elderly individuals are depressed and others are not is that some were admitted to a nursing home and others were not; some were older and some were younger; and other factors, such as level of pain, medical prognosis, and availability of social supports, also had an effect on depression.

One way to increase the precision in this study would be to control age, thereby removing the variability in depression that is the result of differences in the participants' ages. We could do this, for example, by including in our sample only elderly people within a fairly narrow age range (e.g., only those older than 80

---

*The reader should not be concerned at this point with how these numbers can be obtained in a real analysis. The procedure will be explained in Chapter 19.

years of age). By limiting the age of the sample, the variability in levels of depression due to age would be reduced or eliminated. As a result, the effect of nursing home admission on depression becomes greater, relative to the remaining extraneous variability. Thus, we can say that this design has enabled us to get a more precise estimate of the effect of nursing home admission on level of depression. Research designs differ considerably in the sensitivity with which effects under study can be detected with statistical tools. Lipsey (1990) has prepared an excellent guide to assist researchers in enhancing the sensitivity of their research designs.

Power

Power is another desirable feature of a quantitative research design. We use **power** here to describe the ability of a research design to detect relationships among variables. Precision contributes to the power of a design. Power is also increased when a large sample is used. This aspect of power is discussed in Chapters 12 and 19.

One other aspect of a powerful design concerns the construction or definition of the independent variable. For both statistical and theoretical reasons, results are clearer and more conclusive when the differences between groups that are being compared are large. The researcher should generally aim to maximize group differences on the dependent variables by maximizing differences on the independent variable. In other words, the results are likely to be more clearcut if the groups are as different as possible. This advice is more easily followed in experimental than in nonexperimental research. In experiments, the investigator can devise interventions that are distinct and as strong as time, money, ethics, and practicality permit. Even in nonexperimental research, however, there are frequently opportunities to operationalize the independent variables in such a way that power to detect differences is enhanced.

TIPS ON DESIGNING RESEARCH

If you are planning to undertake a study, you will need to make a number of important decisions regarding the study's overall design. These decisions will affect your ability to interpret the data and the overall believability of your findings. In some cases, the decisions will affect whether you receive funding (if you are seeking financial support for your study) or whether you are able to publish your research report (if you plan to submit it to a professional journal). Therefore, a great deal of care and thought should go into these decisions. The following tips may be useful in designing a study:

- When deciding between competing design alternatives, make a written list of the pros and cons of each. For example, in the hypothetical study about the emotional consequences of an abortion, what are the advantages and disadvantages of using as a comparison group women who delivered the baby versus women who had a miscarriage versus those who were not pregnant at all?

- In making design decisions, you will often need to balance a number of considerations, such as time, cost, ethical issues, and the integrity of the study. Try to get a firm understanding of what your upper limits are before making final design decisions. That is, what is the most money that can be spent on the project? What is the maximal amount of time available for conducting the study? What is the limit of acceptability with regard to ethical issues, given the risk/benefit ratio of the study? These limits often eliminate a number of design options. With these constraints in mind, the central focus should be on designing a study that maximizes the validity of the data.

- In designing a study, try to anticipate alternative findings and consider whether design adjustments might affect the results.

For example, suppose we hypothesized that environmental factors such as light and noise affect the incidence of acute confusion among the hospitalized elderly. With a preliminary design for such a study in mind, try to imagine findings that *fail* to support the hypothesis. Then ask yourself what could be done to decrease the possibility of these negative results. Can power be increased by making differences in environmental conditions sharper? Can precision be increased by controlling additional extraneous variables? Can bias be eliminated by better training of research personnel?

- Do not try to make all design decisions single-handedly. Seek the advice of professors, colleagues, research consultants, and so on.
- Once you have made your design decisions, it may be useful to write out a rationale for your choices. Share the rationale with those you have consulted to see if they can find any flaws in your reasoning or if they can make suggestions for further improvements.

RESEARCH EXAMPLES

We conclude this chapter with examples of two research studies that highlight some of the points made. The first example illustrates a structured design that involved the collection of data at two points in time. The second example describes a qualitative study with a flexible design. In reading these brief summaries, consider the strengths and weaknesses of the designs in terms of the study's objectives, referring as needed to the original journal articles.

Example of a Structured, Prospective Design

Winkelstein and Feldman (1993) used a theoretical model that combined elements from the Health Belief Model with psychosocial elements from other models to predict the consumption of sweet-tasting high-calorie foods after smoking cessation. A total of 203 men and women who were participating in Freedom From Smoking programs agreed to participate in the study.

During the first round of data collection, which occurred at the first program session, subjects completed a questionnaire and were observed in a "snack choice" exercise. The questionnaire included measures of the factors hypothesized to be predictive of the consumption of sweets after smoking cessation (e.g., the previous consumption of sweets, intention to avoid sweets, attitudes toward eating sweets, self-efficacy). Follow-up data were obtained at the sixth program session, which was 5 weeks after the first session (2 weeks after smoking cessation). The 114 subjects who were present at the follow-up completed another questionnaire and again made snack choices. The dependent variable was based on three follow-up questions regarding the recent consumption of sweets as well as on the number of sweet snacks consumed in the second snack choice exercise.

The results indicated that subjects who stopped smoking reported eating more sweets than those who did not stop, regardless of prior habit of eating sweets. However, prior habit and self-efficacy as reported in the initial questionnaire were strong predictors of eating sweet-tasting, high-calorie foods after smoking cessation.

Example of a Flexible Research Design

Kidd (1993) conducted a study to understand factors contributing to motor vehicle crashes (MVCs). A flexible design was used to explore qualitatively the variables surrounding an MVC and their interrelationships.

Kidd's design decisions evolved as new data were gathered and interpreted. The basic sample consisted of 18 MVC trauma patients, who were all interviewed during their hospitalization. Kidd decided to reinterview a subset of three informants while they were still in the hospital, to confirm certain of her findings. She also added three former trauma patients to her sample, who were interviewed in the community at varying lengths of time after their MVC injury. Kidd's development of data for comparative purposes also evolved during the course of the study. For example, after reflecting on some of her early data, Kidd decided to make an active effort to include informants with negative as well as positive blood alcohol levels, to determine whether pretrauma perceptions differed between these two groups. She also decided to augment her interview data by analyzing automobile advertisements in several periodicals and by analyzing favorite songs, commercials, and actors cited by her informants.

Based on her various sources of data, Kidd began to develop a theory of self-protection. She found that self-protecting strategies were contingent on the driver evaluating loss of control during the MVC. Kidd's self-protection theory postulates that if motor vehicle control was perceived to have been lost and such control is desired, then self-protecting strategies to enhance future control will be adopted.

SUMMARY

The **research design** is the researcher's overall plan for answering the research question. The design indicates whether there is an intervention and what the intervention is, the nature of any comparisons to be made, the methods to be used to control extraneous variables and enhance the study's interpretability, the timing and frequency of data collection, the site and setting in which the data collection is to take place, and the nature of communications with participants.

Although there is no clearcut typology of research designs, designs can be described along various dimensions, such as whether there is an intervention (experimental versus nonexperi-

mental designs). Another dimension concerns the degree of structure imposed on the design in advance. Most quantitative studies tend to be highly structured, with major features of the design specified before a single piece of data is collected. The designs in most qualitative studies, by contrast, are more fluid, with design changes permitted—and even encouraged—to take advantage of information gathered early in the study.

When a study involves a comparison between different groups of people (e.g., men and women), the design is referred to as a **between-subjects design**. When the same people are compared across time or under different conditions, the design is called a **within-subjects design**.

Another important dimension concerns the handling of the time dimension. **Cross-sectional designs** involve the collection of data at one point in time, whereas **longitudinal designs** collect data at two or more points in time. Research problems that involve trends, changes, or development over time or that intend to demonstrate temporal sequencing of phenomena are best addressed through longitudinal designs. **Trend studies** investigate a particular phenomenon over time by repeatedly drawing different samples from the same general population. **Cohort studies** are ones in which a particular subpopulation (typically a specific age cohort) is studied over time with respect to some phenomenon. Longitudinal studies in which the *same* sample of participants is questioned twice (or more often) are known as **panel studies**. **Follow-up studies** similarly deal with the same people studied at two or more points in time and generally refer to those investigations in which participants who have received a treatment or who have a particular characteristic of interest are followed to study their subsequent development. Longitudinal studies are typically expensive, time-consuming, and beset with such difficulties as **attrition** (loss of participants over time), but they often produce extremely valuable information.

Many quantitative studies attempt to elucidate cause-and-effect relationships. Nonexperimental studies with such an aim use either a retrospective or prospective design. **Retrospective designs** are ones in which the researcher observes the manifestation of some phenomenon (the dependent variable) and tries to identify retrospectively its antecedents or causes (the independent variable). **Prospective designs** start with an observation of presumed causes and then go forward in time longitudinally to observe the consequences. Prospective research is typically initiated after evidence of important relationships is produced by retrospective investigations.

A good research design must be appropriate to the question being asked. It must also minimize or avoid **biases** that can distort the results of the study. Sometimes, **triangulation**, which refers to the use of multiple methods or referents to draw conclusions, is used to address biases. Another feature of a good design for quantitative studies is that it attempts to enhance **precision**, which refers to the sensitivity with which the effects of the independent variable, relative to the effects of extraneous variables, can be detected. Finally, in quantitative studies, the research design should deal adequately with the issue of **power**, which concerns the ability of the design to create maximal contrasts among groups being compared.

🍂 STUDY ACTIVITIES

Chapter 7 of the *Study Guide to Accompany Nursing Research: Principles and Methods, 6th ed.*, offers various exercises and study suggestions for reinforcing the concepts presented in this chapter. Additionally, the following study questions can be addressed:

1. Suppose you were planning to conduct a nonexperimental study concerning the effects of three types of ambulation de-

vices (a cane, a walker, and a crutch) on feelings of control or security for people requiring such assistive devices. What types of extraneous variables relating to characteristics of the participants would be important to consider and, if possible, control?

2. Suppose you wanted to study how nurses' attitudes toward death change as a function of years of nursing experience. Design a cross-sectional study to research this question, specifying the samples that you would want to include. Now design a longitudinal study to research the same problem. Identify the problems and strengths of each approach.

3. Read one of the studies cited in Table 7-4. If you have chosen a prospective study, indicate how the study might have been conducted retrospectively, and vice versa. Compare the strengths and weaknesses of the new design with the design used in the actual study.

🍂 SUGGESTED READINGS

Methodologic References

Given, B. A., Keilman, L. J., Collins, C., & Given, C. W. (1990). Strategies to minimize attrition in longitudinal studies. *Nursing Research, 39*, 184–186.

Kelly, J. R., & McGrath, J. E. (1988). *On time and method.* Newbury Park, CA: Sage.

Kerlinger, F. N. (1986). *Foundations of behavioral research* (3rd ed.). New York: Holt, Rinehart & Winston.

Lipsey, M. W. (1990). *Design sensitivity: Statistical power for experimental research.* Newbury Park, CA: Sage.

Motzer, S.A., Moseley, J.R., & Lewis, F.M. (1997). Recruitment and retention of families in clinical trials with longitudinal designs. *Western Journal of Nursing Research, 19*, 314–333.

Spector, P. E. (1981). *Research designs.* Beverly Hills, CA: Sage.

Weekes, D. P., & Rankin, S. H. (1988). Life-span developmental methods: Application to nursing research. *Nursing Research, 37,* 380–383.

Substantive References

Barroso, J. (1997). Social support and long-term survivors of AIDS. *Western Journal of Nursing Research, 19,* 554–582.

Bearinger, L. H., & Blum, R. W. (1997). The utility of locus of control for predicting adolescent substance use. *Research in Nursing & Health, 20,* 229–245.

Berg, J., Dunbar-Jacob, J., & Sereika, S. M. (1997). An evaluation of a self-management program for adults with asthma. *Clinical Nursing Research, 6,* 225–238.

Courts, N. F., & Boyette, B. G. (1998). Psychosocial adjustment of males on three types of dialysis. *Clinical Nursing Research, 7,* 47–63.

Coyne, M. L., & Hoskins, L. (1997). Improving eating disorders in dementia using behavioral strategies. *Clinical Nursing Research, 6,* 275–290.

Decker, F. H. (1997). Occupational and nonoccupational factors in job satisfaction and psychological distress among nurses. *Research in Nursing & Health, 20,* 453–464.

Dzurec, L. C. (1997). Experiences of fatigue and depression before and after low-dose 1-thyroxine supplementation in essentially euthyroid individuals. *Research in Nursing & Health, 20,* 389–398.

Fogel, C. I. (1993). Pregnant inmates: Risk factors and pregnancy outcomes. *Journal of Obstetric, Gynecologic, and Neonatal Nursing, 22,* 33–39.

Hanneman, S. K. (1994). Multidimensional predictors of success or failure with early weaning from mechanical ventilation after cardiac surgery. *Nursing Research, 43,* 4–10.

Heidrich, S. M. (1996). Mechanisms related to psychological well-being in older women with chronic illnesses: Age and disease comparisons. *Research in Nursing & Health, 19,* 225–235.

Kenney, J. W., Reinholtz, C., & Angelini, P. J. (1998). Sexual abuse, sex before age 16, and high risk behaviors of young females with sexually transmitted diseases. *Journal of Obstetric, Gynecologic, and Neonatal Nursing, 27,* 54–63.

Kidd, P. S. (1993). Self-protection: Trauma patients' perspectives of their motor vehicle crashes. *Qualitative Health Research, 3,* 320–340.

Kinzel, D. (1991). Self-identified health concerns of two homeless groups. *Western Journal of Nursing Research, 13,* 181–190.

Nugent, L. S., Tamlyn-Leaman, K., Isa, N., Reardon, E., & Crumley, J. (1993). Anxiety and the colposcopy experience. *Clinical Nursing Research, 2,* 267–277.

Porter, C. P., Oakley, D., Ronis, D. L., & Neal, R. W. (1996). Pathways of influence on fifth and eighth graders' reports about having had sexual intercourse. *Research in Nursing & Health, 19,* 193–204.

Rogers, A. E., & Aldrich, M. S. (1993). The effect of regularly scheduled naps on sleep attacks and excessive daytime sleepiness associated with narcolepsy. *Nursing Research, 42,* 111–117.

Shiao, S. P. K. (1997). Comparison of continuous versus intermittent sucking in very-low-birth-weight infants. *Journal of Obstetric, Gynecologic, and Neonatal Nursing, 26,* 313–319.

Troy, N. W., & Dalgas-Pelish, P. (1997). The natural evolution of postpartum fatigue among a group of primiparous women. *Clinical Nursing Research, 6,* 126–139.

White, C. L., LeFort, S. M., Amsel, R., & Jeans, M. E. (1997). Predictors of the development of chronic pain. *Research in Nursing & Health, 20,* 309–318.

Williams, R. P. (1988). College freshmen aspiring to nursing careers: Trends from the 1960s to the 1980s. *Western Journal of Nursing Research, 10,* 94–97.

Winkelstein, M. L., & Feldman, R. H. L. (1993). Psychosocial predictors of consumption of sweets following smoking cessation. *Research in Nursing & Health, 16,* 97–105.

Wise, L. C. (1993). The erosion of nursing resources: Employee withdrawal behaviors. *Research in Nursing & Health, 16,* 67–75.

Woods, N. F., & Mitchell, E. S. (1997). Pathways to depressed mood for midlife women: Observations from the Seattle Midlife Women's Health Study. *Research in Nursing & Health, 20,* 119–129.

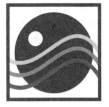

CHAPTER **8**

Research Designs for Quantitative Studies

In Chapter 7, we discussed various aspects of research design. This chapter focuses on research designs for quantitative studies, and Chapter 10 examines the issue of research design for qualitative studies. The sections that follow elaborate on different types of design for quantitative nursing research, with the major emphasis on designs that vary in terms of whether the researcher actively controls the independent variable. We begin with a discussion of research designs that offer the greatest amount of control: experimental studies.

EXPERIMENTAL RESEARCH

Experiments differ from nonexperiments in one important respect: the researcher is an active agent in experimental studies rather than a passive observer. Early physical scientists learned that although observation of natural phenomena is valuable and instructive, the complexity of the events occurring in the natural state often obscures understanding of important relationships. This problem was handled by isolating the phenomenon of interest in a laboratory set-

ting and controlling the conditions under which it occurred. The procedures developed by physical scientists were profitably adopted by biologists during the 19th century, resulting in many achievements in physiology and medicine. The 20th century has witnessed the use of experimental methods by scholars and researchers interested in human behavior and psychological phenomena.

Characteristics of True Experiments

The controlled experiment is considered by many to be the ideal of science. Except for purely descriptive research, the aim of many research studies is to understand the nature of relationships among phenomena. For example, does a certain drug cause the cure of a certain disease? Do certain nursing techniques produce a decrease in patient anxiety? The strength of the true experiment over other methods lies in the fact that the experimenter can achieve greater confidence in the genuineness and interpretability of relationships because they are observed under carefully controlled conditions. As we pointed out in Chapter 3, hypotheses are never ultimately proved or disproved by scientific methods, but true experiments offer the most convincing evidence concerning the effects one variable has on another.

A true experiment is a scientific investigation characterized by the following properties:

- *Manipulation*—the experimenter *does* something to at least some of the subjects in the study
- *Control*—the experimenter introduces one or more controls over the experimental situation, including the use of a control group
- *Randomization*—the experimenter assigns subjects to a control or experimental group on a random basis

Each of these properties is discussed more fully below.

MANIPULATION

Manipulation involves *doing* something to at least one group of subjects. The introduction of that "something" (often referred to as the experimental **treatment** or experimental **intervention**) constitutes the independent variable. The experimenter manipulates the independent variable by administering a treatment to some subjects and withholding it from others (or by administering some other treatment, such as a placebo). The experimenter, in other words, consciously *varies* the independent variable and observes the effect that the manipulation has on the dependent variable of interest.

For example, let us say we have hypothesized that the color of a pediatric nurse's uniform affects the degree to which children display positive affective behaviors, such as smiling and laughing, during hospitalization. The independent or presumed causative variable in this example is uniform color, which could be manipulated by assigning some nurses white uniforms (for instance) and other nurses brightly colored uniforms. Thus, in this study, we might compare, 24 hours after hospitalization, the affective behavior (the dependent variable) of two groups of children: (1) those cared for by white-uniformed nurses, and (2) those cared for by nurses in colored uniforms.

CONTROL

The notion of control in an experimental context actually summarizes all the major experimental activities: control is acquired by manipulating, by randomizing, by carefully preparing the experimental protocols, and by using a control group. This section focuses on the function of the control group in experiments.

Obtaining evidence about relationships requires making at least one comparison. If we were to supplement the diet of a group of premature infants with a particular combination of vitamins and other nutrients every day for 2 weeks, the weight of those infants at the end of the 2-week period would give us absolutely no information about the effectiveness of the treatment. At a bare minimum, we would need to compare their posttreatment weight with their pretreatment weight to determine if, at least, their weight had increased. But let us assume for the moment that we find an average weight gain of 1 pound. Does this finding support the conclusion that there is a causative relationship between the nutritional supplements (the independent variable) and weight gain (the dependent variable)? No, it does not. Babies normally gain weight as they mature. Without a control group—a group that does *not* receive the nutritional supplements—it is impossible to separate the effects of maturation from those of the treatment. The term control group, in other words, refers to a group of subjects whose performance on a dependent variable is used as a basis for evaluating the performance of the experimental group (the group that receives the treatment of interest to the researcher) on the same dependent variable.

In some biologic, medical, and psychological research, the experimenter administers the treatment of interest to the experimental group, whereas the control group receives no treatment at all and is merely observed with respect to behavior on the dependent variable. This kind of situation probably is not feasible for many nursing research projects because it may be impossible to isolate a control group and do nothing to those subjects. For example, if we wanted to evaluate the effectiveness of some nursing intervention on hospital patients, it would be unlikely that we would devise an experiment in which the control group of patients received no nursing care at all. We would have to evaluate our new intervention, not against the total absence of care, but rather against a control group receiving conventional methods of care.

RANDOMIZATION

Randomization (also referred to as **random assignment**) involves the placement of subjects in groups on a random basis. Random essentially means that every subject has an equal chance of being assigned to any group. If subjects are placed in groups randomly, there is no **systematic bias** in the groups with respect to attributes that may affect the dependent variable under investigation.

Before discussing the mechanics of random assignment, we should pause to consider its function. Suppose a researcher wishes to study the effectiveness of a hospital-based contraceptive counseling program for a group of multiparous women who have just given birth. Two groups of subjects are established, one of which will be counseled and the other of which will receive no counseling. The women in the sample may be expected to differ from one another on a number of characteristics, such as age, marital status, financial situation, attitudes toward child-rearing, and the like. Any of these characteristics could have an effect on the diligence with which a woman practices contraception, independent of whether or not she receives counseling. The researcher needs to have the "counsel" and "no counsel" groups

equal with respect to these extraneous characteristics to assess properly the impact of the experimental counseling program on the women's subsequent pregnancies. The random assignment of subjects to one group or the other is designed to perform this equalization function. One method might be to flip a coin for each woman (more elaborate procedures are discussed later). If the coin is "heads," the woman would be assigned to one group; if the coin is "tails," she would be assigned to the other group.

Although randomization is the preferred scientific method for equalizing groups, there is no guarantee that the groups will, in fact, be equal. Let us take as an extreme example the case in which only 10 women, all of whom have given birth to at least four children, constitute the entire sample for the study. Five of the 10 women are aged 35 years or older, and the remaining five are younger than 35 years of age. One would anticipate that a random assignment of women to an experimental or control group would result in about 2 or 3 women from the two age ranges in each group. But let us suppose that, by chance, the older 5 women all ended up in the experimental group. Because these women are nearing the end of their childbearing years, the likelihood of their conceiving is diminished. Thus, follow-up of their subsequent reproductive behavior (the dependent variable) might suggest that the counseling program was effective in reducing subsequent pregnancies; however, a higher pregnancy rate for the control group may only reflect the age and fecundity differences and not the lack of exposure to counseling.

Despite this possibility, randomization remains the most trustworthy and acceptable method of equalizing groups. Unusual or deviant assignments such as this one are rare, and the likelihood of obtaining markedly unequal groups is reduced as the number of subjects increases.

Students often wonder why the researcher does not consciously control those characteristics of subjects that are likely to affect the experimental outcome. The procedure that is sometimes used to accomplish this is known as **matching**. For example, if matching were used in the contraceptive counseling study, the researcher might want to ensure that if there were a married, 38-year-old woman with six children in the experimental group, there would be a married, 38-year-old woman with six children in the control group as well. There are two serious problems with matching, however. First of all, to match effectively, we must know what the characteristics are that are likely to affect the dependent variable. This information is not always known. Second, even if we knew the relevant traits, the complications of matching on more than three or four characteristics simultaneously are prohibitive. With random assignment, on the other hand, *all* possible distinguishing characteristics—age, gender, intelligence, blood type, religious affiliation, and so on—are likely to be equally distributed in all groups. Over the long run, the groups tend to be counterbalanced with respect to an infinite number of biologic, psychological, economic, and social traits.

To demonstrate how random assignment is actually performed, we turn to another example. Suppose we have 15 children who are about to have a tonsillectomy and are interested in testing the effectiveness of two alternative nursing interventions with regard to the child's level of preoperative anxiety. One intervention focuses on structured information regarding the activities of the surgical team (procedural information); the other focuses on structured information regarding what the child will feel (sensation information). A third group will receive no special intervention. Five children will be in each of the three groups. Because there are three groups, we can no longer use the flip of a coin to decide the group to which an individual will be assigned. One possibility would be to write the names of the individuals on slips of paper, put the slips into a hat, and then draw names. The first five individuals whose names were drawn would be assigned

to group I, the second five would be assigned to group II, and the remaining five would be assigned to group III.

Pulling names from a hat involves considerable work, especially if there are many subjects. Researchers typically use a **table of random numbers** to facilitate the randomization process. A portion of such a table is reproduced in Table 8-1. A random number table is set up by using the digits from 0 to 9 in such a way that each number is equally likely to follow any other. These tables are often generated by computers. Going in any direction from any point in the table produces a random sequence.

In our example, we would number the 15 subjects from 1 to 15, as shown in the second column of Table 8-2, and then draw numbers between 1 and 15 from the random number table. A simple procedure for finding a starting point is to close your eyes and let your finger fall at some point on the table. For the sake of following the example, let us assume that we have followed this procedure and that the starting point is at number 52 as circled on Table 8-1. We can now move from that point in any direction in the table. Our task is to select the first five numbers that fall between 01 and 15. Let us move from the starting point to the right, looking at two-digit combinations to be sure to get numbers from 10 to 15. The next number to the right of 52 is 06. The person whose number is 06, that is, Nathan O., is assigned to group I. Moving along in the table, we find that the next number within the range of 01 to 15 is 11. Alana M., whose number is 11, is also assigned to group I. When we get to the end of the row, we move down to the next row, and so forth. To find numbers in the required range, we may have to bypass many numbers. The next three numbers we find are 01, 15, and 14. Thus, Kristina N., Charles T., and Taylor M. are all put into group I. The next five numbers between 01 and 15 that emerge in the random number table are used to assign five individuals to group II in the same fashion, as shown in the third column of Table 8-2. The remaining five

TABLE 8-1	Small Table of Random Digits

46 85 05 23 26	34 67 75 83 00	74 91 06 43 45
69 24 89 34 60	45 30 50 75 21	61 31 83 18 55
14 01 33 17 92	59 74 76 72 77	76 50 33 45 13
56 30 38 73 15	16 (52) 06 96 76	11 65 49 98 93
81 30 44 85 85	68 65 22 73 76	92 85 25 58 66
70 28 42 43 26	79 37 59 52 20	01 15 96 32 67
90 41 59 36 14	33 52 12 66 65	55 82 34 76 41
39 90 40 21 15	59 58 94 90 67	66 82 14 15 75
88 15 20 00 80	20 55 49 14 09	96 27 74 [8]2 57
45 13 46 35 45	59 40 47 20 59	43 94 75 16 80
70 01 41 50 21	41 29 06 73 12	71 85 71 59 57
37 23 93 32 95	05 87 00 11 19	92 78 42 63 40
18 63 73 75 09	82 44 49 90 05	04 92 17 37 01
05 32 78 21 62	20 24 78 17 59	45 19 72 53 32
95 09 66 79 46	48 46 08 55 58	15 19 11 87 82
43 25 38 41 45	60 83 32 59 83	01 29 14 13 49
80 85 40 92 79	43 52 90 63 18	38 38 47 47 61
80 08 87 70 74	88 72 25 67 36	66 16 44 94 31
80 89 07 80 02	94 81 33 19 00	54 15 58 34 36
93 12 81 84 64	74 45 79 05 61	72 84 81 18 34
82 47 42 55 93	48 54 53 52 47	18 61 91 36 74
53 34 24 42 76	75 12 21 17 24	74 62 77 37 07
82 64 12 28 20	92 90 41 31 41	32 39 21 97 63
13 57 41 72 00	69 90 26 37 42	78 46 42 25 01
29 59 38 86 27	94 97 21 15 98	62 09 53 67 87
86 88 75 50 87	19 15 20 00 23	12 30 28 07 83
44 98 91 68 22	36 02 40 08 67	76 37 84 16 05
93 39 94 55 47	94 45 87 42 84	05 04 14 98 07
52 16 29 02 86	54 15 83 42 43	46 97 83 54 82
04 73 72 10 31	75 05 19 30 29	47 66 56 43 82

Reprinted from *A Million Random Digits with 100,000 Normal Deviates.* New York: The Free Press, 1955. Used with permission of the Rand Corporation, Santa Monica, CA.

people are put into group III. Note that numbers that have already been used often reappear in the table before our randomization task is completed. For example, the number 15 appeared four times during the randomization procedure. This is perfectly normal because the numbers are random. After the first time a number appears and is used, subsequent appearances can be ignored.

It might be useful to look at the three groups to see if they are about equal with respect to one readily discernible characteristic,

that is, the gender of the subject. We started out with eight girls and seven boys in the total group. The gender breakdown of the three groups is presented in Table 8-3. As this table shows, the randomization procedure did a good job of allocating boys and girls about equally across the three groups. We must accept on faith the probability that other characteristics are fairly well distributed in the randomized groups as well.

One more step in the randomization process must be completed before the experiment begins.

TABLE 8-2	Example of Random Assignment Procedure	
NAME OF SUBJECT	NUMBER	GROUP ASSIGNMENT
Kristina N.	1	I
Chester Z.	2	III
Claire L.	3	III
Lauren C.	4	II
Rebecca C.	5	II
Nathan O.	6	I
Lindsey S.	7	III
Thomas N.	8	III
Chad C.	9	II
Rosanna D.	10	III
Alana M.	11	I
Emily B.	12	II
Alex H.	13	II
Taylor M.	14	I
Charles T.	15	I

Note that in the previous discussion, we did not state that the five subjects in group I would be assigned to the procedural information group. This is because it is a good strategy to assign groups to treatments as well as individuals to groups randomly. To continue with our example, we give the procedural information, sensation information, and control conditions the numbers 1, 2, and 3, respectively. Finding a new starting point in the random number table, we look for the numbers 1, 2, or 3. This time we can look at one digit at a time, because the range of values we are seeking does not include a two-digit number. Let us say that we start at number

TABLE 8-3	Breakdown of the Gender Composition of the Three Groups		
GENDER	GROUP I	GROUP II	GROUP III
Boys	3	2	2
Girls	2	3	3

8 in the ninth row of the table, which is indicated by a rectangle. Reading *down* this time, we find the number 1. We therefore assign group I to the procedural information condition. Further along in the same column we come to the number 3. Group III, therefore, is assigned to the second condition, sensation information, and the remaining group, group II, is assigned to the control condition.

In most cases, randomization involves the assignment of individual subjects to different groups on a random basis. However, an important alternative is **cluster randomization**, which involves randomly assigning groups or clusters of individuals to different treatment groups (Hauck, Gilliss, Donner, & Gortner, 1991). There are several advantages to such an approach, the most important of which is enhancing the feasibility of conducting a true experiment. Groups of patients who enter a hospital unit at the same time, or groups of patients from different medical practices, can be randomly assigned to a treatment condition as a unit—thus ruling out, in some situations, some practical impediments to randomization. This approach also reduces the possibility of **contamination** between two different treatments, that is, the comingling of subjects in the groups, which could reduce the effectiveness of the manipulation. The main disadvantages of cluster randomization are that the statistical analysis of data obtained through this approach is somewhat more complex, and sample size requirements are usually greater for a given level of accuracy.

Experimental Designs

There are numerous types of experimental design. The most commonly used designs are discussed in this section.

BASIC EXPERIMENTAL DESIGNS

At the beginning of this chapter, we described an example of testing hospitalized children's affective behavior after being cared for by nurses wearing different-colored uniforms. This exam-

TABLE 8-4 Before–After (Pretest–Posttest) Experimental Design		
	BEFORE TREATMENT	**AFTER TREATMENT**
Experimental Group	Pretest	Posttest
Control Group	Pretest	Posttest

ple illustrates a simple design that is sometimes referred to as an **after-only design** or a **posttest-only design** because data on the dependent variable are only collected once—after the experimental treatment has been introduced.

A second basic design is slightly more complex. Let us suppose that we are interested in investigating the effect on heart rate of being physically restrained by a Posey belt. We might choose to begin our experimentation with some subhuman species such as the rat. We decide to use an experimental scheme such as the one shown in Table 8-4. This design involves imposing restraint by Posey belt on one group of rats (the experimental group) while imposing no restraint on another (the control group). In this design, the dependent variable is measured at two points in time: before and after the experimental intervention. This scheme permits us to examine what changes in heart rate were produced as a result of being physically restrained, which is our independent variable. This design, because of its two measurement points, is referred to as a **before–after design** or a **pretest–posttest design**. In such designs, the initial measure of the dependent variable is often referred to as the **baseline measure**. (Some researchers involved in experimental research refer to the posttest measure of the dependent variable as the **outcome measure**—that is, the measure that captures the outcome of the experimental intervention.)

SOLOMON FOUR-GROUP DESIGN

When data are collected both before and after an intervention, the pretest (initial) measure

sometimes has the potential to distort the results. That is, the posttest measures may be affected not only by the treatment but also by exposure to the pretest. For example, if our intervention was a workshop to improve nurses' attitudes toward AIDS patients, a pretest attitudinal measure may in itself constitute a sensitizing treatment and could obscure an analysis of the workshop's effect. Such a situation might call for the **Solomon four-group design**, which consists of two experimental groups and two control groups. One experimental group and one control group would be administered the pretest and the other groups would not, thereby allowing the effects of the pretest measure and intervention to be segregated. Figure 8-1 illustrates the Solomon four-group design.

FACTORIAL DESIGN

The discussion to this point has considered designs in which the experimenter systematically

Group	Data Collection	
	Before	**After**
Experimental—with pretest	X	X
Experimental—without pretest		X
Control—with pretest	X	X
Control—without pretest		X

Figure 8-1. Solomon four-group experimental design.

varies or manipulates only one independent variable at a time. It is possible, however, to manipulate two or more variables simultaneously. Suppose that we were interested in comparing two therapeutic strategies for premature infants: one method involves tactile stimulation, and the second approach involves auditory stimulation. At the same time, we are interested in learning if the daily amount of stimulation is related to the progress of the infant. The dependent variables for the study will be various measures of infant development, such as weight gain, cardiac responsiveness, and so forth. Figure 8-2 illustrates the structure of this experiment.

This type of study, which is an experiment with a **factorial design**, permits the testing of multiple hypotheses in a single experiment. In this example, the three research questions being addressed are as follows:

1. Does auditory stimulation have a more beneficial effect on the development of premature infants than tactile stimulation?
2. Is the duration of stimulation (independent of type) related to infant development?
3. Is auditory stimulation most effective when linked to a certain dose and tactile stimulation most effective when coupled with a different dose?

The third question demonstrates a major strength of factorial designs: they permit us to evaluate not only **main effects** (effects resulting from experimentally manipulated variables, as exemplified in questions 1 and 2) but also **interaction effects** (effects resulting from combining the treatment methods). We may feel that it is insufficient to say that auditory stimulation is preferable to tactile stimulation (or vice versa) and that 45 minutes of stimulation per day is more effective than 15 minutes per day. Rather, it is how these two variables interact (how they behave in combination) that is of interest. Our results may indicate that 15 minutes of tactile stimulation and 45 minutes of auditory stimulation are the most beneficial treatments. We could *not* have obtained these results by conducting two separate experiments that manipulated only one independent variable and held the second one constant.

In factorial experiments, subjects are assigned at random to a specific combination of conditions. In the example that Figure 8-2 illustrates, the premature infants would be assigned randomly to one of the six cells. A **cell** in experimental research refers to a treatment condition; it is represented in a schematic diagram as a box (cell) in the design.

Figure 8-2 can also be used to define some design terminology that may be encountered in the research literature. The two independent variables in a factorial design are referred to as the **factors**. The type-of-stimulation variable is factor A and the amount-of-daily-exposure variable is factor B. Each factor must have two or more **levels** (if there were only one level, the factor would not be a variable). Level one of factor A is auditory and level two of factor A is tactile. When describing the dimensions of the design, researchers refer to the number of levels. The design in Figure 8-2 would be described as a 2 × 3 design: two levels in factor A times three levels in factor B. If a third source of stimulation, such as visual stimulation, were added, and if a daily dosage of 60 minutes were also added, the design would be referred to as a 3 × 4 design.

Factorial experiments can be performed with three or more independent variables (fac-

TYPE OF STIMULATION

		Auditory A1	Tactile A2
	15 Min. B1	A1 B1	A2 B1
DAILY EXPOSURE	30 Min. B2	A1 B2	A2 B2
	45 Min. B3	A1 B3	A2 B3

Figure 8-2. Factorial design.

tors). However, designs with more than three factors are rare because the analysis becomes complex and because the number of subjects required becomes prohibitive.

REPEATED MEASURES DESIGN

Thus far, we have described experimental studies in which the subjects who are randomly assigned to different treatments are different people. For instance, in the previous example, the infants exposed to 15 minutes of auditory stimulation were not the same infants as those exposed to the other five possible treatment conditions. A **repeated measures design** (sometimes called a **crossover design**) involves the exposure of the same subjects to more than one experimental treatment. This type of design has the advantage of ensuring the highest possible equivalence among subjects exposed to different conditions—the groups being compared are obviously equal with respect to age, weight, psychological state, and so on because they are composed of the same people.

In repeated measures experimental designs, the subjects are randomly assigned to different ordering of treatments. For example, if a repeated measures design were used to compare the effects of auditory and tactile stimulation on the development of premature infants, some infants would be randomly assigned to receive auditory stimulation first, whereas others would be randomly assigned to receive tactile stimulation first. In such a study, the three conditions for an experiment have been met: there is manipulation, randomization, and control—with subjects serving as their own control group.

Although repeated measures designs are extremely powerful, they are sometimes inappropriate for certain research questions because of the problems of **carry-over effects**. When subjects are exposed to two different treatments or conditions, they may be influenced in the second condition by their experience in the first condition. As one example, drug studies rarely use a repeated measures design because drug B administered after drug A is not neces-

sarily the same treatment as drug A administered after drug B.

RANDOMIZED CLINICAL TRIALS

Medical researchers and epidemiologists often evaluate an innovative treatment through the use of a randomized clinical trial (sometimes referred to simply as a clinical trial). **Clinical trials** typically use either a before–after or an after-only design. The term clinical trial, then, does not refer so much to a distinctive design as to an application of a design. Clinical trials always involve the testing of a clinical treatment; the random assignment of subjects of experimental and one or more control conditions; the collection of information on outcomes of the treatment from subjects in all groups, sometimes after a long period has elapsed; and generally, the use of a large and heterogeneous sample of subjects, frequently selected from multiple, geographically dispersed sites to ensure that the findings are not unique to a single setting.

When clinical trials involve the withholding of a potentially beneficial treatment from the control group or the administration of a potentially risky new treatment to the experimental group, researchers are sometimes reluctant to allocate subjects to groups on an equal basis. For example, for evaluating a promising new drug for the treatment of AIDS, researchers may randomly allocate 75% of the subjects to the experimental group and 25% to the control group. This unequal allocation has obvious advantages from an ethical point of view, but it is generally more costly because when subjects are not equally divided among treatment groups, the total number of subjects needed is greater to achieve the same level of power in performing statistical tests.

Advantages and Disadvantages of Experiments

Controlled experiments are often considered the ideal of science. In this section, we explore the reasons why experimental methods are held in high esteem and examine some of their limitations.

EXPERIMENTAL ADVANTAGES

True experiments are the most powerful method available to scientists for testing hypotheses of cause-and-effect relationships between variables. Because of its special controlling properties, the scientific experiment offers greater corroboration than any other research approach that, *if* the independent variable (e.g., diet, drug dosage, or teaching approach) is manipulated in a specified way, *then* certain consequences in the dependent variable (e.g., weight loss, recovery of health, or learning) may be expected to ensue. This "if . . . then" type of relationship is important to nursing and medical researchers because of its implications for prediction and control. The great strength of experiments, then, lies in the confidence with which causal relationships can be inferred.

Lazarsfeld (1955) identified three criteria for causality. The first criterion is temporal: a cause must precede an effect in time. If we were testing the hypothesis that saccharin causes bladder cancer, it would obviously be necessary to demonstrate that the subjects had not developed cancer before exposure to saccharin. The second requirement is that there be an empirical relationship between the presumed cause and the presumed effect. In the saccharin and cancer example, the researcher would have to demonstrate an association between the ingestion of saccharin and the presence of a carcinoma, that is, that a higher percentage of saccharin users than nonusers developed cancer. The final criterion for establishing a causal relationship is that the relationship cannot be explained as being the result of the influence of a third variable. Suppose, for instance, that people who use saccharin tend also to drink more coffee than nonusers of saccharin. There would then be a possibility that any empirical relationship between saccharin use and bladder cancer in humans reflects an underlying causal relationship between a substance in coffee and bladder cancer. It is particularly because of this third criterion that the experimental approach is so strong. Through the controls imposed by manipulation, comparison, and randomization, alternative explanations to a causal interpretation can often be ruled out or discredited.

EXPERIMENTAL DISADVANTAGES

Despite the overwhelming advantages of experimental research, this type of design has several limitations. First of all, there are a number of constraints that make an experimental approach impractical or impossible in some situations. These constraints are discussed later in this chapter.

Experiments are sometimes criticized for their artificiality. Part of the difficulty lies in the requirement for randomization and then equal treatment within groups. In ordinary life, the way in which we interact with people is not random. For example, within the nursing field, certain aspects of the patient (e.g., age, physical attractiveness, personality, or severity of illness) will cause us to modify our behavior and, hence, our care. The differences may be extremely subtle, but they undoubtedly are not random. Another aspect of experiments that is sometimes considered artificial by those espousing the naturalistic paradigm is the focus on only a handful of variables while attempting to hold all else constant. This requirement has been criticized as being reductionist and as artificially constraining human experience.

Another problem with experiments is the Hawthorne effect, which is a kind of placebo effect. The term is derived from a series of experiments conducted at the Hawthorne plant of the Western Electric Corporation in which various environmental conditions, such as light and working hours, were varied to determine their effects on worker productivity. Regardless of what change was introduced, that is, whether the light was made better or worse, productivity increased. Thus, it appears that the knowledge of being included in a study may be sufficient to cause people to change their behavior, thereby obscuring the effect of the variable of interest. In a hospital situation, the researcher might have to contend with a double Hawthorne effect. For example, if an experiment to investigate the effect of a new postoperative patient routine were conducted, nurses and hospital staff, as well as patients, might be aware of their participation in a study, and both groups might alter their actions accordingly. It is precisely for this reason

that double-blind experiments, in which neither the subjects nor those who administer the treatment know who is in the experimental or control group, are so powerful. Unfortunately, the double-blind approach is not feasible for some types of nursing research because nursing interventions are more difficult to disguise than medications.

In sum, despite the clearcut superiority of experiments in terms of their ability to test research hypotheses, they are subject to a number of limitations that make them difficult to apply to many real-world problems. Nevertheless, the

---

TABLE 8-5   Examples of Studies Using Experimental Designs

RESEARCH QUESTION	MANIPULATED VARIABLE	SUBJECTS
Design: After Only		
What is the effect of psyllium hydrophilic mucilloid (PHM) on diarrhea in enterally fed patients? (Belknap, Davidson, & Smith, 1997)	PHM versus no PHM	60 patients receiving newly initiated enteral feeding through feeding tube
Design: Before-After		
What are the effects of 8-week cancer support groups with and without adaptation coaching on the quality of relationships with significant others among women with early-stage breast cancer? (Samarel, Fawcett, & Tulman, 1997)	Coaching on adaptation versus no coaching	181 women with newly diagnosed early-stage breast cancer
Design: Factorial		
What are the effects of a patient's family structure on nurses' impressions of the patient and verbal responses to the patient's questions? (Ganong & Coleman, 1997)	Patients' family structure as portrayed in a video-taped interview with a patient	117 female nurses assigned to one of 8 family structure conditions (4 marital status × 2 parental status)
Design: Repeated Measures		
What is the effect of boomerang pillows on the respiratory capacity of hospitalized patients? (Roberts, Brittin, Cook, & deClifford, 1994)	Placement of patients on boomerang pillows versus straight pillows	42 patients exposed to both types of pillow in random order

fact that experimental conditions may be difficult to establish does not mean that all attempts to achieve them should be abandoned.

Research Example of an Experimental Design

Nurse researchers are increasingly using experimental designs to test their hypotheses. Table 8-5 summarizes some recent examples. An experimental study described in more detail follows.

Hastings-Tolsma, Yucha, Tompkins, Robson, and Szeverenyi (1993) used an interesting design to study differences in tissue response to warm versus cold applications to infiltrated intravenous sites. The researchers also wanted to investigate the effect of warm versus cold applications on the resolution of infiltrated solutions of three different levels of osmolarity (½ saline, normal saline, and 3% saline). The dependent variables included measures of pain intensity, erythema and induration, and interstitial fluid volume.

The sample consisted of 18 healthy adults. Six subjects were sequentially assigned to each of the three different solutions, in order of recruitment into the study. The experimental procedure (i.e., infiltration, application of a thermostated pad, and measurements of the dependent variable) was performed twice on each subject—once with a cold application (0°C) and once with a warm application (43°C), on alternate arms. Randomization was used to determine which application would be done first (cold or warm) and which arm would be used first (left or right). Measurements of pain intensity, surface induration, and fluid volume were obtained three times: at 12, 42, and 72 minutes after infiltration.

Given the complexity of the design and measures used, the study yielded many findings. For example, the researchers found that the cold versus warm applications did not yield any significant differences in terms of pain intensity or surface induration, but there were differences in interstitial fluid volume. For all three solutions, the volume was less with warm than with cold application. A difference in pain intensity by solution was found, with the highest pain ratings resulting in the 3% saline condition. There were no interaction effects between type of solution, warm versus cold application, and time of measurement on pain intensity.

QUASI-EXPERIMENTAL RESEARCH

Research that uses a quasi-experimental design often looks much like an experiment. **Quasi-experiments**, like true experiments, involve the manipulation of an independent variable, that is, the institution of an experimental treatment. However, quasi-experimental designs lack at least one of the other two properties that characterize true experiments: randomization or a control group.

Quasi-Experimental Designs

The basic difficulty with the quasi-experimental approach is its weakness, relative to experiments, in allowing us to make causal inferences. The problems inherent in quasi-experiments are most easily discussed using examples of specific designs. Before presenting these examples, however, it is useful to introduce some notation to facilitate our discussion.* Figure 8-3 presents a symbolic representation of a pretest–posttest experimental design, identical to the design shown in Table 8-4. According to the notation used in Figure 8-3, R means that there has been a random assignment to separate treatment groups; O represents an observation, that is, the collection of data on the dependent variable; and X stands for the exposure of a group to an experimental treatment. Thus, the top line in Figure 8-3 represents the experimental group that has had subjects randomly assigned to it

---

*The notation, as well as most of the concepts in this section, are derived from Campbell and Stanley's (1963) classic monograph.

R = Randomization   R O_1 X O_2
O = Observation or measurement
X = Treatment or intervention R O_1 O_2

Figure 8-3. Symbolic representation of a pretest–posttest (before–after) experimental design.

(R), has had both a pretest (O_1) and a posttest (O_2), and has been exposed to the experimental treatment of interest (X). The second row in the figure represents the control group, which differs from the experimental group only by the absence of exposure to the experimental treatment. We are now equipped to examine a few quasi-experimental designs.

NONEQUIVALENT CONTROL GROUP DESIGNS

The most frequently used quasi-experimental design is the **nonequivalent control group design**, which involves an experimental treatment and two or more groups of subjects. Let us consider an example. Suppose that we wished to study the effect of introducing primary nursing as the method of delivering nursing care on nursing staff morale. The system is being implemented in a 600-bed hospital in a large metropolitan area. Because the new system of nursing care delivery is being implemented throughout the hospital, randomization is not possible. Therefore, we decide to find another hospital with similar characteristics (size, geographic location, and the like) that is not instituting primary nursing. We decide to collect baseline data by administering a staff morale questionnaire in both hospitals before the change is made (the pretest). We would again collect data on nurses' morale after the system is installed in the experimental hospital (the posttest).

Figure 8-4 depicts this study symbolically. The top row is our experimental (primary

O_1 X O_2
O_1 O_2

Figure 8-4. Nonequivalent control group pretest–posttest design (quasi-experimental).

nursing) hospital; the second row is the hospital using traditional nursing. A comparison of this diagram with the one in Figure 8-3 shows that they are identical, *except* that subjects have not been randomly assigned to treatment groups in the second diagram. The design in Figure 8-4 is the weaker of the two because *it can no longer be assumed that the experimental and comparison groups are equal.* Because of the inability to randomize subjects, our study is quasi-experimental rather than truly experimental. The design is, nevertheless, a strong one because the collection of pretest data allows us to determine whether the groups were initially similar in terms of their morale. If the morale of the two groups is very different at the start, our interpretation of the posttest data will be difficult, although there are statistical procedures that can help. If the comparison and experimental groups respond similarly, on the average, on the pretest questionnaire, then we can be relatively confident that any posttest differences in self-reported morale were the result of introducing the experimental method of nursing care. (Note that in quasi-experiments, the term **comparison group** is generally used in lieu of *control group* to refer to the group against which outcomes in the treatment group are evaluated.)

Suppose that we had not thought to or had been unable to collect pretest data before the new method of nursing care delivery was introduced. The resulting study could be diagrammed to show the scheme in Figure 8-5. This design has a flaw that is difficult to remedy. We have no basis on which to judge the initial equivalence of the two nursing staffs. If we find that, at the posttest, the morale of the experimental hospital staff is lower than that of the control hospital staff, can we conclude that the new method of delivering care *caused*

X   O
             O

Figure 8-5. Nonequivalent control group posttest-only design (preexperimental).

a decline in staff morale? There could be several alternative explanations for the posttest differences. In particular, it might be that the morale of the employees in the two hospitals differed even at the outset. Campbell and Stanley (1963), in fact, would call the design shown in Figure 8-5 **preexperimental** rather than quasi-experimental because of its essentially irreconcilable weaknesses. Thus, although quasi-experiments lack some of the controlling properties inherent in true experiments, the hallmark of the quasi-experimental approach is the effort to introduce other controls to compensate for the absence of either the randomization or control group component.

TIME SERIES DESIGNS

The designs reviewed in the previous section illustrate studies in which a control group was used but randomization was not, but some designs have neither. In some studies in which both characteristics are absent, there are inherent weaknesses that jeopardize the validity of the findings. However, there are several designs that offer the researcher some measure of protection against these problems.

Let us suppose that a hospital decides to adopt a requirement that all its nurses accrue a certain number of continuing education units before being considered for a promotion or raise. The nursing administrators want to assess some of the positive and negative consequences of this mandate. Some of the indicators they might examine include turnover rate, absentee rate, qualifications of new employee applicants, number of raises and promotions awarded, and so on. For the purposes of this example, let us assume that there is no other comparable hospital that could reasonably serve as a comparison for this study. In such a case, the only kind of comparison that could

be made is a before–after contrast. If the requirement were inaugurated in January, one could compare the turnover rate, for example, for the 3-month period before the new rule with the turnover rate for the subsequent 3-month period. The schematic representation of such a study is shown in Figure 8-6.

Although this design appears logical and straightforward, there actually are numerous problems with it. What if either of the 3-month periods is atypical, apart from the new regulation? What about the effects of any other hospital rules inaugurated during the same period? What about the effects of external factors that influence employment patterns, such as employment opportunities at other nearby hospitals? The design in Figure 8-6 offers no way of controlling for any of these problems. This design is also preexperimental because it fails to control for many possible extraneous factors.

A design that can assist us in this case is known as the **time series design** (sometimes referred to as the **interrupted time series design**) and is diagrammed in Figure 8-7. The basic notion underlying the time series design is the collection of information over an extended period and the introduction of an experimental treatment during the course of the data collection period. In the figure, O_1 through O_4 represent four separate instances of observation or data collection on a dependent variable before treatment; X represents the treatment (the introduction of the independent variable); and O_5 through O_8 represent four posttreatment observations. In our present example, O_1 might be the number of nurses who left the hospital in January through March in the year before the new continuing education rule, O_2 the number of resignations in April through June, and so forth. After the rule is implemented, data on turnover are similarly col-

O_1 X O_2

Figure 8-6. One-group pretest–posttest pie (experimental).

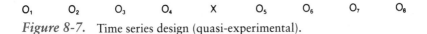

O_1 O_2 O_3 O_4 X O_5 O_6 O_7 O_8

Figure 8-7. Time series design (quasi-experimental).

lected for four consecutive 3-month periods, giving us observations O_5 through O_8.

Even though the time series design does not eliminate all the problems of interpreting changes in turnover rate, the extended time perspective immensely strengthens our ability to attribute any change to the experimental manipulation, which in this case is the continuing education requirement. Figure 8-8 attempts to demonstrate why this is so. The two diagrams (*A* and *B*) in the figure show two possible outcome patterns for the eight measures of nurse turnover. The vertical dotted line in the center represents the time at which

the continuing education rule was implemented. Both *A* and *B* reflect a feature that is common to most time series studies, and this is the fluctuation from one observation or measurement to another. These fluctuations are, of course, perfectly normal. One would not expect that, if 48 nurses resigned from a hospital in 1 year, the resignations would be spaced evenly during the course of the year with exactly four resignations per month. It is precisely because of these fluctuations that the design shown in Figure 8-6, with only one observation before and after the experimental treatment, is so weak.

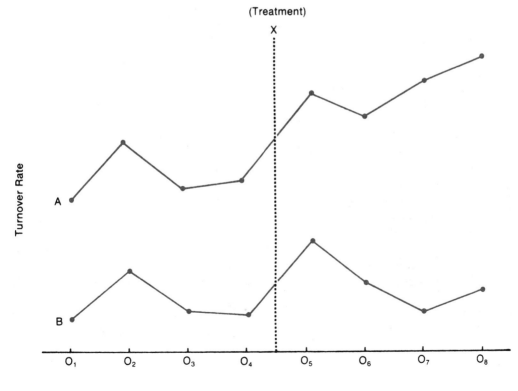

Figure 8-8. Two possible time series outcome patterns.

Figure 8-9. Time series non-equivalent control group design (quasi-experimental).

$$O_1 \quad O_2 \quad O_3 \quad O_4 \quad X \quad O_5 \quad O_6 \quad O_7 \quad O_8$$

$$O_1 \quad O_2 \quad O_3 \quad O_4 \quad\quad O_5 \quad O_6 \quad O_7 \quad O_8$$

Let us compare the kind of interpretations that can be made for the outcomes reflected in Figure 8-8*A* and *B*. In both cases, the number of resignations increases between O_4 and O_5, that is, immediately after the introduction of the continuing education requirement. In *B*, however, the number of resignations falls at O_6 and continues to decrease at O_7. The increase at O_5, therefore, looks similar to other apparently haphazard fluctuations in the turnover rate at other periods. Therefore, it probably would be erroneous to conclude that the treatment had an effect on resignations. In *A*, on the other hand, the number of resignations increases at O_5 and remains relatively high for all subsequent periods of data collection. It is true, of course, that there may be other explanations for a change in turnover rate from one year to the next. The time series design, however, does permit us to rule out the possibility that the data reflect an unstable measurement of resignations made at only two points in time. If we had used the design in Figure 8-6 to study this problem, it would have been analogous to obtaining the measurements at O_4 and O_5 of Figure 8-8 only. The outcomes in both *A* and *B* look similar at these two points in time. Yet the use of a broader time perspective leads us to draw different conclusions about the nature of the changes from one pattern of outcomes to the next.

A particularly powerful quasi-experimental design results when the time series and nonequivalent control group designs are combined, as diagrammed in Figure 8-9. In the example just described, **a time series nonequivalent con-**trol group design would involve the collection of data over an extended period from both the hospital introducing the continuing education mandate and another hospital not imposing the mandate. This use of information from another hospital with similar characteristics would make any inferences regarding the effects of the mandate more convincing because trends influenced by external factors would presumably be observed in both groups.

Numerous variations on the simple time series design are possible and are being used by nurse researchers. For example, additional evidence regarding the effects of a treatment can be achieved by instituting the treatment at several different points in time, strengthening the treatment over time, or instituting the treatment at one point in time and then **withdrawing** the treatment at a later point, sometimes with **reinstitution of treatment**. These three designs are diagrammed in Figures 8-10 through 8-12. Clinical nurse researchers are often in a good position to use such time series designs because measures of patient functioning are generally routinely made at multiple points over an extended period.

Advantages and Disadvantages of the Quasi-Experimental Approach

The great strength of quasi-experiments lies in their practicality, feasibility, and, to a certain extent, generalizability. In the real world, it is often impractical, if not impossible, to conduct true experiments. A good deal of the research that is of interest to nurses occurs in natural

$$O_1 \quad O_2 \quad X \quad O_3 \quad O_4 \quad X \quad O_5 \quad O_6 \quad X \quad O_7 \quad O_8$$

Figure 8-10. Time series with multiple institutions of treatment (quasi-experimental).

$$O_1 \quad O_2 \quad X \quad O_3 \quad O_4 \quad X+1 \quad O_5 \quad O_6 \quad X+2 \quad O_7 \quad O_8$$

Figure 8-11. Time series with intensified treatment (quasi-experimental).

settings. Frequently, it is difficult to deliver an innovative treatment to only half of a group, and randomization may be even less feasible. The inability to randomize, or even to secure a control group, need not force a researcher to abandon all hopes of conducting a rigorous investigation. Quasi-experimental designs are research plans that introduce some controls over extraneous variables when full experimental control is lacking.

It is precisely because the control inherent in true experiments *is* absent in quasi-experiments that the researcher needs to be acquainted with the weaknesses of this approach. When a researcher uses a quasi-experimental design, there may be several **rival hypotheses** competing with the experimental manipulation as explanations for observed results. Take as an example the case in which we administer certain medications to a group of babies whose mothers are heroin addicts to assess whether this treatment results in a weight gain in these typically low-birthweight babies. If we use no comparison group or if we use a nonequivalent control group and then observe a weight gain, we must ask the questions: Is it *plausible* that some other factor caused or influenced the gain? Is it *plausible* that pretreatment differences between the experimental and comparison groups of babies resulted in differential gain? Is it *plausible* that the babies could have gained the weight simply as a result of maturation? If the answer is "yes" to any of these questions, then the inferences we can make about the effect of the experimental treatment are weakened considerably. The plausibility of any one threat cannot, of course, be answered unequivocally. It is generally a situation in which judgment must be exercised. It is because quasi-experiments ultimately depend in part on human judgment, rather than on more objective criteria, that the validity of cause-and-effect inferences can be challenged. We must hasten to add that the quality of a study is not necessarily a function of its design. There are many excellent quasi-experimental investigations as well as weak experiments.

Research Example of a Quasi-Experimental Study

Table 8-6 briefly summarizes the characteristics of several studies conducted by nurse researchers in which a quasi-experimental or pre-experimental design was used. A more detailed description of a quasi-experimental study follows. It may be helpful to consult the full journal article for more information about the research design.

Pickler, Higgins, and Crummette (1993) used a strong quasi-experimental design to examine the effects of nonnutritive sucking on the physiologic and behavioral stress reactions of preterm infants at early bottle feedings. The sample consisted of 20 preterm infants, 10 of whom were provided nonnutritive sucking for 5 minutes before and 5 minutes after an early bottle feeding. The 10 infants who served as a comparison group (and who received no nonnutritive sucking) were matched to the experimental group on the basis of gender, race, birthweight, and gestational age.

Physiologic stress was measured in terms of heart rate and oxygen saturation rate. For

$$O_1 \quad O_2 \quad X \quad O_3 \quad O_4 \quad (-X) \quad O_5 \quad O_6 \quad X \quad O_7 \quad O_8$$

Figure 8-12. Time series with withdrawn and reinstituted treatment (quasi-experimental).

TABLE 8-6   Examples of Studies Using Quasi-Experimental and Preexperimental Designs

RESEARCH QUESTION	MANIPULATED VARIABLE	SUBJECTS
Design: One Group, Before–After (Preexperimental)		
Is a special educational program for nurses concerning causes of noise effective in decreasing noise levels in an intensive care unit for infants? (Elander & Hellstrom, 1995)	Nurses' participation in the special program	52 nurses
Design: Nonequivalent Control Group, After-Only (Preexperimental)		
How do four different methods of securing endotracheal tubes in orally intubated patients compare in terms of tube stability, facial skin integrity, and patient satisfaction? (Kaplow & Bookbinder, 1994)	Method of securing endotracheal tubes (Lillihie, harness, Comfit, Dale, and SecureEasy)	120 intensive care unit patients (30 per method)
Design: Nonequivalent Control Group, Before–After (Quasi-Experimental)		
Does participation in the Cardiovascular Health Education Program (CHEP) improve adolescents' cardiovascular health knowledge? (MacDonald, 1995)	Participation versus nonparticipation in CHEP	22 adolescents in CHEP; 12 in control group
Design: Time Series (Quasi-Experimental)		
What is the effect of 12 weeks of low-impact aerobic exercise program on fatigue, aerobic fitness, and disease activity measures in people with rheumatoid arthritis? (Neuberger et al., 1997)	Participation in the exercise program	32 people with rheumatoid arthritis
Design: Time Series Nonequivalent Control Group (Quasi-Experimental)		
What are the rates of absenteeism and turnover of nurses working in a nurse-managed special care unit (SCU) compared with that of nurses working in a traditional intensive care unit (CUI)? (Song, Daly, Rudy, Douglas, & Dyer, 1997)	Type of unit (ICU versus SCU)	Nurses on the two units over a 4-year period

each, mean rates were computed for three periods: the 5 minutes before feeding, the first 5 minutes of bottle feeding, and the 5 minutes after total feeding. Behavioral stress was mea-

sured by observation of the infants' behavioral state at four points: immediately before the 5-minute prefeeding period, immediately after the initiation of bottle feeding, immediately after the conclusion of bottle feeding, and immediately after the conclusion of the 5-minute postfeeding period.

The results indicated that infants who received nonnutritive sucking before and after bottle feedings were more likely to be in a quiescent behavior state 5 minutes after feeding. However, there were no treatment, time, or time × treatment interaction effects for heart rate. Oxygen saturation was unaffected by the treatment but did change between different measurements in time.

NONEXPERIMENTAL RESEARCH

Many research problems do not lend themselves to an experimental or quasi-experimental design, that is, to experimental manipulation of the independent variable. Let us suppose, for example, that we were interested in studying the effect of widowhood on physical and psychological functioning. We could use as our dependent variables various physiologic and medical measures, such as blood pressure, heart rate, and so on, as well as standard psychological diagnostic tests, such as the Center for Epidemiological Studies Depression Scale. Our independent variable is widowhood versus nonwidowhood. Clearly, we would be unable to manipulate widowhood. Spouses become widows or widowers by a process that is neither random nor subject, ethically, to research control. Thus, we must proceed by taking two groups (widows and nonwidows) as they naturally occur and comparing them in terms of psychological and physical well-being.

Reasons for Undertaking Nonexperimental Research

Many research studies involving human subjects, including most nursing research investigations, are nonexperimental in nature. There are many different reasons for choosing a nonexperimental approach. First, a vast number of human characteristics are inherently not subject to experimental manipulation (e.g., blood type, personality, health beliefs, medical diagnosis), and thus the effects of these characteristics on some phenomenon of interest cannot be studied experimentally.

A second issue is that in nursing research, as in other fields in which human behavior is of primary interest, numerous variables could technically be manipulated but should not be manipulated for ethical reasons. If the nature of the independent variable is such that its manipulation could cause physical or mental harm to subjects, then that variable should not be controlled experimentally. For example, if we were interested in studying the effect of prenatal care on infant mortality, it would be unethical to provide such care to one group of pregnant women but deliberately deprive a second group. What we would need to do is locate a naturally occurring group of mothers-to-be who have not received prenatal care. The birth outcomes of these women could then be compared with those of a group of women who had received appropriate care. The problem, however, is that the two groups of women are likely to differ in terms of a number of other characteristics, such as age, education, nutrition, and health, any of which individually or in combination could have an impact on infant mortality, independent of the absence or presence of prenatal care. This is precisely why experimental designs are so strong in demonstrating cause-and-effect relationships.

Third, there are many research situations in which it is simply not practical to conduct a true experiment. Constraints might involve insufficient time, lack of administrative approval, excessive inconvenience to patients or staff, or lack of adequate funds.

Finally, there are some research questions for which an experimental design is not at all appropriate. This is especially true for descriptive quantitative studies, which seek to capture the characteristics, prevalence, or intensity of phenomena, and, as we discuss in Chapter 10, almost all qualitative studies are nonexperimental because researchers conducting in-depth qualitative studies typically want as little disturbance as possible to the people or groups they are studying. Manipulation is neither attempted nor considered desirable; the emphasis is on the natural everyday world of humans.

Types of Nonexperimental Research

Essentially, there are two broad classes of nonexperimental research: correlational (ex post facto) and descriptive. The characteristics of each are discussed in this section.

EX POST FACTO
OR CORRELATIONAL RESEARCH

The first broad class of nonexperimental research is **ex post facto research**. The literal translation of the Latin term ex post facto is "from after the fact." This expression is meant to indicate that the research in question has been conducted *after* the variations in the independent variable have occurred in the natural course of events. Ex post facto research attempts to understand relationships among phenomena as they naturally occur, without any researcher intervention.

Ex post facto research is sometimes referred to as **correlational research**.* The precise meaning of correlational will become clearer when we have covered some statistical concepts. Basically, a **correlation** is an interrelationship or association between two variables, that is, a tendency for variation in one variable to be related to variation in another. For example, in

human adults, height and weight tend to be correlated because there is a tendency for taller people to weigh more than shorter people.

Ex post facto or correlational studies often share a number of structural and design characteristics with experimental, quasi-experimental, and preexperimental research. If we use the notation scheme outlined in the previous section to represent symbolically the hypothetical study of the effects of widowhood, we find that it bears a strong resemblance to the nonequivalent control group posttest-only design. Both designs are presented in Figure 8-13. As these diagrams show, the preexperimental design is distinguished from the ex post facto study only by the presence of an *X*, the manipulation of an experimental treatment.

The basic purpose of ex post facto research is essentially the same as that of experimental research: to understand relationships among variables. The most important distinction between the two is the difficulty of inferring *causal* relationships in ex post facto studies because of the lack of manipulative control of the independent variables. In experiments, the investigator makes a prediction that a deliberate variation in *X*, the independent variable, will result in the occurrence of some event or behavior, *Y* (the dependent variable). For example, the researcher predicts that if some medication is administered, then patient improvement will ensue. The experimenter has direct control over the *X*; the experimental treatment can be administered to some and withheld from others, and subjects can be randomly assigned to an experimental group and a control group.

In ex post facto research, on the other hand, the investigator does not have control of the independent variable because it has already occurred. The examination of the independent variable—the presumed causative factor—is done after the fact. As a result, attempts to draw any cause-and-effect conclusions are often problematic. For example, we might hypothesize that there is a correlation between the number of cigarettes smoked and

---

*The use of the terms *ex post facto* and *correlational* is not entirely consistent in the literature on research methods. Some authors use ex post facto to refer to all nonexperimental research that examines relationships among variables; others use the term correlational for this purpose. Still other researchers prefer to make a distinction between whether the intent of the study is causal and comparative (ex post facto) or merely descriptive of relationships (correlational). In general, the terms are used roughly equivalently in this chapter to designate studies of relationships among variables when the independent variable is not under the researcher's control.

```
GROUP A        X              O        Nonequivalent control group
               ------------------      (preexperimental) design
GROUP B                       O

GROUP A                       O                                          Figure 8-13. Schematic diagram
               ------------------      Ex post facto design             comparing nonequivalent control
GROUP B                       O                                         group and ex post facto designs.
```

Figure 8-13. Schematic diagram comparing nonequivalent control group and ex post facto designs.

the incidence of lung cancer, and empirical data would most likely corroborate this expectation. The inference we would like to make based on observed relationships is that cigarette smoking *causes* cancer. This kind of inference, however, is a fallacy that has been called *post hoc ergo propter* ("after this, therefore caused by this"). The fallacy lies in the assumption that one thing has caused another merely because it occurred chronologically before the other.

To illustrate why such a cause-and-effect conclusion might not be warranted, let us assume (strictly for the sake of an example) that there is a preponderance of cigarette smokers in urban areas, but people living in rural areas are largely nonsmokers. Let us further assume that bronchogenic carcinoma is actually caused by the poor environmental conditions typically associated with cities and industrial areas. Therefore, we would be incorrect to conclude that cigarette smoking causes lung cancer, despite the strong relationship that might be shown to exist between the two variables. This is because there is *also* a strong relationship between cigarette smoking and the "real" causative agent, living in a polluted environment. (Of course, the cigarette smoking and lung cancer studies in reality have been replicated in so many different places with so many different groups of people that causal inferences are increasingly justified.) This hypothetical example illustrates a famous research dictum: *Correlation does not prove causation.* That is, the mere existence of a relationship—even a strong one—between two variables is not enough to warrant the conclusion that one variable has caused the other.

Although correlational studies are inherently weaker than experimental studies in elucidating

cause-and-effect relationships, different designs offer different degrees of supportive evidence. In the previous chapter, we discussed two types of ex post facto designs—retrospective and prospective. Prospective designs tend to be considerably stronger than retrospective designs with regard to causal inferences because the researcher does at least go forward in time from the independent to the dependent variable. However, the researcher can sometimes strengthen a retrospective design by taking certain steps. For example, one type of retrospective design, referred to as a **case-control design**, involves the comparison of cases or subjects with a certain illness or condition (e.g., lung cancer victims) with controls (e.g., people without lung cancer). To the degree that the researcher can demonstrate similarity between cases and controls with regard to extraneous traits, the inferences regarding the presumed cause of the disease are enhanced.

Researchers interested in testing theories of causation based on nonexperimental data are increasingly using a technique known as **path analysis**. Using sophisticated statistical procedures, the researcher tests a hypothesized causal chain among a set of independent variables, mediating variables, and a dependent variable. Path analytic procedures, which are described more fully in Chapter 20, allow researchers to test whether nonexperimental data conform sufficiently to the underlying model to justify causal inferences.

DESCRIPTIVE RESEARCH

The second broad class of nonexperimental studies is **descriptive research**. The purpose of descriptive studies is to observe, describe, and document aspects of a situation as it naturally occurs and sometimes to serve as a starting point for hypothesis generation or theory development.

Although there is considerable emphasis in scientific research on understanding what causes behaviors, conditions, and situations, researchers can often do little more than describe existing relationships without fully comprehending the complex causal pathways that exist. Thus, many of our research problems are often cast in noncausal terms. We ask, for example, whether men are less likely than women to achieve a bonding with their newborn infants, not whether a particular configuration of sex chromosomes has *caused* differences in parental attachment. As in the case of other types of ex post facto research, the investigator engaged in a **descriptive correlational study** has no control over the independent variables. That is, there is no experimental manipulation or random assignment to groups. However, unlike other types of ex post facto studies—such as the cigarette smoking and lung cancer investigations—the aim of descriptive correlational research is to describe the relationship among variables rather than to infer cause-and-effect relationships.

Other descriptive studies are undertaken to describe what exists in terms of frequency of occurrence (or its presence versus absence) rather than to describe the relationship between variables. For example, an investigator may wish to determine the health care and nutritional practices of pregnant teenagers. **Univariate descriptive studies** are not necessarily focused on only one variable. For example, a researcher might be interested in women's experiences during menopause. The investigation might describe the frequency with which various symptoms are reported, the average age at menopause, the percentage of women seeking formal health care, and the percentage of women using medications to alleviate symptoms. There are multiple variables in this study, but the primary purpose is to describe

the status of each and not to relate them to one another.

Advantages and Disadvantages of Ex Post Facto or Correlational Research

As mentioned earlier, the quality of a study is not necessarily related to its approach; there are many excellent nonexperimental studies as well as seriously flawed experiments and quasi-experiments. Nevertheless, nonexperimental studies suffer from several drawbacks.

DISADVANTAGES OF EX POST FACTO OR CORRELATIONAL RESEARCH

As already noted, the major disadvantage of nonexperimental research is that, relative to experimental and quasi-experimental research, it is weak in its ability to reveal causal relationships. There is a continuum of design types in terms of capacity to reveal causal relationships. True experimental designs are at one end of that continuum, and retrospective correlational research is at the other, as shown in Figure 8-14; descriptive studies are not included on this continuum because they are not intended to elucidate cause-and-effect relationships.

Ex post facto studies are in most instances susceptible to the possibility of faulty interpretation. This situation stems in large part from the fact that in ex post facto studies, the researcher works with preexisting groups that were not formed by a random process but rather by what might be termed a self-selecting process. Kerlinger (1986) offered the following description of **self-selection**:

> Self-selection occurs when the members of the groups being studied are in the groups, in part, because they differentially possess traits or characteristics extraneous to the research problem, characteristics that possibly influence or are otherwise related to the variables of the research problem. (p. 349)

Strongest Design					Weakest Design
True experimental design	Quasi-experimental design	Pre-experimental design	Path analytic design	Prospective correlational design	Retrospective correlational design

Figure 8-14. Continuum of research designs with respect to power to elucidate causal relationships.

As in the case of quasi-experimental or pre-experimental research, the researcher doing a correlational study cannot assume that the groups being compared were similar before the occurrence of the independent variable. Because of this fact, preexisting differences may be a plausible alternative explanation for any observed differences on the dependent variable of interest.

To illustrate this problem, let us consider a hypothetical study in which the researcher is interested in examining the relationship between type of nursing program (the independent variable) and job satisfaction after graduation. If the investigator finds that diploma school graduates are more satisfied with their work than baccalaureate graduates 1 year after graduation, the conclusion that the diploma school program provides better preparation for actual work situations and, hence, leads to increased satisfaction may or may not be accurate. The students in the two programs undoubtedly differed to begin with in terms of a number of important characteristics, such as personality, career goals, personal values, and so forth. That is, students self-selected themselves into one of the two programs; it may be the selection traits themselves that resulted in different job expectations and satisfactions.

The difficulty of interpreting correlational findings stems in large part from the fact that, in the real world, behaviors, states, attitudes, and characteristics are interrelated (correlated) in complex ways. Another example may help to make the problems of interpreting ex post

facto results more clear. Let us suppose we were interested in studying differences in the level of depression of cancer patients who do or do not have adequate social support (i.e., adequate assistance and emotional sustenance through a social network). Our independent variable in this hypothetical study is social support, and our dependent variable is level of depression. Let us say that we find that the patients without social support are significantly more depressed than the patients whose social support is adequate. We could interpret this finding to mean that people's emotional states are influenced by the adequacy of their social supports. This relationship is diagrammed in Figure 8-15A. There are, however, alternative explanations for the findings. Perhaps there is a third variable that influences *both* social support and depression, such as the patients' family configuration (e.g., whether they are married or have children). That is, it may be that the availability or quantity of significant others is a powerful influence on how depressed cancer patients feel *and* on the quality of their social support. This set of relationships is diagramed in Figure 8-15B. A third possibility may be reversed causality, as shown in Figure 8-15C. Depressed cancer patients may find it more difficult to elicit needed social support from others than patients who are more cheerful or sociable. In this interpretation, it is the person's depression that causes the amount of received social support, and not the other way around. Undoubtedly, the reader will be able to invent other alternatives. The point is that interpretations of most ex post facto results

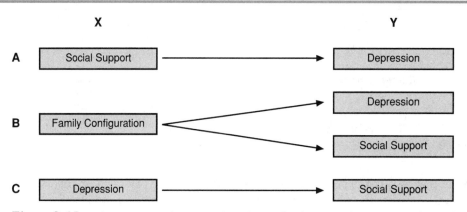

Figure 8-15.   Alternative explanations for relationship between depression and social support in cancer patients.

should be considered tentative, particularly if the research has no theoretical basis.

ADVANTAGES OF EX POST FACTO OR CORRELATIONAL RESEARCH

Earlier, we discussed constraints that limit the possibility of applying experimental designs to some research problems. Ex post facto or correlational research will continue to play a crucial role in nursing, medical, and social science research precisely because many of the interesting problems to be addressed in those fields are not amenable to experimentation.

Despite our emphasis on causality in relationships, it has already been noted that in some kinds of research, such as descriptive research, a full understanding of causal networks may not be important. Furthermore, if the study is testing a hypothesis that has been deduced from an established theory, determining the direction of causation may be relatively straightforward, especially if powerful techniques such as path analysis have been used.

Correlational research is often an efficient and effective means of collecting a large amount of data about a problem area. For example, it would be possible to collect extensive information about the health histories and eating habits of a large number of individuals. Researchers could then examine which health

problems are correlated with which diets. Thus, they could discover a large number of interrelationships in a relatively short amount of time. By contrast, an experimenter usually looks at only a few variables at a time. For example, one experiment might be devoted to manipulating foods high in cholesterol to observe the effects on certain biophysiologic measures, and another experiment could manipulate protein consumption.

Finally, ex post facto research is often strong in realism and therefore has an intrinsic appeal for the solution of many practical problems. Unlike many experimental studies, ex post facto research is seldom criticized for its artificiality.

Research Example of Nonexperimental Research

We have used a number of hypothetical research problems to help explain many of the points made in this chapter. Table 8-7 presents a brief description of several actual nonexperimental studies that have been conducted by nurse researchers. An additional nonexperimental study is described in greater detail below.

Estok, Rudy, Kerr, and Menzel (1993) studied menstrual responses (e.g., duration and amount of menses) to women's running. Their sample consisted of 146 women aged 20 to 36 years who were grouped according to their level of running intensity: group I, nonrunning women who did little exercise; group II, women who ran 1 to 14.9 miles per week; group III, women who ran 15 to 30 miles per week; and group IV, women who ran more than 30 miles per week. Menstrual and running data were recorded by the subjects in a Menstrual/Exercise Diary over 4 months or three menstrual cycles. The subjects also tested themselves for the presence of luteinizing hormone with the self-test, OvuQuick.

The four groups were found to be similar in terms of various background characteristics, such as age, height, weight, ethnicity, education, and age of menarche. The results indicated that the nonrunners had significantly

TABLE 8-7 Examples of Nonexperimental Studies	
RESEARCH QUESTION	**STUDY PARTICIPANTS**
Design: Correlational, Retrospective	
What is the role of self-esteem, depression, and learned helplessness in predicting the health practices of homeless women? (Flynn, 1997)	122 homeless women from six homeless shelters
Design: Correlational, Prospective	
What are the factors that best predict functional status after percutaneous transluminal coronary angioplasty (PTCA)? (Fitzgerald, Zlotnick, & Kolodner, 1996)	135 adults who underwent PTCA, followed for 12 months after the PTCA procedure
Design: Case-Control	
Can assaultive patients be distinguished from nonassaultive patients on the basis of behavioral assessments or sociodemographic variables? (Lanza, Kayne, Pattison, Hicks, & Islam, 1996)	36 patients who were assaultive (cases) and 36 patients randomly selected from patients who were not assaultive (controls)
Design: Descriptive Correlational	
What are the types and intensity levels of elementary school children's leisure time activities in relation to the children's gender, their risk factors for future cardiovascular disease, and their families socioeconomic status? (Harrell, Gansky, Bradley, & McMurray, 1997)	2200 third- and fourth-grade children
Design: Univaritate Descriptive	
To what extent are the handwritten medication orders of physicians legible and complete? (Winslow, Nestor, Davidoff, Thompson, & Borum, 1997)	176 medication orders

more days of menses and larger amounts of menses than the two highest-intensity running groups. Women in all three running groups reported a shorter luteal phase than nonrunners and had significantly more ovulatory disturbances. Across groups, a history of menstrual irregularity before 18 years of age was a strong predictor of menstrual cycle characteristics.

ADDITIONAL TYPES OF QUANTITATIVE RESEARCH

The previous sections discussed different types of quantitative research based on an important dimension of research design, namely whether the researcher manipulates the independent variable. All research studies can be categorized as either experimental, quasi-experimental/preexperimental, or nonexperimental in design. This section describes some additional types of quantitative research that vary according to the study's purpose rather than the dimensions outlined in Table 7-3 in Chapter 7, with the hope that such a presentation will give you a better sense of the full range of nursing research aims. This section describes several types of research that usually involve a quantitative approach, but it is important to note that for certain types of research described here (e.g., evaluation research), qualitative methods may also be used.

Survey Research

A **survey** is designed to obtain information from populations regarding the prevalence, distribution, and interrelations of variables within those populations. The decennial census of the U.S. population is one example of a survey. Political opinion polls, such as those conducted by Gallup or Harris, are other examples. When surveys use samples of individuals, as they usually do, they may be referred to as **sample surveys** (as opposed to a **census**,

which covers the entire population). Surveys obtain information from a sample of people by means of **self-report**—that is, the study participants respond to a series of questions posed by the investigator. Surveys tend to yield data that are primarily quantitative. Surveys may be either cross-sectional or, as in the case of panel studies, longitudinal.

The content of a self-report survey is essentially limited only by the extent to which respondents are able and willing to report on the topic. Any information that can reliably be obtained by directly asking a person for that information is acceptable for inclusion in a survey. Often, a survey focuses on what people do: how or what they eat, how they care for their health needs, their compliance in taking medications, what kinds of family planning behaviors they engage in, and so forth. In some instances, particularly in political surveys, the emphasis is on what people plan to do—how they plan to vote, for example. Surveys also collect information on people's knowledge, opinions, attitudes, and values.

Survey data can be collected in a number of ways. The most respected method of securing survey information is through **personal interviews**, the method in which interviewers meet with individuals face to face and secure information from them. Generally, personal interviews are rather costly: They require considerable planning and interviewer training and tend to involve a lot of personnel time. Nevertheless, personal interviews are regarded as the most useful method of collecting survey data because of the quality of the information they yield. A further advantage of personal interviews is that relatively few people refuse to be interviewed in person.

Telephone interviews are a less costly, but often less effective, method of gathering survey information. When the interviewer is unknown, respondents may be uncooperative and unresponsive in a telephone situation, especially if the interview is long. However, telephoning can be a convenient method of collecting information quickly if the interview is short, specific, and not too personal, or if the researcher has had prior personal contact with the respondents.

Questionnaires differ from interviews primarily in that they are self-administered. That is, the respondent reads the questions on a form and gives an answer in writing. Because respondents differ considerably in their reading levels and in their ability to communicate in writing, questionnaires are *not* merely a printed form of an interview schedule. Great care must be taken in the development of a questionnaire to word questions clearly, simply, and unambiguously. Self-administered questionnaires are economical but are not appropriate for surveying certain populations (e.g., the elderly, children). In survey research, questionnaires are generally distributed through the mail.

The greatest advantage of survey research is its flexibility and broadness of scope. It can be applied to many populations, it can focus on a wide range of topics, and its information can be used for many purposes. However, the information obtained in most surveys tends to be relatively superficial: surveys rarely probe deeply into such complexities as contradictions of human behavior and feelings. Survey research is better suited to extensive rather than intensive analysis. Although surveys can be conducted within the context of large-scale experiments, surveys are usually done as part of a nonexperimental study.

Nurse researchers have used the survey research approach to study a wide range of phenomena. For example, Preski and Walker (1997) used mailed questionnaires to survey mothers about their lifestyles and their children's adjustment. Woods and Mitchell (1997) used personal interviews to examine factors contributing to depressed mood among women in midlife. Stratton, Dunkin, Juhl, and Geller (1993) completed a telephone survey of directors of nursing in rural hospitals to examine barriers to recruiting nurses to rural practice settings.

Evaluation Research

Evaluation research is an applied form of research that involves finding out how well a program, practice, procedure, or policy* is working. Its goal is to assess or evaluate the success of a program. In evaluations, the research objective is utilitarian—the purpose is to answer the practical questions of people who must make decisions: Should a new program be adopted or an existing one discontinued? Do current practices need to be modified, or should they be abandoned altogether? Do the costs of implementing a new program outweigh the benefits?

Evaluation research has an important role to play both in localized settings and in programs at the national level. Evaluations are often the cornerstone of an area of research known as **policy research**; nurses have become increasingly aware of the potential contribution their research can make to the formulation of national and local health policies and thus are undertaking evaluations that have implications for such policies.

In doing an evaluation, the researcher often confronts a set of problems that are organizational, interpersonal, or political in nature. Evaluation research can be threatening to individuals. Even when the focus of an evaluation is on a nontangible entity, such as a program or procedure, it is *people* who developed and implemented it. People tend to think that they, or their work, are being evaluated and may in some cases feel that their job or reputation is at stake. Thus, evaluation researchers need to have more than methodologic skills—they need to be diplomats, adept in interpersonal dealings with people. If the people operating a program are

---

*Although we use the term *program* throughout most of this discussion, this term is meant to include practices, procedures, and policies as well.

defensive and noncooperative, the evaluation could be unproductive.

EVALUATION RESEARCH MODELS

Various schools of thought have developed concerning the conduct of evaluation research. The traditional strategy for the conduct of evaluation research consists of four broad phases: determining the objectives of the program, developing a means of measuring the attainment of those objectives, collecting the data, and interpreting the data in terms of the objectives.

Often, the most difficult task is to spell out the program objectives. Typically, there are numerous objectives of a program, and these objectives may be vague. In response to this issue, the classic evaluation model stresses the importance of developing behavioral objectives. A **behavioral objective** is the intended outcome of a program stated in terms of the behavior of those people at whom the program is aimed, that is, the behavior of the beneficiaries, rather than the agents, of the program. Thus, if the goal is to have patients ambulate after surgery, the behavioral objective might be stated as, "The patient will walk the length of the corridor within 3 days after surgery." The objective should *not* be stated as, "The nurse will *teach* the patient to walk the length of the corridor within 3 days after surgery." An emphasis on behavioral objectives can be taken to extremes, however. An evaluation may be concerned with psychological dimensions such as morale or an emotion (e.g., anxiety) that do not always manifest themselves in behavioral terms. Once the program objectives have been delineated, the evaluator proceeds to design the study, measure the behaviors under study, and compare program objectives to actual outcomes. An evaluation can use either an experimental design (with subjects randomly assigned to either the program being evaluated or a control group), a quasi-experimental design, or a nonexperimental design.

The traditional model of evaluation has sometimes been criticized for a certain narrowness of conceptualization. One alternative evaluation model is the **goal-free approach**. Proponents of this model argue that programs may have a number of consequences besides accomplishing the official objectives of the program and that the classic model is handicapped by its inability to investigate these other effects. Goal-free evaluation represents an attempt to evaluate the outcomes of a program in the absence of information about intended outcomes. The job of the evaluator—a demanding one—is basically that of describing the repercussions of a program or practice on various components of the overall system. The goal-free model can often be a profitable approach, and it certainly leaves more room for creativity on the part of the evaluator. In many cases, however, the model may not be practical because there are seldom unlimited resources (personnel, time, or money) for the conduct of an evaluation. Decision makers may need to know whether objectives are being met so that immediate decisions can be made.

TYPES OF EVALUATIONS

Evaluations are undertaken to answer a variety of questions about a program or policy. This section briefly describes evaluations designed to address different types of questions. In evaluations of large-scale interventions (sometimes called **demonstrations** if they are implemented on a trial basis), the evaluator may well undertake all the evaluation activities discussed here.

Process or Implementation Analysis. A process or **implementation analysis** is undertaken when there is a need for descriptive information about the process by which a program or procedure gets implemented and how it functions in actual operation. A process analysis is typically designed to address such questions as the following: Does the program function in the real world the way its designers intended it? What appear to be the strongest and weakest aspects of the program? What exactly *is* the treatment, and how does it differ (if at all) from traditional practices? What, if any, were the barriers to implementing the program successfully? A process analysis may be undertaken with the aim of improving a new or ongoing program; in such a situation, the evaluation may be referred to as a **formative evaluation**. In other situations, the purpose of the process analysis may be primarily to describe a program carefully so that it can be replicated by others. In either case, a process analysis typically involves an in-depth examination of the operation of a program, often involving the collection of both qualitative and quantitative data. As an example of an implementation analysis, Mitchell, Armstrong, Simpson, and Lentz (1989) studied the implementation of a special critical care nurses demonstration project with regard to nurse–physician collaboration, work and information flow, and staff morale.

Outcome Analysis. Evaluations typically focus on whether a program or policy works, that is, whether it is effective in meeting its objectives. Evaluations that assess the worth of a program are sometimes referred to as **summative evaluations**, in contrast to formative evaluations. The intent of such evaluations is to help people decide whether the program should be discarded, replaced, modified, continued, or replicated. Many evaluation researchers distinguish between an outcome analysis and an impact analysis. An **outcome analysis** tends to be descriptive and does not use a rigorous design. Such an analysis simply documents the extent to which the goals of the program are attained, that is, the extent to which positive outcomes occur. For example, a program may be designed to encourage women in a poor rural community to obtain prenatal care. An outcome analysis would document outcomes without formal comparisons (e.g., the percentage of women delivering babies in the community who had obtained prenatal care, the average month in which prenatal care was begun, and so on). As an actual example, Schirm (1993) evaluated a cholesterol screening program for older people to determine their cholesterol levels and their practices used to lower cholesterol levels.

Impact Analysis. An **impact analysis** attempts to identify the **net impacts** of an intervention, that is, the impacts that can be attributed exclusively to the intervention over and above the effects of other factors (such as the effect of the standard treatment). Impact analyses almost always use an experimental or quasi-experimental design because the aim of such evaluations is to attribute a causal influence to the special intervention. In the example cited earlier, let us suppose that the program to encourage prenatal care involved having nurses make home visits to women in the rural community to explain the benefits of early care during pregnancy. If the visits could be made to pregnant women on a random basis, the labor and delivery outcomes of the group of women receiving the home visits and of those not receiving them could be compared to determine the net impacts of the intervention, that is, the percentage increase in receipt of prenatal care among the experimental group relative to the control group. Most evaluations published in the nursing literature are impact analyses. Rothert and her colleagues (1997) developed a decision support intervention to assist menopausal women in their decision making relating to hormone replacement therapy and tested the impacts of the intervention using an experimental design. Another group of researchers (Beck, Heacock, Mercer, Walls, Rapp, & Vogelpohl, 1997) used a time series design to examine the effects of a behavioral intervention on improved dressing independence among cognitively impaired nursing home residents and on caregiver efficiency.

Cost–Benefit Analysis. New programs or policies are often expensive to implement, and existing programs may be expensive to operate.

Therefore, evaluations sometimes include a **cost–benefit analysis** to determine whether the benefits of the program outweigh the costs, in terms of monetary value. Cost–benefit analyses are typically done in connection with impact analyses, that is, when there is solid evidence regarding the net impacts of an intervention. In the example of home visitation, the evaluator would compare the total cost of operating the new program against the cost that could be incurred in its absence (e.g., for the treatment of low-birthweight infants in the control group). In the previously cited critical care nurses demonstration project (Mitchell, Armstrong, Simpson, & Lentz, 1989), the fiscal costs and benefits of the intervention were carefully assessed. Betz, Traw, and Bostrom (1994) evaluated the cost-effectiveness of two intravenous additive systems, analyzing the effects of each system on nursing productivity.

Needs Assessment

Like evaluation research, a needs assessment represents an effort to provide a decision maker with information for action. As the name implies, a **needs assessment** is a study in which a researcher collects data for estimating the needs of a group, community, or organization. Thus, whereas an evaluation seeks to ascertain if a program is attaining its objectives, the aim of needs assessments is to determine if the objectives of a program are meeting the needs of the individuals who are supposed to benefit from it. Nursing educators may wish to assess the needs of their clients (students); hospital staff members may wish to learn the needs of those they serve (patients); a mental health outreach clinic may wish to gather information on the needs of some target population (e.g., adolescents in the community). Because resources are seldom limitless, information that can help in establishing priorities is almost always valuable.

There are various methods for doing a needs assessment; these methods are not necessarily mutually exclusive. The **key informant** approach, as the name implies, collects information concerning the needs of a group from people who are presumed to be in a key position to know those needs. These key informants could be community leaders, prominent health care workers, agency directors, or other knowledgeable individuals. Questionnaires or interviews are generally used to collect the data. (In some cases, key informant interviews collect narrative, qualitative information that is analyzed qualitatively rather than through statistical procedures.)

Another method is the **survey approach,** in which data are collected from a sample of the target group whose needs are being assessed. In a survey, there would be no attempt to question only people who are in positions of authority or who are knowledgeable. Any member of the group or community could be asked to give his or her viewpoint.

Another alternative is to use an **indicators approach**, which relies on inferences made from statistics available in existing reports or records. For example, a nurse-managed clinic that is interested in analyzing the needs of its clients could examine over a 5-year period the number of appointments that were kept, the employment rate of its clients, the changes in risk appraisal status, methods of payment, and so forth. The indicators approach is flexible and may also be economical because the data are generally available but need organization and interpretation.

Needs assessments almost always involve the development of recommendations. The role of the researcher conducting a needs assessment is often that of making judgments about priorities in light of considerations such as costs and feasibility and of advising on means by which the most highly prioritized needs can be addressed.

Nurse researchers have examined the needs of diverse groups. For example, Silveira and Winstead-Fry (1997) studied the physical and psychological needs of cancer patients and their caretakers living in rural areas. Berk, Baigis-Smith, and Nanda (1995) studied the health care needs of people with HIV or

AIDS in hospital, outpatient, and long-term care settings.

Outcomes Research

Outcomes research, designed to document the effectiveness of health care services, is gaining momentum as a research enterprise in nursing and health care fields. Outcomes research overlaps in some instances with evaluation research, but evaluation research more typically focuses on an appraisal of a specific new intervention, whereas outcomes research represents a more global assessment of health care services. The impetus for outcomes research comes from the quality assessment and quality assurance functions that grew out of the professional standards review organizations (PSROs) in the 1970s. Outcomes research represents a response to the increasing demand from policy makers, insurers, and the public to justify care practices and systems in terms of both improved patient outcomes and costs. The focus of outcomes research in the 1980s was predominantly on patient health status and costs associated with medical care, but there is a growing interest among nurses to study patient outcomes in relation to nursing care.

In appraising quality in health care services, three aspects are relevant: outcome, process, and structure (Donabedian, 1987). *Outcomes* refer to the specific clinical end-results of patient care. Outcomes can be defined in terms of physical or physiologic function (e.g., heart rate, blood pressure), psychological function (e.g., comfort, life quality), or social function (e.g., relations with family members). Outcomes of interest to nurses may be either short-term and temporary (e.g., postoperative body temperature) or more long-term and permanent (e.g., return to regular employment). Furthermore, outcomes may be defined in terms of the end-results to individual patients (i.e., the recipients of care) or to broader units, such as a community or our entire society. Appraising quality of care in terms of *process* involves assessments of such provider-related

factors as clinical judgment, diagnoses, practice styles, management, and cost, as well as such client-related factors as compliance, understanding, and satisfaction. The *structure* of care can be appraised in terms of such attributes as accessibility, range of services, facilities, personnel, organization, and financing.

Outcomes research, then, encompasses a great deal of the areas of inquiry in which nurse researchers are interested. However, specific efforts to appraise and document the quality of nursing care—as distinct from the care provided by the overall health care system—are not numerous. A major obstacle is attribution—that is, linking the outcomes of interest to specific nursing actions or interventions, distinct from the actions or interventions of other members of the health care team. In a broader sense, it is also difficult in some cases to determine a causal connection between outcomes and any health care intervention. Many factors outside the health care system—including patient characteristics and behaviors and environmental factors—affect outcomes in complex ways.

Outcomes research has employed a variety of traditional designs, sampling strategies, and data collection and analysis approaches but is also developing a rich array of methods that are not within the traditional research framework. The complex and multidisciplinary nature of outcomes research suggests that this evolving area will offer opportunities for methodologic creativity in the years to come.

A number of nursing studies are considered outcomes research, including a number of evaluation studies that assess the effects of nursing interventions. Strzalka and Havens (1996) conducted a study that examined the quality of nursing care in a hospital unit provided by unit-hired, float pool, and agency nurses through a comparison of the groups' performance on nine clinical quality indicators. Leveck and Jones (1996) studied the effects of various factors in the nursing practice environment (e.g., management style, job stress, job satisfaction, group cohesiveness) on staff nurse retention and process aspects of quality of care. Williams (1997) explored whether there is a relationship between patients' perceptions of nurse caring and their satisfaction with nursing care.

Secondary Analysis

Secondary analysis involves the use of data gathered in a previous study to test new hypotheses or explore new relationships. The amount of research conducted every year in such fields as nursing, medicine, the life sciences, and the social sciences is overwhelming. In a typical research project, more data are collected than the investigator actually analyzes. Secondary analysis is efficient and economical because data collection is typically the most time-consuming and expensive part of a research project.

A number of avenues are available for making use of an existing set of quantitative data:

1. Variables and relationships among variables that were previously unanalyzed can be examined (e.g., an independent variable in the original study could become the dependent variable in the secondary analysis).
2. The secondary analysis can focus on a particular subgroup rather than on the full original sample (e.g., survey data about health habits from a national sample could be analyzed to study smoking among urban teenagers).
3. The unit of analysis can be changed. A **unit of analysis** is the basic unit that yields data for an analysis; in nursing studies, each individual subject is typically the unit of analysis. However, data are sometimes aggregated to yield information about larger units (e.g., a study of individual nurses drawn from 25 hospitals could be converted to aggregated data about the hospitals).

In recent years, a number of groups, such as university institutes and federal agencies, have

been attempting to organize data and make them available to researchers for secondary analysis. The policies regulating the public use of data vary from one organization to another, but it is not unusual for data to be provided to an interested researcher at about the cost of duplicating files and documentation, plus handling. Thus, in some cases in which the gathering of the data involved an expenditure of hundreds of thousands of dollars, reproduced materials may be supplied for less than 1% of the initial costs. Many universities and research institutes within universities maintain libraries of data sets from large national surveys.

One source of secondary data for nurse researchers is the various surveys sponsored by the National Center for Health Statistics (NCHS). For example, NCHS periodically conducts such national surveys as the National Health Interview Survey and the Health Promotion and Disease Prevention Survey, both of which gather health-related information from thousands of people all over the United States.

The use of available data makes it possible for the researcher to bypass time-consuming and costly steps in the research process, but there are some noteworthy disadvantages in working with existing data. In particular, if an investigator does not play a role in collecting the data, the chances are pretty high that the data set will be deficient or problematic in one or more ways, such as in the sample used, the variables measured, and so forth. The researcher may continuously face "if only" problems: If only they had asked a question about a certain topic or had measured a particular variable differently. Nevertheless, opportunities for secondary analysis are often worth exploring. Note that although most secondary analysis studies involve existing quantitative data sets, the approach can also be used with qualitative data.

Nurse researchers have used a secondary analysis approach with both large national data sets and smaller, more localized sets. For example, Brown, Knapp, & Radke (1997) undertook a secondary analysis with four data sets to determine the extent to which sex, age, height, and weight predict such physiologic outcomes as forced expiratory volume, hemoglobin concentration, and serum glucose concentration; three of the data sets were from local studies, whereas the fourth was from a national data set, the National Health and Nutrition Examination Survey II. Kocher and Thomas (1994) used data from Department of Defense surveys of military personnel in their study of factors that predicted retention among Army nurses. Weaver, Richmond, and Narsavage (1997) used data from a previous study of patients with chronic obstructive pulmonary disease to test an explanatory model of variables affecting functional status in this disorder.

Meta-analysis

Chapter 4 described the function of a literature review as a preliminary step in a research project. However, there is growing recognition of the fact that the careful integration of knowledge on a topic in itself constitutes an important scholarly endeavor that can contribute new knowledge. The procedure known as **meta-analysis** represents an application of statistical procedures to findings from research reports. In essence, meta-analysis treats the findings from one study as a single piece of data—that is, the study is the unit of analysis. The findings from multiple studies on the same topic, therefore, can be combined to yield a data set that can be analyzed in a manner similar to that obtained from individual subjects.

The earliest form of nonnarrative research integration used what has been referred to as the **voting method**. This procedure involves tallying the outcomes of previous studies to determine what outcome has received the greatest empirical support. The voting method has since been superseded by methods of considerable sophistication and complexity. Because beginning researchers may have no statistical background, a discussion of actual statistical procedures cannot be included here. Suffice it

to say that these methods, described in detail by Glass, McGaw, and Smith (1981), generally involve the calculation of an index known as the **effect size**, which quantifies the strength of the relationship between the independent and dependent variables.

Traditional narrative reviews of the literature are handicapped by several factors uncharacteristic of meta-analysis. The first is that if the number of studies on a specific topic is large and if the results are inconsistent, then it is difficult to draw conclusions. Moreover, narrative reviews are often subject to potential biases. The researcher may unwittingly give more weight to findings that are congruent with his or her own viewpoints. Thus, meta-analytic procedures provide a convenient and objective method of integrating a large body of findings and of observing patterns and relationships that might otherwise have gone undetected. Furthermore, meta-analysis provides information about the magnitude of differences and relationships. Meta-analysis can thus serve as an important scholarly tool in theory development as well as in research utilization.

Meta-analysis has also been criticized on a number of grounds. One issue has been called the **fruit problem**, that is, the possibility of combining studies that conceptually do not belong with each other (apples and oranges). Another issue is that there is generally a bias in the studies appearing in published sources. Studies in which no group differences or no relationships between variables have been found are less likely to be published and, therefore, are less likely to be included in the meta-analysis. Narrative literature reviews are subject to the same two problems, but these problems may take on added significance in a meta-analysis because the quantitative results make the conclusions appear more concrete and absolute. Another problem is that a research report could provide general information about the study's findings but might not include sufficient quantitative information for computing an effect size. Despite these potential problems, careful and thorough meta-analyses represent an important advancement to the scientific community.

A number of nurse researchers have published meta-analytic studies in recent years. For example, Labyak and Metzger (1997) did a meta-analysis of studies of the effects of effleurage back rubs on the physiologic components of relaxation. Devine and Reifschneider (1995) conducted a meta-analysis of the literature on the effects of psychoeducational care on such outcomes as blood pressure, medication compliance, weight, and anxiety.

Delphi Surveys

Delphi surveys were developed as a tool for short-term forecasting. The technique involves a panel of experts who are asked to complete a series of questionnaires focusing on the experts' opinions, predictions, or judgment concerning a specific topic of interest.

The Delphi technique differs from other surveys in several respects. First, the Delphi technique consists of several rounds of questionnaires. Each of the cooperating experts is asked to complete at least two (and often more) questionnaires. This multiple iteration approach is used as a means of effecting group consensus of opinion, without the necessity of face-to-face committee work. A second feature is the use of feedback to members of the panel. Responses to each round of questionnaires are analyzed, summarized, and returned to the experts with a new questionnaire. The experts can then reformulate their opinions with the knowledge of the group's viewpoint in mind. The process of response–analysis–feedback–response is usually repeated at least three times until a general consensus is obtained.

The Delphi technique is a relatively efficient and effective method of combining the expertise of a large group of individuals to obtain information for planning and prediction purposes. The experts are spared the necessity of being brought together for a formal meeting, thus saving considerable time and expense for the panel members. Another advantage is that any one persuasive or prestigious expert cannot have an undue influence on the opinions of others, as could happen in a face-to-face situation. Each panel member is on an equal footing with all others. Anonymity probably encourages a greater frankness of opinion than might be expressed in a formal meeting. The feedback–response loops allow for multichanneled communication without any risk of the members being sidetracked from their mission.

At the same time, it must be conceded that the Delphi technique is time-consuming for the researcher. Experts must be solicited, questionnaires prepared and mailed, responses analyzed, results summarized, new questionnaires prepared, and so forth. The cooperation of the panel members may wane in later rounds of the questionnaire mailings. The problem of bias through attrition is a constant threat, although probably less severe than through ordinary questionnaire procedures. On the whole, the Delphi technique represents a significant methodologic tool for solving problems, planning, and forecasting.

A number of studies using the Delphi technique have appeared in the nursing literature. For example, the Delphi technique has been used to identify the competencies needed by nurse leaders in public health programs (Misener et al., 1997); to determine how a multidisciplinary clinical staff viewed the future development of community mental health centers (Beech, 1997); and to identify nursing management diagnoses (Morrison, 1997).

Methodologic Research

Methodologic research refers to controlled investigations of the ways of obtaining, organizing, and analyzing data. Methodologic studies address the development, validation, and evaluation of research tools or techniques. Nurse researchers in recent years have become increasingly interested in methodologic research.

This is not surprising in light of growing demands for sound and reliable measures and for sophisticated procedures for obtaining and analyzing data.

The methodologic researcher may, for example, concentrate on the development of an instrument that accurately measures patients' satisfaction with nursing care. The researcher in such a case does not focus on the level of patient satisfaction nor on how that satisfaction relates to characteristics of the nurses, the hospital, or the patients. The goals of the researcher are to develop an effective, serviceable, and trustworthy instrument that can be used by other researchers and to evaluate his or her success in accomplishing this.

Methodologic research may appear less exciting than substantive research, but it is virtually impossible to conduct high-quality and useful research on a substantive topic with inadequate research tools. Studies of a methodologic nature are indispensable in any scientific discipline, and perhaps especially so in fields that deal with highly complex, intangible phenomena such as human behavior or welfare, as is the case with nursing.

As an example of a recent methodologic study, Froman and Owen (1997) undertook a study to validate the AIDS Attitude Scale, a measure of attitudes toward people with AIDS. Morse, Simon, Besch, and Walker (1995) conducted a study to determine the organizational and client-centered factors that function as barriers for the recruitment, retention, and protocol compliance of subjects in community-based clinical trials.

Content Analysis Studies

The term **content analysis** has traditionally been used to describe the quantification of narrative, qualitative material. Although qualitative researchers who do not quantify their data sometimes refer to their analytic work as a content analysis, the term in its classic sense refers to "a research technique for the objective, systematic, and quantitative description of the manifest content of communication" (Berelson, 1971, p. 18).

Quantitative content analysis is applied to people's written and oral communications. It can be used with such materials as diaries, letters, speeches, books, articles, and other linguistic expressions. In traditional content analysis, the researcher enhances objectivity by proceeding on the basis of explicitly formulated rules. The rules serve as guidelines to enable two or more people analyzing the same materials to obtain the same results. The analysis is rendered systematic by the inclusion or exclusion of materials according to consistently applied selection criteria.

The most common applications of content analysis involve describing the characteristics of the content of the message (as opposed to its style, for example). The investigator must identify the variables to be recorded and the unit of analysis that will be used, that is, the unit that will be used to categorize the content into meaningful groupings. Individual **words**, which are easy to work with, are sometimes the unit. A **theme** is a larger and more inclusive unit of analysis. A theme may be a phrase, sentence, or paragraph embodying ideas or making an assertion about some topic. Some examples of themes that might emerge in patients' accounts of a long-term illness experience include coping with pain, fear of death, loneliness, and loss of motivation for recovery. These are illustrations of themes organized around the content of a message, but it is possible to detect stylistic themes such as different tones (proselytizing, admonishing, or informing), different grammatical structures, and so forth.

Another possible unit of analysis is the **item**. This unit refers to an entire message, document, or other production: a letter, editorial, diary entry, conference presentation, issue of a journal, and the like. The whole item can then be categorized in terms of one or more characteristics. For example, articles appearing in the journal

Nursing Research can be classified according to whether the research problem was clinical in nature, and trends over time could then be analyzed. Finally, the unit may be a **space-and-time measure.** This type of unit consists of a physical measurement of content, such as the number of pages, number of words, number of speakers, amount of time spent in a discussion, and so forth. The units referred to here as item and theme are probably most useful for nurse researchers.

Once the researcher has established the unit of analysis, a method of categorizing the data must be developed. After the individual pieces of communication are sampled and categorized, analysis can proceed. The most common form of quantifying materials is the enumeration of recorded occurrences in each category. A second approach is simply to create a binary index (yes or no) of whether the concepts covered in the category scheme were present or absent in the materials. The ranking of materials according to prespecified criteria is a third possibility. Finally, rating scales can be used to assess various aspects of the communications.

Content analysis suffers from several disadvantages, including the risk of subjectivity and the amount of tedious work involved. However, this technique may be expedient and efficient in its use of available materials, and there may be several research problems for which there are no alternatives.

Quantitative content analysis has been used productively by several nurse researchers. For example, McDougall, Blixen, and Suen (1997) did a content analysis of therapy notes from life review therapy sessions provided by an advanced practice geropsychiatric nurse to older adults discharged from psychiatric hospitals to home health care. Pollack (1993) used content analysis to study the characteristics of group processes that are most important to inpatients with bipolar disorder in group therapy, using transcripts from group therapy sessions.

Research Examples of Various Types of Quantitative Studies

All the types of research described in this section have been reported on in the nursing research literature, and several studies of each type have already been mentioned. Two studies are described in greater detail below.

EXAMPLE OF A SURVEY

Pollow, Stoller, Forster, and Duniho (1994) conducted a survey of elderly people living in community settings and managing their own health to examine their use of over-the-counter (OTC) medications and their consumption of alcohol. A major purpose of the study was to document drug use patterns among community-dwelling elders and their risk of adverse drug reactions.

Data were collected from a sample of 667 people living in community settings in northeastern New York, all of whom were 65 years of age or older. Of the people who were approached for the study, 79% agreed to participate.

Data were gathered through personal interviews in the respondents' homes. The interview covered a wide range of topics, including the respondents' health and disabilities, use of prescription and OTC medications, consumption of alcohol, and other health-related behaviors (e.g., smoking, exercise, eating patterns). Respondents who had difficulty remembering the names or therapeutic intent of any medications were asked to show the medicine to the interviewers, who recorded the names of the medications.

The findings indicated that almost two thirds of the respondents reported one or more drug–drug or drug–alcohol combination associated with a possible adverse reaction. The potential for risk was highest among people taking psychoactive drugs, antidiabetic agents, anticoagulants, and ulcer medications. The results suggest the need for health care practitioners to obtain more detailed drug histories when treating elderly clients who are taking certain categories of medications.

EXAMPLE OF AN EVALUATION

York and her colleagues (1997) conducted a clinical trial to evaluate an intervention for high-risk child-bearing women—pregnant women diagnosed with diabetes or hypertension. Women meeting the study criteria and agreeing to participate were randomly assigned to either a control or an experimental intervention group after signing informed consent forms. The sample consisted of 52 women in the control group and 42 women in the intervention group. Women in the control group were discharged normally from the hospital. Those in the experimental group had an early hospital discharge, combined with in-hospital education and follow-up care in the form of home visits and telephone contacts from a clinical nurse specialist.

The research team was interested in evaluating the effect of the intervention in terms of three broad areas: (1) maternal outcomes, such as acute care visits, rehospitalizations, return to normal activities, and satisfaction with care; (2) infant outcomes, such as birthweight, acute care visits, and rehospitalizations; and (3) costs of care.

The results indicated that the intervention group had fewer rehospitalizations than the control group during pregnancy and that diabetic women in the control group were three times more likely to have a low-birthweight infant (less than 2500 g) than those in the intervention group. The two groups were similar in terms of postpartum hospitalizations, acute care visits, postpartum functional status, and satisfaction with care. However, the cost analysis revealed that a net savings of $13,327 was realized for each mother–infant dyad in the intervention group.

TIPS FOR DESIGNING QUANTITATIVE STUDIES

Because research design has profound implications for the interpretability of study findings, we offer the following suggestions for strengthening designs for quantitative studies:

- It is usually advantageous to design a study with as many relevant comparisons as possible. Preexperimental designs are weak in part because the comparative information they yield is limited. A one-group, before–after design is strengthened considerably by the addition of a second group. Sometimes, having two or more comparison groups greatly enhances the value of a study. In an experimental context, for example, the comparison of treatment A to treatment B yields much less information than the comparison of both treatments to no treatment (or to a placebo). In a nonexperimental context, having multiple comparison groups is often an effective way to address the problem of self-selection, especially if the comparison groups are selected to address competing biases. For example, in case-control studies of patients with lung cancer, one comparison group could comprise people with a respiratory disease other than lung cancer and a second could comprise those with no respiratory disorder.
- Another way to maximize comparative possibilities is to design a study with more than one data collection point, as in before–after experimental designs. In such a design, the experimental and control groups can be compared not only with respect to differences in posttest status but also with respect to changes over time. Moreover, the availability of pretest data typically greatly enhances the precision of the statistical analyses. Data collection before the introduction of a treatment may be unwise when the researcher suspects that the data collection itself would have an effect on the dependent variable, but this is rarely the case. The major deterrents to the collection of pretest data

are typically practical considerations such as time and cost.

- In general, it is wise to randomize whenever possible, to reduce the possibility of biases. In an experimental context, this means randomly assigning subjects to groups, groups to treatments, and conditions to subjects (in a repeated measures design). It also means looking for other opportunities to randomize whenever other conditions vary across subjects, such as randomly assigning patients to rooms or nursing staff to patients. In a nonexperimental context, there may also be opportunities to randomize, such as randomly assigning data collection staff to study participants, or participants to different times for data collection (morning versus afternoon).
- When using an experimental design that involves the collection of data both before and after the intervention, it is considered good practice to collect the pretest data *before* randomization to groups. This ensures that subjects (and researchers) will not be biased in any way by knowledge of the group assignments.

SUMMARY

Experiments are characterized by three fundamental properties: manipulation, control, and randomization. **Manipulation** involves doing something to or acting on at least some of the subjects in a research study. The experimenter manipulates, or varies, the independent variable (often referred to as the experimental **treatment** or **intervention**) to see if the manipulation has an effect on the dependent variable. True experiments always require the use of a **control group**, whose performance on the dependent variable is used as a basis for assessing the performance of the experimental group. Subjects are assigned to control and experimental groups by a process known as **randomization**. The random assignment proce-

dure can be accomplished by any method that allows every subject an equal chance of being included in any group, such as by flipping a coin or using a **table of random numbers**. Randomization is the most reliable method for equating groups on all possible characteristics that could affect the outcome of the study.

The most basic experimental design is the **after-only** or **posttest-only design**, which involves collecting data from subjects after the experimental treatment has been introduced. When data are also collected before treatment (i.e., at **baseline**), the design is a **before–after** or **pretest–posttest design**. When a researcher manipulates more than one variable at a time, the design is known as a **factorial experiment**. Factorial designs permit testing of both **main effects** (effects resulting from the experimentally manipulated variables) and **interaction effects** (effects resulting from combining the treatments). In **repeated measures (crossover)** designs, one group of subjects is exposed to two or more conditions in random order, thereby allowing subjects to serve as their own controls. When an experimental design is used to test the efficacy of a clinical treatment in a large, heterogeneous population, the study is often referred to as a **clinical trial**. True experiments are considered by many to be the ideal of science because they come closer than any other type of research approach to meeting the criteria for inferring causal relationships.

Quasi-experimental and preexperimental designs involve manipulation but lack a comparison group or randomization. **Quasi-experimental designs** are designs in which efforts are made to introduce controls into the study to compensate in part for the absence of one or both of these important characteristics. In contrast, **preexperimental designs** have no such safeguards and, therefore, are subject to ambiguity and multiple interpretations of results.

A commonly used quasi-experimental design is the **nonequivalent control group design**, which involves the use of a **comparison group** that is not created through random assignment. The problem with the use of such a comparison group is the possibility that the groups are initially different in ways that will affect the research outcomes, and so the collection of pretest data becomes an important means of assessing their initial equivalence. In studies in which there is no control group, a method for overcoming some of the difficulties in the interpretation of results is the collection of information over time before and after the treatment is instituted. Such a study is known as a **time series design**. Quasi-experimental designs may in some cases be more practical in the nursing field than experimental designs; however, in evaluating the results of quasi-experiments, it is important to ask whether it is plausible that factors other than the experimental treatment caused or affected the obtained outcomes (i.e., whether there are **rival hypotheses** for explaining the results).

Three types of constraints preclude experimentation and make **nonexperimental research** useful or necessary. First, a number of independent variables, such as height and gender, are characteristics that are not amenable to control and randomization. Second, other variables are technically manipulable but cannot ethically be manipulated in studies with human subjects. Third, it may often be impractical or impossible to manipulate variables. Finally, researchers sometimes deliberately choose not to manipulate variables, to achieve a more realistic understanding of phenomena as they operate in naturalistic settings.

Nonexperimental research includes two broad categories: ex post facto or correlational research and descriptive research. **Ex post facto** or **correlational studies** are investigations designed to examine the relationships among variables, without active manipulation of the independent variable. Because the scrutiny of the independent variable is done after the fact—that is, after it has occurred in the natural course of events—it becomes difficult to draw cause-and-effect conclusions. **Descriptive research** is designed to summarize the status of phenomena of interest as they currently exist. **Descriptive correlational studies** do not focus on cause-and-effect relationships, but rather on a description of how one phenomenon is related to another. **Univariate descriptive research** provides information on the occurrence, frequency of occurrence, or average value of the research variables without examining how variables are interrelated. The primary weakness of ex post facto or correlational studies is that they can harbor biases due to **self-selection** into groups being compared. Ex post facto or correlational research is thus more vulnerable to the risk of erroneous interpretation of results than experimental research.

Quantitative studies vary according to purpose as well as design. **Survey research** is the branch of research that examines the characteristics, behaviors, attitudes, and intentions of a group of people by asking individuals belonging to that group to answer a series of questions. The preferred method of collecting survey information is through **personal interviews**, in which interviewers meet with participants in a face-to-face situation and question them directly. **Telephone interviews** are convenient and economical, but they are not recommended when the interview is long or detailed or when the questions are sensitive or highly personal. **Questionnaires** are self-administered; that is, questions are read by the respondent, who then gives a written response.

Evaluation research assesses the effectiveness of a program, policy, or procedure to assist decision makers in choosing a course of action. The classic evaluation model assesses the congruence between the goals of the program and actual outcomes. Goals are typically phrased in the form of **behavioral objectives**, which delineate the intended outcomes of a program in terms of the behaviors of the program's beneficiaries. The **goal-free model** attempts to understand all the effects of a program, whether or not they were intended. Evaluations can answer a variety of questions. **Process** or **implementation analyses** are undertaken to describe the process by which a program gets implemented and how it is functioning in practice. **Outcome analyses**

basically *describe* the status of some condition after the introduction of an intervention. **Impact analyses,** which typically use rigorous comparative designs, test whether an intervention caused any **net impacts. Cost–benefit analyses** attempt to answer the question of whether the monetary costs of a program are outweighed by the monetary benefits.

Needs assessments, which are investigations of the needs of a group, community, or organization for certain types of services or policies, are another form of applied research aimed at providing useful information for planners and decision makers. Several techniques or approaches are used in the conduct of needs assessments, notably the **key informant,** survey, or **indicator approach.**

Outcomes research is designed to document the effectiveness and quality of health care services. Outcomes research considers three aspects of health care quality: outcomes (the specific end-results of patient care in terms of patient functioning); process (provider-related factors, such as clinical judgment and diagnoses, and client-related factors, such as compliance and satisfaction); and structure (factors such as accessibility, personnel, and facilities).

Secondary analysis refers to research projects in which the investigator analyzes previously collected data. The secondary analyst may examine unanalyzed variables, test unexplored relationships, focus on a particular subsample, or change the **unit of analysis.** The use of existing data offers the potential of saving time and resources, but the researcher may be unable to find a data set with exactly the kinds of data needed.

Meta-analysis is a method of integrating the findings of prior research using statistical procedures. Meta-analyses typically involve the calculation of an **effect size** that quantifies relationships between variables in each study in the analysis. Effect sizes from numerous studies can then be averaged to provide a numeric estimate of the magnitude of relationships.

The **Delphi technique** is a method in which several rounds of questionnaires are mailed to a panel of experts. Feedback from previous questionnaires is provided with each new questionnaire so that the experts can converge on a consensus opinion in subsequent rounds. Delphi studies are used for problem solving, planning, and forecasting.

In **methodologic research,** the investigator is concerned with the development, validation, and assessment of methodologic tools or strategies. The researcher conducting a methodologic study focuses primarily on increasing knowledge with respect to the methods used in performing scientific research rather than contributing to some substantive area.

Content analysis is a method for quantifying the content of narrative communications in a systematic and objective fashion. Communications include diaries, speeches, letters, and other verbal expressions. A variety of units of analysis exist for verbal expressions. The most useful units for nurse researchers are **themes,** which embody ideas or concepts, and **items,** which refer to the entire message.

STUDY ACTIVITIES

Chapter 8 of the *Study Guide to Accompany Nursing Research: Principles and Methods, 6th ed.,* offers various exercises and study suggestions for reinforcing the concepts presented in this chapter. Additionally, the following study questions can be addressed:

1. A researcher is interested in studying the effect of sensitivity training for nurses on their behavior in crisis intervention situations. Describe how you would set up an experiment to investigate this problem. Now describe two quasi-experimental or preexperimental designs that could be used to study the same problem. Discuss what the weaknesses of each would be.

2. Assume that you have 10 individuals— Z, Y, X, W, V, U, T, S, R, and Q—who are going to participate in an experiment

you are conducting. Using a table of random numbers, assign five individuals to group I and five to group II. Then randomly assign the groups to an experimental or control treatment.

3. Using the notation presented in Figures 8-4 to 8-13, diagram a few of the research examples described in the text that are not already shown.

4. A nurse researcher is interested in studying the success of several different approaches to feeding patients with dysphagia. Can the researcher use an ex post facto design to examine this problem? Why or why not? Could an experimental or quasi-experimental approach be used? How?

5. A nurse researcher is planning to investigate the relationship between the social class of hospitalized children and the frequency and content of children-initiated communications with the nursing staff. Which is the independent variable, and which is the dependent variable? Would you classify this research as basically experimental or correlational, or could both approaches be used?

6. Suppose you were interested in doing a survey of nurses' attitudes toward caring for cancer patients. Would you use a personal interview, telephone interview, or questionnaire to collect your data? Defend your decision.

7. A psychiatric nurse therapist working with emotionally disturbed children is interested in evaluating a program of play therapy. Explain how you might proceed if you were to use (a) the classic evaluation model and (b) a goal-free approach. Which approach do you think would be more useful, and why?

8. Explain how you would use the key informant, survey, and indicator approaches to assess the need to teach Spanish to nurses in a given community.

9. What units of analysis might be especially appropriate for performing a content analysis of the following materials: letters from nurses stationed in Europe during World War II, the diary of an adolescent dying from leukemia, the minutes of meetings from a state nurses' association, and the articles appearing in the *American Journal of Nursing?*

SUGGESTED READINGS

Methodologic References

Berelson, B. (1971). *Content analysis in communication research.* New York: Free Press.

Brown, J. S., & Semradek, J. (1992). Secondary data on health-related subjects: Major sources, uses, and limitations. *Public Health Nursing, 3,* 162–171.

Brown, S. A. (1991). Measurement of quality of primary studies for meta-analysis. *Nursing Research, 40,* 352–355.

Campbell, D. T., & Stanley, J. C. (1963). *Experimental and quasi-experimental designs for research.* Chicago: Rand McNally.

Christensen, L. M. (1996). *Experimental methodology.* (7th ed.). Boston: Allyn and Bacon.

Clinton, J., Beck, R., Radjenovic, D., Taylor, L., Westlake, S., & Wilson, S. E. (1986). Time series designs in clinical nursing research. *Nursing Research, 35,* 188–191.

Cook, T., & Campbell, D. T. (1979). *Quasi-experimental design and analysis issues for field settings.* Chicago: Rand McNally.

Crisp, J., Pelletier, D., Duffield, C., Adams, A., & Nagy, S. (1997). The Delphi method? *Nursing Research, 46,* 116–118.

Dillman, D. (1978). *Mail and telephone surveys: The Total Design Method.* New York: John Wiley and Sons.

Donabedian, A. (1987). Some basic issues in evaluating the quality of health care. In L. T. Rinke (Ed.), *Outcome measures in home care* (Vol. I, pp. 3–28). New York: National League for Nursing.

Fetter, M. S., Feetham, S. L., D'Apolito, K., Chaze, B. A., Fink, A., Frink, B., Hougart, M., & Rushton, C. (1989). Randomized clinical trials: Issues for researchers. *Nursing Research, 38,* 117–120.

Fowler, F. J. (1993). *Survey research methods* (2nd ed.). Beverly Hills: Sage.

Glass, G. V., McGaw, B., & Smith, M. L. (1981). *Meta-analysis in social research*. Beverly Hills: Sage.

Hauck, W. W., Gilliss, C. L., Donner, A., & Gortner, S. (1991). Randomization by cluster. *Nursing Research, 40*, 356–358.

Jacobson, A. F., Hamilton, P., & Galloway, J. (1993). Obtaining and evaluating data sets for secondary analysis in nursing research. *Western Journal of Nursing Research, 15*, 483–494.

Kerlinger, F. N. (1986). *Foundations of behavioral research* (3rd ed.). New York: Holt, Rinehart & Winston.

Kirchoff, K. T., & Dille, C. A. (1994). Issues in intervention research: Maintaining integrity. *Applied Nursing Research, 7*, 32–37.

Krippendorff, K. (1980). *Content analysis: An introduction to its methodology*. Beverly Hills: Sage.

Lavrakas, P. J. (1993). *Telephone survey methods*. Thousand Oaks, CA: Sage.

Lazarsfeld, P. (1955). Foreword. In H. Hyman (Ed.), *Survey design and analysis*. New York: The Free Press.

McCain, N. L., Smith, M. C., & Abraham, I. L. (1986). Meta-analysis of nursing interventions. *Western Journal of Nursing Research, 8*, 155–167.

McKillip, J. (1986). *Needs analysis: Tools for the human services and education*. Beverly Hills: Sage.

Reynolds, N. R., Timmerman, G., Anderson, J., & Stevenson, J. S. (1992). Meta-analysis for descriptive research. *Research in Nursing & Health, 15*, 467–475.

Rossi, P. H., & Freeman, H. E. (1993). *Evaluation: A systematic approach*. (5th ed.). Beverly Hills: Sage.

Stewart, D. W., & Kamins, M. A. (1993). *Secondary research: Information sources and methods*. (2nd ed.). Thousand Oaks, CA: Sage.

Warheit, G. J., Bell, R. A., & Schwab, J. J. (1975). *Planning for change: Needs assessment approaches*. Washington, DC: National Institute of Mental Health.

Witkin, B. R., & Altschuld, J. W. (1995). *Planning and conducting needs assessments*. Thousand Oaks, CA: Sage.

Substantive References

Beck, C., Heacock, P., Mercer, S. O., Walls, R. C., Rapp, C. G., & Vogelpohl, T. S. (1997). Improving dressing behavior in cognitively impaired nursing home residents. *Nursing Research, 46*, 126–132.

Beech, B. (1997). Studying the future. *Journal of Advanced Nursing, 25*, 331–338.

Belknap, D., Davidson, L. J., & Smith, C. R. (1997). The effects of psyllium hydrophilic mucilloid on diarrhea in enterally fed patients. *Heart and Lung, 26*, 229–237.

Berk, R. A., Baigis-Smith, J., & Nanda, J. P. (1995). Health care needs of persons with HIV/AIDS in various settings. *Western Journal of Nursing Research, 17*, 647–671.

Betz, M. L., Traw, B., & Bostrom, J. (1994). The cost-effectiveness of two intravenous additive systems. *Applied Nursing Research, 7*, 59–66.

Brown, J. K., Knapp, T. R., & Radke, K. J. (1997). Sex, age, height, and weight as predictors of selected physiologic outcomes. *Nursing Research, 46*, 101–104.

Devine, E. C., & Reifschneider, E. (1995). A meta-analysis of the effects of psychoeducational care in adults with hypertension. *Nursing Research, 44*, 237–243.

Elander, G., & Hellstrom, G. (1995). Reduction of noise levels in intensive care units for infants: Evaluation of an intervention program. *Heart & Lung, 24*, 376–379.

Estok, P. J., Rudy, E. B., Kerr, M. E., & Menzel, L. (1993). Menstrual response to running: Nursing implications. *Nursing Research, 42*, 158–165.

Fitzgerald, S. T., Zlotnick, C., & Kolodner, K. B. (1996). Factors relate to functional status after percutaneous transluminal coronary angioplasty. *Heart & Lung, 25*, 24–30.

Flynn, L. (1997) The health practices of homeless women: A causal model. *Nursing Research, 46*, 72–77.

Froman, R. D., & Owen, S. V. (1997). Further validation of the AIDS Attitude Scale. *Research in Nursing & Health, 20*, 161–167.

Ganong, L. H., & Coleman, M. (1997). Effects of family structure information on nurses' impression formation and verbal responses. *Research in Nursing & Health, 20*, 139–151.

Harrell, J. S., Gansky, S. A., Bradley, C. B., & McMurray, R. G. (1997). Leisure time activities of elementary school children. *Nursing Research, 46*, 246–253.

Hastings-Tolsma, M. T., Yucha, C. B., Tompkins, J., Robson, L., & Szeverenyi, N. (1993). Effect of warm and cold applications on the resolution of IV infiltrations. *Research in Nursing & Health, 16,* 171–178.

Kaplow, R., & Bookbinder, M. (1994). A comparison of four endotracheal tube holders. *Heart & Lung, 23,* 59–66.

Kocher, K. M., & Thomas, G. W. (1994). Retaining Army nurses: A longitudinal model. *Research in Nursing & Health, 17,* 59–65.

Labyak, S. E., & Metzger, B. L. (1997). The effects of effleurage backrub on the physiological components of relaxation: A meta-analysis. *Nursing Research, 46,* 59–62.

Lanza, M. L., Kayne, H. L., Pattison, I., Hicks, C., & Islam, S. (1996). The relationship of behavioral cues to assaultive behavior. *Clinical Nursing Research, 5,* 6–27.

Leveck, M. L., & Jones, C. B. (1996). The nursing practice environment, staff retention, and quality of care. *Research in Nursing & Health, 19,* 331–343.

MacDonald, S. A. (1995). An assessment of the Cardiovascular Health Education Program in primary health care. *Applied Nursing Research, 8,* 114–117.

McDougall, G. J., Blixen, C. E., & Suen, L. J. (1997). The process and outcome of life review psychotherapy with depressed homebound older adults. *Nursing Research, 46,* 277–283.

Misener, T. R., Alexander, J. W., Blaha, A. J., Clarke, P. N., Cover, C. M., Felton, G. M., Fuller, S. G., Herman, J., Rodes, M. M., & Sharp, H. F. (1997). National Delphi study to determine competencies for nursing leadership in public health. *Image— The Journal of Nursing Scholarship, 29,* 47–51.

Mitchell, P. H., Armstrong, S., Simpson, T. F., & Lentz, M. (1989). American Association of Critical-Care Nurses Demonstration Project: Profile of excellence in critical care nursing *Heart & Lung, 18,* 219–237.

Morrison, R. S. (1997). Identification of nursing management diagnoses. *Journal of Advanced Nursing, 25,* 324–330.

Morse, E. V., Simon, P. M., Besch, C. L., & Walker, J. (1995). Issues of recruitment, retention, and compliance in community-based clinical trials with traditionally underserved populations. *Applied Nursing Research, 8,* 8–14.

Neuberger, G. B., Press, A. N., Lindsley, H. B., Hinton, R., Cagle, P. E., Carlson, K., Scott, S., Dahl, J., & Kramer, B. (1997). Effects of exercise on fatigue, aerobic fitness, and disease activity

measures in persons with rheumatoid arthritis. *Research in Nursing & Health, 20,* 195–204.

Pickler, R. H., Higgins, K. E., & Crummette, B. D. (1993). The effect of nonnutritive sucking on bottle-feeding stress in preterm infants. *Journal of Obstetric, Gynecologic, and Neonatal Nursing, 22,* 230–234.

Pollack, L. E. (1993). Content analysis of groups for inpatients with bipolar disorder. *Applied Nursing Research, 6,* 19–27.

Pollow, R. L., Stoller, E. P., Forster, L. E., & Duniho, T. S. (1994). Drug combinations and potential for risk of adverse drug reaction among community-dwelling elderly. *Nursing Research, 43,* 44–49.

Preski, S., & Walker, L. O. (1997). Contributions of maternal identity and lifestyle to young children's adjustment. *Research in Nursing & Health, 20,* 107–117.

Roberts, K. L., Brittin, M., Cook, M. A., & de-Clifford, J. (1994). Boomerang pillows and respiratory capacity. *Clinical Nursing Research, 3,* 157–165.

Rothert, M. L., Holmes-Rovner, M., Rovner, D., Kroll, J., Breer, L., Talaczyk, G., Schmitt, N., Padonu, G., & Wills, C. (1997). An educational intervention as decision support for menopausal women. *Research in Nursing & Health, 20,* 377–387.

Samarel, N., Fawcett, J., & Tulman, L. (1997). Effect of support groups with coaching on adaptation to early stage breast cancer. *Research in Nursing & Health, 20,* 15–26.

Schirm, V. (1993). Cholesterol screening of older persons. *Applied Nursing Research, 6,* 119–124.

Silveira, J. M., & Winstead-Fry, P. (1997). The needs of patients with cancer and their caregivers in rural areas. *Oncology Nursing Forum, 24,* 71–76.

Song, R., Daly, B. J., Rudy, E. B., Douglas, S., & Dyer, M. A. (1997). Nurses' job satisfaction, absenteeism, and turnover after implementing a special care unit practice model. *Research in Nursing & Health, 20,* 443–452.

Stratton, T. D., Dunkin, J. W., Juhl, N., & Geller, J. M. (1993). Recruiting registered nurses to rural practice settings. *Applied Nursing Research, 6,* 64–70.

Strzalka, A., & Havens, D. S. (1996). Nursing care quality: Comparison of unit-hired, hospital float pool, and agency nurses. *Journal of Nursing Care Quality, 10,* 59–65.

Weaver, T. E., Richmond, T. S., & Narsavage, G. L. (1997). An explanatory model of functional status in chronic obstructive pulmonary disease. *Nursing Research, 46,* 26–31.

Williams, S. A. (1997). The relationship of patients' perceptions of holistic nurse caring to satisfaction with nursing care. *Journal of Nursing Care Quality, 11,* 15–29.

Winslow, E. H., Nestor, V., Davidoff, S., Thompson, P., & Borum, J. (1997). Legibility and completeness of physicians' handwritten medication orders. *Heart & Lung, 26,* 158–164.

Woods, N. F., & Mitchell, E. S. (1997). Pathways to depressed mood for midlife women. *Research in Nursing & Health, 20,* 119–129.

York, R., Brown, L. P., Samuels, P., Finkler, S. A., Jacobsen, B., Persely, C. A., Swank, A., & Robbins, D. (1997). A randomized trial of early discharge and nurse specialist transitional follow-up care of high-risk childbearing women. *Nursing Research, 46,* 254–261.

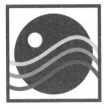

CHAPTER 9

Research Control in Quantitative Research

A major function of research design for most research questions addressed through structured, quantitative procedures is to maximize the amount of control that an investigator has over the research situation and variables. The researcher strives to control extraneous variables to determine the true nature of the relationship between the independent and dependent variables under investigation. Extraneous variables are variables that have an irrelevant association with the dependent variable and that can confound the testing of the research hypothesis. This chapter discusses various methods of controlling extraneous variables in quantitative studies.*

There are two basic types of extraneous variables: those that are intrinsic to the subjects of the study and those that are external factors stemming from the research situation.

---

*Many of the control techniques outlined in this chapter are not normally used in qualitative studies, in which the aim is for the research setting to be as natural as possible. The qualitative researcher often wants to study, rather than control, extraneous variables to understand better the context of the phenomena under investigation.

We begin with a discussion of methods of controlling external factors.

CONTROLLING EXTERNAL FACTORS

In quantitative studies, the researcher often takes a number of steps to minimize situational contaminants. That is, he or she tries to make the conditions under which the data are collected as similar as possible for every participant in the study. The control that a researcher imposes on a study by attempting to maintain **constancy of conditions** probably represents one of the earliest forms of scientific control.

The environment has been found to exert a powerful influence on people's emotions and behavior. In designing a quantitative study, therefore, the investigator needs to pay attention to the environmental context within which the study is to be conducted. Control over the environment is most easily achieved in laboratory experiments in which all subjects are brought into an environment that the experimenter is in a position to arrange. Researchers have much less freedom in controlling the environment in studies that occur in natural settings. This does not mean that the researcher should abandon all efforts to make the environments as similar as possible. For example, in conducting a survey in which the information is to be gathered by means of an interview, the researcher should attempt to conduct all interviews in basically the same kind of environment. That is, it would not be desirable to interview some of the respondents in their own homes, some in their places of work, some in the researcher's office, and so forth. In each of these settings, the participant normally assumes different roles (e.g., wife, husband, parent; employee; and client or patient), and responses to questions may be influenced to some degree by the role in which the respondent is operating.

One of the advantages of conducting a study in an artificial setting such as a laboratory is that the researcher has greater confidence of having control over the independent and extraneous variables. In real-life settings, even when subjects are randomly assigned to groups, the differentiation between groups may be difficult to control. Let us look at another example to see why this is so. Suppose we were planning to teach nursing students a unit on dyspnea, and we have used a lecture-type approach in the past. If we were interested in trying an individualized, autotutorial approach to cover the same material and wanted to evaluate the effectiveness of this method before adopting it for all students, we might randomly assign students to one of the two methods. Scores on a test covering the content of the unit could be used as the dependent or criterion variable. But now, suppose the students in the two groups talk to one another about their learning experiences. Some of the lecture-group students might go through parts of the programmed text. Perhaps some of the students in the autotutorial group will sit in on some of the lectures. In short, field experiments are often subject to the problem of **contamination of treatments**. In the same study, it would also be

difficult to control other variables, such as the time or place in which the learning occurs for the individualized group.

Another external factor that is often controlled is the time factor. Depending on the topic of the study, the dependent variable may be influenced by the time of day or time of year in which the data are collected, or both. It would, in such cases, be desirable for the researcher to strive for constancy of times across subjects. If an investigator were studying fatigue or perceptions of physical well-being, it would probably matter a great deal whether the data were gathered in the morning, afternoon, or evening, or in the summer as opposed to the winter. Although time constancy is not always critical, it is often relatively easy for the researcher to control and should, therefore, be sought whenever possible.

Another aspect of maintaining constancy of conditions concerns constancy in the communications to the subjects and in the treatment itself in the case of experiments or quasi-experiments. In most research efforts, the researcher informs participants about the purpose of the study, what use will be made of the data, under whose auspices the study is being conducted, and so forth. This information generally should be prepared ahead of time, and the same message should be delivered to all subjects. Generally, there should be as little ad-libbing as possible in a quantitative study.

In studies involving the implementation of a treatment, care should be taken to adhere to the specifications (often referred to as **research protocols**) for that treatment. For example, in experiments to test the effectiveness of a new drug to cure a medical problem, the researcher would have to take great care to ensure that the subjects in the experimental group received the same chemical substance and the same dosage, that the substance was administered in the same way, and so forth. Some treatments are much "fuzzier" than in the case of administering a drug, as is the case for most nursing interventions. In such a situation, the investigator should spell out in detail the exact behaviors required of the personnel responsible for delivering or administering the treatment.

One of the features that distinguishes non-experimental research from experimental and quasi-experimental studies is that if the researcher has not manipulated the independent variable, then there is no means of ensuring constancy of conditions. Let us take as an example an ex post facto study that attempts to determine if there is a relationship between a person's knowledge of nutrition and his or her own eating habits. Suppose the investigator finds no relationship between nutritional knowledge and eating patterns. That is, the investigator finds that people who are well-informed about nutrition are just as likely as uninformed people to maintain inadequate diets. In this case, however, the researcher has had no control over the source of a person's nutritional knowledge (the independent variable). This knowledge was measured after the fact (post facto), and the conditions under which the information was obtained cannot be assumed to be constant or even similar. The researcher may conclude from the study that it is not meaningful to teach nutrition to people because knowledge has no impact on their eating behavior. It may be, however, that different methods of providing nutritional information vary in their ability to motivate people to alter their nutritional habits. Thus, the ability of the investigator to control or manipulate the independent variable of interest may be extremely important in understanding the relationships between variables, or the absence of relationships.

CONTROLLING INTRINSIC FACTORS

Characteristics of the participants in a quantitative scientific study almost always need to be controlled for the findings to be interpretable. This section describes six specific ways of controlling extraneous variables associated with subject characteristics.

Randomization

We have already discussed the most effective method of controlling individual extraneous variables—randomization. The primary function of randomization is to secure comparable groups, that is, to equalize the groups with respect to the extraneous variables. A distinct advantage of random assignment, compared with other methods of controlling extraneous variables, is that randomization controls *all* possible sources of extraneous variation, without any conscious decision on the researcher's part about which variables need to be controlled.

Suppose, for example, that we were interested in assessing the effect of a physical training program on cardiovascular functioning among nursing home residents. Characteristics such as the individual's age, gender, prior occupation, history of smoking, and length of stay in the nursing home could all affect the patient's cardiovascular system, independently of the physical training program. The effects of these other variables are extraneous to the research problem and should be controlled. Through randomization, we could expect that an experimental group (receiving the physical training program) and control group (not receiving the program) would be comparable in terms of these as well as any other factors that influence cardiovascular functioning.

Repeated Measures

Randomization within the context of a repeated measures design is an especially powerful method of ensuring equivalence between groups being compared, that is, of controlling all extraneous subject characteristics. However, such a design is not appropriate for all studies because of the problem of carry-over effects. When subjects are exposed to two different treatments or conditions, they may be influenced in the second condition by their experience in the first condition. In our example of the physical training program, a repeated measures design is unsuitable because the no-program-followed-by-program condition would not be the same as the program-followed-by-no-program condition: Those subjects who were in the program in the first condition might independently decide to exercise more during the time they are not in the program.

Thus, because the two (or more) treatments are not applied simultaneously in repeated measures designs, the order of the treatment may be important in affecting the subject's performance. The best approach is to use randomization to determine the ordering. When there are only two conditions in a repeated measures design, the researcher simply designates that half the subjects, at random, will receive treatment A first and that the other half will receive treatment B first. When there are three or more conditions to which each subject will be exposed, the procedure of **counterbalancing** is frequently used to minimize the impact of ordering effects. For example, if there were three conditions (A, B, C), subjects would be randomly assigned to six different orderings in a counterbalanced scheme:

A,	B,	C	A,	C,	B
B,	C,	A	B,	A,	C
C,	A,	B	C,	B,	A

Note that, in addition to their potential for excellent control over extraneous subject characteristics, repeated measures designs offer another important advantage: fewer research subjects are needed. Fifty subjects exposed to two treatments in random order yield 100 pieces of data (50×2); 50 subjects randomly assigned to two different treatment groups yield only 50 pieces of data (25×2).

In sum, repeated measures can be a useful, rigorous, and efficient design for eliminating extraneous variables. When carry-over effects from one condition to another are anticipated, however, as might be the case in many medical or nursing interventions, the researcher will need to seek other designs.

Homogeneity

When randomization and repeated measures are not feasible, there are alternative methods of controlling intrinsic subject characteristics that could contaminate the relationships under investigation. One such method is to use only subjects who are homogeneous with respect to those variables that are considered extraneous. The extraneous variables, in this case, are not allowed to vary. In the example of the physical training program, suppose that the subjects were in two separate nursing homes and that those in one nursing home received the physical training program and those in the other nursing home did not receive the program. If gender were considered to be an important confounding variable, the researcher might wish to use only men (or only women) as subjects. Similarly, if the researcher were concerned about the effects of the subjects' age on cardiovascular functioning, participation in the study could be limited to those within a specified age range.

This method of utilizing a homogeneous subject pool is fairly easy and offers considerable control. The limitation of this approach lies in the fact that the research findings can only be generalized to the type of subjects who participated in the study. If the physical training program were found to have beneficial effects on the cardiovascular status of a sample of men 65 to 75 years of age, its usefulness for improving the cardiovascular status of women in their 80s would be strictly a matter of conjecture.

Blocking

A fourth approach to controlling extraneous variables is to include them in the design of a study as independent variables. To pursue our example of the physical training program, if gender were thought to be a confounding variable, it could be built into the study design, as illustrated in Figure 9-1. This procedure would allow us to make an assessment of the impact

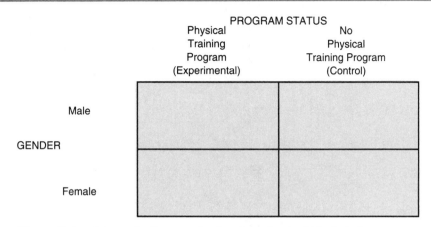

Figure 9-1. Schematic diagram of a 2 × 2 randomized block design.

of our training program on the cardiovascular functioning of both elderly men and women. Furthermore, this approach has the advantage of adding greater precision and enhancing the likelihood of detecting differences between our experimental and control groups because the effect of the extraneous variable on the dependent variable can be assessed.

Let us consider this third approach in greater detail. We refer to the design shown in Figure 9-1 as a **randomized block design.*** The variable of gender, which cannot be manipulated by the researcher, is known as a **blocking variable.** In an experiment to test the effectiveness of the physical training program, the experimenter obviously could not randomly assign subjects to one of four cells, as in a factorial experiment, because the gender of the subjects is a given. However, the experimenter can randomly assign men and women separately to the experimental and control conditions. Let us say that there are 40 men and 40 women available for the randomized block study. The researcher would not take the 80 subjects and assign half to the physi-

cal training program group and the other half to the control group. Rather, the randomization procedure would be performed separately for men and women, thereby guaranteeing 20 subjects in each cell of the four-cell design.

The design can be extended to include more than one blocking variable, as shown in Figure 9-2. In this design, the age of the subject has been included in the design to control for this second extraneous variable. Once again, the experimenter would randomly assign subjects from each block to either the experimental or control conditions. In other words, half the men 66 to 70 years of age would randomly be assigned to the program, as would half the men 71 to 75 years of age, and so forth. Although in theory, the number of blocks that could be added is unlimited, practical concerns usually dictate a relatively small number of blocks (and, hence, a small number of extraneous variables that can be controlled). Expansion of the design usually requires that a larger subject pool be used. As a general rule of thumb, a minimum of 20 to 30 subjects per cell is often recommended. This means that, whereas a minimum of 80 subjects would be needed for the design in Figure 9-1, 240 subjects would be needed for the design in Figure 9-2. This suggests that, if a decision is made to

---

*The terminology for this design varies from text to text. Some authors refer to this as a factorial design; others call it a levels-by-treatment design. We have chosen not to use the term factorial because gender is not under experimental control, and hence, complete randomization is impossible.

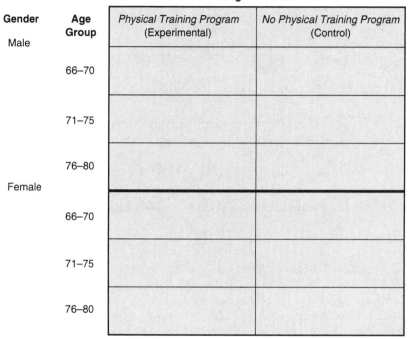

Figure 9-2.   Schematic diagram of a 2 × 2 × 3 randomized block design.

introduce extraneous variables into the design of a study, great care should be taken to choose the most relevant subject characteristics as the blocking variables.

Strictly speaking, the type of design we have discussed is appropriate only in experimental studies, but in reality, it is used commonly in quasi-experimental and ex post facto studies as well. If an investigator were studying the effects of a physical training program on cardiovascular functioning after the fact (i.e., subjects self-selected themselves into one of the two groups, and the researcher had no control over who was included in each group), the investigator might want to set up the analysis in such a way that differential effects for men and women would be analyzed. The design structure would look the same as the one presented in Figure 9-1, although the implications and conclusions that could be drawn from the results would be different than if the researcher had been in con-

trol of the manipulation and randomization procedures.

Matching

A fifth method of dealing with extraneous variables is known as matching. **Matching** (also referred to as **pair matching**) involves using knowledge of subject characteristics to form comparison groups. If a matching procedure were to be adopted for our physical training program example, and age and gender were the extraneous variables of interest, we would need to match each subject in the experimental group with one in the control group with respect to age and gender. If the subjects could be assigned on a random basis, we would actually have a special type of randomized block design with one subject per cell.

Pair matching, however, is usually a post hoc attempt to approximate this experimental blocking design. That is, the researcher may begin with 20 subjects who participate in the training program and then create a comparison group by matching, one by one, the training group participants with nonparticipating nursing home residents in terms of age and gender.

Despite the intuitive appeal of such a design, there are reasons why matching is problematic. First, to match effectively, the researcher must know in advance what the relevant extraneous variables are. Second, after two or three variables, it often becomes impossible to pair match adequately. Let us say that we are interested in controlling for the age, gender, race, and length of nursing home stay of the subjects. Thus, if subject 1 in the physical training program were an African American woman, aged 80 years, whose length of stay is 5 years, the researcher would need to seek another woman with these same or similar characteristics as a comparison group counterpart. With more than three variables, the matching procedure becomes extremely cumbersome, if not impossible. For these reasons, matching as a technique for controlling extraneous variables should, in general, be used only when other, more powerful procedures are not feasible, as might be the case for some ex post facto studies.

Sometimes, as an alternative to pair matching, in which subjects are matched on a one-to-one basis for each matching variable, researchers choose to have a **balanced design** with regard to key extraneous variables. In such situations, the researcher attempts only to ensure that the composition of the groups being compared have proportional representation with regard to variables believed to be correlated with the dependent variable. For example, if gender and race were the two extraneous variables of interest in our example of the physical training program, the researcher adopting a balanced design would strive to ensure that the same percentage of men and women (and the same percentage of white and African American subjects) were in the group participating in the physical training program as were in a comparison group of nonpartici-

pants. Such an approach is much less cumbersome than pair matching, but it also has similar limitations. Nevertheless, both pair matching and balancing are preferable to failing to control for intrinsic subject characteristics at all.

Statistical Control

A sixth method of controlling unwanted variables is through statistical procedures. We recognize that, at this point, many readers may be unfamiliar with basic statistical procedures, let alone the sophisticated techniques referred to here. Therefore, a detailed description of powerful **statistical control** mechanisms will not be attempted. If you have a background in statistics, you should consult Chapter 20 or a textbook on advanced statistics for fuller coverage of this topic. However, because the possibility of statistical control may mystify readers, we explain the underlying principle with a simple illustration of a procedure called **analysis of covariance**.

Returning to the physical training program example, suppose we have a group that is participating in the physical training program and another group that is not. The groups represent intact groups (e.g., residents of two different nursing homes, only one of which is offering the physical training program), and therefore randomization is impossible. As our measures of cardiovascular functioning, suppose we use maximal oxygen consumption and resting heart rate. As with most things in life, there undoubtedly will be individual differences on these two measures—that is, heart rate and oxygen consumption will vary from one person to the next. The research question is, Can some of the individual differences be attributed to a person's participation in the physical training program? Unfortunately, the individual differences in cardiovascular functioning are also related to other, extraneous characteristics of the subjects, such as age. The large circles in Figure 9-3 may be taken to represent the total variability (extent of individual differences) for both groups on, say, resting

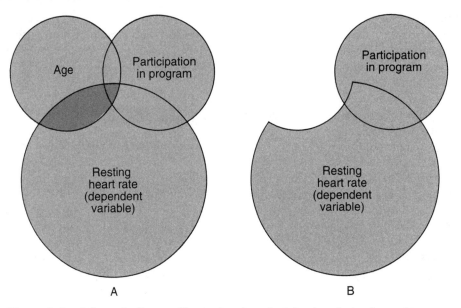

Figure 9-3. Schematic diagram illustrating the principle of analysis of covariance.

heart rate. A certain amount of that total variability can be explained simply by virtue of the subject's age, which is schematized in the figure as the small circle on the left in Figure 9-3A. Another part of the variability can be explained by the subject's participation or nonparticipation in the physical training program, represented as the small circle on the right in A. In A, the fact that the two small circles (age and participation in program) overlap indicates that there is a relationship between those two variables. In other words, subjects in the group receiving the physical training program are, on average, either older or younger than members of the comparison group. Therefore, age should be controlled. Otherwise, it will be impossible to determine whether differences in resting heart rate should be attributed to age differences or to differences in program participation.

Analysis of covariance can accomplish this control function by statistically removing the effect of the extraneous variable on the dependent variable. In the illustration, that portion of heart rate variability that is attributable to

age could be removed through the analysis of covariance technique. This is designated in Figure 9-3A by the darkened area in the large circle; *B* illustrates that the final analysis would examine the effect of program participation on heart rate after removing the effect of age. By controlling the variability of heart rate resulting from age, we can have a much more precise estimate of the effect of the training program on heart rate. Note that even after removing the variability resulting from age, there is still individual variability not associated with the program treatment—the bottom half of the large circle in B. This means that the precision of the study can probably be further enhanced by controlling additional extraneous variables, such as gender, type of previous occupation, and so forth. Analysis of covariance, as well as other sophisticated procedures, can accommodate multiple extraneous variables.

When pretest measures of the dependent variables have been obtained, these are often controlled statistically, which greatly enhances the precision of the estimates of the effect of an intervention. In our example, controlling pre-program measures of cardiovascular functioning through analysis of covariance would be especially powerful because it would remove the effect of most individual variation stemming from a host of other extraneous factors.

Evaluation of Control Methods

Overall, the random assignment of subjects to groups is the most effective approach to managing extraneous variables because randomization tends to cancel out individual variation on all possible extraneous variables. Repeated measures designs, although extremely useful in controlling all possible sources of extraneous variation, cannot be applied to most nursing research problems. The remaining alternatives to randomization—homogeneity, blocking, matching, and analysis of covariance—have one disadvantage in common: the researcher must know or predict in advance the relevant extraneous variables. To select homogeneous samples, develop a blocking design, match, or perform an analysis of covariance, the researcher must make a decision about what variables need to be measured and controlled. This constraint may pose severe limitations on the degree of control that is possible, particularly because the researcher can seldom deal explicitly with more than two or three extraneous variables at one time (except in the case of analysis of covariance).

Although we have repeatedly hailed randomization as the ideal mechanism for controlling extraneous subject characteristics, it is clear that randomization is not always possible. For example, if the independent variable cannot be manipulated, then other techniques must be used. In ex post facto and quasi-experimental studies, the control options available to researchers include homogeneity, blocking, matching, and analysis of covariance. In quantitative research, the use of any of the control procedures discussed here is far preferable to the absence of any attempt to control intrinsic extraneous variables.

INTERNAL VALIDITY

One method of evaluating the adequacy of research control mechanisms and overall research design is to assess its internal and external validity. Campbell and Stanley (1963), in a classic monograph, use the term **internal validity** to refer to the extent to which it is possible to make an inference that the independent variable is truly influencing the dependent variable and that the relationship is not spurious. **External validity**, which is discussed in the next section, is achieved when the results can confidently be generalized to situations outside the specific research setting.

The control mechanisms reviewed in the previous sections are all strategies for improving the internal validity of research studies. If the researcher is not careful in managing extraneous variables and in other ways controlling the design of the study, there may be reason to challenge the conclusion that the subjects' performance on the dependent measure resulted from the effect of the independent variable.

Threats to Internal Validity

True experiments possess a high degree of internal validity because the use of control procedures (manipulation and randomization) enables the researcher to rule out most alternative explanations for the results. With quasi-experimental, pre-experimental, or ex post facto designs, the investigator must always contend with competing explanations for the obtained results. These competing explanations, referred to as **threats to internal validity**, have been grouped into several classes, a few of which are examined here.

HISTORY

The threat of **history** refers to the occurrence of external events that take place concurrently with the independent variable that can affect the dependent variables of interest. For example, suppose we were studying the effectiveness of a county-wide nurse outreach program designed to encourage pregnant women in rural areas to improve their health-related practices before delivery (e.g., better nutritional practices, cessation of smoking and drinking, and earlier prenatal care). The program might be evaluated by comparing the average birthweight of infants born in the 12 months before the outreach program with the average birthweight of those born in the 12 months after the program was introduced. However, suppose that 1 month after the new program was launched, a highly publicized docudrama regarding the inadequacies of prenatal care for poor women was aired on national television. Our dependent variable in this case, infants' birthweight, might now be affected by both the intervention and the messages in the docudrama, and it becomes impossible for us to disentangle the two effects.

In a true experiment, history generally is not a threat to the internal validity of a study because we can often assume that external events are as likely to affect the experimental as the control group. When this is the case, any group differences that emerge at the end of the study represent effects over and above those created by external factors. An exception, however, is when a repeated measures design is used. If an external event that has an effect on the dependent variable occurs during the first half (or second half) of the experiment, then the treatments would be contaminated by the effect of that event. That is, some people would receive treatment A with the event and others would receive treatment A without it, and the same would be true for treatment B.

SELECTION

The term **selection** encompasses biases resulting from preexisting differences between groups. When individuals are not assigned randomly to groups, we must always be alert to the possibility that the groups are nonequivalent. They may differ, in fact, in ways that are subtle and difficult to detect. If the groups are nonequivalent, the researcher is faced with the possibility that any group difference on the dependent variable is the result of initial differences rather than the effect of the independent variable. For example, if a researcher found that women with a fertility problem were more likely to be depressed than women who were mothers, it would be impossible to conclude that the two groups differed in terms of depression *because* of their differences in reproductive status; the women in the two groups might have been different in terms of psychological adjustment to begin with. The problem of selection is clearly reduced when the researcher can collect data regarding the characteristics of the subjects before the occurrence of the independent variable, but this is often difficult to accomplish. In the example relating to the fertility problem, the best design would involve the collection of information on the women's level of depression even before their attempts to become pregnant. Selection bias is one of the most problematic and frequently encountered threats to the internal validity of studies not using an experimental design.

Selection biases also often interact with other biases to compound the threat to the internal validity of the study. For example, if the comparison group is different from the experimental group or main group of interest, then the characteristics of the members of the comparison group could lead them to have different intervening experiences, thereby introducing both history and selection biases into the design.

MATURATION

In a research context, **maturation** refers to processes occurring within the subjects during the course of the study as a result of the passage of time rather than as a result of a treatment or independent variable. Examples of such processes include physical growth, emotional maturity, fatigue, and the like. For instance, if we wanted to evaluate the effects of a special sensorimotor development program for developmentally retarded children, we would have to consider that progress does occur in these children even without special assistance. A design such as a one-group pretest–posttest design (see Figure 8-6 in Chapter 8), for example, would be highly susceptible to this threat to internal validity.

Maturation would be a relevant consideration in many areas of nursing research. Remember that maturation here does not refer to aging or developmental changes exclusively but rather to any kind of change that occurs with the individual as a function of time. Thus, wound-healing, postoperative recovery, and many other bodily changes that can occur with little or no nursing or medical intervention must be considered as an explanation for outcomes in subjects that rivals an explanation based on the effects of the independent variable.

TESTING

The effects of taking a pretest on the participants' performance on a posttest are known as **testing** effects. It has been documented in numerous studies, particularly in those dealing with opinions and attitudes, that the mere act of collecting information from people changes them. Let us say that we administer to a group of nursing students a questionnaire dealing with their attitudes toward euthanasia. We then proceed to acquaint the students with various arguments that have been made for and against euthanasia, outcomes of court cases, and the like. At the end of instruction, we give them the same attitude measure as before and observe whether their attitudes have changed as a function of the instruction. The problem here is that the first administration of the questionnaire might sensitize the students to issues that they had not contemplated before. The sensitization may, in fact, result in attitude changes regardless of whether instruction follows. If a comparison group is not used in the study, it becomes

impossible to segregate the effects of the instruction from the effects of having taken the pretest (as well as from the effects of history, maturation, and so forth). In true experiments, testing may not be a problem because its effects would be expected to be about equal in all groups, but the Solomon four-group design (discussed in Chapter 8) could be used if the researcher wanted to segregate the effects of the intervention from those of the pretest.

Sensitization, or testing, problems are typically much more likely to occur when the pretest involves information that subjects provide through self-report (e.g., in a questionnaire), especially if we are exposing the subjects to controversial or novel material. For many nursing studies (e.g., those that involve the collection of biophysiologic information), testing effects are not a major concern.

INSTRUMENTATION

Another threat that is related to the researcher's measurements is referred to as the threat of **instrumentation**. This bias reflects changes in the researcher's measuring instruments between an initial point of data collection and a subsequent point. For example, if the researcher uses one measure of stress at baseline and a different measure at follow-up, then any changes might reflect changes in the measuring tool rather than the effects of the independent variable.

Instrumentation effects can occur even if the same measure is used. For example, if the measuring tool yields more accurate measures on the second administration (e.g., if the people collecting the data are more experienced) or less accurate measures the second time (e.g., if the subjects become bored or fatigued), then these differences could bias the results.

MORTALITY

Mortality refers to the threat that arises from differential attrition from the groups being compared. The loss of subjects during the course of a study may differ from one group to another because of a priori differences in interest, motivation, health, and so on. For example, suppose we used a nonequivalent control group design to assess the morale of the nursing personnel from two different hospitals, one of which was initiating primary nursing. The dependent variable, nursing staff morale, is measured in both hospitals before and after the intervention. Comparison group members, who may have no particular commitment to the study, may decline to complete a posttest questionnaire because of lack of incentive. Those who do fill it out may be unrepresentative of the group as a whole—they may be those who are most enthusiastic about their work environment, for example. If this were the case, it might appear that the morale of the nurses in the comparison hospital had improved over time, but this improvement might only be an artifact of the attrition from the study of a biased segment of this group.

The threat of mortality is apt to be especially high when the length of time between points of data collection is long. A 12-month follow-up of subjects, for example, is likely to produce higher rates of attrition than a 1-month follow-up. In clinical nursing studies, the problem of attrition may be especially acute because of patient death or disability.

Note that if attrition is random (i.e., those dropping out of the study are highly similar to those remaining in the study with respect to characteristics that are related to the dependent variable), then the risk of bias is low. However, attrition is rarely totally random. In general, the higher the rate of attrition, the greater the likelihood of bias. Although there is no absolute standard for acceptable attrition rates, biases are generally of concern if the rate exceeds 20%.

Internal Validity and Research Design

Quasi-experimental and ex post facto studies are especially susceptible to threats to internal validity. The threats just described (as well as

others, which are less frequently of concern to nurse researchers) represent alternative explanations that compete with the independent variable as a cause of the dependent variable. The aim of a good research design is to rule out these competing explanations.

An experimental design normally controls for these factors, but it must not be assumed that in a true experiment the researcher need not worry about them. For example, if constancy of conditions is not maintained for experimental and control groups, then history might be a rival explanation for any group differences. Mortality is, in particular, a salient threat in true experiments. Because the experimenter does things differently with the experimental and control groups, subjects in the groups may drop out of the study differentially. This is particularly apt to happen if the experimental treatment is painful, inconvenient, or time-consuming, or if the control condition is boring or considered a nuisance. When this happens, the subjects remaining in the study may differ from those who left in important ways, thereby nullifying the initial equivalence of the groups.

Internal Validity and Data Analysis

A researcher's best strategy for enhancing the internal validity of a study is to use a strong research design that includes the use of the control mechanisms discussed earlier in this chapter. Even when this is possible (and, certainly, when this is *not* possible), it is highly advisable to analyze the data to determine the nature and extent of any biases. When biases are detected, the information can be used to interpret the results of the substantive analyses, and in some cases, the biases can be statistically controlled.

The researcher must essentially be a self-critic and consider the types of biases that could have arisen within the context of the chosen design—and then systematically search for evidence of their existence (while hoping, of course, that no evidence can be found). A few examples should illustrate how the researcher should proceed.

Selection biases are the most prevalent of the threats to internal validity and should be examined whenever possible. Typically, this involves the comparison of subjects on pretest measures, when pretest data have been collected. For example, if we were studying depression in women who delivered a baby by cesarean section versus those who delivered vaginally, an ideal way to evaluate selection bias would be to compare the level of depression in these two groups during or before the pregnancy. If there are significant predelivery differences, then postdelivery differences would have to be interpreted with these initial differences in mind (or with these differences controlled). In after-only designs or in cross-sectional ex post facto studies in which there is no pretest information on the dependent variable, the researcher should nevertheless search for selection biases by comparing groups with respect to important background variables, such as age, gender, ethnicity, social class, health status, and so on. When group differences are detected, they should be controlled if possible (through analysis of covariance) or at least taken into account in the interpretation of the findings. Selection biases should be analyzed even when random assignment has been used to form groups because there is no absolute guarantee that randomization will yield perfectly equivalent groups.

Whenever the research design involves multiple points of data collection, the researcher should analyze attrition biases. This is typically achieved through a comparison of those who did and did not complete the study with regard to initial measures of the dependent variable or other characteristics measured at the first point of data collection.

In a repeated measures design, history is a potential threat both because an external event could differentially affect subjects in different treatment orderings and because the different orderings are in themselves a kind of differential history. The substantive analysis of the data would involve a comparison of the dependent variable under treatment A versus treatment B. The analysis for evidence of bias, by contrast, would involve a comparison of subjects in the different orderings (e.g., A then B versus B then A). If there are significant differences between the two orderings, then the researcher would have evidence of an ordering bias.

In summary, efforts to enhance the internal validity of a study should not end once the design strategy has been put in place. The researcher should seek additional opportunities to understand (and possibly to correct) the various threats to internal validity that can arise.

EXTERNAL VALIDITY

The term **external validity** refers to the generalizability of the research findings to other settings or samples. Research is almost never conducted with the intention of discovering relationships among variables for one group of people at one point in time. The aim of research is typically to reveal enduring relationships, the understanding of which can be used to improve the human condition. If a nursing intervention under investigation is found to be successful, others will want to adopt the procedure. Therefore, an important question is whether the intervention will work in another setting and with different patients. Researchers should routinely ask themselves, To what populations, environments, and conditions can the results of the study be applied?

External Validity and Sampling

One aspect of a study's external validity concerns the adequacy of the sampling design. If the characteristics of the sample are representative of those of the population, then generalization is straightforward. Sampling designs are described at length in Chapter 12.

Strictly speaking, the findings of a study can only be generalized to the population of subjects from which a study sample has been selected at random. If an investigator were studying the effects of a newly developed therapeutic treatment for heroin addicts, then the researcher might begin with a population of addicts in a particular clinic or drug treatment center. From this population, a random sample of drug users could be selected for participation in the study. Individuals from the sample would then be randomly assigned to one of two or more conditions, assuming that an experiment were possible. If the results revealed that the new therapeutic treatment was highly effective in reducing recidivism among the sample of addicts, could it be concluded that all addicts in the United States would benefit from the treatment? Unfortunately, no. The population of heroin addicts undergoing treatment in one particular facility may not be representative of all addicts. For example, the facility in question may attract drug users from certain ethnic, socioeconomic, or age groups. Perhaps the new treatment is only effective with individuals from such groups.

Of relevance here is Kempthorne's (1961) distinction between accessible populations and target populations. The **accessible population** is the population of subjects available for a particular study. In our drug treatment example, all of the heroin addicts in treatment at a particular treatment center would constitute the accessible population. When random procedures have been used to select a sample from an accessible population, there is no difficulty in generalizing the results to that group.

The **target population** is the total group of subjects about whom the investigator is interested and to whom the results could reasonably be generalized. This second type of generalization is considerably more risky and cannot be done with as much confidence as in the case of generalizations to the accessible population. The adequacy and utility of this type of inference hinge strongly on the similarity of the characteristics of the two populations. Thus, the researcher must be aware of the characteristics of the accessible population and, in turn, define the target population to be like the accessible population. In the drug treatment example, the accessible population might predominantly comprise voluntarily admitted white men in their 20s living in New York City. Although we might ideally like to generalize our results to all drug addicts, we would be on much safer ground if we defined our target population as young, urban, white men who present themselves for treatment.

Threats to External Validity

In addition to characteristics of the sample that limit the generalizability of research findings, there are various characteristics of the environment or research situation that affect the study's representativeness and, hence, its external validity. These characteristics should be taken into consideration in developing a research design and in interpreting results once the data have been collected. Among the most noteworthy threats to the external validity of studies are the following five effects:

1. *The Hawthorne effect.* As discussed in Chapter 8, subjects in an investigation may behave in a particular manner largely because they are aware of their participation in a study. If a certain type of behavior or performance is elicited only in a research context, then the results cannot be generalized to more natural settings.

2. *Novelty effects.* When a treatment is new, subjects and research agents alike might alter their behavior in a variety of ways. People may be either enthusiastic or skeptical about new methods of doing things. The results may reflect these reactions to the novelty; once the treatment is more familiar, the same results may fail to appear.

3. *Interaction of history and treatment effect.* The results may reflect the impact of the treatment *and* some other events external to the study. When the treatment is implemented again in the absence of the

other events, different results may be obtained. For example, if a dietary intervention for people with high cholesterol levels was being evaluated shortly after extensive media coverage of research demonstrating a link between consumption of oat bran and reduction in cholesterol levels, it would be difficult to know whether any observed effects would be observed again if the intervention were implemented several months later with a new group of people.

4. *Experimenter effects.* The performance of the subjects may be affected by characteristics of the researchers. The investigators often have an emotional or intellectual investment in demonstrating that their hypotheses are correct and may unconsciously communicate their expectations to the subjects, or they may be somewhat biased in their observations. If this is the case, any observed relationships in the original study might be difficult to replicate in a more neutral situation.

5. *Measurement effects.* In research studies, the investigators collect a considerable amount of data, such as pretest information, background data, and so forth. The results may not apply to another group of people who are not also exposed to the same data collection procedures.

EXTERNAL VERSUS INTERNAL VALIDITY

Ideally, the researcher strives to design studies that are strong with respect to both internal and external validity. In some instances, however, the requirements for ensuring one type of validity may interfere with the possibility of achieving the second.

As one example of why this is so, consider a researcher who uses the principle of homogeneity to enhance the internal validity of a study. By controlling extraneous variables through the selection of a homogeneous sample with respect to those variables, the researcher has limited his or her ability to generalize the study results to the entire population of interest.

As another example of the conflict between internal and external validity, if the researcher exerts a high degree of control over a study through constancy of conditions in an effort to maximize internal validity, the setting may become highly artificial and pose a threat to the generalizability of the findings to more naturalistic environments. Thus, it is often necessary to reach a compromise by introducing sufficient controls while maintaining some semblance of realism.

When there is a conflict between internal and external validity, it is often preferable to opt for stronger internal validity. Indeed, it has been argued that if the findings are not internally valid, they cannot possibly be externally valid. That is, it makes little sense to generalize the findings when the findings are themselves uninterpretable. Whenever a compromise is necessary, the concept of replication, or the repetition of a study in a new setting with new subjects, is an extremely important one. Much greater confidence can be placed in the findings of a study if it can be demonstrated that the results can be replicated in other settings and with new subjects.

TIPS FOR ENHANCING RESEARCH CONTROL

In most quantitative studies, it is extremely important to control for the effects of extraneous variables. When external factors or intrinsic subject characteristics confound the relationship between the independent and dependent variables, the results of the study are likely to be ambiguous. We offer the following suggestions for enhancing research control:

- Whenever constancy of research conditions cannot be achieved, the researcher should consider controlling external factors by using some of the same strategies we suggested for controlling intrinsic subject characteristics. For example, if the researcher suspects that the time of day may influence measurement of the dependent variable but cannot collect all the data at the same time of day, perhaps it is possible to assign subjects randomly to morning versus afternoon sessions.

- Achieving constancy of conditions is not always easy, especially in clinical studies, but various steps can be taken. For example, in addition to having standard protocols, it is important to train thoroughly the people who will be collecting the data and, in the case of an experiment or quasi-experiment, the personnel responsible for implementing the intervention. The extent to which the protocols are followed should also be monitored.

- This chapter offered various strategies for controlling the most important source of extraneous variation: the study participants themselves. These alternative strategies are not mutually exclusive; whenever possible, multiple methods should be used. For example, statistical methods of control, such as analysis of covariance, can be used in conjunction with blocking or matching. Even when randomization has been used, analysis of covariance increases the precision of the design.

- The first and best defense against threats to internal validity is a strong research design. As noted earlier, the next line of defense is through analysis. The researcher must, therefore, plan the study in such a way that opportunities to analyze bias are possible. This means giving careful consideration to variables that should be measured. Information on characteristics of the subjects that are likely to have a strong effect on the dependent variable should be collected whenever possible. In a longitudinal study, variables that are likely to be related to attrition should also be measured.

- The extraneous variables that need to be controlled obviously vary from one study to another, but we can nevertheless offer some guidance in identifying variables that should be measured. The single best variable to measure and control is the dependent variable itself, before the introduction of the independent variable. Major demographic variables—age, race/ ethnicity, gender, educational attainment, income level, marital status—should almost always be measured because these variables are related to many other variables of a social or psychological nature (including willingness to participate and remain in a scientific study). When the dependent variable is biophysiologic, measures of health status, medication, hospitalization history, and so on are likely to be important. Extraneous variables that are particular to the research problem should be identified through the review of the research literature.

- In longitudinal studies, the best method of avoiding attrition is to implement procedures to relocate subjects. Attrition typically occurs because of the researcher's inability to find participants, not because of their refusal to continue in the study. There are many sophisticated (and costly) methods of tracing subjects, but the simplest and most effective is to obtain **contact information** from participants at each major point of data collection. Contact information includes, at a minimum, the names, addresses, and telephone numbers of two or three people with whom the subject is close (e.g., his or her mother, father, siblings, or good friends)—people who would be likely to know how to contact the subject if he or she moved between points of data collection.

RESEARCH EXAMPLE

All the control techniques discussed in this chapter have been profitably used by nurse researchers. Table 9-1 presents some research examples of the use of these procedures. We conclude this chapter with a more detailed example of a study that was especially careful in exercising research control.

Gilliss, Gortner, Hauck, Shinn, Sparacino, and Tompkins (1993) undertook a randomized clinical trial in two hospitals. The researchers were testing the effect of a psychoeducational nursing intervention on several posthospital recovery outcomes (e.g., self-efficacy expectations, mood, quality of life) after cardiac surgery. To avoid contamination of treatments, the subjects were randomly assigned to the experimental or control group using cluster randomization, in groups of 8 to 10 patients. For patients in the experimental group, standard care was supplemented with in-hospital education on emotional reactions to surgery and follow-up telephone contact for 2 months.

The subjects were English-speaking cardiac patients between the ages of 25 and 75 years. Patients with certain conditions (e.g., aneurysms, aortic arch repairs, chronic ventricular arrhythmia) were excluded from the sample. A total of 91% of the subjects originally

---

TABLE 9-1   Examples of Studies Using Various Control Techniques

RESEARCH QUESTION	CONTROL TECHNIQUE	EXTRANEOUS VARIABLES CONTROLLED
What is the effect of a special coping intervention program on the coping outcomes of critically ill children and their mothers? (Melnyk, Alpert-Gillis, Hensel, Cable-Beiling, & Rubenstein, 1997)	Randomization	All characteristics of mothers and children
What is the effect of activity intensity on the sensitivity and reproducibility of dual-mode actigraphy? (Leidy, Abbott, & Fedenko, 1997)	Repeated measures	All characteristics
How effective are various comfort measures in alleviating nipple soreness in breastfeeding women? (Buchko, Pugh, Bishop, Cochran, Smith, & Lerew, 1994)	Homogeneity	Parity, riskiness of pregnancy, method of delivery, gestational age
What are the effects of a patient's family structure on nurses' impressions of the patient and verbal responses to the patient's questions? (Ganong & Coleman, 1997)	Blocking Randomization	Nurses' age All other characteristics
What is the impact of the perceived quality of parental relationships on coping strategies, received support, and well-being in adolescents from separated/divorced versus married households? (Grossman & Rowat, 1995)	Matching	Adolescents' gender, age class, and parents' occupation
Do women who receive different treatments for breast cancer (mastectomy, mastectomy with delayed or immediate reconstruction, conservative surgery) differ with respect to body image? (Mock, 1993)	Analysis of covariance	Age

recruited into the study were retained through the in-hospital treatment period, and of these, 95% remained in the study for the 6-month period of follow-up. The instruments used to measure patient outcomes were administered at baseline (before the intervention) and again at 4, 12, and 24 weeks after discharge. The follow-up data were analyzed through a statistical procedure that controlled the baseline measures.

The data analysis revealed that the experimental and control groups were comparable with respect to age, gender, history of previous myocardial infarction, functional status, surgery type, and education. They were also comparable with respect to baseline measures of the dependent variables. The results indicated that the subjects in the experimental group reported greater expectations regarding their self-efficacy for walking and also in actual walking behavior after surgery.

SUMMARY

A major function of research designs for structured, quantitative studies is to control extraneous variables, that is, the variables irrelevant to the study that could affect the dependent variable. Extraneous variables include both factors in the research setting and characteristics of the study participants.

One important type of control relates to the **constancy of conditions** under which a study is performed, as a means of controlling external factors. A number of aspects of the study, such as the environment, timing, communications, and the implementation of treatment, should be held constant or kept as similar as possible for each participant.

The most problematic and pervasive extraneous variables are intrinsic characteristics of the subjects. Several techniques are available to control such characteristics. First, the ideal method of control is through the **random assignment** of subjects to groups, which effectively controls for all possible extraneous variables. Second, in some types of studies, subjects can be exposed to more than one level of a treatment and thus serve as their own controls, although such **repeated measures** designs may be unsuitable because of the potential problem of carry-over effects. The third principle is **homogeneity**—the use of a homogeneous sample of subjects such that there is no variability on the characteristics that could affect the outcome of a study. Fourth, the extraneous variables can be built into the design of a study, as in the case of a **randomized block design**. The fifth approach, **matching**, is essentially an after-the-fact attempt to approximate a randomized block design. This procedure matches subjects (either through **pair matching** or **balancing** groups) on the basis of one or more extraneous variables in an attempt to secure comparable groups. Finally, another technique is to control extraneous variables by means of **statistical control**. One such procedure is known as **analysis of covariance**. Four of the procedures for controlling extraneous individual characteristics—homogeneity, blocking, matching, and statistical control—share one disadvantage: the researcher must know which variables need to be controlled.

The control mechanisms reviewed here help to improve the **internal validity** of studies. Internal validity is concerned with the question of whether the results of a project are attributable to the independent variable of interest or to other, extraneous factors. **Threats to the internal validity** of a study, which represent rival hypotheses, include **history, selection, maturation, testing, instrumentation**, and **mortality**.

External validity refers to the generalizability of the research findings to other individuals and other settings. A research study possesses external validity to the extent that the sample is representative of the broader population and to the extent that the study setting and experimental arrangements are representative of other environments. A useful distinction can be made between the **accessible population**, the population from which a sample is drawn, and the **target population**, which represents a larger group of individuals in whom the investigator is interested. The researcher should define the target population in terms of those characteristics that are present in the accessible population. A research design must balance the need for internal and external validity to produce useful scientific results.

STUDY ACTIVITIES

Chapter 9 of the *Study Guide to Accompany Nursing Research: Principles and Methods, 6th ed.,* offers various exercises and study suggestions for reinforcing the concepts presented in this chapter. Additionally, the following study questions can be addressed:

1. How do you suppose the use of identical twins in a research study can enhance control?
2. Read a research report suggested under Substantive References in Chapters 8. Assess the adequacy of the control mechanisms used by the investigator, and recommend additional controls if appropriate.
3. For each of the examples below, indicate the types of research approach that could be used to study the problem (e.g., experimental, quasi-experimental, and so forth), the type of approach you would recommend using, and how you would go about controlling extraneous variables.
   a. What effect does the presence of the newborn's father in the delivery room have on the mother's subjective report of pain?
   b. What is the effect of different types of bowel evacuation regimes for quadriplegics?
   c. Does the reinforcement of intensive care unit nonsmoking behavior in smokers affect postintensive care unit behaviors?
   d. Is the degree of change in body image of surgical patients related to their need for touch?

SUGGESTED READINGS

Methodologic References

Beck, S. L. (1989). The crossover design in clinical nursing research. *Nursing Research, 38,* 291–293.

Braucht, G. H., & Glass, G. V. (1968). The external validity of experiments. *American Educational Research Journal, 5,* 437–473.

Campbell, D. T., & Stanley, J. C. (1963). *Experimental and quasi-experimental designs for research.* Chicago: Rand McNally.

Conlon, M., & Anderson, G. C. (1991). Three methods of random assignment: Comparison of balance achieved on potentially confounding variables. *Nursing Research, 39,* 376–378.

Gilliss, C. L., & Kulkin, I. L. (1991). Technical notes: Monitoring nursing interventions and data collection in a randomized clinical trial. *Western Journal of Nursing Research, 13,* 416–422.

Kempthorne, O. (1961). The design and analysis of experiments with some reference to educational research. In R. O. Collier & S. M. Elan (Eds.), *Research design and analysis* (pp. 97–126). Bloomington, IN: Phi Delta Kappa.

Kerlinger, F. N. (1986). *Foundations of behavioral research* (3rd ed.). New York: Holt, Rinehart & Winston.

Kirk, R. E. (1995). *Experimental design: Procedures for the behavioral sciences* (3rd ed.). Pacific Grove, CA: Brooks-Cole.

Lipsey, M. W. (1990). *Design sensitivity: Statistical power for experimental research.* Newbury Park, CA: Sage.

Rosenthal, R. (1976). *Experimenter effects in behavioral research.* New York: Halsted Press.

Substantive References

Buchko, B. L., Pugh, L. C., Bishop, B. A., Cochran, J. F., Smith, L. R., & Lerew, D. J. (1994). Comfort measures in breastfeeding, primiparous women. *Journal of Obstetric, Gynecologic and Neonatal Nursing, 23,* 46–52.

Ganong, L. H., & Coleman, M. (1997). Effects of family structure information on nurses' impression formation and verbal responses. *Research in Nursing & Health, 20,* 139–151.

Gilliss, C. L., Gortner, S. R., Hauck, W. W., Shinn, J. A., Sparacino, P. A., & Tompkins, C. (1993). A randomized clinical trial of nursing care for recovery from cardiac surgery. *Heart & Lung,* 22, 125–133.

Grossman, M., & Rowat, K. M. (1995). Parental relationships, coping strategies, received support, and well-being in adolescents of separated or divorced and married parents. *Research in Nursing & Health, 18,* 249–261.

Leidy, N. K., Abbott, R. D., & Fedenko, K. M. (1997). Sensitivity and reproducibility of the dual-mode actigraph under controlled levels of activity intensity. *Nursing Research, 46,* 5–11.

Melnyk, B. M., Alpert-Gillis, L. J., Hensel, P. B., Cable-Beiling, R. C., & Rubenstein, J. S. (1997). Helping mothers cope with a critically ill child: A pilot test of the COPE intervention. *Research in Nursing & Health, 20,* 3–14.

Mock, V. (1993). Body image in women treated for breast cancer. *Nursing Research, 42,* 153–157.

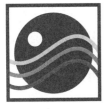

Qualitative Research Design and Approaches

THE DESIGN OF QUALITATIVE STUDIES

As we have seen, quantitative researchers carefully specify a research design before collecting even one piece of data, and rarely depart from that design once the study is underway. In qualitative research, by contrast, the study design typically evolves over the course of the project. Decisions about how best to obtain data, whom to obtain data from, how to schedule data collection, and how long each data collection session should last are made in the field as the study unfolds. The design for a qualitative study is often referred to as an **emergent design**—a design that emerges as the researcher makes ongoing decisions reflecting what has already been learned. As noted by Lincoln and Guba (1985), an emergent design in qualitative studies is not the result of sloppiness or laziness on the part of the researcher, but rather a reflection of the researcher's desire to have the inquiry based on the realities and viewpoints of those under study—realities and viewpoints that are not known or understood at the outset of the study.

Characteristics of Qualitative Research Design

As we discuss in a later section of this chapter, qualitative inquiry has been guided by a number of different disciplines, and each has developed different methods best suited to address questions of particular interest. However, there are some general characteristics of qualitative research design that tend to apply across disciplines, as noted by Janesick (1994). These characteristics include the following:

1. Qualitative design is flexible and elastic, capable of adjusting to what is being learned during the course of data collection.
2. Qualitative design typically involves a merging together of various methodologies.
3. Qualitative design tends to be holistic, striving for an understanding of the whole.
4. Qualitative design is focused on understanding a phenomenon or social setting, not necessarily on making predictions about the setting or phenomenon.

5. Qualitative design requires that the researcher become intensely involved, usually remaining in the field for lengthy periods of time.

6. Qualitative design requires the researcher to become the research instrument.

7. Qualitative design requires ongoing analysis of the data in order to formulate subsequent strategies and to determine when field work is done.

8. Qualitative design pushes the researcher to develop a model of what is transpiring in the social setting or what the phenomenon of interest is about.

9. Qualitative design provides opportunities for description of the researcher's role as well as description of his her own biases.

With regard to the second characteristic, qualitative researchers tend to put together a complex array of data, derived from a variety of sources and using a variety of methods. This tendency has sometimes been described as **bricolage,** and the qualitative researcher has been referred to as a **bricoleur,** a person who "is adept at performing a large number of diverse tasks, ranging from interviewing to observing, to interpreting personal and historical documents, to intensive self-reflection and introspection" (Denzin and Lincoln, 1994, p. 2).

Qualitative Design and Planning

Although design decisions are not specified in advance, the qualitative researcher typically does considerable advance planning that can support an emergent design. In the total absence of planning, flexibility in the design might actually be constrained. For example, the researcher initially might anticipate a 6-month period for data collection but may need to be prepared (financially and emotionally) to spend even longer periods of time in the field to pursue data collection opportunities that could not have been foreseen. In other words, the qualitative researcher plans for broad contingencies that may be expected to pose decision opportunities once the study has begun. Examples of the areas in which advanced planning is especially useful include the following:

- Identification of potential study collaborators and reviewers of the research plans
- Selection of the site where the study will take place
- Arrangements for gaining entrée into the site
- Collection of relevant written or photographic materials about the site (e.g., maps, organizational charts, resource directories)
- Identification of the types of settings within the site that are likely to be especially fruitful for the collection of meaningful data
- Identification of the names and roles of key gatekeepers who can provide (or deny) access to important sources of data
- Determination of the maximum amount of time available for the study, given costs and other constraints
- Identification of all foreseeable types of equipment that could aid in the collection and analysis of data in the field (e.g., audio and video recording equipment, lap-top computers)
- Determination of the number and type of assistants needed (if any) to complete the project
- Training of any assistants and self-training
- Identification of appropriate informed-consent procedures, including contingencies for dealing with ethical issues as they present themselves during data collection

Thus, a qualitative researcher needs to plan for a variety of potential circumstances, but decisions about how he or she will deal with them must be resolved when the social context of time, place, and human interactions are better understood. By both allowing for and anticipating an evolution of strategies, procedures, and data-gathering mechanisms, qualitative researchers seek to make their research design responsive to the situation and to the phenomenon under study.

One further task that qualitative researchers typically undertake before collecting data is an analysis of their own biases and ideology. Probably to a greater extent than quantitative researchers, qualitative researchers tend to accept that research is subjective and may be ideologically driven. Decisions about research design and research approaches are not value free. Qualitative researchers, then, are more inclined to take on as an early research challenge the identification of their own biases. Such an identification is particularly important in qualitative inquiry because of the intensely personal nature of the data collection and data analysis experience.

Phases in Qualitative Design

Although the exact form of a qualitative study cannot be known and specified in advance, Lincoln and Guba (1985) have noted that a naturalistic inquiry typically progresses through three broad phases while in the field:

1. *Orientation and overview.* Quantitative researchers generally believe that they know what they do not know—that is, they know exactly what type of knowledge they expect to obtain by doing a study, and then strive to obtain it. A qualitative researcher, by contrast, enters the study not knowing what is not known—that is, not knowing what it is about the phenomenon that will drive the inquiry forward. Therefore, the first phase of many qualitative studies is to get a handle on what *is* salient about the phenomenon of interest.
2. *Focused exploration.* The second phase of the study is a more focused scrutiny and in-depth exploration of those aspects of the phenomenon that are judged to be salient. The questions asked and

the types of people invited to participate in the study are shaped by the understandings developed in the first phase.
3. *Confirmation and closure.* In the final phase, qualitative researchers undertake efforts to establish that their findings are trustworthy, often by going back and discussing their understanding with study participants. Phase 3 activities are described at greater length in Chapter 17.

The three phases are not discrete events. Rather, they overlap to a greater or lesser degree in different projects. For example, even the first few interviews or observations are typically used as a basis for selecting subsequent informants, even though the researcher is still striving to understand the full scope of the phenomenon and to identify its major dimensions. The various phases might take only a few days to complete, or they may take many months.

Qualitative Design Features

Some of the design features described in connection with quantitative studies (see Chapter 7) also apply to qualitative studies. However, the design features are often post hoc characterizations of *what happened* in the field rather than features specifically planned in advance. As a further means of clarifying the important differences between qualitative and quantitative research design, we refer to the design elements identified in Chapter 7:

- *Intervention or control over independent variable.* Qualitative research is almost always nonexperimental.* Researchers conducting a study within the naturalistic paradigm do not normally conceptualize their studies as having independent and dependent variables, and they rarely control or manipulate any aspect of the people or environment under study. The goal

---

*As we discuss in a subsequent chapter, however, a qualitative study can be embedded within an experimental project.

of most qualitative studies is to develop a rich understanding of a phenomenon as it exists in the real world and as it is constructed by individuals within the context of that world.

- *Type of group comparisons.* Qualitative researchers typically do not plan in advance to focus on group comparisons. Nevertheless, patterns emerging in the data sometimes suggest that certain comparisons are relevant and illuminating. For example, Astrom, Furaker, and Norberg (1995) studied nurses' skills in managing ethically difficult care situations with cancer patients. Their analysis revealed that interesting patterns emerged when nurses with limited experience in managing ethically difficult care situations were compared with nurses with extensive experience.

- *Number of data collection points.* Qualitative research, like quantitative research, can be either cross-sectional (one data collection point per study participant) or longitudinal (multiple data collection points over an extended time period, to observe the evolution of some phenomenon). Sometimes, a qualitative researcher plans in advance for multiple sessions, but in other cases, the decision to study a phenomenon longitudinally may be made in the field after preliminary data have been collected and analyzed. As an example of a cross-sectional qualitative study in which the researcher gathered information about a time-related event, Dickerson (1998) studied in a single session the help-seeking experiences of cardiac patients' spouses over the course of the illness, from the patients' diagnosis to homecoming from hospitalization. Doolittle and Sauve (1995), on the other hand, conducted a longitudinal study that addressed the personal struggles of aborted sudden cardiac death survivors and their spouses during recovery, collecting data at 6- to 8-week intervals for about 6 months after the arrest.

- *Occurrence of independent and dependent variables.* Qualitative researchers typically would not apply the terms retrospective or prospective to their studies—nor are they typically focused on establishing a causal chain. Nevertheless, in trying to elucidate the full nature of a particular phenomenon, they may look back retrospectively (with the assistance of study participants) for antecedent factors leading up to the occurrence of that phenomenon. For example, Kerr (1994) studied adult women's perceptions of how the death of a parent, which had occurred years earlier, resulted in changes in their lifestyle. Qualitative researchers may also study the evolution of development of a phenomenon prospectively. For example, Reutter, Field, Campbell, and Day (1997) studied how baccalaureate nursing students became professionally socialized over the 4 years of nursing school.

- *Setting.* Qualitative researchers almost always collect their data in real-world, naturalistic settings. Whereas a quantitative researcher usually strives to collect data in one type of setting to maintain constancy of conditions (e.g., conducting all interviews with study participants in their homes), qualitative researchers may deliberately strive to study their phenomena in a variety of natural contexts. For example, Hatton (1994) conducted an in-depth study of health perceptions among older urbanized American Indians. The investigator made a conscious effort to conduct the study in numerous settings, including sessions in the study participants' homes, on fishing trips, at senior citizen lunches, and on outings to outlying reservations.

QUALITATIVE RESEARCH TRADITIONS

Despite the fact that there are some features common to all qualitative research designs, there is nevertheless a wide variety of overall approaches. Unfortunately, there is no readily agreed-upon classification system or taxonomy for the various approaches. Some authors have categorized qualitative studies in terms of analysis styles, others have classified studies according to their broad focus. We believe that one useful system is to describe various types of qualitative research according to disciplinary traditions. These traditions vary in their conceptualization of what types of questions are important to ask in understanding the world in which we live. The section that follows provides an overview of several qualitative research traditions, and subsequent sections describe in greater detail three traditions that have been especially useful for nurse researchers.

Overview of Qualitative Research Traditions

The research traditions that have provided a theoretical underpinning for qualitative studies come primarily from the disciplines of anthropology, psychology, and sociology. As shown in Table 10-1, each discipline has tended to focus on one or two broad domains of inquiry.

The discipline of anthropology is concerned with human cultures. **Ethnography** is the primary research tradition within anthropology and provides a framework for studying the meanings, patterns, and experiences of a defined cultural group in a holistic fashion. Ethnographic research is described at greater length in the next section. **Ethnoscience** (sometimes referred to as **cognitive anthropology**)

TABLE 10-1 Overview of Qualitative Research Traditions

DISCIPLINE	DOMAIN	RESEARCH TRADITION	AREA OF INQUIRY
Anthropology	Culture	Ethnography Ethnoscience (cognitive anthropology)	Holistic view of a culture Mapping of the cognitive world of a culture; a culture's shared meanings, semantic rules
Psychology/ Philosophy	Lived experience	Phenomenology Hermeneutics	Experiences of individuals within their "life-worlds" Experiences of individuals as access to sociocultural context
Psychology	Behavior and events	Ethology Ecological psychology	Behavior observed over time in natural context Behavior as influenced by the environment
Sociology	Social settings	Grounded theory Ethnomethodology Symbolic interaction (semiotics)	Social structural processes within a social setting Manner by which shared agreement is achieved in social settings Manner by which people make sense of social interactions
Sociolinguistics	Human communication	Discourse analysis	Forms and rules of conversation

focuses on the cognitive world of a culture, with particular emphasis on the semantic rules and the shared meanings that shape behavior. Ethnoscience often relies on quantitative as well as qualitative data.

Phenomenology, which has its disciplinary roots in both philosophy and psychology, is concerned with the lived experiences of humans. Because many nursing studies have adopted a phenomenologic approach, this research tradition is described more fully in a subsequent section. A closely related research tradition is **hermeneutics**, which uses the lived experiences of people as a tool for better understanding the social, cultural, political, or historical context in which those experiences occur. Hermeneutic inquiry almost always focuses on *meaning* and interpretation—how socially and historically conditioned individuals interpret their world within their given context.

The discipline of psychology has several other qualitative research traditions that focus on human *behavior*. Human **ethology**, which is sometimes described as the biology of human behavior, studies human behavior as it evolves in its natural context. Human ethologists use primarily observational methods in an attempt to discover universal behavioral structures. **Ecological psychology** focuses more specifically on the influence of the environment on human behavior and attempts to identify principles that explain the interdependence of humans and their environmental context.

Sociologists study the social world in which we live and have developed several research traditions of importance to qualitative researchers. The **grounded theory** tradition (described briefly in Chapter 5 and elaborated upon in a later section of this chapter) seeks to describe and understand the key social psychological and structural processes that occur in a social setting.

Ethnomethodology seeks to discover how people make sense of their everyday activities and interpret their social worlds so as to behave in socially acceptable ways. Within this tradition, researchers attempt to understand a social group's norms and assumptions that are so deeply ingrained that the members no longer think about the underlying reasons for their behaviors. Unlike most other qualitative researchers, ethnomethodologists occasionally engage in **ethnomethodologic experiments**. During these experiments, the researcher disrupts ordinary activity by doing something that violates the group's norms and assumptions. The researcher then observes what the group members do and how they try to make sense of what is happening. An example is going into the library and deliberately sitting next to someone at a table when there are plenty of empty tables, to observe how people make sense of and deal with this mild violation of social expectations about personal space.

Symbolic interaction is a sociologic and social psychological tradition with roots in American pragmatism. Like other qualitative frameworks, symbolic interaction has been defined and specified in various ways and is therefore difficult to describe briefly. Basically, symbolic interaction focuses on the manner in which people make sense of social interactions and the interpretations they attach to social symbols, such as language. There are three basic premises underlying this tradition: first, that people act and react on the basis of the meanings that objects and other people in their environment have for them; second, that these meanings are based on social interaction and communication; and third, that these meanings are established through an interpretive process undertaken by each individual. Symbolic interactionists sometimes use **semiotics**, which refers to the study of signs and their meanings. A sign is any entity or object that carries information (e.g., a diagram, map, or picture).

Finally, the domain of inquiry for sociolinguists is human communication. The tradition often referred to as **discourse analysis** seeks to understand the rules, mechanisms, and structure of conversations. Discourse analysts are interested in understanding the action that a given kind of talk "performs." The data for discourse analysis typically are transcripts from naturally occurring conversations, such as those between nurses and their patients.

Researchers in each of these traditions have developed methodologic guidelines for the design and conduct of relevant studies. Thus, once a researcher has identified what aspect of the human experience is of greatest interest, there is typically a wealth of advice available with regard to methods likely to be productive and design issues that need to be handled in the field.

Ethnography

Ethnography is a type of qualitative inquiry that involves the description and interpretation of cultural behavior. Ethnographies are a blend of a process and a product: field work and a written text. Field work is the process by which the ethnographer inevitably comes to understand a culture, and the ethnographic text is how that culture is communicated and portrayed. Because culture is, in itself, not visible or tangible, it must be constructed through ethnographic writing.

Ethnographic research is in some cases concerned with broadly defined cultures (e.g., a Samoan village culture) in what is sometimes referred to as a **macroethnography.** However, ethnographies sometimes focus on more narrowly defined cultures in a **microethnography.** *
Microethnographies are exhaustive, fine-grained studies of either small units within a group or culture (e.g., the culture of homeless shelters) or of specific activities within an organizational unit (e.g., how nurses communicate with children in an emergency room). An underlying assumption of the ethnographer is that every

human group eventually evolves a culture that guides the members' view of the world and the way they structure their experiences.

The aim of the ethnographer is to learn from (rather than to study) members of a cultural group—to understand their world view as they define it. Ethnographic researchers sometimes refer to emic and etic perspectives (terms that originate in linguistics, i.e., phone*mic* versus phon*etic*). An **emic perspective** refers to the way the members of the culture envision their world—it is the insiders' view. The emic is the local language, concepts, or means of expression that are used by the members of the group under study to name and characterize their experiences. The **etic perspective**, by contrast, is the outsiders' interpretation of the experiences of that culture; it is the language used by those doing the research to refer to the same phenomena. Ethnographers strive to acquire an emic perspective of a culture under study. Moreover, they strive to reveal what has been referred to as **tacit knowledge**, information about the culture that is so deeply embedded in cultural experiences that members do not talk about it or may not even be consciously aware of it. Although it is important to grasp the insider's perspective, it is also important for the ethnographer to illuminate the connection between the emic and the second-order, integrative and interpretational concepts that advance the aims of knowledge.

Ethnographers almost invariably undertake extensive field work to learn about the cultural group in which they are interested. Ethnographic research typically is a labor-intensive endeavor that requires long periods of time in the field—months and even years of field work may be required. In most cases, the researcher strives to participate actively in cultural events and activities. The study of a culture requires a certain level of intimacy with members of the cultural group, and such intimacy can only be developed over time and by working directly with those members as an active participant. The concept of **researcher as**

---

*Ethnographers sometimes engage in what has been called a **meta-ethnography**, which refers to the process of creating new interpretations from the synthesis of multiple ethnographic studies. Unlike meta-analysis, which is primarily a method of aggregating information, meta-ethnography is focused primarily on interpretation.

instrument is frequently used by anthropologists to describe the significant role the ethnographer plays in analyzing and interpreting a culture.

Three broad types of information are usually sought by ethnographers: cultural behavior (what members of the culture do), cultural artifacts (what members of the culture make and use), and cultural speech (what people say). This implies that the ethnographer relies on a wide variety of data sources, including observations, in-depth interviews, records, charts, and other types of physical evidence (e.g., photographs, diaries, letters). Ethnographers typically conduct in-depth interviews with about 25 to 50 informants.

The product of ethnographic research usually includes rich and holistic descriptions of the culture under study. Ethnographers also make interpretations of the culture, describing normative behavioral and social patterns. Among health care researchers, ethnography provides access to the health beliefs and health practices of a culture or subculture. Ethnographic inquiry can thus help to facilitate understanding of behaviors affecting health and illness. Many nurse researchers have undertaken ethnographic studies. Indeed, Leininger has coined the phrase **ethnonursing research,** which she defines as "the study and analysis of the local or indigenous people's viewpoints, beliefs, and practices about nursing care behavior and processes of designated cultures" (1985, p. 38).

A rich array of ethnographic methods have been developed and cannot be fully explicated in this general textbook. More detailed information may be found in Hammersley and Atkinson (1995), Spradley and McCurdy (1972), Fetterman (1989), and LeCompte and Preissle (1993).

Phenomenology

Phenomenology, rooted in a philosophical tradition developed by Husserl and Heidegger, is an approach to thinking about what the life experiences of people are like. The phenomenologic researcher asks the question: What is the *essence* of this phenomenon as experienced by these people? The phenomenologist assumes there is an essence that can be understood, in much the same way that the ethnographer assumes that cultures exist. The phenomenologist investigates subjective phenomena in the belief that essential truths about reality are grounded in people's lived experiences.

The focus of phenomenologic inquiry, then, is what people experience in regard to some phenomenon and how they interpret those experiences. The phenomenologist believes that lived experience gives meaning to each person's perception of a particular phenomenon. The goal of phenomenologic inquiry is to describe fully the lived experience and the perceptions to which it gives rise. Four aspects of lived experience that are of interest to phenomenologists are **lived space** or **spatiality, lived body** or **corporeality, lived time** or **temporality,** and **lived human relation** or **relationality** (Van Manen, 1990).

Phenomenologists assume that human existence is meaningful and interesting because of people's consciousness of that existence. The phrase **being-in-the-world** (or **embodiment**) is a concept that acknowledges that people have physical ties to their world—they think, see, hear, feel, and are conscious through their bodies' interaction with the world.

In a phenomenologic inquiry, the main source of data typically is in-depth conversations in which the researcher and the informant are full coparticipants. The researcher helps the informant to describe lived experiences without leading the discussion. Through in-depth conversations, the researcher strives to gain entrance into the informants' world, to have full access to their experiences as lived. Sometimes, two separate interviews or conversations may be needed. Typically, phenomenologic studies involve a small number of study participants—often fewer than 10. For some phenomenologic researchers, the inquiry includes not only learning about the experience by gathering information from those people under study but also efforts to experience the phenomenon in the same way, typically through participation, observation, and introspective reflection.

There have been a number of methodologic interpretations of phenomenology, and hence different authors suggest different steps in the conduct of a phenomenologic inquiry. However, a phenomenologic study often involves the following four steps: bracketing, intuiting, analyzing, and describing. **Bracketing** refers to the process of identifying and holding in abeyance any preconceived beliefs and opinions one might have about the phenomenon under investigation. The researcher brackets out the world and any presuppositions in an effort to confront the data in pure form. Bracketing is sometimes considered a central component of what is referred to as **phenomenologic reduction**; the isolation of the pure phenomenon, versus what is already known of the phenomenon, is the goal of the reductive process.

Intuiting occurs when the researcher remains open to the meanings attributed to the phenomenon by those who have experienced it. The intuitive process results in a common understanding about the phenomenon under study. Intuiting requires that the researcher creatively vary the data until such understanding emerges. That is, the researcher must wonder and be imaginative about the phenomenon in relationship to other descriptions that have been generated. Intuiting requires that the researcher become totally immersed in the phenomenon under investigation.

Phenomenologic researchers then proceed to the analysis phase (i.e., coding, categorizing, and making sense of the essential meanings of the phenomenon). As the researchers "dwell" with the rich descriptive data, common themes or essences begin to emerge. Dwelling with the data is essentially total immersion for as long as needed to ensure pure and thorough description.

Finally, the descriptive phase occurs when the researcher comes to understand and de-fine the phenomenon. The aims of the final step are to communicate and to offer distinct, critical description in written and verbal form.

The phenomenologic approach is especially useful when a phenomenon of interest has been poorly defined or conceptualized. The topics appropriate to phenomenology are ones that are fundamental to the life experiences of humans; for health researchers, these include such topics as the meaning of stress, the experience of bereavement, and the quality of life with a chronic illness.

A wealth of resources are available on the phenomenologic approach. Interested readers may wish to consult Spiegelberg (1975), Giorgi (1985), Colaizzi (1978), or Van Manen (1990).

Grounded Theory

Grounded theory has become a strong research tradition that began more as a systematic method of qualitative research than as a philosophy. Grounded theory was developed in the 1960s by two sociologists, Glaser and Strauss (1967), whose own theoretical links were in symbolic interactionism.

Grounded theory is an approach to the study of social processes and social structures. The focus of most grounded theory studies is the development and evolution of a social experience—the social and psychological stages and phases that characterize a particular event or episode. As noted in Chapter 5, the primary purpose of the grounded theory approach is to generate comprehensive explanations of phenomena that are grounded in reality.

Grounded theory methods constitute an entire approach to the conduct of field research. For example, a study that truly follows Glaser and Strauss's precepts does not begin with a highly focused research problem; the problem emerges from the data. One of the fundamental features of the grounded theory approach is that data collection, data analysis, and sampling of study participants occur simultaneously.

Grounded theory methods are inherently non-linear in nature and therefore difficult to characterize. The process is recursive because the researchers must systematically collect and categorize data, describe a core category, and recycle earlier steps.

A procedure referred to as **constant comparison** is used to develop and refine theoretically relevant categories. The categories elicited from the data are constantly compared with data obtained earlier in the data collection process so that commonalities and variations can be determined. As data collection proceeds, the inquiry becomes increasingly focused on emerging theoretical concerns. Data analysis within a grounded theory framework is described in greater depth in Chapter 22.

Data for a grounded theory study may come from many sources. In-depth interviews are the most common data source, but observational methods and existing documents may also be used. Typically, a grounded theory study involves interviews with a sample of about 25 to 50 informants.

Grounded theory has become an important research method for the study of nursing phenomena and has contributed to the development of many middle-range theories of phenomena relevant to nurses. Most qualitative nursing studies that identify a research tradition claim grounded theory as the tradition to which they are linked.

OTHER TYPES OF QUALITATIVE RESEARCH

Most qualitative studies can be characterized and described in terms of the disciplinary research traditions discussed in the previous section. However, two other important types of qualitative research also deserve mention: historical research and case studies. A final subsection discusses qualitative research that is not associated with any particular research tradition but that is sometimes referred to generally as a content analysis.

Historical Research

Historical research is the systematic collection and critical evaluation of data relating to past occurrences. Generally, historical research is undertaken to answer questions concerning causes, effects, or trends relating to past events that may shed light on present behaviors or practices. An understanding of contemporary nursing theories, practices, or issues can often be enhanced by an investigation of a specified segment of the past. Historical data are usually qualitative, although in some cases, quantitative data may be available.

Nurses have used historical research methods to examine a wide range of phenomena in both the recent and more distant past. Lusk (1997) studied nursing's claim to professional status by examining classifications of American nurses as professionals or nonprofessionals from 1910 to 1935. Widerquist (1992) examined Florence Nightingale's spirituality and its influence on the development of early modern nursing. Stuart (1992) examined the ways in which gender became an important variable in the articulation of power among public health nurses in Ontario in the 1920s.

It is important not to confuse historical research with a review of the literature about historical events. Like other types of research, historical inquiry has as its goal the discovery of new knowledge, not the summary of existing knowledge. One important difference between historical research and a literature review is that a historical researcher is often guided by specific hypotheses or questions. The hypotheses represent attempts to explain and interpret the conditions, events, or phenomena under investigation. Hypotheses in historical research are not tested statistically; rather, they are broadly stated conjectures about relationships among historical events, trends, and phenomena. For example, it might be hypothesized that a relationship exists between the presence or absence of war and the amount of research-based nursing knowledge generated. This hypothesis could be tested by analyzing research trends in nursing in relation to political conflicts.

The steps involved in performing historical research are similar to those for other types of research: The historical researcher defines a problem area, develops specific questions, collects data, analyzes the data, and interprets the findings. However, historical researchers typically need to devote considerable effort to identifying and evaluating data sources on events, situations, and human behavior that occurred in the past.

COLLECTION OF HISTORICAL DATA

Data for historical research are usually in the form of written records of the past: periodicals, diaries, books, letters, newspapers, minutes of meetings, medical or legal documents, and so forth. However, a number of nonwritten materials may also be of interest. For example, physical remains and objects are potential sources of information. Visual materials, such as photographs and films, are forms of data, as are audio materials, such as records and tapes.

Many of these materials may be difficult to obtain—even written materials are not always conveniently indexed by subject, author, or title. The identification of appropriate historical materials may require a considerable amount of time, effort, and detective work. Fortunately, there are several archives of historical nursing documents, such as the collections at Boston University and Columbia University, as well as the collections of the National Library of Medicine, the Nursing Museum in Philadelphia, the American Journal of Nursing, and the National League for Nursing.

Historical materials generally are classified as either primary or secondary sources. A **primary source** is first-hand information, such as original documents, relics, or artifacts. Examples are Louisa May Alcott's book *Hospital*

Sketches, minutes of early American Nurses' Association meetings, hospital records, and so forth. Primary sources represent the most direct link with historical events or situations: only the narrator (in the case of written materials) intrudes between original events and the historical researcher.

Secondary sources are second- or third-hand accounts of historical events or experiences. For example, textbooks, encyclopedias, or other reference books are generally secondary sources. Secondary sources, in other words, are discussions of events written by individuals who are summarizing or interpreting primary source materials. Primary sources should be used whenever possible in historical research. The further removed from the historical event the information is, the less reliable, objective, and comprehensive the data are likely to be.

EVALUATION OF HISTORICAL DATA

Historical evidence is usually subjected to two types of evaluation, which historians refer to as external and internal criticism. **External criticism** is concerned basically with the authenticity and genuineness of the data. For example, a nursing historian might have a diary presumed to be written by Dorothea Dix. External criticism would involve asking such questions as: Is this the handwriting of Ms. Dix? Is the paper on which the diary is written of the right age? Are the writing style and ideas expressed consistent with her other writings? There are various scientific techniques available to determine the age of materials, such as x-ray and radioactive procedures. Other flaws, however, may be less easy to detect. For example, there is the possibility that material of interest may have been written by a ghost writer, that is, by someone other than the person in whom we are really interested. There is also the potential problem of mechanical errors associated with transcriptions, translations, or typed versions of historical materials.

Internal criticism of historical data refers to the evaluation of the worth of the evidence. The focus of internal criticism is not so much on the physical aspects of the materials as on their content. An important issue here is the accuracy or truth of the data. For example, the historical researcher must question whether a writer's representations of historical events are unbiased. It may also be appropriate to ask if the author of a document was in a position to make a valid report of an event or occurrence or whether the writer was competent as a recorder of fact. Evidence bearing on the accuracy of historical data might include comparisons with other people's accounts of the same event to determine the degree of agreement, knowledge of the time at which the document was produced (reports of events or situations tend to be more accurate if they are written immediately after the event), knowledge of the point of view or biases of the writer, and knowledge of the degree of competence of the writer to record events authoritatively and accurately.

Those interested in historical research should consult Lewenson (1995) or Matejski (1986) for further information.

Case Studies

Case studies are in-depth investigations of a single entity or a small series of entities. Typically, the entity is an individual, but families, groups, institutions, or other social units may also be the focus. The researcher conducting a case study attempts to analyze and understand the phenomena that are important to the history, development, or care of an individual or an individual's problems.

One way to think of a case study is to consider what is center stage. In most studies, whether qualitative or quantitative, a certain phenomenon or variable (or set of variables) is the core of the inquiry. In a case study, the *case* itself is central to the researcher. As befits an intensive analysis, the focus of case studies is typically on determining the dynamics of *why* the individual thinks, behaves, or develops in a particular manner rather than on *what* his or her status, progress, actions, or thoughts are. It

is not unusual for probing research of this type to require a detailed study over a considerable period. Data are often collected that relate not only to the person's present state but also to past experiences and situational and environmental factors relevant to the problem being examined. The data for in-depth case studies are usually (but not always) qualitative.*

Although the foremost concern of a case study is to generate knowledge of the particular case, case studies are sometimes a useful way to explore phenomena that have not been rigorously researched. The information obtained in case studies can be extremely useful in the production of hypotheses to be tested more rigorously in subsequent research. The intensive probing that characterizes case studies often leads to insights concerning previously unsuspected relationships. Furthermore, in-depth case studies may serve the important role of clarifying concepts or of elucidating ways to capture them.

The greatest advantage of case studies is the depth that is possible when a limited number of individuals, institutions, or groups is being investigated. A common complaint leveled at other types of research is that the data tend to be superficial. Case studies provide the researcher with the opportunity of having an intimate knowledge of a person's condition, thoughts, feelings, actions (past and present), intentions, and environment. On the other hand, this same strength is a potential weakness because the familiarity of the researcher with the person may make objectivity more difficult—especially if the data are collected by observational techniques for which the researcher is the main (or only) observer. Perhaps the most serious disadvantage of the case study

---

*Most case studies are nonexperimental; in such studies, the researcher obtains a wealth of descriptive information and may examine relationships among different variables or trends over time. Some case studies, however, involve the administration of a treatment and analysis of ensuing consequences of that treatment on the individual. Such studies are sometimes referred to as **single-subject experiments**. Time series designs are often especially appropriate in such situations (i.e., repeated observations before and after the initiation of an intervention).

method is its lack of generalizability. That is, if the researcher reveals the existence of important relationships, it is generally difficult to know whether the same relationships would manifest themselves in other subjects (or in other institutions). It may be perfectly reasonable, however, to make predictions about the future behavior of an individual who is the subject of the case study, based on events or relationships experienced by the person in the past.

Case study research has been used by nurses to study individuals, families, and larger organizational units. For example, Reese and Murray (1996) conducted multiple case studies at the individual level, examining the issue of how being a great-grandmother enhanced possibilities for meaning and transcendence. Perry and Olshansky (1996) engaged in an in-depth case study of a family in which one member had Alzheimer's disease, studying the ways in which the family members made meaning of the situation. Twinn and Lee (1997) studied health education in two different settings (a medical ward and a surgical ward) using case study methods. Two excellent resources for further reading on case study methods are the books by Yin (1994) and Stake (1995).

Qualitative Content Analysis

Qualitative researchers generally identify their studies as being rooted in one of the research traditions discussed in this chapter. There are a number of qualitative studies, however, that claim no particular disciplinary or methodologic roots. The researchers may simply say in their reports that they have conducted a qualitative study or a naturalistic inquiry. Or they may say that they have done a content analysis (without implying that they have quantified their data, as in the classical content analyses described in Chapter 8) or a **qualitative content analysis**.

Thus, a number of legitimate qualitative studies do not have a formal name or do not fit into the typology we have presented in this chapter. The term content analysis that is some-

times used for such studies is less a description of the research design than of the broad approach to analyzing the narrative data—that is, the researcher analyzes the content of the narrative to determine themes or patterns. Sometimes, these studies tend to look like quantitative studies in that the researcher begins to collect data with a definite data collection and sampling plan in mind—and with specific questions to be asked of each respondent. In such a situation, the study may look formally like a descriptive quantitative study, except that the data being gathered are narrative and qualitative rather than numeric.

As an example, Brink and Ferguson (1998) conducted unstructured interviews with 162 men and women in an exploratory qualitative study concerning the decision to lose weight. In a study that relied on written diaries rather than interviews, O'Brien, Relyea, and Lidstone (1997) did a qualitative content analysis of women's experiences with nausea and vomiting during pregnancy.

RESEARCH EXAMPLES

Nurse researchers have conducted studies within all of the qualitative research traditions described in this chapter. Table 10-2 provides several examples of research questions addressed within various traditions. Below we present more detailed descriptions of three qualitative nursing studies.

Example of an Ethnographic Study

Dreher and Hayes (1993) conducted an in-depth ethnographic study of perinatal use of marijuana in rural Jamaican communities. They spent 6 years in the field (starting in 1983) studying marijuana use among pregnant Jamaican women and subsequent effects on the offspring. The field researchers lived in a rural parish of St. Thomas for most of the 6-year period. This particular parish, in the

TABLE 10-2	Examples of Qualitative Studies Within Various Traditions
RESEARCH TRADITION	**RESEARCH QUESTION**
Ethnography	What are the critical health-related, social, and economic issues of the Afghan refugee community? (Lipson & Omidian, 1997)
Phenomenology	What is the lived experience of the diagnosis and treatment of a malignant brain tumor? (Ward-Smith, 1997)
Hermeneutics	How do patients who have had a near-death experience (NDE) understand and experience the early aftermath of the NDE? (Orne, 1995)
Ethology	What are the interaction dynamics between nurses and patients at transitions from one type of nurse attending to another? (Bottorff & Varcoe, 1995)
Grounded theory	What is the social process underlying a nurse's experience with implementing developmental care in a neonatal intensive care unit? (Premji & Chapman, 1997)
Ethnomethodology	How do nurses define and redefine medication error? (Baker, 1997)
Symbolic interactionism	How is responsibility for health generated in a primary nursing care clinic for stress management? (Lowenberg, 1997)
Discourse analysis	What are some of the major ways in which a cancer patient and her oncologist claim power in a medical encounter? (Ainsworth-Vaughn, 1995)

southeastern part of Jamaica, was known for its widespread use of marijuana (called *ganja* in Jamaica). A sample of gravid women was recruited from six different locations within the parish, constituting a range of rural communities and neighborhoods.

The ethnographers had regular, ongoing contact with each of the families in the study. The ethnographic data involved general observations and interviews with the women relating to perinatal use of ganja. Because of the longitudinal nature of the study, the researchers were also able to do focused observations of each child in the study, both in their homes and in their communities. By conducting the study in a rural parish, the researchers had an opportunity to compare users and nonusers "drawn from a culturally and socioeconomically homogeneous population in which there was not significant varia-

tion in nutritional intake and perinatal care" (p. 219).

The researchers found that most female users prepared and consumed ganja for themselves and their families in the form of teas and tonics for medicinal or health-rendering purposes. Ganja smoking was less common among Jamaican women than Jamaican men, although the researchers found that smoking increased among women over the course of the field work. Women who smoked ganja often smoked throughout pregnancy, during labor, and into the breastfeeding period.

The researchers included a clinical component in their 6-year ethnographic study. In the clinical portion, the researchers compared the offspring of 30 ganja users and 30 nonusers using standardized measures of development (e.g., the Bayley Scales of Infant Development). The ethnographic work proved to be critical in suggesting adaptations that made these instruments appropriate for a different culture.

Example of a Phenomenologic Study

Coward (1995) used a phenomenologic approach to studying the lived experience of self-transcendence in women with AIDS. Coward defined self-transcendence as reaching out beyond the boundaries of the self—either outward beyond personal concern or inward toward increased understanding—to achieve broader perspectives and behaviors that facilitate the discovery of meaning.

Coward obtained her data primarily through unstructured interviews with 10 women with class IV HIV infection (AIDS), recruited through support groups and a family clinic. The women were asked to describe fully situations in which they experienced self-transcendence, including all their thoughts, feelings, and perceptions.

The audiotaped interviews were transcribed verbatim, and phenomenologic analysis techniques were used to organize and synthesize the descriptions. The analysis revealed eight central themes: experiencing fear and aloneness, experiencing uncertainty, using others as role models, finding inner strength, reaching out to give and to receive, making a difference/having purpose, viewing AIDS as opportunity, and having hope. Here is an excerpt that contributed to the theme of "making a difference":

> I've not always been a strong person. As a matter of fact, I was a follower more than a leader. But now that I have this AIDS, it's like, I'm not going to follow no more. I want people to know—teenagers especially—that AIDS is out there and no one can hide from it.

Example of a Case Study

Price (1992) undertook a series of case studies in highland Ecuador to analyze the processes by which people cope with serious illness. The case studies were used as a vehicle for illuminating psychological coping mechanisms within family and sociocultural contexts.

Price conducted eight in-depth case studies of families who were involved in a serious illness over a 2-year period. Data were gathered by observation and in-depth interviewing. A complete story of the illness was obtained from individuals with caretaking responsibility and from others associated with the family. Price also used interviews to address specific questions on coping, interactions with health specialists, and illness meanings. Two case study examples were described in Price's report. The following is a summary of the first case study:

> Susana was a 6-year-old who suffered from severe hip malformation. The first symptoms appeared when she was 1 year old after she had been hospitalized for an acute intestinal infection. The family consulted many different health care specialists and tried many therapies to prevent total disability. Ultimately, Susana underwent surgery in the public children's hospital, then physical therapy in the same hospital; finally, she received treatment from a spiritualist healer, including a spiritualist operation performed from a distance.

Price noted that Susana's mother, Maria, was able to cope effectively with her daughter's illness because she took steps to preserve her self-esteem and sense of participation, both of which were undermined by the traditional health care practitioners at the hospital. The researcher concluded that Maria achieved a renewal of faith in herself as caretaker, which allowed the family to transform the experience of illness.

Based on the case analyses, Price concluded that two mechanisms are critical in constructive psychological coping in an illness situation. First, coping functions to preserve and strengthen self-esteem. And second, patients and their caretakers must maintain a sense of participation in shaping the outcome of events.

SUMMARY

Qualitative research typically involves an **emergent design**—a design that emerges in the field once the study is underway. As **bricoleurs**, qualitative researchers tend to be creative and intuitive, putting together an array of data drawn from many sources in an effort to arrive at a holistic understanding of some phenomenon. Although qualitative design is often elastic and flexible, the qualitative researcher nevertheless can plan for broad contingencies that can be expected to pose decision-making opportunities about the design of the study in the field. Although the exact form of a qualitative study is not known in advance, a naturalistic inquiry typically progresses through three broad phases in the field: an orientation and overview phase to determine what it is about the phenomenon under investigation that is salient, a focused exploration phase that closely examines important aspects of the phenomenon, and a confirmation and closure phase to confirm findings.

A variety of research traditions stemming from several disciplines fall within the broad umbrella of qualitative research. These traditions have their roots in anthropology (**ethnography** and **ethnoscience**), philosophy (**phenomenology** and **hermeneutics**), psychology (**ethology, ecological psychology**), sociology (**grounded theory, ethnomethodology, symbolic interaction**), and sociolinguistics (**discourse analysis**). The various research traditions vary in their conceptualization of what types of questions are important to ask about humans and our social contexts.

Ethnography, which has been used by many nurse researchers, focuses on the culture of a group of people and relies on extensive field work. The ethnographer strives to acquire an **emic**, or insider's, perspective of the culture under study; the outsider's perspective is known as **etic**. The concept of **researcher as instrument** is frequently used by ethnographers to describe the significant role the researcher plays in analyzing and interpreting a culture. Nurses doing ethnographic work sometimes refer to their studies as **ethnonursing research**.

Phenomenology strives to discover the *essence* of a phenomenon as it is experienced by

some people. Four aspects of lived experience that are of interest to phenomenologists are **lived space** or **spatiality, lived body** or **corporeality, lived time** or **temporality,** and **lived human relation** or **relationality**. The phenomenologic researcher strives to **bracket** out any preconceived views so that the data can be confronted in pure form and to **intuit** the essence of the phenomenon by remaining open to the meanings attributed to it by those who have experienced it.

Grounded theory is a research tradition that began as a systematic method of conducting qualitative research. Grounded theory is an approach to studying social psychological processes and social structures. The aim of grounded theory studies is to discover theoretical precepts grounded in the data. This approach makes use of a technique called **constant comparison**: categories elicited from the data are constantly compared with data obtained earlier so that shared themes and variations can be determined.

In addition to qualitative designs associated with disciplinary traditions, there are other types of qualitative studies. **Historical research** is the systematic attempt to establish facts and relationships concerning past events. The historical researcher uses the scientific method insofar as possible to answer questions or test hypotheses by objectively evaluating and interpreting available historical evidence. Historical data are normally subjected to two forms of evaluation: **external criticism**, which is concerned with the authenticity of the source, and **internal criticism**, which assesses the worth of the evidence.

Case studies are intensive investigations of a single entity or a small number of entities. Typically, that entity is an individual, but groups, organizations, families, or communities may sometimes be the focus of concern. Such studies generally involve collecting data over an extended period. The case study offers the potential of great depth but runs the risk of subjectivity and limited generalizability.

Finally, a number of qualitative studies have no formal name or do not fit into any disciplinary tradition. Such studies may simply be referred to as qualitative studies, naturalistic inquiries, or **qualitative content analyses**.

STUDY ACTIVITIES

Chapter 10 of the *Study Guide to Accompany Nursing Research: Principles and Methods, 6th ed.*, offers various exercises for reinforcing concepts presented in this chapter. Additionally, the following study questions can be addressed:

1. Develop a research question for a nursing research macroethnography. Then develop a research question that would be appropriate for a microethnography.
2. Suppose a researcher gets onto a crowded elevator and deliberately faces the back, and then observes people's reactions. What type of study would this be?
3. Which of the following topics is best suited to a phenomenologic inquiry? to an ethnography? to a grounded theory study? Provide a rationale for each response.
    a. The passage through menarche among Haitian refugees
    b. The process of coping among AIDS patients
    c. The experience of having a child with leukemia
    d. Rituals relating to dying among nursing home residents
    e. The experience of waiting for service in a hospital emergency room
    f. The decision-making process among nurses regarding do-not-resuscitate orders
4. Why is it that most qualitative researchers do not know in advance how many weeks or months will be required in the field to complete an investigation?

SUGGESTED READINGS

Methodologic References

Chenitz, W. C., & Swanson, J. (Eds.). (1985). *Qualitative research in nursing: From practice to grounded theory*. Menlo-Park, CA: Addison-Wesley.

Colaizzi, P. F. (1978). Psychological research as the phenomenologist views it. In R. Valle & M. King (Eds.). *Existential phenomenological alternative for psychology*. New York: Oxford University Press.

Denzin, N. K. (1988). *The research act* (3rd ed.). Englewood Cliffs, NJ: Prentice Hall.

Denzin, N. K., & Lincoln, Y. S. (Eds.). (1994). *Handbook of qualitative research*. Thousand Oaks, CA; Sage.

Fetterman, D. M. (1989). *Ethnography: Step by step*. Newbury Park, CA: Sage.

Giorgi, A. (1985). *Phenomenology and psychological research*. Pittsburgh: Duquesne University Press.

Glaser, B. G., & Strauss, A. L. (1967). *The discovery of grounded theory: Strategies for qualitative research*. Chicago: Aldine.

Hammersley, M., & Atkinson, P. (1995). *Ethnography: Principles in practice* (2nd ed.). New York: Routledge.

Janesick, V. J. (1994). The dance of qualitative research design. In N. K. Denzin & Y. S. Lincoln (Eds.). *Handbook of qualitative research*. Thousand Oaks, CA: Sage.

LeCompte, M. D. & Preissle, J. (1993). *Ethnography and qualitative design in educational research* (2nd ed.). Orlando: Academic Press.

Leininger, M. M. (Ed.). (1985). *Qualitative research methods in nursing*. New York: Grune and Stratton.

Lewenson, S. B. (1995). Historical research approach. In H. J. Streubert & D. R. Carpenter (Eds.). *Qualitative research in nursing: Advancing the humanistic perspective*. Philadelphia: J. B. Lippincott.

Lincoln, Y. S., & Guba, E. G. (1985). *Naturalistic inquiry*. Newbury Park, CA: Sage.

Matejski, M. (1986). Historical research: The method. In P. L. Munhall & C. J. Oiler (Eds.). *Nursing research: A qualitative perspective*. Norwalk, CT: Appleton-Century-Crofts.

Morse, J. M. (1991). *Qualitative nursing research: A contemporary dialogue*. Newbury Park, CA: Sage.

Morse, J. M., & Field, P. A. (1995). *Qualitative research methods for health professionals* (2nd ed.). Thousand Oaks, CA: Sage.

Spiegelberg, H. (1975). *Doing phenomenology*. The Hague: Nijhoff.

Spradley, J. P., & McCurdy, D.W. (1972). *The cultural experience: Ethnography in complex society*. Prospect Heights, IL: Waveland.

Stake, R. (1995). *The art of case study research*. Thousand Oaks, CA: Sage.

Streubert, H. J., & Carpenter, D. R. (1995). *Qualitative research in nursing: Advancing the humanistic imperative*. Philadelphia: J. B. Lippincott.

Van Manen, M. (1990). *Researching lived experience: Human science for an action sensitive pedagogy*. London, Ontario: Althouse.

Yin, R. (1994). *Case study research: Design and methods* (2nd ed.). Thousand Oaks, CA: Sage.

Substantive References

Ainsworth-Vaughn, N. (1995). Claiming power in the medical encounter: The whirlpool discourse. *Qualitative Health Research, 5,* 270–291.

Astrom, G., Furaker, C., & Norberg, A. (1995). Nurses' skills in managing ethically difficult care situations: Interpretations of nurses' narratives. *Journal of Advanced Nursing, 21,* 1073–1080.

Baker, H. M. (1997). Rules outside the rules for administration of medication. *Image: The Journal of Nursing Scholarship, 29,* 155–158.

Bottorff, J. L., & Varcoe, C. (1995). Transitions in nurse-patient interactions: A qualitative ethology. *Qualitative Health Research, 5,* 315–331.

Brink, P. J., & Ferguson, K. (1998). The decision to lose weight. *Western Journal of Nursing Research, 20,* 84–102.

Coward, D. D. (1995). The lived experience of self-transcendence in women with AIDS. *Journal of Obstetric, Gynecologic, and Neonatal Nursing, 24,* 314–318.

Dickerson, S. S. (1998). Cardiac spouses' help-seeking experiences. *Clinical Nursing Research, 7,* 6–28.

Doolittle, N. D., & Sauve, M. J. (1995). Impact of aborted sudden cardiac death on survivors and their spouses. *American Journal of Critical Care, 45,* 389–396.

Dreher, M. C., & Hayes, J. S. (1993). Triangulation in cross-cultural research of child development in Jamaica. *Western Journal of Nursing Research, 15,* 216–229.

Hatton, D. C. (1994). Health perceptions among older urban American Indians. *Western Journal of Nursing Research, 16,* 392–403.

Kerr, R. B. (1994). Meanings adult daughters attach to a parent's death. *Western Journal of Nursing Research, 16,* 347–365.

Lipson, J. G., & Omidian, P. A. (1997). Afghan refugee issues in the U.S. social environment. *Western Journal of Nursing Research, 19,* 110–126.

Lowenberg, J. S. (1997). Who's responsible? Clients in a stress management clinic. *Qualitative Health Research, 7,* 448–467.

Lusk, B. (1997). Professional classification of American nurses, 1910 to 1935. *Western Journal of Nursing Research, 19,* 227–242.

O'Brien, B., Relyea, J., & Lidstone, T. (1997). Diary reports of nausea and vomiting during pregnancy. *Clinical Nursing Research, 6,* 239–252.

Orne, R. M. (1995). The meaning of survival: The early aftermath of a near-death experience. *Research in Nursing & Health, 18,* 239–247.

Perry, J., & Olshansky, E. F. (1996). A family's coming to terms with Alzheimer's disease. *Western Journal of Nursing Research, 18,* 12–28.

Premji, S. S. J., & Chapman, J. S. (1997). Nurses' experience with implementing developmental care in NICU's. *Western Journal of Nursing Research, 19,* 97–109.

Price, L. J. (1992). Metalogue on coping with illness: Cases from Ecuador. *Qualitative Health Research, 2,* 135–158.

Reese, C. G., & Murray, R. B. (1996). Transcendence: The meaning of great-grandmothering. *Archives of Psychiatric Nursing, 10,* 245–251.

Reutter, L., Field, P. A., Campbell, I. E., & Day, R. (1997). Socialization into nursing: Nursing students as learners. *Journal of Nursing Education, 36,* 149–155.

Stuart, M. (1992). "Half a loaf is better than no bread": Public health nurses and physicians in Ontario, 1920–1925. *Nursing Research, 41,* 21–27.

Twinn, S. F., & Lee, D. T. F. (1997). The practice of health education in acute care settings in Hong Kong. *Journal of Advanced Nursing, 25,* 178–185.

Ward-Smith, P. (1997). Stereotactic radiosurgery for malignant brain tumours. *Journal of Neuroscience Nursing, 29,* 117–122.

Widerquist, J. G. (1992). The spirituality of Florence Nightingale. *Nursing Research, 41,* 49–55.

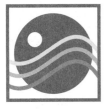

CHAPTER **11**

Integration of Qualitative and Quantitative Designs

Until recently, nursing research was dominated by quantitatively oriented studies. However, consistent with the overall expansion of nursing research inquiry and with the generally increased acceptance of methodologic pluralism, qualitative studies gained considerable ground during the 1980s. An emerging trend, and one that we believe will gain momentum in the years to come, is the blending of qualitative and quantitative data within single studies or coordinated clusters of studies. This chapter discusses the reasons and some strategies for undertaking such integrated designs.

RATIONALE FOR MULTIMETHOD RESEARCH

The dichotomy between quantitative and qualitative data represents the key epistemologic and methodologic distinction within the social and behavioral sciences. Some people, whom Rossman and Wilson (1985) have characterized as purists, argue that qualitative and quantitative research are based on totally incompatible paradigms. Thus, there are people who will disagree with the fundamental premise of

this chapter, namely that some areas of inquiry can be enriched through the judicious blending of qualitative and quantitative data—that is, by undertaking what is generally referred to as **multimethod** (or **mixed-method**) **research**. It would be imprudent to argue that all (or even most) research problems could be enhanced by such integration of methods or that all (or most) researchers should strive to collect and blend both types of data. However, we believe that there are many noteworthy advantages of combining various types of data in a single investigation and that these advantages will increasingly come to be recognized by nurse researchers in the years ahead. Our stance has been called a "pragmatist" view on integration, which sees paradigms more as descriptions of, rather than prescriptions for, research practices (Rossman & Wilson, 1985). Some of the major advantages are reviewed in the following sections.

Complementarity

One argument in support of blending qualitative and quantitative data in a single research project is that they are complementary; they represent words and numbers, the two fundamental languages of human communication. Webster's* defines *complementary* as "mutually supplying each other's lack," and this characterizes the two methodologic strategies well. Researchers address their problems with methods and measures that are invariably fallible. By integrating different methods and modes of analysis, the weaknesses of a single approach may be diminished or overcome.

Quantitative data derived from relatively large or representative samples have many strengths. Quantitative studies are often strong in terms of generalizability, precision, and control over extraneous variables. However, a major problem with quantitative research is that its validity is sometimes called into question. By introducing tight controls, quantitative studies may fail to capture the full context of a situation. Moreover, by reducing complex human experiences, behavior, and characteristics to numbers, such studies sometimes suffer from superficiality. Another issue is that the use of tightly structured questions or instruments may lead to biases in capturing constructs under study. All these weaknesses are aspects of the study's ability to yield valid and meaningful answers to the research questions.

Qualitative research, by contrast, has strengths and weaknesses that are diametrically opposite. The strength of qualitative research lies in its flexibility and its potential to yield insights into the true nature of complex phenomena through a wealth of in-depth information. However, such insights are not gratuitous. Because qualitative research is almost always based on small and unrepresentative samples and is often engaged in by a solitary researcher or small team of researchers using data collection and analytic procedures that rely on subjective judgments, qualitative research may suffer in terms of reliability and generalizability.

This discussion suggests that *neither of the two styles of research can fully deliver on its promise to establish the truth about phenomena of interest to nurse researchers.* However, the strengths and weaknesses of quantitative and qualitative data are complementary. Haase and Myers (1988) also noted the complementarity of the assumptions underlying the two approaches. Combined judiciously in a single study, qualitative and quantitative data can "supply each other's lack." By using multiple methods, the researcher can allow each method to do what it does best, with the possibility of avoiding the limitations of a single approach.

Enhanced Theoretical Insights

Most theories do not have paradigmatic or methodologic boundaries. As discussed in Chapter 5, the major nursing theories embrace four broad concepts: (1) person, (2) environment, (3) health, and (4) nursing. There is nothing inherent in these concepts that demands (or excludes) a qualitative or quantitative orientation.

The world in which we live is complex and multidimensional, as are most of the theories we have developed to make sense of it. Qualitative and quantitative research constitute alternative ways of viewing and interpreting the world. These alternatives are not necessarily correct or incorrect; rather, they reflect and reveal different aspects of reality. To be maximally useful, nursing research should strive to understand these multiple aspects. We believe that the blending of quantitative and qualitative data in a single study can lead to insights on these multiple aspects that might be unattainable without such integration. Denzin (1989), who has been a staunch advocate of combining methods, coined the term **triangulation** to refer to the use of multiple sources to converge on the truth. He expressed the value of triangulation eloquently:

> Each method implies a different line of action toward reality—and hence each will reveal different aspects of it, much as a kaleidoscope,

---

*From Webster's Ninth New Collegiate Dictionary © 1985 by G. & C. Merriam Company, publishers of the Merriam-Webster® Dictionaries, with permission.

depending on the angle at which it is held, will reveal different colors and configurations of objects to the viewer. Methods are like the kaleidoscope: depending on how they are approached, held, and acted toward, different observations will be revealed. This is not to imply that reality has the shifting qualities of the colored prism, but that it too is an object that moves and that will not permit one interpretation to be stamped upon it. (p. 235)

Incrementality

It is sometimes argued that different approaches are especially appropriate for different phases in the evolution of a theory or problem area. In particular, it has been said that qualitative methods are well suited to exploratory or hypothesis-generating research early in the development of a research problem area, and quantitative methods are needed as the problem area matures for the purposes of verification.

It is certainly true that in-depth qualitative research can be highly productive in revealing theoretically relevant aspects of a phenomenon and suggesting lines for further inquiry. It is also true that statistical analysis provides a useful framework for the testing of hypotheses. However, the evolution of a theory or problem area is rarely linear and unidirectional. The need for exploration and in-depth insights is rarely confined to the beginning of an area of research inquiry, and subjective impressions may need to be checked for accuracy early and continually.

Thus, progress in a developing area tends to be incremental and to rely on multiple feedback loops. It therefore can be productive to build a loop into the design of a single study, potentially speeding the progress toward understanding. This point is illustrated by inquiry in the area of work-related stress and coping. Bargagliotti and Trygstad (1987) conducted two separate studies of job stress among nurses, one using quantitative procedures and the other using qualitative procedures. The quantitative study identified discrete events as sources of

stress, and the qualitative study revealed stress-related processes over time. The discrepant findings, because they were derived from different samples of nurses working in different settings, could not be easily integrated and reconciled. The investigators noted, "Comparison of findings from the two studies suggests that the questions raised by the findings in each study might have been more fully addressed by using a combined quantitative/qualitative methodology" (p. 172).

Enhanced Validity

Another advantage of designing multimethod research lies in the potential for enhancements to the validity of the study findings. When a researcher's hypothesis or model is supported by multiple and complementary types of data, the researcher can be much more confident about the validity of the results. Scientists are basically skeptics, constantly seeking evidence to validate their theories and models. Evidence derived from different approaches can be especially persuasive. As Brewer and Hunter (1989) noted, "Although each type of method is relatively stronger than the others in certain respects, none of the methods is so perfect even in its area of greatest strength that it cannot benefit from corroboration by other methods' findings" (p. 51).

In Chapter 9, we discussed various types of validity problems—such problems as rival hypotheses to explain the data (internal validity) and difficulties of generalizing beyond the study circumstances (external validity); in Chapter 17, we will discuss validity issues relating to measures that fail to capture the constructs under investigation. The use of a single approach leaves the study vulnerable to at least one (and often more) of these validity problems. The integration of qualitative and quantitative data can provide better opportunities for testing alternative interpretations of the data, for examining the extent to which the context helped to shape the results, and for arriving at convergence in tapping a construct. For example, Hinds (1989), in her study of adolescents' change in hope-fulness as they progressed through a program for substance abuse, used qualitative findings as a means of validating her quantitative find-ings. As Hinds noted, "Using both methods together results in an increased ability to rule out rival explanations of observed change and reduces skepticism of change-related findings" (p. 442). Ersek, Ferrell, Dow, and Melancon (1997), in their study of quality of life in women with ovarian cancer, similarly used qualitative data to validate their quantitative quality-of-life measures.

Creating New Frontiers

Inevitably, researchers will sometimes find that qualitative and quantitative data are inconsis-tent with each other. This lack of congruity—when it happens in the context of a single investigation—can actually lead to insights that can push a line of inquiry further than would otherwise have been possible.

When separate investigations yield incon-sistent results, the differences are difficult to reconcile and interpret because they may reflect differences in the people being studied and in the circumstances under which they are studied, rather than theoretically meaningful distinc-tions that merit further investigation. In a sin-gle study, any discrepancies that emerge can be tackled head on. By probing into the reasons for any observed incongruities, the researchers can help to rethink the constructs under investi-gation and possibly to redirect the research pro-cess. The incongruent findings, in other words, can be used as a springboard for the investiga-tion of the reasons for the discrepancies and for a thoughtful analysis of both the methodologic and theoretical underpinnings of the study.

APPLICATIONS OF MULTIMETHOD RESEARCH

Researchers make decisions about the types of data to collect and analyze based on the specific objectives of their investigation. In this section, we illustrate how multimethod research can be used to address a variety of research goals.

Instrument Development

One of the most frequent uses of an integrated approach in nursing research involves the de-velopment of instruments, particularly self-report instruments that involve questions to be posed to respondents. When a researcher be-comes aware of the need for a new measuring tool, where do the items come from? The item pool is sometimes generated by the researcher based on theory, his or her clinical experience, readings in the field, or prior research. When a construct is new, however, these mechanisms may be inadequate to capture its full complex-ity and dimensionality. No matter how rich the researcher's experience or knowledge base, the fact remains that this base is highly per-sonal and inevitably biased by the researcher's values and world view.

In recognition of this situation, many nurse researchers have begun to use data obtained from qualitative inquiries as the basis for gener-ating items for quantitative instruments that are subsequently subjected to rigorous quantitative assessment in methodologic studies. For exam-ple, Melillo, Williamson, Futrell, and Chamber-lain (1997) developed the Physical Fitness and Exercise Activity Level of Older Adults Scale, an instrument that measures self-perceived physi-cal fitness and perceived barriers to exercise of community-dwelling older adults. During the first phase, the researchers conducted in-depth interviews with 23 men and women aged 63 to 82 years. Based on the qualitative findings, 50 items were generated and incorporated into a scale that was tested in a second phase of the re-search. After the pilot testing, 41 items were re-tained in the final instrument.

Explicating and Validating Constructs

Multimethod research is often used to develop a comprehensive understanding of a construct or to validate the construct's dimensions. Such research may be undertaken when a little-researched phenomenon has been identified as worthy of further scrutiny (usually in an in-depth qualitative study) or when there is a body of existing research in which some serious gaps have been identified or doubts have been raised about the prevailing conceptualization.

As an example of this application, Reece and Harkless (1996) conducted a multimethod study to examine the maternal experiences of women older than 35 years. The researchers administered a previously developed quantitative measure of maternal experience, the revised "What Being the Parent of a Baby is Like" (WPL-R) scale, which involves three subscales: Self-Evaluation in Parenting, Centrality, and Life Change. The researchers also asked their respondents broad, probing questions about their motherhood experience and qualitatively analyzed the themes that emerged. The investigators found that several new dimensions arose in the qualitative portion of the research, including loss of control, fatigue and the need to heal, and the sense of mortality and the passage of time.

This application of integrated analysis is also used to refine research instruments or to assess the validity of existing ones. For example, Nyamathi and Flaskerud (1992) developed an instrument designed to document the concerns of highly disadvantaged groups of women. After a pilot testing of the initial 50 items, which were derived on the basis of the literature, a qualitative study was undertaken to verify the concerns and stresses experienced by low-income women. The in-depth discussions validated 34 of the initial 50 concerns and suggested 6 others that needed to be added to the instrument.

These examples illustrate the important role that the integration of qualitative and quantitative data can play in enhancing the measurement of and in validating important nursing constructs.

Illustration

Qualitative data are sometimes combined with quantitative data to illustrate the meaning of constructs or relationships. Such illustrations often help to clarify important results or to corroborate the understandings gleaned from the statistical analysis. In this sense, these illustrations often help to illuminate the analyses and give guidance to the interpretation of results.

As an example, Hough and her colleagues (Hough, Lewis, & Woods, 1991; Lewis, Woods, Hough, & Bensley, 1989) conducted a study on family coping and adaptation to a mother's chronic illness. Using structured self-report information, the researchers performed a sophisticated statistical analysis to test a theoretical model of family functioning under stress. The quantitative analysis suggested that the mother's illness had an impact on the spouse and on the quality of his relationship with his wife. Qualitative data were also gathered in the course of the same study (through observations and unstructured interview). The following excerpt illustrating a family that adjusted poorly after the mother's diagnosis of breast cancer adds a perspective that the quantitative results alone could not provide:

> It was a tremendous surprise how I felt about myself after losing part of my body. The fact that this is a life-threatening disease and you could die is quite sobering. The relationships within the family have been difficult. My husband's a denier—he can't understand why I can't forget about it. He left the house when he knew I was going to get a call regarding the lab results. The denial and the sexuality change is a strain on our relationship. (Hough, Lewis, & Woods, 1991, p. 577)

Qualitative materials can be used to illustrate specific statistical findings or to provide more global and dynamic views of the phenomena under study, often in the form of illustrative case studies. For example, Polit and her colleagues (Polit, Morton, & White, 1989; Polit, White, & Morton, 1990), in their study of the sexual and contraceptive behavior of teenagers who had been abused as children, used quantitative data to model statistically the probability of a premarital pregnancy in this high-risk sample. In addition, their report included several case studies illustrating the emotional and social problems these teenagers faced and the evolution and resolution of these problems over time. The case studies were based on interviews with the teenagers, their parents or foster parents, and their social workers as well as on information available in their case records.

Understanding Relationships and Causal Processes

Quantitative methods often demonstrate that variables are systematically related to one another, but they often fail to provide insights about *why* the variables are related. This situation is especially likely to occur with ex post facto research.

Typically, the discussion section of research reports is devoted to an interpretation of the findings. In quantitatively oriented studies, the interpretations are often speculative, representing the researcher's best guess (a guess that may, of course, be built on solid theory or prior research) about what the findings mean. In essence, the interpretations represent a new set of hypotheses that could be tested in another study. When a study integrates both qualitative and quantitative data, however, the researcher may be in a much stronger position to derive meaning immediately from the statistical findings. A collaborative study by a group of researchers (Meleis, Norbeck, & Laffrey, 1989; Hall, Stevens, & Meleis, 1992) provides a good illustration of this application of blended data collection methods. These researchers examined how married, low-income working women from different cultural backgrounds integrate their multiple roles on a daily basis. The data were collected by means of lengthy interviews that included both structured questions and in-depth, probing questions that focused on role integration. In the quantitative analysis, these researchers learned that role integration was important in predicting health outcomes—but not *why* this was so. By means of an analysis of the qualitative data, the researchers developed a theoretical understanding of the construct of role integration. The theoretical framework identified and related the aspects, processes, and patterns of role integration as they are experienced in women's everyday lives. The framework provided insights into how health could be affected by role integration.

Quantitative analyses can also help to clarify and give shape to findings obtained in qualitative analyses. For example, a thematic analysis of interviews with infertile couples could reveal various aspects of the emotional consequences of infertility and shed light on the meaning of those consequences to individuals; the administration of a standardized scale (such as the Center for Epidemiological Studies Depression, or CES-D, Scale) to the same subjects could indicate more precisely the distribution of depressive symptoms and their magnitude among the infertile couples. A study by Lipson (1992) illustrates this approach. Lipson conducted an in-depth field study to investigate the health and adjustment of Iranians who had immigrated to the United States. The primary data were qualitative, gathered by means of detailed qualitative observations and in-depth interviews. After a dozen interviews, Lipson observed that many of the immigrants reported various stress-related physical symptoms. Thereafter, interview respondents were also asked to complete a structured scale (the Health Opinion Survey, or HOS) that measured in a more systematic fashion the symptoms that are common reactions to stress.

The integration of qualitative and quantitative materials for the purpose of enhancing the interpretability of study results is essentially a mechanism of substantive validation. In some studies, it may be useful to use multiple data sources as a methodologic check. For example, if a researcher is concerned with biases that could result from attrition in a longitudinal survey, it might be profitable to undertake a small number of in-depth interviews with non-respondents (if feasible) to evaluate the direction and magnitude of such biases.

Theory Building, Testing, and Refinement

The most ambitious application of multi-method research is in the area of theory development. As we have pointed out repeatedly, a theory is never proved nor confirmed but rather is supported to a greater or lesser extent. A theory gains acceptance as it escapes

disconfirmation. The use of multiple methods provides greater opportunity for potential disconfirmation of the theory. If the theory can survive these assaults, it can provide a substantially stronger context for the organization of our clinical and intellectual work. Brewer and Hunter (1989), in their discussion of the role of multimethod research in theory development, made the following observation:

> Theory building and theory testing clearly require variety. In building theories, the more varied the empirical generalizations to be explained, the easier it will be to discriminate between the many possible theories that might explain any one of the generalizations. And in testing theories, the more varied the predictions, the more sharply the ensuing

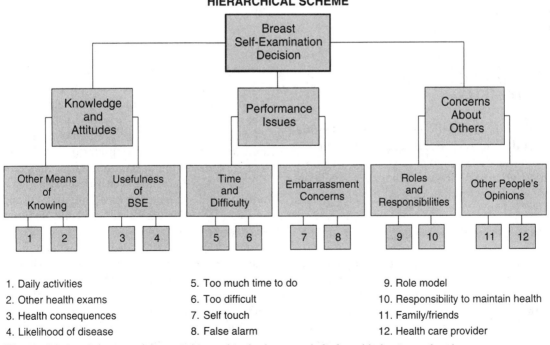

Figure 11-1. Salazar and Carter's hierarchical scheme on beliefs and behaviors related to breast self-examination. (Reprinted with permission from Salazar, M. K., & Carter, W. B. [1993]. Evaluation of breast self-examination beliefs using a decision model. *Western Journal of Nursing Research, 15,* 403–418.)

research will discriminate among competing theories. (p. 36)

Salazar and Carter (1993) conducted a study that promotes the development of theory in the area of decision making. These researchers sought to identify the factors that influence the decision of working women to practice breast self-examination (BSE). The first phase of the study involved in-depth interviews with 19 women, purposively selected on the basis of how frequently the women said they practiced BSE. The transcribed interviews were qualitatively analyzed and led to the development of a hierarchical scheme of factors influencing the BSE decision. This scheme is presented in Figure 11-1. In the next phase of the research, the researchers used the hierarchy as the basis for developing a survey questionnaire, which was administered to 52 women. BSE performers and nonperformers were compared, and a powerful statistical analysis was used to identify factors in the decision hierarchy that best distinguished the two groups.

MULTIMETHOD RESEARCH DESIGNS

Green and Caracelli (1997) have identified several types of research designs that involve a multimethod approach. The designs cluster into two broad categories that they label component designs and integrated designs.

Multimethod Component Designs

In studies that can be described as having a **component design**, the qualitative and quantitative aspects are implemented as discrete components of the overall inquiry and remain distinct during data collection and analysis. The combining of the qualitative and quantitative components occurs during the interpretation and reporting phases of the project.

Green and Caracelli (1997) classify three types of designs as component designs. The first is what they call a **triangulated design**, in which both qualitative and quantitative methods are used to capture the same phenomenon, with a focus on convergence and increased validity. This type of design fits the application described in the previous section as "explicating and validating constructs." Second, in **complementarity designs**, the results from one dominant method type are enhanced or clarified by results from the other type. The use of case studies to illustrate important relationships discerned in quantitative analyses exemplifies this type of design. The third type of component design is the **expansion design**, in which different methods are used for distinct inquiry components—as might be the case in an evaluation that involved both an implementation and an impact analysis. The results from such studies are often presented in a side-by-side fashion, rather than woven together into a single story.

Multimethod Integrated Designs

In studies that Green and Caracelli (1997) refer to as having an **integrated design**, there is greater integration of the method types at all phases of the project, from the development of research questions, through data collection and analysis, to the interpretation of the results. The blending of data occurs in ways that integrate the elements from the different paradigms and offers the possibility of yielding more insightful understandings of the phenomenon under study.

Four types of integrated designs have been identified. **Iterative designs** involve a dynamic in which the findings from one method are used as a basis for moving forward with further research using the alternative method (as is typically the case with instrument development and refinement). In some studies, there is a single iteration, moving from qualitative to quantitative (or vice versa); in other studies, there might be multiple iterations, with a progressive reconfiguration of data collection, data analysis, and interpretation in a spiraling pattern of findings and insights. In **embedded designs** (or **nested designs**), one methodologic approach is embedded within the other, "interlocking contrasting inquiry characteristics in a framework of creative tension" (Green & Caracelli, 1997, p. 24). **Holistic designs** feature the essential interdependence of alternative methods for gaining a full understanding of complex phenomena. In holistic designs, the methods are integrated simultaneously rather than co-linearly or hierarchically. Finally, in **transformative designs**, the emphasis is on blending the value commitments of different research traditions to arrive at a better representation of the multiple interests in the larger social context. In general, integrated designs are better suited to the application of theory building and testing than are component designs.

STRATEGIES FOR MULTIMETHOD RESEARCH

The ways in which a researcher might choose to combine qualitative and quantitative methods in a single study are almost limitless—or rather, are limited only by the ingenuity of the investigator. Therefore, it is impossible to develop a catalog of multimethod strategies. However, some of the following scenarios are apt to be especially common.

Embedding Qualitative Approaches Within a Survey

By far the most common form of data collection method currently used by nurse researchers is structured self-reports, which are discussed at some length in Chapter 14. Once the researcher has gained the cooperation of the sample for the structured portion of a study, he or she is in an ideal position to move

into a second in-depth stage with a subset of the initial respondents. The second stage might involve such approaches as in-depth or focus group interviews, unstructured observations in a naturalistic environment such as a hospital or nursing home, or the use of health diaries.

From a practical point of view, it is efficient to have the two forms of data collection occurring simultaneously. For example, the researcher could administer a structured questionnaire and an in-depth interview on the same day for a subset of the entire sample. In some studies, this procedure is likely to work well. However, a two-stage (iterative) approach has two distinct advantages. First, if the second-stage data collection can be postponed until after the quantitative data have been collected and analyzed, then the researcher will have greater opportunity to probe deeply into the reasons for any obtained results. This is especially likely to be beneficial if the quantitative analyses did not confirm the researcher's hypotheses or if there were any inconsistencies in the results. The second-stage respondents, in other words, can be used as informants to help the researcher interpret the outcomes. A second reason for using an iterative approach is that the researcher can use information from the first stage to select a useful subsample for the second. For example, the researcher might want to use information from the first round to select respondents with certain characteristics, such as those who are most knowledgeable about the phenomena under investigation, those who represent "typical" cases, or those who are at opposite extremes with regard to the key constructs.

Murphy's (1989) longitudinal study of the consequences and processes relating to a natural disaster (the eruption of Mt. St. Helens in southwestern Washington state in 1980) provides an example of multimethod research in which qualitative interviews were embedded within a larger survey. In the study, the bulk of the data were collected by way of structured self-report instruments administered to three groups of individuals: (1) a bereaved group (individuals who experienced the loss of a family member or close friend); (2) a property-loss group (individuals who experienced serious damage or destruction to their homes); and (3) a matched no-disaster-loss group for comparison purposes. Complex multivariate analyses of the quantitative data were undertaken to test alternative theories regarding disaster-related effects. In addition, in-depth interviews were conducted with subsets of the study group participants to obtain richer information regarding disaster-induced stress, coping strategies, and processes of recovery.

Embedding Quantitative Measures Into Field Work

Qualitative research conducted in the field (e.g., ethnographies) has a long history of using multiple methods of data collection. Generally, the methods used in field studies yield a rich array of data amenable to qualitative analysis, such as notes from qualitative observations, in-depth interviews, and narrative documents such as diaries and letters. However, field researchers can in some cases profit from the collection of more structured information from a larger or more representative sample than is possible in collecting the qualitative data. The secondary data might be in the form of structured self-reports from a survey, or quantifiable records. For example, if the researcher's field work focused on family violence, police and hospital records could be used to gather systematic data amenable to statistical analysis.

As field work progresses, researchers typically gain considerable insight into the communities, organizations, or social groups under study. With this knowledge, the researcher can generate hypotheses that can be subjected to more systematic scrutiny through structured data collection methods. Alternatively, the quantitative

portion of the study could be used to gather descriptive information about the characteristics of the community or group so that the qualitative findings could be understood in a broader context. In either case, having already gained entrée into the community and the trust and cooperation of its members, the field researcher may be in an ideal position to pursue a survey or a record-extraction activity.

A study by Grau and Wellin (1992) provides an example of a field study that included the use of structured, quantitative data. Their ethnographic study focused on the question of how nursing homes cope with the demands of government regulation for state licensure and Medicaid and Medicare certification. Two skilled-care nursing facilities were studied over a 6-month period. The field work included detailed observations in the two nursing homes and in-depth interviews with the nursing home staff, residents, and residents' families. The researchers provided a context for interpreting the qualitative data by administering structured interviews to all administrative personnel, social workers, registered nurses, and licensed practical nurses working in the two facilities. The structured interviews obtained information on the employees' backgrounds, daily work routines, knowledge of regulatory strategies, and experience with regulatory surveys.

Other examples of building quantitative methods into field work are provided by studies that use the GENESIS model. GENESIS (General Ethnographic and Nursing Evaluation Studies In the State) is a community analysis strategy that integrates ethnographic and epidemiologic data to develop a comprehensive, holistic description of the health of a community and its residents, and the needs of those residents. The GENESIS model, which has been implemented mainly in rural settings, has been extended to urban, multicultural communities in a model referred to as ACTION, or Assessing Communities Together in the Identification of

Needs (Russell, Gregory, Wotton, Mordoch, & Counts, 1996).

Qualitative and Quantitative Data in Experimental Research

Because experimental research involves highly controlled designs and the testing of causal hypotheses, it is easy to get the impression that only quantitative data are appropriate. However, qualitative data can greatly enrich studies that use an experimental or quasi-experimental design. Through in-depth, unstructured approaches, the researcher can better understand qualitative differences between groups, including differences in the reactions of subjects to the experimental conditions and in experiences and processes underlying experimental effects.

Qualitative data collection methods may be especially useful when the researcher is evaluating complex interventions. When an experimental treatment is simple and straightforward (e.g., a new drug), it might be relatively easy to interpret the results. Any posttreatment group differences (assuming that sufficient controls have been instituted) can be attributed to the intervention. However, many nursing interventions are not so straightforward. They may involve new ways of interacting with patients or new approaches to organizing the delivery of care. Sometimes, the intervention is multidimensional, involving several different components. At the end of the experiment, even when hypothesized results are obtained, people may ask, What *is* it that really caused the group differences? (If there were no group differences, then the important question would be, *Why* was the intervention unsuccessful?) In-depth qualitative interviews with subjects could help to address these questions. In other words, qualitative data may help researchers to address the **black box** question—understanding what it is about the complex intervention that is driving any observed effects. This knowledge can be helpful for theoretical purposes and can also help to streamline an intervention and make it more efficient and cost-effective.

Another reason for gathering qualitative data in evaluations of complex interventions is that there is often a need to understand exactly what the intervention was like in practice and how people reacted to it. Unstructured observations and interviews with people with different perspectives (e.g., nurses, physicians, hospital administrators, patients, or patients' family members) are especially well suited for such process evaluations.

A study in which one of the authors was a coinvestigator (Quint, Bos, & Polit, 1997; Quint & Musick, 1994; Quint, Fink, & Rowser, 1991) provides an example of using both qualitative and quantitative data collection and analysis in an experimental study. The study was a multifaceted evaluation of a comprehensive program for poor teenage mothers, implemented in 16 sites nationwide. The intervention, known as New Chance, included educational, health, employment, parenting, and social services for participating young mothers and their children. Data were collected over a 4-year period from a sample of more than 2000 young mothers. The quantitative data were obtained through several structured interviews with young mothers in the experimental and control groups, various psychosocial scales and tests administered to the mothers and their young children, and structured observations of the home environment. The evaluation also involved in-depth ethnographic interviews with a small sample of the mothers, unstructured observations of program operations, and unstructured interviews with program staff and participants.

OBSTACLES TO MULTIMETHOD RESEARCH

Throughout this chapter, we have stressed the advantages of designing studies that blend qualitative and quantitative data in a single investigation. We believe that the potential for advancing nursing science through such integration is great and is as yet relatively untapped. We also believe that integration efforts such as those proposed are inevitable because, at the level of the problem, almost all research questions are inherently multimethod.

Nevertheless, we recognize that there are various obstacles that may constrain the gathering of qualitative and quantitative data in a single investigation. Among the most salient are the following:

- *Epistemologic biases.* Qualitative and quantitative researchers often operate with a different set of assumptions about the world and ways of learning about it. For those with a hard-line, purist view, these assumptions may be seen as inevitably irreconcilable. According to a survey of nurses with doctorates, however, extreme positions of this type are atypical among nurse researchers (Damrosch & Strasser, 1988).
- *Costs.* A major obstacle facing researchers who would like to gather qualitative and quantitative data is that such multimethod research is usually expensive. Agencies that sponsor research activities may need to be "educated" about the contribution that multimethod designs can make. In addition to the many substantive advantages that integration offers, it can also be argued that blending qualitative and quantitative data in a single study is actually less costly and more efficient than two discrete research projects on the same topic.
- *Researcher training.* Most researchers obtain graduate-level training that stresses either qualitative or (more typically) quantitative research methods. According to a survey by Damrosch and Strasser (1988), only about one third of doctorally prepared academic nurses have training in both qualitative and quantitative methods. Thus, investigator skills may pose an obstacle to multimethod research. However,

there is nothing about such research that suggests that all phases of the investigation must be done by a single researcher. Collaboration among researchers might, indeed, be an important byproduct of the decision to use a multimethod approach. Such collaboration provides opportunities for triangulation in terms of both methods and investigator perspectives.
- *Analytic challenges.* Despite the many advantages of doing multimethod research, it is nevertheless true that a successful integrated data analysis is a challenging task. The researcher may be confronted with issues about how best to combine numeric and narrative data or about how to resolve and interpret inconsistent or contradictory findings. However, the outcome of such challenges may well be clearer or more refined conceptualizations of the phenomenon under study.
- *Publication biases.* Some journals have a distinct preference for studies that are qualitative, and others lean toward quantitative studies. Because of this, researchers might be concerned that they would need to write up the qualitative and quantitative results separately, foregoing many of the advantages of multimethod research. However, publication biases are much less evident today than they were a decade ago. All of the major nursing journals devoted to research publish qualitative and quantitative studies, and they are increasingly publishing reports of multimethod studies.

In conclusion, although it is recognized that there are various obstacles to multimethod research, we believe that the simultaneous use of qualitative and quantitative data to address problems of interest to the nursing profession represents a powerful methodologic strategy. We are confident that nurse researchers will develop mechanisms for dealing with the obstacles.

TIPS FOR CONDUCTING MULTIMETHOD RESEARCH

The blending of qualitative and quantitative data in a single study is not always feasible, nor necessarily desirable. However, we offer the following suggestions for those contemplating the possibility of a multimethod study:

- In many situations, a researcher comes to the final stage of a study—the interpretation of the findings—realizing that the interpretation is hampered by the absence of information on some issues. In some cases, this "if only" situation involves the wish that additional information were available using the same data collection method already used (e.g., the addition of another structured scale or question). In many other cases, however, the researcher's interpretation would be enhanced by data of a different sort, such as in-depth questioning. This suggests that many studies would benefit from additional planning. It is often wise to consider in advance a wide variety of scenarios with regard to the findings (especially in studies that are primarily quantitative, which tend to be somewhat less flexible once the study is underway). For example, if you knew in advance that the hypotheses would *not* be supported, what else might you want to ask respondents? If you knew that the hypotheses were supported only for certain types of people or in certain types of conditions, what kinds of data would you like to have to help explain this pattern? In many situations, the information you will want will not be of the same type used to test the hypotheses. Integrated methods may be the obvious and natural strategy among researchers who use their imaginations—and who are thoughtful in anticipating alternative findings.
- If you are considering the possibility of doing a multimethod research study, try to find someone whose research skills complement yours to collaborate with you. It is almost always useful to have two (or more) minds working on a common problem, and this is especially true when the methods are varied. Top-notch qualitative researchers are rarely top-notch quantitative researchers, and vice versa. It is usually wise to do what you do best and to brainstorm with a person whose talents are different.
- Many multimethod studies are conducted in two or more phases, for example, conducting in-depth interviews with a subsample of patients from whom biophysiologic data were obtained after analysis of those data has been done. If there is a possibility that you *might* go back to research subjects to obtain more data, be sure to structure your consent form in such a way that subjects are aware of any potential future demands on their time. Also, be sure to obtain contact information to facilitate finding the subjects at a later date.

RESEARCH EXAMPLES

We have provided examples of multimethod studies throughout this chapter in an effort to demonstrate the advantages of such an approach as well as to illustrate different applications to which such integration has been put. Table 11-1 identifies some other studies in which qualitative and quantitative data were blended, and two additional examples are described in greater detail.

Example of Construct Explication and Understanding Relationships

Reed (1991) studied the link between developmental resources on the one hand and mental health on the other among the oldest-old (those over 80 years of age). Specifically, Reed

TABLE 11-1   Examples of Multimethod Studies

RESEARCH QUESTION	DATA SOURCES	
	Quantitative	Qualitative
How do the Appalachian culture and rural living influence illness experiences and health recovery behaviors? (Rosswurm, Dent, Armstrong-Persily, Woodburn, & Davis, 1996)	Structured interviews	In-depth interviews
What are the knowledge, perceptions, and attitudes of critical care nurses toward caring for potential and actual organ donors? (Watkinson, 1995)	Structured questionnaires	In-depth interviews
What is the perception of loneliness among adults receiving treatment in a psychiatric facility? (Lee, Coenen, & Heim, 1994)	Structured scales	In-depth interviews
What is the effect of marijuana consumption during pregnancy and lactation on offspring from birth to school age? (Dreher & Hayes, 1993)	Structured scales	In-depth interviews and observation
What is the effect of a neonate's breastfeeding competence on the mother's satisfaction with and perception of the experience? (Matthews, 1993)	Hospital records Structured scales	In-depth questions
What are the nurses' judgments of pain in newborns, and what cues do they use to assess the possible presence of pain? (Shapiro, 1993)	Structured scale (visual analogue scale)	In-depth interviews

was interested in a resource that she labeled self-transcendence—the expansion of one's conceptual boundaries inwardly through introspective activities, outwardly through concerns about the welfare of others, and temporally by integrating perceptions of one's past and future.

Reed collected a variety of both quantitative and qualitative data from a sample of 55 older adults living independently. Several structured scales were administered, including the CES-D Scale, the Self-Transcendence Scale (STS) that the author herself developed, and the Lang-

ner Scale of Mental Health Symptomatology (MHS). Additionally, because the construct of self-transcendence had not previously been widely studied, Reed used a loosely structured interview designed to elicit the respondents' own descriptions of self-transcendence perspectives and behaviors that promoted their sense of well-being. The questions addressed the respondents' perspectives about their past, present, and future and about the bodily changes they were experiencing. The questions also probed the respondents' tendency and ability to focus on things beyond themselves.

Reed used a highly systematic, iterative process to analyze the qualitative data. A conceptually clustered matrix was constructed to answer questions about patterns of variables across respondents. Cases were listed in the matrix by rows; the columns were arranged to bring together conceptually similar clusters of data. This analysis revealed four conceptual clusters that the researcher labeled Generativity, Introjectivity, Temporal Integration, and Body-Transcendence. Table 11-2 presents Reed's clusters and categories for the qualitative data.

The relationship between self-transcendence and depression was examined by juxtaposing the qualitatively generated self-transcendence patterns and quantitative depression scores for each respondent. Using correlational procedures, Reed found a relationship between self-transcendence and positive mental health among the very elderly.

It may be noted that Coward (1995), whose phenomenologic study was described as a research example in the previous chapter, built on Reed's concepts and framework in her research.

Example of Theory Building

Connelly, Bott, Hoffart, and Taunton (1997) conducted a multimethod research project that focused on the retention of staff nurses. Their basic study was primarily quantitative and involved the development of a sophisticated statistical model designed to predict nurse retention. The researchers measured four types of factors that they believed could predict retention: characteristics of the managers (e.g., leadership style); characteristics of the organization (e.g., promotional opportunity); work characteristics (e.g., group cohesion); and characteristics of the nurses themselves (e.g., education, marital status). The variables in the model had all been verified in the research literature; nevertheless, their cumulative predictive power was relatively low.

In the final year of the project, the researchers did a qualitative study to examine whether a different research approach might produce an additional construct that belonged in the retention model. A total of 21 staff nurses who had low scores on an "Intent to Stay" scale that had been administered to them in the first year of the project—but who had nevertheless remained working in the same hospital—were interviewed in depth about their reasons for staying, their possible reasons for leaving, and the positive and negative aspects of their employment.

The researchers found that there was some correspondence between the information obtained through the in-depth interviews and the variables included in their model, thereby validating aspects of the model. However, new themes also emerged during the qualitative interviews—for example, such variables as location close to home, fringe benefits, ability to provide high-quality care, and ability to transfer among units within the hospital. The advantages of having used a multimethod design were described as follows:

> Triangulation helped us attain three benefits. First, the careful comparison of quantitative and qualitative data added support for the variables in the retention model. Second, the comparison also showed new dimensions about nurse retention, thereby contributing to a more complete understanding of nurse retention. . . . Third, the researchers were able to make suggestions for revision of the quantitative instrument. (Connelly, Bott, Hoffart, & Taunton, 1997, p. 301)

🌀 SUMMARY

The judicious blending of qualitative and quantitative data collection and analysis in a single project offers many advantages. The most obvious advantage to a **multimethod** (or **mixed-method) research** is that the two methods have complementary strengths and weaknesses and offer the possibility of "mutually supplying each other's lack." Second, an integrated approach can lead to theoretical and substantive insights into the multidimensional nature of reality that might otherwise be unattainable. Third, multi-

TABLE 11-2   Reed's Clusters and Categories of Self-Transcendence

CLUSTER, CATEGORIES	SAMPLE RESPONSES
I. Generativity	
(1)* Helping others	Visiting the sick; volunteer work; teaching; church work
(1) Family involvement	Visiting siblings, helping children
II. Introjectivity	
(1) Interiority	Hobbies; travel; housework
(1) Lifelong learning	Reading; taking formal courses; spiritual or self-reflection
III. Temporal Integration	
Past	
(2) Active acceptance	Sense of pride in past; feelings of joy about past
(1) Passive acceptance	The past is gone; I have no regrets
(0) Negative acceptance	It saddens me; I regret it
Present	
(2) Active positive	I make the best of it; I am happy; one must change to grow
(1) Passive positive	Take one day at a time; you have to roll with the punches
(0) Negative	I am existing, not living; it is worrisome; discouraging
Future	
(2) Active anticipation	I look forward to it; I am at peace; I have hope
(1) Passive anticipation	Que sera sera; I don't think about it
(0) Negative anticipation	I worry about my health then; I have fears about it
IV. Body Transcendence	
(2) Flexibility	Learn how to live with it; have to accept it; don't dwell on it
(1) Maybe or unsure	Never thought about it; I think I'm able to accept the changes
(0) Negative	I get disgusted; I feel trapped by my body; I hate my body

*Indicates weighting used to code the score for each cluster.

Reprinted with permission from Reed, P. G. (1991). Self-transcendence and mental health in oldest-old adults. *Nursing Research, 40,* 5–11.

method research can provide feedback loops that augment the incremental gains in knowledge that a single-method study could achieve. Fourth, the potential for confirmation of the study hypotheses through multiple and complementary types of data can strengthen the researcher's confidence in the validity of the findings. Fifth, when the multiple methods yield inconsistent findings, a careful scrutiny of the discrepancies could push the line of inquiry further than might otherwise have been possible.

The blending of qualitative and quantitative data can be used in many applications. In nursing, one of the most frequent uses of multimethod research has been in the area of instrument development and refinement. Qualitative data are also used in some studies to illustrate the meaning of quantified descriptions or relationships. Multimethod studies are also used in efforts to explicate constructs or to interpret and give shape to relationships and causal processes. Finally, the most ambitious application of an integrated approach is in the area of theory development.

There are two broad categories of designs in multimethod research. In studies with a **component design**, the qualitative and quantitative aspects of the study are implemented as discrete components and are distinct during data collection and data analysis. Examples of component designs include **triangulated designs, complementarity designs**, and **expansion designs**. The second broad category are **integrated designs**, in which there is greater integration of methods throughout the research process. The four major types of integrated designs are **iterative designs, embedded (nested) designs, holistic designs**, and **transformative designs**.

Researchers can implement a multimethod study in a variety of ways, but three strategies are especially likely to be common. The first is to embed qualitative methods (such as in-depth interviews or unstructured observations) within a survey. The second is to add structured data collection (such as a survey or a systematic analysis of records data) into qualitative studies involving field work. The third is to collect both types of data within the context of an experimental or quasi-experimental design. In some studies, the simultaneous collection and analysis of qualitative and quantitative data may address the objectives of integration, but in many studies, a multistage approach is likely to yield more insights.

Despite the advantages of blending both types of data in a single study, there are several obstacles to doing so. These obstacles include epistemologic biases, high costs, inadequate researcher training, and publication biases. However, these obstacles are not insurmountable; the potential contribution that integration would afford nursing science makes the effort to surmount them a worthwhile investment.

STUDY ACTIVITIES

Chapter 11 of the *Study Guide to Accompany Nursing Research: Principles and Methods, 6th ed.*, offers various exercises and study suggestions for reinforcing the concepts presented in this chapter. Additionally, the following study questions can be addressed:

1. Suppose you were interested in studying the psychological consequences of miscarriage. Suggest ways in which qualitative and quantitative data could be gathered for such a study.

2. Read an article in a recent issue of a nursing research journal in which the researcher collected only quantitative data. Suggest some possibilities for how qualitative data might have enhanced the validity or interpretability of the findings.

3. Read one of the studies cited under Substantive References at the end of this chapter. To what extent were the qualitative and quantitative analyses integrated? Describe how the absence of either the quantitative or qualitative portions of the study might have affected the study quality and the study conclusions.

SUGGESTED READINGS

Methodologic References

Brewer, J., & Hunter, A. (1989). *Multimethod research: A synthesis of styles.* Newbury Park, CA: Sage.

Bryman, A. (1988). *Quantity and quality in social research.* London: Unwin Hyman.

Carey, J. W. (1993). Linking qualitative and quantitative methods: Integrating cultural factors into public health. *Qualitative Health Research, 3,* 298–318.

Chesla, C. A. (1992). When qualitative and quantitative findings do not converge. *Western Journal of Nursing Research, 14,* 681–685.

Damrosch, S. P., & Strasser, J. A. (1988). A survey of doctorally prepared academic nurses on qualitative and quantitative research issues. *Nursing Research, 37,* 176–180.

Denzin, N. K. (1989). *The research act* (3rd ed.). Englewood Cliffs, NJ: Prentice-Hall.

Duffy, M. (1987). Methodological triangulation: A vehicle for merging quantitative and qualitative research methods. *Image—The Journal of Nursing Scholarship, 19,* 130–133.

Ford-Gilboe, M., Campbell, J., & Berman, H. (1995). Stories and numbers: Coexistence without compromise. *Advances in Nursing Science, 18,* 14–26.

Green, J. C., & Caracelli, V. J. (Eds.). (1997). *Advances in mixed method evaluation: The challenges and benefits of integrating diverse paradigms.* San Francisco: Jossey-Bass Publishers.

Haase, J. E., & Myers, S. T. (1988). Reconciling paradigm assumptions of qualitative and quantitative research. *Western Journal of Nursing Research, 10,* 128–137.

Jicks, T. D. (1979). Mixing qualitative and quantitative methods: Triangulation in action. *Administrative Science Quarterly, 24,* 602–611.

Mitchell, E. S. (1986). Multiple triangulation: A methodology for nursing science. *Advances in Nursing Science, 8,* 18–26.

Morse, J. M. (1991). Approaches to qualitative-quantitative methodological triangulation. *Nursing Research, 40,* 120–122.

Murphy, S. A. (1989a). Multiple triangulation: Applications in a program of nursing research. *Nursing Research, 38,* 294–298.

Myers, S. T., & Haase, J. E. (1989). Guidelines for integration of quantitative and qualitative approaches. *Nursing Research, 38,* 299–301.

Rossman, G. B., & Wilson, B. L. (1985). Numbers and words: Combining quantitative and qualitative methods is a single large-scale evaluation study. *Evaluation Review, 9,* 627–643.

Seiber, S. D. (1973). Integrating field work and survey methods. *American Journal of Sociology, 78,* 1335–1359.

Tilden, V. P., Nelson, C. A., & May, B. A. (1990). Use of qualitative methods to enhance content validity. *Nursing Research, 39,* 172–175.

Tripp-Reimer, T. (1985). Combining qualitative and quantitative methodologies. In M. Leininger (Ed.), *Qualitative research methods in nursing.* New York: Grune & Stratton.

Substantive References

Bargagliotti, L. A., & Trygstad, L. N. (1987). Differences in stress and coping findings: A reflection of social realities or methodologies. *Nursing Research, 36,* 170–173.

Connelly, L. M., Bott, M., Hoffart, N., & Taunton, R. L. (1997). Methodological triangulation in a study of nurse retention. *Nursing Research, 46,* 299–302.

Coward, D. D. (1995). The lived experience of self-transcendence in women with AIDS. *Journal of Obstetric, Gynecologic, and Neonatal Nursing, 24,* 314–318.

Dreher, M. C., & Hayes, J. S. (1993). Triangulation in cross-cultural research of child development in Jamaica. *Western Journal of Nursing Research, 15,* 216–229.

Ersek, M., Ferrell, B. R., Dow, K. H., & Melancon, C. H. (1997). Quality of life in women with ovarian cancer. *Western Journal of Nursing Research, 19,* 334–350.

Grau, L., & Wellin, E. (1992). The organizational cultures of nursing homes: Influences on responses to external regulatory controls. *Qualitative Health Research, 2,* 42–60.

Hall, J. M., Stevens, P. E., & Meleis, A. I. (1992). Developing the construct of role integration: A narrative analysis of women clerical workers' daily lives. *Research in Nursing & Health, 15,* 447–457.

Hinds, P. S. (1989). Method triangulation to index change in clinical phenomena. *Western Journal of Nursing Research, 11,* 440–447.

Hough, E. E., Lewis, F. M., & Woods, N. F. (1991). Family response to mother's chronic illness: Case studies of well- and poorly-adjusted families. *Western Journal of Nursing Research, 13*, 568–596.

Lee, H., Coenen, A., & Heim, K. (1994). Island living: The experience of loneliness in a psychiatric hospital. *Applied Nursing Research, 7*, 7–13.

Lewis, F. M., Woods, N. F., Hough, E. E., & Bensley, L. (1989). The family's functioning with chronic illness in the mother. *Social Science and Medicine, 29*, 1261–1269.

Lipson, J. G. (1992). The health and adjustment of Iranian immigrants. *Western Journal of Nursing Research, 14*, 10–24.

Matthews, M. K. (1993). Experiences of primiparous breast-feeding mothers in the first days following birth. *Clinical Nursing Research, 2*, 309–326.

Meleis, A. I., Norbeck, J. S., Laffrey, S. (1989). Role integration and health among female clerical workers. *Research in Nursing & Health, 12*, 355–364.

Melillo, K. D., Williamson, E., Futrell, M., & Chamberlain, C. (1997). A self-assessment tool to measure older adults' perceptions regarding physical fitness and exercise activity. *Journal of Advanced Nursing, 25*, 220–226.

Murphy, S. A. (1989). An explanatory model of recovery from disaster loss. *Research in Nursing & Health, 12*, 67–76.

Nyamathi, A. M., & Flaskerud, J. (1992). A community-based inventory of current concerns of impoverished homeless and drug-addicted minority women. *Research in Nursing & Health, 15*, 121–129.

Polit, D. F., Morton, T., & White, C. M. (1989). Sex, contraception, and pregnancy among children in foster care. *Family Planning Perspectives, 21*, 203–206.

Polit, D. F., White, C. M., & Morton, T. (1990). Child sexual abuse and premarital intercourse among high-risk adolescents. *Journal of Adolescent Health Care, 11*, 231–234.

Quint, J. C., Fink, B. L., & Rowser, S. L. (1991). *New Chance: Implementing a comprehensive program for disadvantaged young mothers and their children.* New York: Manpower Demonstration Research Corporation.

Quint, J. C., & Musick, S. J. (1994). *Lives of promise, lives of pain: Young mothers after New Chance.* New York: Manpower Demonstration Research Corporation.

Quint, J. C., Bos, H., & Polit, D. F. (1997). *New Chance: Final report on on a comprehensive program for young mothers in poverty and their children.* New York: Manpower Demonstration Research Corporation.

Reece, S. M., & Harkless, G. (1996). Divergent themes in maternal experience in women older than 35 years of age. *Applied Nursing Research, 9*, 148–153.

Reed, P. G. (1991). Self-transcendence and mental health in oldest-old adults. *Nursing Research, 40*, 5–11.

Rosswurm, M. E., Dent, D. M., Armstrong-Persily, C., Woodburn, P., & Davis, B. (1996). Illness experiences and health recovery behaviors of patients in southern Appalachia. *Western Journal of Nursing Research, 18*, 441–459.

Russell, C. K., Gregory, D. M., Wotton, D., Mordoch, E., & Counts, M. M. (1996). ACTION: Application and extension of the GENESIS community analysis model. *Public Health Nursing, 13*, 187–194.

Salazar, M. K., & Carter, W. B. (1993). Evaluation of breast self-examination beliefs using a decision model. *Western Journal of Nursing Research, 15*, 403–418.

Shapiro, C. R. (1993). Nurses' judgments of pain in term and preterm newborns. *Journal of Obstetric, Gynecologic, and Neonatal Nursing, 22*, 41–47.

Watkinson, G. E. (1995). A study of the perception and experiences of critical care nurses in caring for potential and actual organ donors. *Journal of Advanced Nursing, 22*, 929–940.

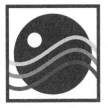

CHAPTER 12

Sampling Designs

Sampling is a complex and technical topic to which entire texts have been devoted. At the same time, the basic features of sampling are familiar to us all. In the course of our daily activities, we gather knowledge, make decisions, and make predictions through sampling. A nursing student may decide on an elective course for a semester by sampling two or three classes on the first day of the semester. Patients may generalize about the competence of nurses in a particular hospital as a result of the care they received from a sample of nurses during a 1-week hospital stay. We all come to conclusions about phenomena based on exposure to a limited portion of those phenomena.

Researchers, too, generally derive knowledge from samples. For example, in testing the efficacy of a medication for asthma patients, a researcher must reach a conclusion without administering the drug to every asthmatic patient. However, researchers cannot afford to draw conclusions about the effectiveness of interventions or the validity of relationships based on a sample of only three or four subjects. The consequences of making erroneous decisions are much more momentous in disciplined inquiries than in private decision making.

Quantitative and qualitative researchers have very different approaches to the issue of sampling. Quantitative researchers seek to select samples that will allow them to generalize their results to much broader groups. They are therefore careful in developing a **sampling plan** that specifies in advance how study participants are to be selected and how many to include. Qualitative researchers are not concerned with issues of generalizability but rather with an in-depth, holistic understanding of the phenomenon of interest. They often allow sampling decisions to emerge during the course of data collection based on informational and theoretical needs and typically do not develop a formal sampling plan in advance.

Because formal sampling designs are more relevant to quantitative than to qualitative research, most of this chapter is devoted to sampling plans for quantitative studies. However, a section of the chapter discusses sampling issues for qualitative research.

❧ BASIC SAMPLING CONCEPTS IN QUANTITATIVE STUDIES

Sampling is an important step in the research process for quantitative studies. Let us first consider some terms associated with sampling—

terms that are used primarily (but not exclusively) in connection with quantitative studies.

Populations

A **population** is the entire aggregation of cases that meet a designated set of criteria. For instance, if a nurse researcher were studying American nurses with doctoral degrees, the population could be defined as all U.S. citizens who are registered nurses (RNs) and who have acquired a Ph.D., D.Sc.N., D.Ed., or other doctoral-level degree. Other possible populations might be all the male patients who underwent cardiac surgery in St. Peter's Hospital during 1997, all the women over 60 years of age who are under psychiatric care in Boston, or all the children in England with cystic fibrosis. As this list illustrates, a population may be broadly defined, involving thousands of individuals, or may be narrowly specified to include only several hundred people.

Populations are not restricted to human subjects. A population might consist of all the hospital records on file in a particular hospital, all the blood samples taken from clients of a health maintenance organization, or all the high schools in the United States with a school-based clinic that dispenses contraceptives. Whatever the basic unit, the population always comprises the entire aggregate of elements in which the researcher is interested.

As noted in Chapter 9, it is sometimes useful to make a distinction between target and accessible populations. The **accessible population** is the aggregate of cases that conform to the designated criteria *and* that are accessible to the researcher as a pool of subjects for a study. The **target population** is the aggregate of cases about which the researcher would like to make generalizations. A target population might consist of all diabetic people in the United States, but the more modest accessible population might consist of all diabetic people who are members of a particular health plan. Researchers usually sample from an accessible

population and hope to generalize to a target population.

Eligibility Criteria

In identifying a population, the researcher should be specific about the criteria that define who is included. Consider the population of American nursing students. Does this population include students in all types of basic nursing programs? Are part-time students included? How about RNs returning to school for a bachelor's degree? Or students who dropped out of school for a semester? Do foreign students enrolled in American nursing programs qualify? Insofar as possible, the researcher must consider the exact criteria by which it could be decided whether an individual would or would not be classified as a member of the population in question. The criteria that specified the characteristics that people in the population must possess are sometimes referred to as **eligibility criteria** or **inclusion criteria**. The eligibility criteria specified in one nursing study are presented in Table 12-1. Sometimes, a population is defined in terms of characteristics that people must *not* possess, which involves stipulating the **exclusion criteria**. For example, the population may be defined to exclude people who cannot speak English. Inclusion or exclusion criteria for a study often reflect considerations other than a substantive or theoretical interest in certain types of people. The criteria for defining the population may reflect one or more of the following:

- *Costs.* Some criteria reflect cost constraints. For example, when non–English-speaking people are excluded, this does not necessarily mean that the researcher is not interested in non–English speakers, but may rather reflect the fact that the researcher cannot afford to hire translators and people who can collect data in other languages.

TABLE 12-1 Eligibility Criteria Specified in a Quantitative Nursing Study	
RESEARCH QUESTION	**ELIGIBILITY CRITERIA**
What are the perceptions about the causes of coronary artery disease (CAD) among patients diagnosed with CAD? (Zerwic, King, & Wlasowicz, 1997)	To be eligible for the study, the patient must be hospitalized because of myocardial infarction or for coronary angiography; have no prior history of CAD; be older than 18 years of age; be in hemodynamically stable condition and free of pain for 24 hours; be oriented to person, place, and time; and be able to speak and understand English.

- *Practical concerns.* Sometimes, there are other practical constraints, such as difficulty in including people from rural areas, people who are hearing impaired, and so on.
- *People's ability to participate in a study.* The health condition of some people may preclude their participation. For example, people with mental impairments, who are in a coma, or who are in an unstable medical condition may need to be excluded.
- *Design considerations.* As noted in Chapter 9, it is sometimes advantageous to define a fairly homogeneous sample as a means of controlling extraneous variables.

The criteria used to define a population for a research project have implications for the interpretation of the results and the generalizability of the findings. Therefore, it is important to give adequate consideration to the implications of the eligibility criteria. There should be a meaningful and justifiable rationale for all criteria that include or exclude people from the population.

Samples and Sampling

Sampling refers to the process of selecting a portion of the population to represent the entire population. A **sample**, then, consists of a subset of the units that compose the population. In sampling terminology, the units that make up the samples and populations are referred to as elements. The **element** is the most basic unit about which information is collected. In nursing research, the elements are usually humans.

Samples and sampling plans vary considerably in quality. *The overriding consideration in assessing a sample in a quantitative study is its* **representativeness**. A representative sample is one whose key characteristics closely approximate those of the population. If a population in a study of family planning practices consists of women 15 to 44 years of age, 40% of whom were using oral contraception and 10% of whom were using Norplant, then a representative sample would reflect these attributes in similar proportions.

Unfortunately, there is no method for making certain that a sample is representative without obtaining the information from the entire population. Certain sampling procedures are less likely to result in biased samples than others, but there is never any guarantee of a representative sample. This may sound somewhat discouraging, but it must be remembered that researchers always operate under conditions in which error is possible. An important role of the quantitative researcher is to minimize or control those errors and, if possible, to estimate the magnitude of their effects. With certain types of sampling plans, it is possible to estimate through statistical procedures the **margin of error** in the data obtained from samples. Advanced textbooks on sampling elaborate on the procedures for making such estimates.

Sampling designs can be grouped into two categories: probability sampling and nonprobability sampling. **Probability sampling** involves some form of random selection in choosing the elements. The hallmark of a probability sample is that a researcher is in a position to specify the probability that each element of the population will be included in the sample. Probability sampling is the more respected of the two approaches because greater confidence can be placed in the representativeness of probability samples. In **nonprobability samples**, elements are selected by nonrandom methods. There is no way to estimate the probability that each element has of being included in a nonprobability sample, and every element usually does *not* have a chance for inclusion.

Strata

Sometimes, it is useful to think of populations as consisting of two or more subpopulations, or **strata**. A stratum refers to a mutually exclusive segment of a population established by one or more characteristics. For instance, suppose our population consisted of all RNs currently employed in the United States. This population could be divided into two strata based on the gender of the nurse. Alternatively, we could specify three strata consisting of nurses younger than 30 years of age, nurses aged 30 to 45 years, and nurses 46 years of age or older. Strata are often identified and used in the sample selection process to enhance the representativeness of the sample.

Sampling Bias

Researchers work with samples rather than with populations because it is more economi-

cal and efficient to do so. The typical researcher has neither the time nor the resources to study all members of a population. Furthermore, it is usually unnecessary to gather data on some phenomenon from an entire population—it is almost always possible to obtain a reasonably accurate understanding of the phenomenon by securing information from a sample. Samples, thus, are practical and efficient means of collecting data.

Still, the data obtained from samples *can* lead to erroneous conclusions. Finding 100 willing subjects to participate in a research project seldom poses difficulty, even to a novice researcher. It is considerably more problematic to select 100 subjects who are not a biased subset of the population. **Sampling bias** refers to the systematic overrepresentation or underrepresentation of some segment of the population in terms of a characteristic relevant to the research question.

As an example of consciously biased selection, suppose a nurse researcher is investigating patients' responsiveness to touch by nurses and decides to use as a sample the first 50 patients meeting certain criteria who are admitted to a specific hospital unit. The researcher decides to omit Mr. Z from the sample because of his hostility to nurses. Mrs. X, who has just lost a spouse, is also excluded from the study out of consideration for her psychological discomfort. The researcher has made conscious decisions to exclude certain types of individuals, and the decisions do not reflect bona fide criteria for selection. This can lead to bias because responsiveness to touch by nurses (the dependent variable) may be affected by patients' feelings about nurses or their psychological state.

Sampling bias is more likely to occur unconsciously than consciously, however. If a researcher studying nursing students systematically interviews every 10th student who enters the nursing school library, the sample of students will be biased in favor of library-goers, even if the researcher exerted a conscientious effort to include every 10th entrant irrespective of the person's appearance, gender, or other characteristics.

The extent to which sampling bias is likely to cause concern is a function of the homogeneity of the population with respect to the attributes under investigation. If the elements in a population were all identical with respect to the critical attributes, then any sample would be as good as any other. Indeed, if the population were completely homogeneous, that is, exhibited no variability at all, then a *single* element would constitute a sufficient sample for drawing conclusions about the population. With regard to many physical or physiologic attributes, it may be safe to assume a reasonably high degree of homogeneity and to proceed in selecting a sample on the basis of this assumption. For example, the blood in a person's veins is relatively homogeneous. A single blood sample chosen haphazardly is usually adequate for clinical purposes. As another illustration, the physiology of laboratory rats is sufficiently similar that elaborate sampling procedures are unnecessary when testing physiologic processes with a sample of rats. For most human attributes, however, homogeneity is the exception rather than the rule. Variables, after all, derive their name from the fact that traits vary from one individual to the next. Age, income, health condition, stress, attitudes, needs, habits—all of these attributes reflect the heterogeneity of humans. The researcher must be concerned with the problem of sampling bias to the degree that a population is heterogeneous on key variables. Whenever variation occurs in the population, then similar variation ideally should be reflected in a sample.

NONPROBABILITY SAMPLING

Nonprobability sampling is less likely than probability sampling to produce accurate and representative samples. Despite this fact, most research samples in most disciplines, including nursing, are nonprobability samples. There are three primary methods of nonprobability sampling: convenience, quota, and purposive.

Convenience Sampling

Convenience sampling entails the use of the most conveniently available people or objects as subjects in a study. The faculty member who distributes questionnaires to the nursing students in class is using a convenience sample, or an **accidental sample,** as it is sometimes called. The nurse who conducts an observational study of husbands whose wives are delivering a baby at the local hospital is also relying on a convenience sample. The problem with convenience sampling is that available subjects might be atypical of the population with regard to the critical variables being measured.

Convenience samples do not necessarily comprise individuals known to the researchers. Stopping people at a street corner to conduct an interview is sampling by convenience. Sometimes, a researcher seeking individuals with certain characteristics will place an advertisement in a newspaper or place signs in clinics, supermarkets, or community centers. These approaches are subject to problems of bias because people self-select themselves as pedestrians on certain streets or as volunteers in response to public notices.

Another type of convenience sampling is known as **snowball sampling** or **network sampling.** With this approach, early sample members are asked to identify and refer other people who meet the eligibility criteria. This method of sampling is most likely to be used when the research population consists of people with specific traits who might otherwise be difficult to identify (e.g., women who stopped breastfeeding within 1 month of delivery; people who are afraid of hospitals). The snowballing process begins with a few eligible study participants and then continues on the basis of referrals from those participants until the desired sample size has been obtained. Like other types of convenience sampling, snowball sampling is often expedient but runs the risk of sampling bias.

Convenience sampling is the weakest form of sampling. It is also the most commonly used sampling method in nursing studies. In cases in which the phenomena under investigation are fairly homogeneous within the population, the risks of bias may be minimal. In heterogeneous populations, there is no other sampling approach in which the risk of bias is greater.

Quota Sampling

Quota sampling is another form of nonprobability sampling. The **quota sample** is one in which the researcher identifies strata of the population and determines the proportions of elements needed from the various segments of the population. By using information about the composition of a population, the investigator can ensure that diverse segments are represented in the sample in the proportions in which they occur in the population. Quota sampling gets its name from the procedure of establishing quotas for the various strata from which data are to be collected.

Let us consider the example of a researcher interested in studying the attitudes of under-graduate nursing students toward working with AIDS patients. The accessible population is a single school of nursing that has an undergraduate enrollment of 1000 students. A sample size of 200 students is desired. The easiest procedure would be to use a convenience sample by distributing questionnaires in classrooms or catching students as they enter or leave the library. Suppose, however, that the researcher suspects that male and female students, as well as members of the four classes, have different attitudes toward working with AIDS victims. A convenience sample could easily sample too many or too few students from these subgroups. Table 12-2 presents some fictitious data showing the proportions of each stratum for the population and for a convenience sample. As this table shows, the convenience sample seriously overrepresents freshmen and women and underrepresents men and members of the sophomore, junior, and senior classes. In anticipation of a problem of this type, the researcher can guide the selection of subjects such that the final sample includes the correct number of cases from each stratum. The bottom panel of Table 12-2 shows the number of cases that would be required for each stratum in a quota sample for this example.

TABLE 12-2 Numbers and Percentages of Students in Strata of a Population, Convenience Sample, and Quota Sample

GROUP	GENDER	FRESHMEN	SOPHOMORES	JUNIORS	SENIORS	TOTAL
Population	Males	25 (2.5%)	25 (2.5%)	25 (2.5%)	25 (2.5%)	100 (10%)
	Females	225 (22.5%)	225 (22.5%)	225 (22.5%)	225 (22.5%)	900 (90%)
	TOTAL	250 (25%)	250 (25%)	250 (25%)	250 (25%)	1000 (100%)
Convenience sample	Males	2 (1%)	4 (2%)	3 (1.5%)	1 (.5%)	10 (5%)
	Females	98 (49%)	36 (18%)	37 (18.5%)	19 (9.5%)	190 (95%)
	TOTAL	100 (50%)	40 (20%)	40 (20%)	20 (10%)	200 (100%)
Quota sample	Males	5 (2.5%)	5 (2.5%)	5 (2.5%)	5 (2.5%)	20 (10%)
	Females	45 (22.5%)	45 (22.5%)	45 (22.5%)	45 (22.5%)	180 (90%)
	TOTAL	50 (25%)	50 (25%)	50 (25%)	50 (25%)	200 (100%)

TABLE 12-3 Students Willing to Work on an AIDS Unit			
SAMPLE	NUMBER IN POPULATION	NUMBER IN CONVENIENCE SAMPLE	NUMBER IN QUOTA SAMPLE
Freshmen males	2	0	0
Sophomore males	6	1	1
Junior males	8	1	2
Senior males	12	0	3
Freshmen females	6	2	1
Sophomore females	16	2	3
Junior females	30	4	7
Senior females	45	3	9
Number of willing students	125	13	26
Total number of students	1000	200	200
Percentage	12.5%	6.5%	13.0%

If we pursue this same example a bit further, the reader may better appreciate the dangers of inadequate representation of the various strata. Suppose that one of the key questions in this study was, Would you be willing to work on a unit that cared exclusively for AIDS patients? The percentage of students in the population who would respond "yes" to this inquiry is shown in the first column of Table 12-3. Of course, these values would not be known by the researcher; they are displayed to illustrate a point. Within the population, males and older students are more likely than females and younger students to express willingness to work on a unit with AIDS patients, yet these are the very groups that are underrepresented in the convenience sample. As a result, there is a sizable discrepancy between the population and sample values: nearly twice as many students are favorable toward working with AIDS victims (12.5%) than one would suspect based on the results obtained from the convenience sample (6.5%). The quota sample, on the other hand, does a reasonably good job of reflecting the viewpoint of

the population. In actual research situations, the distortions introduced by convenience sampling may be much smaller than in this fictitious example but, conceivably, could be larger as well.

Quota sampling does not require sophisticated skills or an inordinate amount of time or effort. Many researchers who claim that the use of a convenience sample is unavoidable for their projects could probably design a quota sampling plan, and it would be to their advantage to do so. The characteristics chosen to form the strata are necessarily selected according to the researcher's judgment. The basis of stratification should be some variable that would reflect important differences in the dependent variable under investigation. Such variables as age, gender, ethnicity, educational attainment, and medical diagnosis are often good stratifying variables in nursing research investigations.

Except for the identification of the strata and the proportional representation for each, quota sampling is procedurally similar to convenience sampling. The subjects in any particular cell constitute, in essence, a convenience sample from that stratum of the population. Referring back to the example in Table 12-2, the initial sample of 200 students constituted a sample chosen by convenience from the population of 1000. In the quota sample, the 45 female seniors would constitute a convenience sample of the 225 female seniors in the population. Because of this fact, quota sampling shares many of the same weaknesses as convenience sampling. For instance, if a researcher is required by a quota sampling plan to interview 10 men between the ages of 65 and 80 years, a trip to a nursing home might be the most convenient method of obtaining those subjects. Yet this approach would fail to give any representation to those many senior citizens who are living independently in the community. Despite its problems, quota sampling represents an important improvement over convenience sampling and should be considered by quantitative researchers whose resources prevent the use of a probability sampling plan.

Purposive Sampling

Purposive sampling or **judgmental sampling** is based on the belief that a researcher's knowledge about the population can be used to hand pick the cases to be included in the sample. The researcher might decide purposely to select the widest possible variety of respondents or might choose subjects who are judged to be typical of the population in question or particularly knowledgeable about the issues under study. Sampling in this subjective manner, however, provides no external, objective method for assessing the typicalness of the selected subjects. Nevertheless, this method can be used to advantage in certain situations. Newly developed instruments can be effectively pretested and evaluated with a purposive sample of diverse types of people. Purposive sampling is often used when the researcher wants a sample of experts, as in the case of a needs assessment using the key informant approach or in Delphi surveys.

Evaluation of Nonprobability Sampling

Although a nonprobability sample is often acceptable for pilot, exploratory, or in-depth qualitative research, for most quantitative studies, the use of nonprobability samples is problematic. Nonprobability samples are rarely representative of the researcher's target population. The difficulty stems from the fact that not every element in the population has a chance of being included in the sample. Therefore, it is likely that some segment of the population will be systematically underrepresented.

Why, then, are nonprobability samples used in most nursing studies? Clearly, the advantage of these sampling designs lies in their convenience and economy. Probability sampling, which is discussed in the next section, requires skill, resources, time, and opportunity. There is often no option but to use a nonprobability approach or to abandon the project altogether. Even hard-nosed research methodologists would hesitate to advocate a total abandonment of one's ideas in the absence of a random sample. The quantitative researcher using a nonprobability sample out of necessity must be cautious about the inferences and conclusions drawn from the data. With care in the selection of the sample, a conservative interpretation of the results, and replication of the study with new samples, researchers may find that nonprobability samples work reasonably well.

PROBABILITY SAMPLING

The hallmark of probability sampling is the random selection of elements from the population. Random selection should not be confused with random assignment, which was described in connection with experimental research in Chapter 8. Random assignment refers to the process of allocating subjects to different treatment conditions on a random basis. Random assignment has no bearing on how the subjects participating in an experiment are selected in the first place. **Random sampling** involves a selection process in which each element in the population has an equal, independent chance of being selected. The four most commonly used probability sampling methods are simple random, stratified random, cluster, and systematic sampling.

Simple Random Sampling

Simple random sampling is the most basic of the probability sampling designs. Because the more complex probability sampling designs incorporate the features of simple random sampling, the procedures involved are described here in some detail.

In simple random sampling, the researcher establishes what is known as a sampling frame. The term **sampling frame** is the technical name for the actual list of the sampling units or elements from which the sample will be chosen. If nursing students attending Wayne State University constituted the accessible population, then a roster of those students would be the sampling frame. If the sampling unit were 400-bed (or larger) general hospitals in the United States, then a list of all such hospitals would be the sampling frame. In actual practice, a population may be defined in terms of an existing sampling frame rather than starting with a population and then developing a list of elements. For example, if we wanted to use a telephone directory as a sampling frame, we would have to define the population as the residents of a certain community who are clients of the telephone company *and* who had a number listed at the time the directory was published. Because not all members of a community own a telephone and others fail to have their numbers listed, it would be inappropriate to consider a telephone directory to be the sampling frame for the entire community population.

Once a listing of the population elements has been developed or located, the elements must be numbered consecutively. A table of random numbers would then be used to draw a sample of the desired size. An example of a sampling frame with 50 individuals is presented in Table 12-4. Let us assume that a sample of 20 people is sufficient for our purposes. As in the case of random assignment, we would find a starting place in a table of random numbers by blindly placing our finger at some point on the page. To include all numbers between 1 and 50, two-digit combinations would be read. Suppose, for the sake of the example, that we began the random selection with the very first number in the random number table of Table 8–1 in Chapter 8, which is 46. The person corresponding to the number, D. Abraham, is the first subject selected to participate in the study. Number 05, C. Eldred, is the second selection, and number 23, R. Yun, is the third. This process would continue until the 20 subjects were chosen. The selected elements are circled in Table 12-4.

It should be clear that a sample selected randomly in this fashion is not subject to the biases of the researcher. There is no chance for the operation of personal preferences. Although there is no guarantee that a randomly drawn sample will be representative, random selection does ensure that differences in the attributes of the sample and the population are purely a function of chance. The probability of selecting a markedly deviant sample is low, and this probability decreases as the size of the sample increases.

Simple random sampling tends to be a laborious process. The development of the sampling frame, enumeration of all the elements, and selection of the sample elements are time-consuming chores, particularly if the population is large. Imagine enumerating all the telephone subscribers listed in the New York City telephone directory! If the elements can be arranged in computer-readable form, then the computer can be programmed to select the sample automatically. In actual practice, simple random sampling is not used frequently because it is a relatively inefficient procedure. Furthermore, it is rarely possible to get a com-

TABLE 12-4   Sampling Frame for Simple Random Sampling Example

(1.) N. Alexander	(26.) G. Berlin
2. H. Bos	27. G. Cave
3. R. Cytron	28. R. De los Santos
4. F. Doolittle	29. D. Edelstein
(5.) C. Eldred	(30.) D. Friedlander
(6.) R. Fellerath	(31.) J. Gueron
7. R. Granger	32. G. Hoerz
8. G. Hamilton	(33.) D. Jones-Brown
9. R. Ivry	(34.) J. Kemple
10. S. James	35. L. London
11. V. Knox	36. L. Miyazaki
12. S. Lynn	37. C. Nicholson
(13.) C. Michalopoulos	(38.) K. Ofosuhene
(14.) S. Nelson	39. K. Paget
15. J. O'Brien	40. G. Queto
16. M. Price	41. J. Riccio
(17.) J. Quint	42. M. Salmon
(18.) I. Robling	(43.) L. Traeger
19. B. Schall	44. E. Vallejo
20. K. Trister	(45.) J. Wallace
(21.) M. Valmont	(46.) D. Abraham
22. J. Walter	47. D. Butler
(23.) R. Yun	48. O. Cardenas
(24.) M. Zaslow	49. F. Derocher
25. M. Agudelo	(50.) J. Edison

plete listing of every element in the population, so other methods may be required.

Stratified Random Sampling

Stratified random sampling is a variant of simple random sampling in which the population is first divided into two or more strata or subgroups. As in the case of quota sampling, the aim of stratified sampling is to enhance representativeness. Stratified sampling designs subdivide the population into homogeneous subsets from which an appropriate number of elements can be selected at random.

The stratification may be based on a wide variety of attributes, such as age, gender, occupation, and so forth. The chosen variable should be one that will result in internally homogeneous strata on the attributes about which information is being sought. The diffi-

culty lies in the fact that the attributes of interest may not be readily discernible or available for stratification purposes. If one is working with a telephone directory, it would be risky to make decisions about a person's gender, and certainly age, ethnicity, or other personal information that is not listed could not be used as the stratifying variables. Patient listings, student rosters, or organizational directories might contain the information needed for a meaningful stratification. Quota sampling does not have the same problem because the researcher can ask the prospective subject questions that determine his or her eligibility for a particular stratum. In stratified sampling, however, a decision about a person's status in a stratum is made before a sample is randomly selected.

Various procedures for drawing a stratified sample have been used. The most common is to group together those elements that belong to a stratum and to select randomly the desired number of elements. The researcher either may take an equal number of elements from each stratum or may decide to select unequal numbers, for reasons discussed later in this section. To illustrate the procedure used in the simplest case, suppose that the list in Table 12-4 consisted of 25 males (numbers 1 through 25) and 25 females (numbers 26 through 50). Using gender as the stratifying variable, we could guarantee a sample of 10 males and 10 females by randomly sampling 10 numbers from the first half of the list and 10 from the second half. As it turns out, our simple random sampling did result in 10 elements being chosen from each half of the list, but this was purely by chance. It would not have been unusual to draw, say, 8 names from one half and 12 from the other. Stratified sampling can guarantee the appropriate representation of different segments of the population.

In many cases, the stratifying variables divide the population into unequal subpopulations. For example, if the person's race were used to stratify the population of U.S. citizens, the subpopulation of white people would be larger than that of African American and other nonwhite people. In such a situation, the researcher might decide to select subjects in proportion to the size of the stratum in the population. This procedure is referred to as **proportionate stratified sampling**. If the population was students in a school of nursing with 10% African American students, 5% Hispanic students, and 85% white students, then a proportionate stratified sample of 100 students, with racial/ethnic background as the stratifying variable, would consist of 10, 5, and 85 students from the respective subpopulations.

When the researcher is interested in understanding differences among the strata, proportionate sampling may result in an insufficient base for making comparisons. In the previous example, would the researcher be justified in coming to conclusions about the characteristics of Hispanic nursing students based on

only five cases? It would be extremely unwise to do so in most types of research. When random selection procedures are used, the probability of obtaining a representative sample increases as the sample size increases. For this reason, researchers often adopt a **disproportionate sampling design** whenever interstratum comparisons are sought between strata of greatly unequal membership size. In the example, the sampling proportions might be altered to select 20 African American students, 20 Hispanic students, and 60 white students. This design would ensure a more adequate representation of the two racial/ethnic minorities. When disproportionate sampling is used, however, it is necessary to make an adjustment to the data to arrive at the best estimate of overall population values. This adjustment process, known as **weighting**, is a simple mathematic computation that is described in detail in most texts on sampling.

Stratified random sampling offers the researcher the opportunity to sharpen the precision and representativeness of the final sample. When it is desirable to obtain reliable information about subpopulations whose memberships are relatively small, stratification provides a means of including a sufficient number of cases in the sample by oversampling for that stratum. Stratified sampling, however, may be impossible if information on the critical variables is unavailable. Furthermore, a stratified sample requires even more labor and effort than simple random sampling because the sample must be drawn from multiple enumerated listings.

Cluster Sampling

For many populations, it is simply impossible to obtain a listing of all the elements. For example, the population consisting of all full-time nursing students in the United States would be difficult to list and enumerate for the purpose of drawing a simple or stratified random sample. In addition, it would often be prohibitively expensive to sample nursing students in this way because the resulting sample would include no more than one or two students per institution. If personal interviews were involved, the interviewers would have to travel to individuals scattered throughout the country. Because of these considerations, large-scale studies almost never use simple or stratified random sampling. The most common procedure for large-scale surveys is cluster sampling.

In **cluster sampling**, there is a successive random sampling of units. The first unit to be sampled is large groupings, or clusters. In drawing a sample of nursing students, the researcher might first draw a random sample of nursing schools and then draw a sample of students from the selected schools. The usual procedure for selecting a general sample of citizens is to sample successively such administrative units as states, cities, districts, blocks, and then households. Because of the successive stages in cluster sampling, this approach is often referred to as **multistage sampling**.

The clusters can be selected either by simple or stratified methods. For instance, in selecting clusters of nursing schools, it may be advisable to stratify on program type. The final selection from within a cluster may also be performed by simple or stratified random sampling.

For a specified number of cases, cluster sampling tends to contain more sampling errors than simple or stratified random sampling. Despite these disadvantages, cluster sampling is considerably more economical and practical than other types of probability sampling, particularly when the population is large and widely dispersed.

Systematic Sampling

The final type of sampling design to be discussed can be classified as either a probability or nonprobability sampling approach, depending on the exact procedure used. **Systematic sampling** involves the selection of every *k*th case from some list or group, such as every 10th person on a patient list or every 100th person listed in a directory of American Nurses' Association members. Systematic sampling is sometimes used to sample every *k*th person entering a bookstore, or passing down the street, or leaving a hospital, and so forth. In such situations, unless the population is narrowly defined as consisting of all those people entering, passing by, or leaving, the sampling is nonprobability in nature.

Systematic sampling designs can be applied in such a way that an essentially random sample is drawn. If the researcher has a list, or sampling frame, the following procedure can be adopted. The desired sample size is established at some number (n). The size of the population must be known or estimated (N). By dividing N by n, the sampling interval width (k) is established. The **sampling interval** is the standard distance between the elements chosen for the sample. For instance, if we were seeking a sample of 200 from a population of 40,000, then our sampling interval would be as follows:

$$k = \frac{40{,}000}{200} = 200$$

In other words, every 200th element on the list would be sampled. The first element should be selected randomly, using a table of random numbers. Let us say that we randomly selected number 73 from a table. The people corresponding to numbers 73, 273, 473, 673, and so forth would be included in the sample.

In actual practice, systematic sampling conducted in this manner is essentially identical to simple random sampling. Problems would arise if the list were arranged in such a way that a certain type of element is listed at intervals coinciding with the sampling interval. For instance, if every 10th nurse listed in a nursing personnel roster were a head nurse and the sampling interval was 10, then head nurses would either always or never be included in the sample. Problems of this type are rare, fortunately. In most cases, systematic sampling is preferable to simple random sampling because the same results are obtained in a more convenient and efficient manner. Systematic sampling procedures can also be applied to lists that have been stratified.

Evaluation of Probability Sampling

Probability sampling is really the only viable method of obtaining representative samples in quantitative studies. If all the elements in the population have an equal probability of being selected, then the likelihood is high that the resulting sample will do a good job of representing the population. A further advantage is that probability sampling allows the researcher to estimate the magnitude of sampling error. **Sampling error** refers to differences between population values (such as the average age of the population) and sample values (such as the average age of the sample). It is a rare sample that is perfectly representative of a population and contains no sampling error on any of the attributes under investigation. Probability sampling does, however, permit estimates of the degree of expected error.*

The great drawbacks of probability sampling are its expense and inconvenience. Unless the population is narrowly defined, it is usually beyond the scope of most research projects to sample using a probability design. A researcher using nonprobability sampling might well be able to argue that the homogeneity of the attribute under consideration makes an elaborate sampling scheme unnecessary. This justification will probably be implausible, however, if psychological, social, or economic attributes are being studied.

In sum, probability sampling is the preferred and most respected method of obtaining

---

*Probability sampling is at the heart of most statistical testing. Strictly speaking, it is inappropriate to apply inferential statistics to data obtained from nonprobability samples, although most researchers ignore this issue in their treatment of data.

sample elements, but it may in some cases be impractical or unnecessary.

SAMPLE SIZE IN QUANTITATIVE STUDIES

A major concern to beginning researchers is the number of subjects needed in a sample. There are sophisticated methods for developing sample size estimates for quantitative studies, using a procedure known as **power analysis**, but some statistical knowledge is needed before this procedure can be explained. Below we offer guidelines to beginning researchers; the advanced student should review the discussion of power analysis in Chapter 19 or consult an advanced sampling or statistical textbook.

Although there are no simple formulas that can tell you how large a sample is needed in a given quantitative study, we can offer a simple piece of advice: You generally should use the largest sample possible. The larger the sample, the more representative of the population it is likely to be. Every time a researcher calculates a percentage or an average based on sample data, the purpose is to estimate a population value. Smaller samples tend to produce less accurate estimates than larger samples. In other words, the larger the sample, the smaller is the sampling error.

Let us illustrate this notion with a simple example of, say, monthly aspirin consumption in a nursing home facility, as shown in Table 12-5. The population consists of 15 residents whose aspirin consumption averages 16 aspirins per month. Eight simple random samples—two each with sample sizes of 2, 3, 5, and 10—have been drawn. Each sample average represents an estimate of the population average, which is 16. Under ordinary circumstances, of course, the population value would be unknown to us, and we would draw only one sample. With a sample size of two, our estimate might have been wrong by as many as

NUMBER IN GROUP	GROUP	VALUES (MONTHLY NUMBER OF ASPIRINS CONSUMED)	AVERAGE
15	Population	2, 4, 6, 8, 10, 12, 14, 16, 18, 20, 22, 24, 26, 28, 30	16.0
2	Sample 1A	6, 14	10.0
2	Sample 1B	20, 28	24.0
3	Sample 2A	16, 18, 8	14.0
3	Sample 2B	20, 14, 26	20.0
5	Sample 3A	26, 14, 18, 2, 28	17.6
5	Sample 3B	30, 2, 26, 10, 4	14.4
10	Sample 4A	22, 16, 24, 22, 2, 8, 14, 28, 20, 2	15.8
10	Sample 4B	14, 18, 12, 20, 6, 14, 28, 12, 24, 16	16.4

TABLE 12-5 Comparison of Population and Sample Values and Averages

eight aspirins (sample 1B), which is a 50% error. As the sample size increases, the averages get closer to the true population value, and the differences in the estimates between samples A and B get smaller as well. As the sample size increases, the probability of getting a markedly deviant sample diminishes. Large samples provide an opportunity to counterbalance atypical values. The safest procedure in most circumstances is to obtain data from as large a sample as is economically and practically feasible.

Large samples are no assurance of accuracy, however. When nonprobability sampling methods are used, even a large sample can harbor extensive bias. The famous example illustrating this point is the 1936 presidential poll conducted by the magazine *Literary Digest,* which predicted that Alfred M. Landon would defeat Franklin D. Roosevelt by a landslide. About 2.5 million individuals participated in this poll—a substantial sample. Biases resulted from the fact that the sample was drawn from telephone directories and automobile registrations during a depression year when only the well-to-do had a car or telephone. Thus, a large sample cannot correct for a faulty sampling design. In quantitative studies, the researcher should make decisions about the sample size and design based primarily on how representative of the population the sample is likely to be.

Because practical constraints such as time, availability of subjects, and resources often limit the number of subjects included in nursing studies, many are based on relatively small samples. In a survey of nursing studies published over four decades (the 1950s to the 1980s), Brown, Tanner, and Padrick (1984) found that the average sample size was under 100 subjects in all four decades, and similar results were reported in a more recent analysis (Moody, Wilson, Smyth, Schwartz, Tittle, & VanCott, 1988). In many cases, a small sample is problematic and can lead to misleading results. In some cases, however, a small sample size may be justifiable. Below we discuss some considerations that affect sample size decisions in quantitative studies.

Homogeneity of the Population

When the researcher has reason to believe that the population is relatively homogeneous with respect to the variables of interest, then a small sample may be adequate for research purposes. Let us demonstrate that this is so. The top half of Table 12-6 presents hypothetical population values for three different populations, with only 10 people in each population. These values could reflect, for example, scores on a measure of anxiety. In all the populations, the average anxiety score is 100. In population A, however,

TABLE 12-6	Three Populations of Different Homogeneity	
POPULATION	**POPULATION VALUES**	**POPULATION AVERAGE**
A	100 110 105 95 90 110 105 95 90 100	100
B	100 120 115 85 80 120 115 85 80 100	100
C	100 130 125 75 70 130 125 75 70 100	100
SAMPLE	**SAMPLE VALUES**	**SAMPLE AVERAGE**
A	110 90 95	98.33
B	120 80 85	95.00
C	130 70 75	91.67

the individuals have fairly similar anxiety scores: the scores range in value from a low of 90 to a high of 110. In population B, the scores are more variable, and in population C, the scores are more variable still, ranging from 70 to 130.

The second half of Table 12-6 presents three sample values from the three populations. In the most homogeneous population (A), the average anxiety score for the sample is 98.33, which is close to the population value of 100. As the population becomes less homogeneous with regard to anxiety scores, the average sample values reflect less accurately the population values. In other words, there is greater sampling error when the population is heterogeneous on the key variable. By increasing the sample size, the risk of sampling error would be reduced. For example, if sample C consisted of five values rather than three (say, all the even-numbered values), then the average would be closer to the population value (i.e., 102.0 rather than 91.67).

For clinical studies that deal with biophysiologic processes in which variation is limited, a small sample may adequately represent the population. For most nursing studies, however, it is probably safer to assume a fair degree of heterogeneity, unless there is evidence from prior research or from experience to the contrary.

Effect Size

Power analysis builds on the concept of effect size, a term that we mentioned briefly in connection with meta-analyses. **Effect size** is concerned with the strength of the relationships among research variables. If the researcher has reason to believe that the independent and dependent variables are strongly interrelated, then a relatively small sample is generally adequate to demonstrate the relationship statistically. For example, if a researcher were testing a powerful new drug to treat AIDS, it might be possible to demonstrate the drug's effectiveness with a small number of subjects. Typically, however, interventions have modest effects, and variables are usually only moderately correlated with one another. When the researcher has no a priori reason for believing that relationships will be strong (i.e., when the effect size is expected to be modest), then small samples are risky.

Attrition

In many longitudinal studies, the number of subjects recruited to participate in a study declines over time. This is most likely to occur if the time lag between data collection points is great; if the population is a mobile or a hard-to-locate one; or if the population is a high-risk, vulnerable one at risk of death or disability. If resources are devoted to tracing subjects in longitudinal studies, or if the researcher has an ongoing relationship with subjects (as might be true in many clinical studies), then the rate of attrition might be low. It is the rare longitudinal study, however, that maintains the entire research sample. Therefore, in estimating sample size needs, the researcher should factor in anticipated loss of subjects from the sample.

Attrition problems are not restricted to longitudinal studies. People who initially agree to cooperate in a study may be subsequently unable or unwilling to participate for a number of reasons, such as death, deteriorating health, early discharge, discontinued need for a particular intervention, or simply a change of heart. Researchers should attempt to anticipate a certain amount of subject loss and to recruit subjects accordingly.

Other Considerations

Several other factors should be considered in deciding how large the research sample should be. These include the following:

Number of variables. In general, the greater the number of independent and extraneous variables, the larger the sample should be. If the research design can be laid out such that the number of "cells" can be determined, then the study should aim to have at least 20 to 30 subjects for each cell of the design. For example, a study of the effects of gender (male/female); race/ethnicity (white/African American/Hispanic); and marital status (married/not married)—2 × 3 × 2—on success in an alcohol treatment program should ideally have at least 140 to 210 subjects. This requirement enhances the likelihood of obtaining a stable estimate for each cell but does not ensure that relationships between variables will be de-

tected. A power analysis may indicate that even more subjects should be included.

Subgroup analyses. A related point is that a researcher is sometimes interested in testing hypotheses not only for an entire population of subjects but also for specific subgroups. For example, a researcher might be interested in determining whether a structured exercise program is effective in improving infants' motor skills. After the researcher has tested this general hypothesis with a sample of infants, it might be useful to test whether the intervention is more effective for certain types of infants than for others (e.g., low-birthweight and normal-birthweight infants). When a sample is divided to test for effects in specific subgroups, the sample must be large enough to support these divisions of the sample.

Sensitivity of the measures. Different measures vary in their ability to measure precisely the concepts under study. Biophysiologic measures are generally very sensitive—they measure phenomena accurately, and they can often make fine discriminations in values. Measures that are psychological in nature often contain a fair amount of error and are typically not precise. In general, when the measuring tool is imprecise and susceptible to errors, larger samples are needed to test hypotheses adequately.

IMPLEMENTING A SAMPLING PLAN IN QUANTITATIVE STUDIES

Once you have made decisions about the sampling design and the sample size, the overall sampling plan must be implemented. This section provides some practical information about such implementation.

Steps in Sampling in Quantitative Studies

The steps to be undertaken in drawing a sample vary somewhat from one sampling design to the next. However, a general outline of procedures for most quantitative studies can be described.

1. *Identify the target population.* The first phase of the sampling process usually involves the general identification of the target population. This is the group to which you want to be able to generalize your results. For example, the target population could consist of all RNs currently unemployed in the United States, or all diabetic people, or all women who have had a miscarriage.

2. *Identify the accessible population.* Unless you have extensive resources at your disposal, you are unlikely to have access to the entire target population. Therefore, you should identify the portion of the target population that is accessible to you. In essence, an accessible population is a sample from the larger target population. An accessible population might consist of unemployed RNs in metropolitan Atlanta, or all diabetic patients under the care of a specific health maintenance organization, or women who had a miscarriage in a particular hospital in the past year. Sometimes, researchers *begin* by defining an accessible population and then decide how best to define the target population.

3. *Specify the eligibility criteria.* The criteria for eligibility in the sample should then be spelled out, preferably in writing. The criteria should be as specific as possible with respect to characteristics that might exclude potential subjects (e.g., extremes of poor health, inability to read English, and so on). The criteria might lead you to redefine your target and accessible populations.

4. *Specify the sampling plan.* Once the accessible population has been identified, you must decide the method of drawing the sample and how large it will be. The sample size specification should consider the various aspects of the study that were discussed in the previous section. If you can perform a power analysis to determine the desired number of subjects, it is highly recommended that you do so. Similarly, if probability sampling is an option for selecting a sample, that option should generally be exercised. The typical nurse researcher is not in a position to do either. In such a situation, we recommend using as large a sample as possible and taking steps to build representativeness into the design (e.g., by using quota sampling).

5. *Recruit the sample.* Once the sampling design has been specified, the next step is to recruit prospective study participants according to the designated plan (after any needed institutional permissions have been obtained) and ask for their cooperation. Issues relating to recruiting subjects is discussed next.

Sample Recruitment

Recruiting subjects for participation in a study involves two major tasks: identifying eligible candidates and persuading them to participate. Researchers may in some cases need to spend time early in the project deciding the best sources for recruiting potential participants. The researcher must ask such questions as, Where do people with the characteristics I want live or obtain care in large numbers? Will I have direct access to subjects, or will I need administrative approval? Will there be sufficiently large numbers in one location, or will multiple referral sources be necessary? During the recruitment phase, it may be necessary to develop a **screening instrument**, which is a brief interview or form that allows the researcher to determine whether a prospective subject meets all the eligibility criteria for the study.

The next task involves actually gaining the cooperation of people who have been deemed eligible for the study. It is critical to have an effective recruitment strategy. Some people, for various reasons, do not ever want to participate in a research project. Most people, however, given the right circumstances, will agree to cooperate. Researchers should ask themselves, What will make this research experience enjoyable, worthwhile, convenient, pleasant, and nonthreatening for the subjects? Factors over which researchers have control that can influence the rate of cooperation include the following:

- *Method of recruitment.* Face-to-face recruitment is almost always preferable to solicitation by a telephone call or a letter.
- *Pleasantness of the recruiters.* A key to successful recruitment is using recruiters who are pleasant, courteous, respectful, and nonthreatening. In some cases, cooperation is enhanced if the characteristics of the recruiters are similar to those of prospective subjects—particularly with regard to gender, race, and ethnicity.
- *Persistence.* Although high-pressure tactics are never acceptable, persistence may sometimes be needed. When prospective subjects are first approached, their initial reaction may be to decline participation, without giving the matter much thought. If a person hesitates or gives an equivocal answer at the first attempt, recruiters should ask if they could come back at a later time.
- *Payment of an incentive.* Gifts and, especially, monetary incentives have been found to increase the participation rate.
- *Explanation of research benefits.* The benefits of participating to the individual and to society should be carefully explained, without exaggeration or misleading information.

- *Offers of a research summary.* Sometimes, it is useful to offer people tangible evidence of their contribution or to assuage their curiosity about the study. Thus, some researchers offer to send participants a brief summary of the results of the study.
- *Making participation convenient.* Every effort should be made to collect data at a time and location that is convenient for the subjects. In some cases, this may mean making arrangements for transportation or for the care of young children.
- *Endorsements.* Prospective participants may be suspicious about a study, about what the "real" agenda is, or about who will have access to information. In some cases, it is extremely valuable to have the study endorsed or acknowledged by a person, group, or organization that has the subjects' confidence and to communicate this to prospective subjects. Endorsements might come from the institution serving as the research setting, from a funding agency, or from a respected community group or person, such as a church leader. Press releases in advance of recruitment are sometimes advantageous.
- *Assurances of research integrity.* Prospective subjects should be told who will see the data, what use will be made of the data, how confidentiality will be maintained, and so on.

Generalizing From Samples

Ideally, the sample is representative of the accessible population, and the accessible population is representative of the target population. By using an appropriate sample size and sampling plan, the researcher can be reasonably confident that the first part of this ideal has been realized. A greater risk is involved in assuming that the second part of the ideal is also realized. Are the unemployed nurses in Atlanta representative of all unemployed nurses in the United States? One can never be sure. The researcher must exercise judgment in assessing the degree of similarity.

The best advice is to be realistic and somewhat conservative. The researcher should interpret the findings and come to conclusions after asking, Is it reasonable to assume that the accessible population is representative of the target population? In what ways might they be expected to differ? How would such differences affect the conclusions? If the researcher decides that the differences in the two populations are too great, it would be prudent to identify a more restricted target population to which the findings could be meaningfully generalized.

Tips for Sampling in Quantitative Studies

Many quantitative nursing studies use less-than-optimal sampling plans that run the risk of yielding erroneous or inconclusive results. We offer below some suggestions on how to strengthen the sampling design in quantitative studies:

- If, in designing a study, you decide that there is no alternative to convenience sampling, you should take several steps to enhance the likelihood of achieving a representative sample. First, identify important extraneous variables. That is, identify the factors that influence the heterogeneity of the population with respect to the dependent variable. For example, in a study of the relationship between stress and health, a person's socioeconomic status is likely to be an important extraneous variable because poor people are likely to be less healthy *and* more stressed than more affluent ones. Then, decide how to account for this source of variation in the sampling design. One solution is to define the population such that variation resulting from extraneous variables is minimized, as discussed in Chapter 9. In the stress and health example, we might, for

instance, restrict the population to middle-class people. Alternatively, we could select the sample from communities known to differ in socioeconomic characteristics so that our sample would be known to reflect the experiences of both lower- and middle-class subjects. This approaches using a quota sampling method. In other words, if the population is known to be heterogeneous, you should take steps to either make it more homogeneous or to capture the full variation in the sample.

- One fairly simple way to increase the generalizability of a study is to select study participants from two or more sites, such as from different hospitals, nursing homes, communities, and so on. Ideally, the two different sites would be sufficiently divergent that broader representation of the population would be obtained (e.g., in a study of compliance with a medication regimen, using patients from an inner-city health clinic and a suburban health maintenance organization). The major issue in using multiple sites is taking steps to ensure that constancy of conditions is maintained across sites insofar as possible.

- Regardless of the type of sampling plan used, it is important to understand and document who the participants are so that biases can be identified and taken into consideration in interpreting the results and developing recommendations. It is particularly helpful to compare sample characteristics with population characteristics whenever possible. Published information about the characteristics of many groups of interest to nurses is usually available to help provide an important context for evaluating sampling bias. For example, if you are studying teenage mothers, obtain information in the library about the characteristics of the population of teenage mothers—for example, their marital status, family income, ethnic distribution, and so on. This information can then be compared with sample characteristics, and differences can be taken into account in interpreting the findings.

- As you recruit your sample, it is wise to document thoroughly. The more information you have about who the sample is and who it is not, the better able you will be to identify potential biases. Biases can occur even in probability sampling because the *selection* of elements that are representative of the population does not guarantee the participation of all those elements, and refusals to participate in a study are rarely random. Thus, you should calculate a **response rate** (the number of people participating in the study relative to the number of people sampled) and document the **nonresponse bias**, that is, differences between the characteristics of participants and those of people who refused to participate in the study. Also, those who remain in a study should be compared with those who drop out to document any attrition biases. It may also be useful to document the reasons people give for not cooperating (or not continuing to cooperate) in a study.

- Subject recruitment often proceeds at a slower pace than researchers anticipate, in part because not everybody who is approached agrees to cooperate. Once you have determined your sample size needs, it is a good idea to develop contingency plans for recruiting more subjects, should the initial plan prove overly optimistic. For example, a contingency plan might involve relaxation of some of the eligibility criteria, the identification of another institution through which participants could be recruited, the payment of a stipend to make participation in the study more attractive, or the lengthening of the time for recruitment into the study. When contingency plans are developed at the outset, it reduces the likelihood that you will have to settle for a less-than-desirable sample size.

SAMPLING IN QUALITATIVE RESEARCH

Qualitative studies almost always use small, nonrandom samples. This does not mean that qualitative researchers are unconcerned with the quality of their samples, but rather that they use different criteria for selecting study participants. This section examines considerations that apply to sampling in qualitative studies.

The Logic of Qualitative Sampling

Quantitative research is concerned with measuring attributes and relationships in a population, and therefore a representative sample is needed to ensure that the measurements accurately reflect and can be generalized to the population. The aim of most qualitative studies is to discover *meaning* and to uncover multiple realities, and so generalizability is not a guiding criterion.

The qualitative researcher begins a study with the following types of sampling question in mind: Who would be an information-rich data source for my study? Who should I talk to, or what should I observe first so as to maximize my understanding of the phenomenon? Clearly, with these types of question, a critical first step in qualitative sampling is the selection of a setting with high potential for information richness.

As the study progresses, new sampling questions emerge, such as the following: Who can I talk to or observe that would confirm my understandings? challenge or modify my understandings? enrich my understandings? Thus, as with the overall design in qualitative studies, sampling design is an emergent design that capitalizes on early learning to guide subsequent direction.

Types of Qualitative Sampling

Qualitative researchers usually eschew probability samples. A random sample is not the best method of selecting people who will make good informants—that is, people who are knowledgeable, articulate, reflective, and willing to talk at length with the researcher. Various nonprobability sampling designs have been used by qualitative researchers.

CONVENIENCE SAMPLING

Qualitative researchers sometimes use or begin with a convenience sample, which is sometimes referred to in qualitative studies as a **volunteer sample.** Volunteer samples are especially likely to be used if the researcher needs to have potential participants come forward and identify themselves. For example, if we wanted to study the experiences of people with frequent nightmares, we might have difficulty readily identifying a sufficient number of potential participants. In such a situation, we might recruit sample members by placing a notice on a bulletin board or in a newspaper, requesting people with frequent nightmares to contact us. In this situation, we would be less interested in obtaining a representative sample of *people* with nightmares than in obtaining a broad and diverse group that represents various experiences with nightmares.

Sampling by convenience may be easy and efficient, but it is not a preferred sampling approach, even in qualitative studies. Particularly because qualitative researchers use rather small samples, it does make a difference how the sample members are chosen. The key in qualitative studies is to extract the greatest possible information from the few cases in the sample, and a convenience sample may not provide the most information-rich sources. However, convenience sample may be an economical and easy way to *begin* the sampling process, relying on other methods as data are collected.

SNOWBALL SAMPLING

Qualitative researchers also use snowball sampling, asking early informants to make refer-

rals to other study participants. This method of sampling is also sometimes referred to as **nominated sampling** (because the method relies on the nominations of others already in the sample), **network sampling,** or **chain sampling.** The researcher may use this method to gain access to people who are difficult to identify. Snowball sampling has distinct advantages over convenience sampling. The first is that it may be more cost-efficient and practical. The researcher may need to spend less time "screening" people to determine if they are appropriate for the study, for example. Furthermore, with an introduction from the referring person, the researcher may have an easier time establishing a trusting relationship with the new participants. Finally, the researcher can more readily specify the characteristics that he or she wants the new participants to have. For example, in our study of people with nightmares, we could ask early respondents if they knew anyone else who had the same problem *and* who was articulate and informative. We could also ask for referrals to people who would add other dimensions to the sample, such as people who vary in age, race, socioeconomic status, and so on.

A weakness of this approach is that the eventual sample might be restricted to a rather small network of acquaintances. Moreover, the quality of the referrals may be affected by whether the referring sample member trusted the researcher and truly wanted to cooperate.

THEORETICAL SAMPLING

Whereas qualitative sampling may begin with volunteer informants and may be supplemented with new participants through snowballing, most qualitative studies eventually evolve to a purposive sampling strategy. In qualitative research, purposive sampling is often referred to as **theoretical sampling** or **purposeful sampling.** Regardless of how initial participants are selected, the researcher usually strives to purposefully select sample members based on the information needs emerging from the early findings. Who to sample next depends on who has been sampled already and what information has been obtained.

Within theoretical sampling, several strategies have been identified (Patton, 1990), only some of which are mentioned here:

- *Maximum variation sampling* involves purposefully selecting cases with a wide range of variation on dimensions of interest. By selecting participants who represent diverse views and perspectives, the researcher is inviting challenges to his or her preconceived notions about the phenomenon of interest. Maximum variation sampling might involve ensuring that people with diverse backgrounds are represented in the sample (e.g., ensuring that there are men and women, poor and affluent people, and so on.) It might also involve deliberate attempts to include people with different viewpoints about the phenomenon under study. For example, the researcher might use snowballing to ask early participants for referrals to people who hold a very different point of view.
- *Homogeneous sampling* deliberately reduces variation and permits a more focused inquiry. Researchers may use this approach if they wish to understand a particular group of people especially well. One advantage of homogenous sampling is that it opens up the possibility of conducting group interviewing with groups of similar individuals.
- *Extreme (deviant) case sampling* provides opportunities for learning from the most unusual and extreme informants (e.g., outstanding successes and notable failures). The assumption underlying this sampling approach is that the extreme cases are rich in information because they are special in some way. In some cases, more can be learned by intensively studying extreme cases, but extreme cases can also distort understanding of a phenomenon.

- *Intensity sampling* is similar to extreme case sampling, but with less emphasis on the extremes. Intensity samples involve information-rich cases that manifest the phenomenon of interest intensely, but not as extreme or potentially distorting manifestations. Thus, the goal in intensity sampling is to select excellent and rich cases that offer strong examples of the phenomenon.
- *Typical case sampling* involves the selection of participants who will illustrate or highlight what is typical or average. The information resulting from such an approach can be used to create a qualitative profile that can be very helpful in illustrating typical manifestations of the phenomenon being studied.
- *Critical case sampling* selects cases that are particularly important regarding the phenomenon of interest. With this approach, the researcher looks for the particularly good story that illuminates critical aspects of the phenomenon.
- *Theory-based sampling* involves the selection of people or incidents on the basis of their potential representation of important theoretical constructs. Theory-based sampling is a very focused approach that is usually based on an a priori theory that is being examined qualitatively.
- *Sampling confirming and disconfirming cases* is an approach that is often used toward the end of data collection in a qualitative study. As the researcher begins to see trends and patterns in the data, there is a need to check the emerging conceptualizations. **Confirming cases** are additional cases that fit the researcher's conceptualizations and offer enhanced credibility. **Disconfirming cases** are examples that do not fit and serve to challenge the researcher's interpretations. These "negative" cases may offer new insights about how the original conceptualization needs to be revised or expanded.

Maximum variation sampling is often the sampling mode of choice in qualitative research because it is useful in documenting the scope of a phenomenon and in identifying important patterns that cut across variations. Other strategies, however, can also be used advantageously, depending on the nature of the research question. It is important to note that almost all of these sampling strategies require that the researcher have a solid base of knowledge about the setting in which the study is taking place. For example, to choose extreme cases, typical cases, or critical cases, the researcher must have information about the range of variation of the phenomenon and how it manifests itself. Key informants are often crucial for implementing these sampling strategies.

Sample Size in Qualitative Research

There are no firmly established criteria or rules for sample size in qualitative research. Sample size is largely a function of the purpose of the inquiry, the quality of the informants, and the type of sampling strategy used. For example, a larger sample is likely to be needed with maximum variation sampling than with typical case sampling. Patton (1990) argues that theoretical samples "be judged on the basis of the purpose and rationale of each study and the sampling strategy used to achieve the study's purpose. The sample, like all other aspects of qualitative inquiry, must be judged in context. . ." (p. 185).

In qualitative research, sample size should be determined on the basis of informational needs. Hence, a guiding principle in sampling is **data saturation**—that is, sampling to the point at which no new information is obtained and redundancy is achieved. Redundancy can typically be achieved with a fairly small number of cases, if the information from each is of sufficient depth. With a fairly homogeneous sample, fewer than 10 cases may suffice. However, when maximum variation is desired or when the researcher is interested in seeking potentially disconfirming evidence, a larger sample is usually required.

In general, phenomenologic studies are based on samples of 10 or fewer study participants. Grounded theory or ethnographic studies are more likely to involve samples of 20 to 40 people.

The Sampling Process in Qualitative Research

Like other aspects of qualitative research, sampling decisions typically emerge in the field on the basis of what has already been learned. The key characteristic of qualitative sampling is that it is responsive to context, previously collected data, and ongoing interpretations. The sampling process might evolve as follows:

1. The researcher begins with a general notion of where and with whom to start. The first few cases may be solicited on the basis of convenience, through snowballing procedures, or by both methods.
2. The sample is selected serially rather than up-front, as is often the case in a quantitative study. That is, successive sample members are chosen based on who has already been chosen and what information they provided.
3. Informants are often used to facilitate the selection of appropriate and information-rich cases for certain types of sampling approaches. Early study participants may sometimes serve as such informants.
4. The sample is adjusted in an ongoing fashion. Emerging conceptualizations help to focus the sampling process.
5. Sampling continues until saturation is achieved.
6. Final sampling includes a search for confirming and disconfirming cases.

Sampling in qualitative studies is thus guided by information goals that help the researcher to formulate purposeful strategies while in the field. Unlike quantitative research, however, there are few methodologic rules.

In a qualitative study, the sampling plan is evaluated in terms of adequacy and appropriateness (Morse, 1991). Adequacy refers to the sufficiency and quality of the data the sample yields. An adequate sample provides the researcher with data without any "thin" spots. When the researcher has truly obtained saturation with a sample, informational adequacy has been achieved, and the resulting description or theory is richly textured and complete. Appropriateness concerns the methods used to select the sample. An appropriate sample is one resulting from the identification and use of participants who can best supply information according to the conceptual requirements of the study. For example, a sampling plan that does not include disconfirming cases may not meet the information needs of the research.

◢ RESEARCH EXAMPLES

Table 12-7 presents some examples of quantitative nursing studies with various sampling designs, and Table 12-8 has examples of sampling approaches used in qualitative studies. Below, we describe at greater length the sampling plans of two nursing studies, one quantitative and the other qualitative.

Research Example From a Quantitative Study

Ferrans and Powers (1992) conducted a methodologic study to appraise a data collection instrument known as the Quality of Life Index (QLI), which measures people's satisfaction with various domains of life. The study involved administering the QLI to a sample of subjects and analyzing the results to determine if the QLI is a good measure of a

person's overall quality of life so that the instrument could be used by other researchers interested in the quality of life construct.

The selected sample consisted of 800 subjects randomly selected from an accessible population of nearly 3000 adult, in-unit hemodialysis patients. The population represented all in-unit hemodialysis patients from 93% of the counties in Illinois, excluding patients undergoing treatment in Veterans Administration hospitals.

Of the 800 sampled patients, 36 had died or had undergone kidney transplantation. Of the 764 remaining subjects, 57% (434) returned a questionnaire. Eighty-five subjects were dropped from the study because they left too many questions blank. The final sample consisted of 349 subjects, which represented a 46% response rate (i.e., 349/764).

The representativeness of the research sample was evaluated by comparing the sample and the population in terms of a number of characteristics about which information was available: gender, number of months on dialysis, presence of diabetes mellitus, primary cause of renal failure, age, and race. The sample and population were comparable with respect to the first four characteristics. However, the sample had a higher proportion of white patients and older patients than the population, although the differences were relatively small. Ferrans and Powers concluded that the sample was adequately representative of the population for the purposes of their study.

Research Example From a Qualitative Study

Quinn (1993) conducted an in-depth study to examine how nurses explain their use of physical restraints with elderly patients and the extent to which the nurses perceive the restraint decision as a moral problem. A sample of nurses was recruited from the medical-surgical unit of a hospital. Nurses were eligible to participate in Quinn's study if they were women, were direct caregivers on the medical-

TABLE 12-7 Examples of Sampling Designs Used in Quantitative Nursing Studies	
RESEARCH QUESTION	SAMPLE DESCRIPTION
Design: Convenience (Nonprobability)	
Does breastfeeding incidence differ among mothers with a usual versus shortened length of hospital stay? (Quinn, Koepsell, & Haller, 1997)	101 primiparous breastfeeding women chosen from an obstetric unit log
Design: Quota (Nonprobability)	
To what extent can nursing home staff members accurately screen residents for competence? (Williams & Engle, 1995)	100 nursing home residents, 25 in each of four types of nursing home (for-profit homes, not-for-profit homes, home for veterans, home for indigent county residents)
Design: Simple Random (Probability)	
What are the values influencing neonatal nurses' perceptions and choice of behavior in a clinical situation? (Raines, 1994)	331 neonatal nurses randomly sampled from members of the National Association of Neonatal Nurses
Design: Stratified Random (Probability)	
What are the factors contributing to job satisfaction and organizational commitment among doctorally prepared nurses? (Gurney, Mueller, & Price, 1997)	National sample of doctorally prepared nurses drawn from membership list of Sigma Theta Tau, stratified by academic versus health service work setting (931 nurses)
Design: Multistage (Probability)	
What are the work situation characteristics, levels of satisfaction, and individual characteristics of intensive care unit (ICU) and non-ICU nurses? (Boumans & Landeweerd, 1994)	Nurses in randomly selected ICU and non-ICU units from 16 randomly selected hospitals in the Netherlands
Design: Systematic (Probability)	
What is the extent to which nurses in a wide variety of practice settings discuss sexual concerns with their patients? (Matocha & Waterhouse, 1993)	Every 17th nurse listed by a state Board of Nursing in a south Atlantic state (500 nurses)

TABLE 12-8　Examples of Sampling Designs Used in Qualitative Nursing Studies

RESEARCH QUESTION	SAMPLE DESCRIPTION
Design: Maximum Variation Sampling	
What are the perceptions of the process of nurse–physician collaboration among intensive care unit nurses and medical resident physicians? (Baggs & Schmitt, 1997)	10 nurses varying in age, gender, education, certification in critical care, and administrative role; 10 physicians varying in gender and year of residency
Design: Snowball, Quota, and Purposive	
What are the weight management methods used by African American and Euro-American women? (Tyler, Allan, & Alcozer, 1977)	40 African American and 40 Euro-American women; half of each group were of higher social status, the other half were of lower social status; deliberate variation on other characteristics
Design: Theoretical	
What are hospitalized young children's perceptions of acute pain? (Woodgate & Kristjanson, 1996)	11 hospitalized children aged 2 to 7 years old
Design: Convenience	
What is the meaning of tuberculosis infection among Latino immigrants? (Ailinger & Dear, 1977)	65 Latino immigrant clients referred from health clinics

surgical unit, and had cared for a restrained elderly patient (65 years of age or older) within the previous 48 hours.

After the first few interviews were completed, theoretical sampling was used to guide the recruitment of subsequent respondents. For example, analysis of the early interviews revealed that nurses made a distinction between initiating physical restraint and continuing restraint that had been initiated by a previous caregiver. Thus, the researcher took care to include respondents with sufficient experience with both types of restraint. As another example, it was noted early in the study that respondents identified time of day as a factor in the use of restraint. Thereafter, Quinn made sure her sample included nurses who cared for restrained patients during all three tours of duty. The final sample consisted of 20 nurses ranging in age from 21 to 58 years, representing a wide range of nursing experience and educational preparation.

SUMMARY

Sampling is the process of selecting a portion of the population to represent the entire population. Both qualitative and quantitative researchers use samples, but their approaches to sampling differ markedly.

Quantitative researchers use a sample to generalize about a **population**, which is the entire aggregate of cases that meet a designated set of criteria. In a sampling context, an **element** is the most basic unit about which information is collected. An element can be sampled from the population if it meets the researcher's **eligibility criteria**. Quantitative researchers usually sample from an **accessible population** rather than from an entire **target population**. The overriding consideration in assessing the adequacy of a sample in a quantitative study is the degree to which it is **representative** of the population and avoids bias. **Sampling bias** refers to the systematic overrepresentation or underrepresentation of some segment of the population.

Sampling designs for quantitative research vary in their ability to reflect adequately the population from which the sample was drawn. In **nonprobability sampling**, elements are selected by nonrandom methods. Convenience, quota, and purposive sampling are the principal nonprobability methods. **Convenience sampling** (sometimes referred to as **accidental sampling**) consists of using the most readily available or most convenient group of people for the sample. **Snowball sampling** is a type of convenience sampling in which referrals for potential participants are made by those already in the sample. **Quota sampling** divides the population into homogeneous **strata** or subgroups to ensure representation of various subgroups in the sample. Within each stratum, the researcher selects participants by convenience sampling. In **purposive** (or **judgmental**) **sampling**, participants are handpicked to be included in the sample based on the researcher's knowledge about the population. Nonprobability sampling designs are convenient and economical; a major disadvantage is their potential for biases.

Probability sampling designs involve the random selection of elements from the population. **Simple random sampling** involves the selection on a random basis of elements from a **sampling frame** that enumerates all the elements. **Stratified random sampling** divides the population into homogeneous subgroups from which elements are selected at random. **Cluster sampling** or (**multistage sampling**) involves the successive selection of random samples from larger to smaller units by either simple random or stratified random methods. **Systematic sampling** is the selection of every *k*th case from some list or group. By dividing the population size by the desired sample size, the researcher is able to establish the **sampling interval**, which is the standard distance between the elements chosen for the systematic sample. Probability sampling designs are the preferred type of design for quantitative studies because they tend to result in more representative samples and because they permit the researcher to estimate the magnitude of sampling error. Probability samples, however, are time-consuming, expensive, inconvenient, and, in some cases, impossible to obtain.

There is no simple equation that can be used to determine how large a sample is needed for a particular quantitative study, but advanced researchers use a procedure known as **power analysis** to estimate **sample size** requirements. Large samples are usually preferable to small ones because, in general, the larger the sample, the more representative of the population it is likely to be. Even a large sample, however, does not guarantee representativeness.

In a qualitative study, sampling design is an emergent one that capitalizes on early learning to guide subsequent direction. Qualitative researchers use the theoretical demands of the study as a framework for selecting articulate and reflective informants with certain types of experience. Qualitative researchers thus most often use purposive sampling—or **theoretical sampling** as it is often called—to guide them in using data sources that maximize the richness of the information obtained.

Various strategies can be used to sample purposively. Among the sampling approaches used by qualitative researchers are **maximum variation sampling** (purposely selecting cases with a wide range of variation); **homogeneous sampling** (deliberately reducing variation); **extreme case sampling** (selecting the most unusual or extreme cases); **intensity sampling** (selecting cases that are intense but not extreme); **typical case sampling** (selecting cases that illustrate what is typical); **critical case sampling** (selecting cases that are especially important or illustrative); **theory-based sampling** (selecting cases on the basis of their representation of important constructs); and **sampling confirming and disconfirming cases** (selecting cases that enrich and challenge the researchers' conceptualizations).

Samples in qualitative studies are typically small. The size of the sample is typically based on information needs. A guiding principle is **data saturation**, which involves sampling to the point at which no new information is obtained and redundancy is achieved. The criteria for evaluating qualitative sampling plans are informational adequacy and appropriateness.

STUDY ACTIVITIES

Chapter 12 of the *Study Guide to Accompany Nursing Research: Principles and Methods, 6th ed.*, offers various exercises and study suggestions for reinforcing the concepts presented in this chapter. Additionally, the following study questions can be addressed:

1. Draw a simple random sample of 15 people from the sampling frame of Table 12-4, using the table of random numbers that appears in Table 8–1 in Chapter 8. Begin your selection by blindly placing your finger at some point on the table.

2. Suppose you have decided to use a systematic sampling design for a research project. The known population size is 5000, and the sample size desired is 250. What is the sampling interval? If the first element selected is 23, what would be the second, third, and fourth elements selected?

3. Suppose a researcher is interested in studying the attitude of clinical specialists toward autonomy in the work situation. Suggest a possible target and accessible population. What strata might be identified by the researcher if quota sampling were used?

4. What type of sampling design was used to obtain the following samples?
   a. 25 experts in critical care nursing
   b. 60 couples attending a particular prenatal class
   c. 100 nurses from a list of nurses registered in the state of Pennsylvania, using a table of random numbers
   d. 20 adult patients randomly selected from a random selection of 10 hospitals located in one state
   e. Every fifth article published in *Nursing Research* during the 1980s, beginning with the first article.

5. Suppose you wanted to study the experiences of nursing students during their first clinical assignment. Describe what you would need to do to select a sample using maximum variation sampling, critical case sampling, typical case sampling, and homogenous sampling.

SUGGESTED READINGS

Methodologic References

Babbie, E. (1990). *Survey research methods.* (2nd ed.). Belmont, CA: Wadsworth.

Brown, J. S., Tanner, C. A., & Padrick, K. P. (1984). Nursing's search for scientific knowledge. *Nursing Research, 33,* 26–32.

Cochran, W. G. (1977). *Sampling techniques* (3rd ed.). New York: John Wiley and Sons.

Cohen, J. (1988). *Statistical power analysis for the behavioral sciences* (2nd ed.). Mahwah, NJ: L. Erlbaum.

Diekmann, J. M., & Smith, J. M. (1989). Strategies for accessment and recruitment of subjects for nursing research. *Western Journal of Nursing Research, 11,* 418–430.

Kish, L. (1965). *Survey sampling.* New York: John Wiley and Sons.

Levey, P. S., & Lemeshow, S. (1980). *Sampling for health professionals.* New York: Lifetime Learning.

Moody, L. E., Wilson, M. E., Smyth, K., Schwartz, R., Tittle, M., & VanCott, M. L. (1988). Analysis of a decade of nursing practice research: 1977–1986. *Nursing Research, 37,* 374–379.

Morse, J. M. (1991). Strategies for sampling. In J. M. Morse (Ed.), *Qualitative nursing research: A contemporary dialogue.* Newbury Park, CA: Sage.

Patton, M. Q. (1990). *Qualitative evaluation and research methods* (2nd ed.). Newbury Park, CA: Sage.

Polit, D. F., & Sherman, R. (1990). Statistical power analysis in nursing research. *Nursing Research, 39,* 365–369.

Sandelowski, M. (1995). Sample size in qualitative research. *Research in Nursing & Health, 18,* 179–183.

Sudman, S. (1976). *Applied sampling.* New York: Academic Press.

Trinkoff, A. M., & Storr, C. L. (1997). Incorporating auxiliary variables into probability sampling designs. *Nursing Research, 46,* 182–185.

Williams, B. (1978). *A sampler on sampling.* New York: John Wiley and Sons.

Substantive References

Ailinger, R. L., & Dear, M. R. (1997) Latino immigrants' explanatory models of tuberculosis infection. *Qualitative Health Research, 7,* 521–531.

Baggs, J. G., & Schmitt, M. H. (1997). Nurses' and resident physicians' perceptions of the process of collaboration in an MICU. *Research in Nursing & Health, 20,* 71–80.

Boumans, N. P. G., & Landeweerd, J. A. (1994). Working in an intensive or non-intensive care unit: Does it make a difference? *Heart & Lung, 23,* 71–79.

Ferrans, E. E., & Powers, M. J. (1992). Psychometric assessment of the Quality of Life Index. *Research in Nursing & Health, 15,* 29–38.

Gurney, C. A., Mueller, C. W., & Price, J. L. (1997). Job satisfaction and organizational attachment of nurses holding doctoral degrees. *Nursing Research, 46,* 163–171.

Matocha, L. K., and Waterhouse, J. K. (1993). Current nursing practice related to sexuality. *Research in Nursing & Health, 16,* 371–378.

Quinn, A. O., Koepsell, D., & Haller, S. (1997). Breastfeeding incidence after early discharge and factors influencing breastfeeding cessation. *Journal of Obstetric, Gynecologic, and Neonatal Nursing, 26,* 289–294.

Quinn, C. A. (1993). Nurses' perceptions about physical restraints. *Western Journal of Nursing Research, 15,* 148–158.

Raines, D. A. (1994). Values influencing neonatal nurses' perceptions and choices. *Western Journal of Nursing Research, 16,* 675–691.

Tyler, D. O., Allan, J. D., & Alcozer, F. R. (1997). Weight loss methods used by African American, and Euro-American women. *Research in Nursing & Health, 20,* 413–423.

Williams, J. S., & Engle, V. F. (1995). Staff evaluations of nursing home residents' competence. *Applied Nursing Research, 8,* 18–22.

Woodgate, R., & Kristjanson, L. J. (1996). "My hurts": Hospitalized young children's perceptions of acute pain. *Qualitative Health Research, 6,* 184–201.

Zerwic, J. J., King, K. B., & Wlasowicz, G. S. (1997). Perceptions of patients with cardiovascular disease about the causes of coronary artery disease. *Heart & Lung, 26,* 92–98.

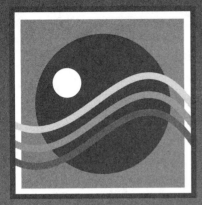

PART IV

Measurement and Data Collection

CHAPTER **13**

Designing and Implementing a Data Collection Plan

The phenomena in which a researcher is interested must ultimately be translated into data that can be analyzed. The tasks of defining the research variables and selecting or developing appropriate methods for collecting data are among the most challenging in the research process. Without high-quality data collection methods, the accuracy and robustness of the conclusions are always subject to challenge. As in the case of research designs and sampling plans, the researcher must often choose from an array of alternatives in deciding how to collect data. This chapter provides an overview of various alternative methods of data collection and discusses the development of a **data collection plan**.

EXISTING DATA VERSUS NEW DATA

One of the first decisions that an investigator makes with regard to research data concerns whether to use existing data or to collect new data that are generated specifically for the research project. Most of the chapters in this part of the book are devoted to methods for generating new data, but it is important to note that researchers often can take advantage of existing information.

Existing **records** represent a very important source of data for nurse researchers. A wealth of data is gathered for nonresearch purposes and can be fruitfully exploited to answer research questions. Nurse researchers are particularly fortunate in the amount and quality of existing data available to them for exploration. Hospital records, patient charts, physicians' order sheets, care plan statements, and so forth all constitute rich data sources to which nurse researchers may have access. The use of records data is discussed at greater length in Chapter 16.

Historical research also typically relies exclusively on available data. As noted in Chapter 10, data for historical research are usually in the form of written records of the past: periodicals, diaries, letters, newspapers, minutes of meetings, medical documents, reports, and so forth. The historical researcher must locate the available records, evaluate the authenticity and accuracy of the data, and then assemble the "data set" of historical information.

As discussed in Chapter 8, researchers sometimes perform a secondary analysis, which is the use of data gathered in a previous study (often by other researchers) to test new hypotheses or address new research questions. The difference between using records and doing a secondary analysis is that the researcher performing a secondary analysis typically has an intact data set that is ready to analyze, whereas the researcher using records has to assemble the data set from records, and considerable coding and data manipulation are usually necessary. A secondary analysis can be performed with either quantitative or qualitative data. For example, Rajan (1994) did a secondary analysis of data from a large-scale quantitative study of pain relief during childbirth to study the effect of obstetric procedures on breastfeeding 6 weeks after delivery. Logan and Jenny (1990) did a secondary analysis of data from a grounded theory study of nurses' perceptions of weaning patients from mechanical ventilation; the secondary analysis yielded a new nursing diagnosis—dysfunctional ventilatory weaning response.

Finally, meta-analyses make use of existing data—that is, data derived from available research reports. As with records information, the researcher doing a meta-analysis does not have to collect new data but must ferret out appropriate data, code or manipulate them, and assemble them into a data set for analysis.

The primary advantages of using existing data are that they are economical and time-saving. The collection of original data is typically costly and time-consuming. On the other hand, it may be difficult to find existing data that are ideally suited to answering a research question.

DIMENSIONS OF DATA COLLECTION APPROACHES

If existing data are not available or not suitable for the research question, the researcher must collect new data. Many methods of collecting new data are used for nursing studies. For example, study participants can be interviewed, observed by the researcher, or tested

with measures of physiologic functioning. Regardless of what specific approach is used, data collection methods vary along four important dimensions: structure, quantifiability, researcher obtrusiveness, and objectivity.

Structure

Research data, particularly in quantitative studies, are often collected according to a structured plan that indicates what information is to be gathered and how to gather it. For example, most self-administered questionnaires are highly structured: they include a fixed set of questions that are generally answered in a specified sequence and with predesignated response options (e.g., agree or disagree). In such structured methods, there is little opportunity for participants to qualify their answers or to explain the underlying meaning of their responses.

In some studies, however, it is more appropriate to impose a minimum of structure and to provide study participants with opportunities to reveal relevant information in a naturalistic way. Most qualitative studies rely almost exclusively on unstructured or loosely structured methods of data collection.

There are advantages and disadvantages to both structured and unstructured approaches. Structured methods often take considerable effort to develop and refine, but they yield data that are relatively easy to analyze. Structured methods are seldom appropriate for an in-depth examination of a phenomenon, however. Consider the following two methods of asking people about their levels of stress:

Structured: During the past week, would you say you felt stressed
  1. rarely or none of the time,
  2. some or a little of the time,
  3. occasionally or a moderate amount of the time, or
  4. most or all of the time?
Unstructured: How stressed or anxious have you been this past week? Tell me

about the kinds of tensions and stresses you have been experiencing.

The structured approach would allow the researcher to compute exactly what percentage of respondents felt highly stressed most of the time but would provide no information about the intensity, cause, or circumstances of the stress. The unstructured question, while allowing for deeper and more thoughtful responses, may pose difficulties for people who are not good at expressing themselves verbally. Moreover, the unstructured question is likely to yield data that are considerably more difficult to analyze.

When data are collected in a highly structured fashion, the researcher must develop (or borrow) what is referred to as the data collection **instrument** (or **tool**), which is the formal written document used to collect and record information, such as a questionnaire. When unstructured methods are used, there is typically no formal instrument, although there may be a list of the types of information needed.

Quantifiability

Data that will be subjected to statistical analysis must be gathered in such a way that they can be quantified. For statistical analysis, all variables must be quantitatively measured—even though the variables are abstract and intangible phenomena that represent *qualities* of humans, such as hope, loneliness, pain, and body image. Data that are to be analyzed qualitatively are typically collected in narrative form.

Structured data collection approaches generally yield data that are easily quantified. It is often possible (and it is sometimes useful), however, to quantify unstructured information as well. For example, responses to the unstructured question concerning stress could be categorized after the fact according to the four levels of stress indicated in the structured question. Whether it is *wise* to do so depends on the nature of the research problem, the philosophical orientation of the researcher, and the nature of the responses.

Researcher Obtrusiveness

Data collection methods differ in terms of the degree to which people are aware of their status as study participants. If participants are fully aware of their role in a study, their behavior and responses may not be normal. When participants distort the data, the entire value of the research can be undermined. When data are collected unobtrusively, however, ethical problems may emerge, as discussed in Chapter 6.

Study participants are most likely to distort their behavior and their responses to questions under certain circumstances. In particular, researcher obtrusiveness is likely to be most problematic when a program is being evaluated and participants have a vested interest in the evaluation outcome, the participants are engaged in socially unacceptable or atypical behavior, the participants have not complied with medical and nursing instructions, or the participants are the type of people who have a strong need to "look good." When researcher obtrusiveness is unavoidable under these circumstances, the researcher should make a strong effort to put participants at ease, to stress the importance of candor and naturalistic behavior, and to use research personnel trained to convey a neutral and nonjudgmental demeanor.

Objectivity

Objectivity refers to the degree to which two independent researchers can arrive at similar "scores" or make similar observations regarding the concepts of interest, that is, make judgments regarding participants' attributes or behavior that are not biased by personal feelings or beliefs. Some data collection approaches require more subjective judgment than others, and some research problems require a higher degree of objectivity than others.

Researchers whose paradigmatic orientation lies in logical positivism generally strive for a reasonable amount of objectivity. However, in some research (especially research based in the naturalistic paradigm), the subjective judgment of the investigator is considered a valuable component of data collection because subjectivity is thought to be essential for the understanding of human experiences.

MAJOR TYPES OF DATA COLLECTION METHODS

In addition to making decisions regarding these four dimensions, nurse researchers must select the form of data collection to use. Three types of approach have been used most frequently by nurse researchers: self-reports, observation, and biophysiologic measures. This section presents an overview of these methods, and subsequent chapters provide more in-depth guidance.

Self-Reports

In the human sciences, a good deal of information can be gathered by questioning people directly, a method known as **self-report**. If, for example, we are interested in learning about patients' perceptions of hospital care, patients' preoperative fears, or nursing students' attitudes toward gerontologic nursing, then we are likely to try to find answers by questioning a group of relevant people. For some research variables, alternatives to direct questions exist. However, the unique ability of humans to communicate verbally on a sophisticated level makes it unlikely that systematic questioning will ever be eliminated from the repertoire of data collection techniques. Most nursing studies involve data collected by means of self-reports.

The self-report method is strong with respect to its directness and versatility. If we want to know what people think, feel, or believe, the most direct means of gathering the information is to ask them about it. Perhaps the strongest argument that can be made for

the self-report method is that it frequently yields information that would be difficult, if not impossible, to gather by any other means. Current behaviors can be directly observed, but only if participants are willing to manifest them publicly. For example, it is usually impossible for a researcher to observe such behaviors as child abuse, contraceptive practices, or drug usage. Furthermore, observers can observe only behaviors occurring at the time of the study; through self-reports, a researcher can gather retrospective data about activities and events occurring in the past or gather projections about behaviors in which people plan to engage in the future. Information about feelings, values, opinions, and motives can sometimes be inferred through observation, but behaviors and feelings do not always correspond exactly. People's actions do not always indicate their state of mind. Here again, self-report instruments can be designed to measure psychological characteristics through direct communication with the participant.

Self-reports are also versatile with respect to content coverage. People can be asked to report on facts about their personal backgrounds; facts about other people known to them; facts about events or environmental conditions; beliefs about what the facts are; attitudes, feelings, and opinions; reasons for opinions, attitudes, or behaviors; level of knowledge about conditions, situations, or practices; and intentions for future behaviors.

Despite these advantages, verbal report instruments share a number of weaknesses. The most serious issue is the question of the validity and accuracy of self-reports: How can we really be sure that respondents feel or act the way they say they do? How can we trust the information that respondents provide, particularly if the questions could potentially require them to reveal an unpopular position on a controversial issue or to admit to socially unacceptable behavior? Investigators often have no alternative but to assume that most of their respondents have been frank. Yet we all have a tendency to want to present ourselves in the best light, and this may conflict with the truth. Researchers who find it necessary or appropriate to gather self-report data should be cognizant of the limitations of this method and should be prepared to take these shortcomings into consideration when interpreting the results. Likewise, consumers of research reports should be alert to potential biases introduced when people are asked to describe themselves, particularly with respect to behaviors or feelings that our society judges to be wrong or unusual.

Observation

For certain types of research problems, an alternative to self-reports is direct observation of people's behavior. Various types of information required by nurse researchers as evidence of nursing effectiveness or as clues to improving nursing practices can be obtained through direct observation. Suppose, for instance, that we were interested in studying mental patients' methods of defending their personal territory, or children's reactions to the removal of a leg cast, or a patient's mode of emergence from anesthesia. These phenomena are all amenable to direct observation. Within nursing research, observational methods have broad applicability, particularly for clinical inquiries. Observational methods can be used fruitfully to gather a variety of information, including information on characteristics and conditions of individuals (e.g., the sleep–wake state of patients); verbal communication behaviors (e.g., exchange of information during medication administration); nonverbal communication behaviors (e.g., facial expressions); activities (e.g., geriatric patients' self-grooming activities); and environmental conditions (e.g., architectural barriers in the homes of disabled people).

Observations can be made in laboratory or in natural settings. In addition, observation can be done directly through the human senses or with the aid of technical apparatus, such as video equipment and tape recorders. Thus, observational methods are an extremely versatile approach to data collection.

Like self-report techniques, observational methods can vary in the degree of structure the researcher imposes. That is, a researcher could observe nurses' methods of touching patients in an unstructured manner, taking detailed narrative notes regarding their use of touch. Alternatively, the researcher could tabulate the frequency of the nurses' use of specific types of touching.

The field of nursing is particularly well suited for observational research. Nurses are in an advantageous position to observe, relatively unobtrusively, the behaviors and activities of patients, their families, and hospital staff. Moreover, nurses may by training be especially sensitive observers. Many nursing problems are better suited to an observational approach than to self-report techniques. Whenever people cannot be expected to describe adequately their own behaviors, observational methods may be needed. This may be the case when people are unaware of their own behavior (e.g., manifesting preoperative symptoms of anxiety), when people are embarrassed to report their activities (e.g., displays of aggression or hostility), when behaviors are emotionally laden (e.g., grieving behavior among the bereaved), or when people are not capable of articulating their actions (e.g., young children or the mentally ill). Observational methods have an intrinsic appeal with respect to their ability to capture a record of behaviors and events directly. Furthermore, with an observational approach, humans—the observers—are used as measuring instruments and provide a uniquely sensitive and intelligent tool.

Several of the shortcomings of the observational approach include possible ethical difficulties, distorted behavior on the part of the person being observed when the observer is conspicuous, and a high rate of refusals to being observed. One of the most pervasive problems, however, is the vulnerability of observational data to **observer biases**. A number of factors interfere with objective observations, including the following:

- Emotions, prejudices, attitudes, and values of the observer may result in faulty inference.
- Personal interest and commitment may color what is seen in the direction of what the observer wants to see.
- Anticipation of what is to be observed may affect what is observed.
- Hasty decisions before adequate information is collected may result in erroneous classifications or conclusions.

Observational biases probably cannot be eliminated completely, but they can be minimized through the careful training of observers.

Biophysiologic Measures

The trend in nursing research has been toward increased clinical, patient-centered investigations, and this trend is likely to continue in years to come. One result of this trend is an expanded use of measures to assess the physiologic status of research subjects—typically through quantitative **biophysiologic measures**. Physiologic and physical variables typically require specialized technical instruments and equipment for their measurement and, generally, specialized training for the interpretation of results. Settings in which nurses operate are usually filled with a wide variety of technical instruments for measuring physiologic functions. In comparison with other types of data collection tools, the equipment for obtaining physiologic measurements is costly. However, because such equipment is generally available in health care settings, the costs to nurse researchers may be small or nonexistent.

A major strength of biophysiologic measures is their objectivity. Nurse A and nurse B, reading from the same spirometer output, are likely to record the same or highly similar tidal volume measurements for a patient. Furthermore, barring the possibility of equipment malfunctioning, two different spirometers are likely to produce identical tidal volume readouts. Another advantage of physiologic measurements is the relative precision and sensitivity that they normally offer. By relative, we are implicitly comparing physiologic instruments with devices for obtaining various psychological measurements, such as self-report measures of anxiety, pain, attitudes, and so forth. Patients are unlikely to be able to distort deliberately measurements of physiologic functioning. Furthermore, researchers are generally confident that physiologic instrumentation provides measures of those variables in which they are interested: thermometers can be depended on to measure temperature and not blood volume, and so forth. For nonphysiologic measurements, the question of whether a quantitative measuring tool is really measuring the target concept is a continuously perplexing problem.

Physiologic measures also have some disadvantages. For example, the highly technical nature of the equipment may constitute a difficulty because the failure of nonengineers to understand the limitations of the instruments may result in greater faith in their accuracy than is warranted. Another problem, which physiologic measures share with other data collection approaches, is the effect that the measuring tool itself has on the variables it is attempting to measure. For instance, a flow transducer located in a blood vessel partially blocks that vessel and, hence, alters the pressure–flow characteristics being measured. Another difficulty is that there are normally interferences that create artifacts in physiologic measurements. For example, the subjects may create artifactual signals, particularly when their movements result in movements of sensing devices. Finally, energy must often be applied to the organism when making the physiologic measurements, which means that extreme caution must always be exercised to avoid the risk of damaging cells by high-energy concentrations. Any researcher utilizing electrical equipment should be thoroughly familiar with safety rules and considerations such as grounding specifications.

DEVELOPING A DATA COLLECTION PLAN

The decisions that a researcher makes about the design of a study are totally independent of his or her decision about which data collection method (or methods) to use. A researcher implementing an experimental repeated measures design can rely on self-report data, as can a researcher doing an ethnography. Biophysiologic data can be used in experimental, quasi-experimental, and nonexperimental studies. Moreover, the three main types of data collection methods—self-reports, observation, and biophysiologic measures—can involve either existing data sources or data created specifically for research purposes. Sometimes, the nature of the research *question* dictates which specific method of data collection to use—and where along the four continua described in the first section the methods should lie. Often, however, the researcher has considerable latitude in selecting or designing a data collection plan. In all cases, the plan should strive to yield accurate, trustworthy, and meaningful data that are maximally effective in answering the research questions. These are rigorous requirements, and to be successful, the researcher usually needs to devote considerable time and effort. This section discusses steps that are often undertaken in the development of a data collection plan. Figure 13-1 provides an overview of the procedures often used in developing such a plan for quantitative studies. In qualitative studies, the data collection strategy emerges while the researcher is in the field, and therefore a structured, orderly plan cannot usually be specified at the outset. Therefore, most of this section presents the development of a data collection plan for quantitative nursing studies.

Identifying Data Needs

The researcher must generally begin by identifying the types of data that are needed to complete the study successfully. Typically, the researcher needs to gather information about more than just the main study variables. Advance planning may help the researcher avoid "if only" disappointments at the analysis stage.

In a quantitative study, the researcher should give thoughtful consideration to what the data needs are for accomplishing the following:

1. *Testing the hypotheses or addressing all the research questions.* The researcher must include one or more measures of all the independent and dependent variables. Multiple measures of some variables may be required if a variable is complex and multifaceted or if there are concerns about the accuracy of a single measure.

2. *Describing the main characteristics of the sample.* Information should normally be gathered about major demographic characteristics of the sample and about relevant aspects of the participants' health status. It is almost always advisable to gather information about the participants' age, gender, race or ethnicity, educational background, marital status, and income level or type of occupation. This information is critical in interpreting the results and in understanding the population to whom the findings can be generalized. If the sample includes study participants with a health problem, data on the nature of that problem also should be gathered (e.g., length of illness, severity of health problem, types of treatment obtained, length of stay in hospital, and so on).

3. *Controlling for important sources of extraneous variables.* As discussed in Chapter 9, various approaches can be used to control extraneous variables, and many of them require the measurement of those variables. For example, when analysis of covariance is used, each of the variables that is statistically controlled

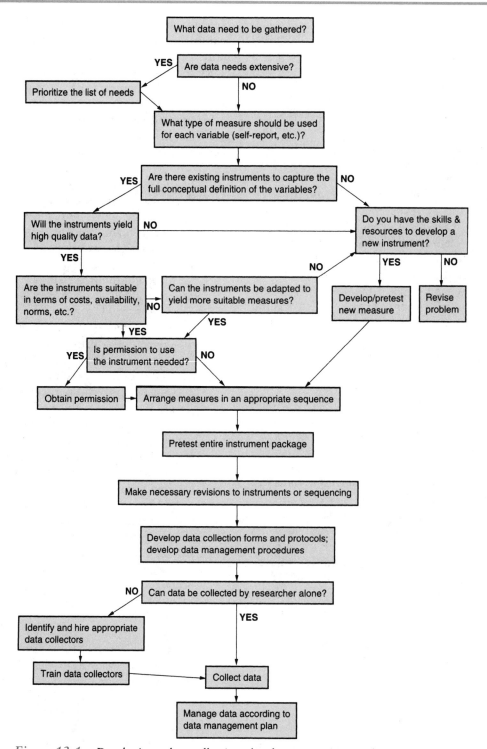

Figure 13-1. Developing a data collection plan for quantitative studies.

must be measured. Even if a researcher uses a design that does not control all important extraneous variables, it is usually a good idea to measure them because then their relationship with the key research variables can be examined. Thought should be given to gathering data on both external and intrinsic factors that could influence the outcomes.

4. *Analyzing potential biases.* Ideally, data that can help the researcher to identify potential biases should be collected. For example, in a nonequivalent control group design, the researcher should gather information that would help to identify selection biases. As another example, if the researcher is collecting self-report data about a socially unacceptable characteristic or behavior, it might be advisable to administer a special test (e.g., the Marlowe-Crowne Social Desirability Scale) to determine whether respondents have a tendency to give responses that are biased in the direction of "looking good." In general, the researcher should give some thought to what potential sources of biases might arise and then determine whether they can be measured.

5. *Understanding subgroup effects.* It is often desirable to answer the research questions not only for the entire sample but also for certain subgroups of participants. For example, we may wish to know if a special intervention for indigent pregnant women is equally effective for primiparas and multiparas. In such a situation, we would need to collect information about the participants' childbearing history so that we could divide the sample and analyze for separate **subgroup effects**.

6. *Interpreting the results.* The researcher should try to anticipate alternative patterns of results and then determine what types of data would best help in interpreting those results. For example, if we hypothesized that the presence of school-based clinics in high schools would lower the incidence of sexually transmitted diseases among students but found that the incidence remained constant after the clinic was established, what type of information would we want to have to help us interpret this result (e.g., information about the students' frequency of intercourse, number of partners, use of condoms, and so on)?

7. *Checking on the manipulation.* When a researcher manipulates the independent variable, it is sometimes advisable to gather information to determine if the manipulation was actually achieved. Such a **manipulation check** provides a mechanism for interpreting negative results. As an example, if a researcher were studying the impact of a new hospital policy on the morale of the nursing staff, it might be important to determine the nurses' level of awareness of the new policy because if the results indicate no change in staff morale, this could reflect lack of awareness of the policy rather than complacency about it.

8. *Obtaining administrative information.* It is almost always necessary to gather various types of administrative information to help in the management of the project. For example, if there are multiple observers, it is desirable to record separate identification numbers for each one on all observational forms. Other types of administrative information might include participant identification numbers, dates of attempted contact with participants, dates of actual data collection, where the data collection occurred, when the data collection session began and ended, reasons that a potential subject did not participate in the study, and contact information if the study is longitudinal.

The list of possible data needs may seem daunting, but in actuality, many categories overlap. For example, variables that are useful in describing participant characteristics are often important extraneous variables or are useful in the creation of subgroups. If time or resource constraints make it impossible to collect the full range of variables, then the researcher should prioritize data needs and be aware of how the absence of certain variables will affect the study's integrity. The important point here is that researchers should understand what their data needs are and take steps to ensure the fullest possible coverage.

In qualitative studies, the data collection plan usually is more fluid, with decisions about types of data to collect evolving in the field. For example, as the researcher begins to gather and digest information, it may become apparent that it would be fruitful to pursue a certain line of questioning that had not originally been anticipated. However, even while allowing and profiting from this flexibility, qualitative researchers should make some upfront decisions about the type of data they will need to obtain initially (e.g., data on sample characteristics, administrative information, and so on).

Selecting Types of Measures

After data needs have been identified, the next step is to select a method to gather information on each concept and to determine where on the four dimensions mentioned earlier (structure, quantifiability, obtrusiveness, and objectivity) the variables will lie. It is common, and often advantageous, to use a multimethod approach. Researchers have profitably combined self-reports, observations, and physiologic measures in a single study. Researchers have also combined measures that vary in terms of the four basic dimensions. In reviewing the data needs, the researcher should determine how best to capture each of the variables of interest in terms of its conceptual or theoretical definition.

Research considerations, unfortunately, are not the only factors that drive decisions about the specific methods to use in collecting data. The decisions must also be guided by ethical considerations, cost constraints, the availability of appropriate staff to help with data collection, time constraints on the researcher's part, and the anticipated burden to the participants and to others not associated with the project, such as hospital staff or the participants' families.

Data collection is typically the costliest and most time-consuming portion of a study. Because of this, the researcher is likely to have to make a number of compromises about the type or amount of data collected.

Selecting and Developing Instruments

Once preliminary decisions have been made regarding the basic data collection methods to be used, the researcher should determine if there are instruments already available to measure the constructs of interest for those variables being measured in a structured fashion. For most constructs, existing instruments will be available and should be reviewed. In the next three chapters, we provide sources for locating existing self-report, observational, and other measures.

After potential data collection instruments have been identified and retrieved, they should be carefully reviewed to determine their appropriateness for the study. The primary consideration is whether the instrument is conceptually relevant: Does the instrument capture your conceptual definition of the variable? The next factor to consider is whether the instrument is likely to yield data of a sufficiently high quality. Approaches to evaluating data quality for both qualitative and quantitative data collection methods are discussed in detail in Chapter 17. In addition to data quality, six other criteria that often affect the researcher's decisions in selecting an instrument are as follows:

1. *Resources.* Resource constraints sometimes make it impossible to use the highest-quality measures. There may be some direct costs associated with the measure (e.g., some psychological tests must be purchased from publishers, or some physiologic equipment may have to be rented), but the biggest data collection cost often involves compensation to the people who are collecting data if you cannot do it single-handedly (e.g., hired interviewers or observers). In such a situation, the length of the instrument and the time it takes to administer may determine whether it can be used. Also, if the data collection procedures are considered burdensome, it may be necessary to pay a respondent stipend. All of the associated costs of data collection should be carefully considered, especially if the use of time-consuming or expensive methods means that the investigator will be forced to cut costs elsewhere (e.g., by using a smaller sample).

2. *Availability and familiarity.* In selecting measures, you may need to consider how readily available or accessible various tools are, especially if they are biophysiologic in nature. Similarly, data collection strategies with which you are familiar or have had experience are generally preferable to new measures because administration is generally smoother and more efficient in such cases.

3. *Norms and comparability.* You may find it desirable to select a measure for which there are relevant norms. **Norms** indicate the "normal" values and distribution of values on the measure with respect to a specified population. For example, most standardized tests (such as the Scholastic Assessment Test) have national norms. The availability of norms is often useful because norms offer, in essence, a built-in comparison group. For similar reasons, you may find it advantageous to adopt a specific instrument because it was used in other similar studies and therefore offers a supplementary basis for putting the study findings in context. Indeed, when a study is an intentional replication, it is often essential to use the same instruments as were used in the original study, even if higher-quality measures are available.

4. *Population appropriateness.* The measure should be chosen with the characteristics of the target population in mind. Characteristics of special importance include the age of the participants, their intellectual abilities or reading skills, and their cultural or ethnic backgrounds. If there is concern about the reading skills of the research sample, it may be necessary to calculate the **readability** of a prospective instrument using procedures such as those described in Gunning (1968) or Fry (1968). If the participants include members of minority groups, you should strive to identify instruments that are not culturally biased, especially if racial or ethnic comparisons will be made. If non–English-speaking participants are included in the sample, then the selection of a measure may be based, in part, on the availability of a translated version of the measure.

5. *Administration issues.* An important consideration often relates to the instrument's requirements for obtaining high-quality data. For example, in obtaining information about the developmental status of children, you may have to consider whether the administration of a given measure requires the skills of a professional psychologist or whether an interviewer with adequate training can obtain high-quality data. Another administration issue concerns constraints on where the data must be collected. Certain instruments may require or assume stringent conditions with regard to the time of administration, privacy of the setting, and so on. In such a case, re-

quirements for obtaining valid measures must match the characteristics of the intended research setting.

6. *Reputation.* Instruments designed to measure the same construct often differ in the kinds of reputation they enjoy among specialists working in a field, even if they are comparable with regard to quality. Therefore, it may be useful to seek the advice of knowledgeable individuals, preferably people with personal, direct experience in using the instruments.

Based on such considerations, you may conclude that existing instruments are not suitable for all your research variables. In such a situation, you will be faced with either adapting an existing instrument to make it more appropriate or developing a new one. The development of a new instrument should be considered a last resort, especially for novice researchers, because it is extremely difficult to develop accurate and valid measuring tools. However, there are situations in which there is no acceptable alternative. In the next few chapters, we provide some guidance for those who elect to construct a new instrument, but in some cases, it may make more sense to modify the research question so that existing instruments can be used.

If you are fortunate in identifying an existing instrument that is suitable for your study, it is likely that your next step will be to obtain written permission from the person who developed it (or from the publisher, if it is a commercially distributed instrument) to use or adapt it. In general, copyrighted materials always require permission. Instruments that have been developed under a federal grant are usually in the public domain, and so do not require permission, because they have been supported with taxpayers' dollars. When in doubt, however, it is best to obtain permission. By contacting the author of an instrument to obtain permission, it is likely that you will also obtain more detailed information about the instrument and its quality than was available in a published report.

Pretesting the Data Collection Package

Researchers who develop their own instrument typically subject it to rigorous **pretesting** so that it can be evaluated and refined. However, even when the data collection plan involves the use of existing instruments, it is usually wise to conduct a small pretest.*

One purpose of a pretest is to determine the length of time it takes to administer the entire instrument package and whether participants feel that the time burden is too great. Typically, researchers use more than one instrument because there are usually many variables to be measured. It is often difficult to estimate in advance how long it will take to administer a complete package of instruments, and such estimates may be required for informed consent purposes or for developing a realistic project budget. If the pretest instruments require more time than is considered acceptable, it may be necessary to eliminate certain variables or instruments, guided by the prioritization list established early in the process.

Pretests can serve many other purposes, including the following:

- Identifying any parts of the instrument package that are difficult for the particular population of participants to read or understand or that may have been misinterpreted by them
- Identifying any parts of the data collection package that the participants find objectionable or offensive

---

*Some writers use the terms *pretest* and *pilot study* interchangeably. That is, some researchers say that they undertook a pilot study to test their instruments, whereas others say that they pretested their instruments. However, a pilot study often involves a small-scale test of the entire study, testing not only instruments but also the sampling plan, the intervention, the study procedures, and so on.

- Determining whether the sequencing of instruments within the data collection package is smooth and effective
- Determining needs for the training of the data collection staff
- Determining if the measures yield data with sufficient variability

The last purpose requires a bit of explanation. For most research questions, the instruments should ideally discriminate among participants with different levels of an attribute. If we are asking, for example, whether women experience greater depression than men when they learn of a cancer diagnosis, we need an instrument capable of distinguishing between people with higher and lower levels of depression. If an instrument yields data with limited variability, then it will be impossible to detect a difference in depression between men and women—even when such a difference actually exists. Thus, a researcher should look at pretest variation in key research variables. If, to pursue the example, the entire pretest sample looks very depressed (or not at all depressed), it may be necessary to modify the instruments.

Developing Data Collection Forms and Procedures

After the instrument package has been finalized, researchers are faced with a number of tasks that are primarily administrative in nature. First, appropriate forms for the collection of the instrument must be developed for data collected in a structured manner. In some studies, many forms have to be developed, for example, forms for screening potential participants to determine their eligibility for the sample, informed consent forms, forms for explaining the study to prospective participants, records of attempted contacts with participants, forms for recording actual research data, contact information forms, and administrative logs for recording the receipt of research forms. It is prudent to design forms that are attractively formatted, legible, and inviting to use. Care should also be taken to design forms in such a way that confidentiality can be ensured. For example, identification information such as names and addresses is often recorded on a separate page that can be detached and kept separate from other types of data.

In most quantitative studies, the researcher also develops protocols that spell out the procedures to be used in data collection. These protocols describe such considerations as the following:

- Conditions that must be met for collecting the data (e.g., Can others be present at the time of data collection? Where must data collection occur?)
- Specific procedures for collecting the data, including requirements for sequencing instruments and recording information
- Standard information to provide participants who ask routine questions about the study. These questions may include the following: How will the information from this study be used? How did you get my name, and why are you asking me? How long will this take? Who will have access to this information? What are the possible benefits and risks?
- Procedures to follow in the event that a participant becomes distraught, disoriented, or for any other reason cannot complete the data collection

Finally, procedures and forms may need to be developed for managing data as they are gathered, especially if data are being gathered from multiple sites or over an extended period. For example, in an observational study, a data management form might record, for each case, the date the observation was scheduled to take place, the date it actually took place, the date the observation form was received back in some central location, and the date the data were coded and entered onto a computer file.

Large-scale surveys are increasingly using new technologic tools to assist in the collection of data. Most major telephone surveys now use **computer-assisted telephone interviewing (CATI)**, and growing numbers of in-person surveys are using **computer-assisted personal interviewing (CAPI)**. Both of these procedures involve the development of computer programs that will present the interviewer with the questions to be asked on the screen of a computer (on a lap-top computer in the case of CAPI). CATI and CAPI surveys greatly facilitate data collection and generally improve data quality because there is less opportunity for interviewer error. However, it clearly requires considerable resources to substitute a computer program for paper-and-pencil forms.

In qualitative studies, there is usually considerably less emphasis on the development of specific forms and protocols because data collection strategies evolve in the field. Nevertheless, the researcher may need to develop a few forms, such as a form for gathering demographic and administrative information or logbook forms for recording narrative information. Also, a preliminary list of questions to be asked or types of observation to be made during the initial data collection is usually useful. Finally, the researcher should make a list of everything that will be needed during data collection, including forms, clipboards, pencils, recording equipment such as tape recorders or cameras, gifts or stipends, and computer equipment. To ensure that interview data are the actual verbatim responses of study participants, it is strongly recommended that qualitative interviews be tape recorded (or video recorded) and subsequently transcribed, rather than relying on interviewer notes. Notes tend to be incomplete and may be biased by the interviewer's memory and personal views.

IMPLEMENTING A DATA COLLECTION PLAN

The quality of data for a research project is affected by the decisions that shape the data col-

lection plan. Data quality is also affected by how the plan is actually implemented.

Selecting Research Personnel

An important decision concerns who will actually collect the research data. In many small research projects, the researchers in charge of the study collect the data themselves. In larger studies, however, this may not be feasible. When data are to be collected by others, great care must be taken to select appropriate research staff. In most studies, the research staff should be neutral agents through whom the data will pass—that is, the characteristics or behavior of the research personnel should not alter or affect the substantive nature of the data. Some of the considerations that should be kept in mind when selecting research personnel are as follows:

- *Experience*. Ideally, the research staff should have prior experience with data collection. For example, for a self-report study, it is advantageous to use data collectors who have experience conducting interviews. This is especially true for qualitative studies, where the interviewer must be especially skilled in soliciting information and directing the flow of the interview. If it is necessary to use an inexperienced person, it is important to look for someone who can readily acquire the necessary skills (e.g., an interviewer should have good verbal and social skills).

- *Congruity with sample characteristics*. To the extent possible, data collectors should match the backgrounds of the study participants with respect to such characteristics as racial or cultural background and gender. In some studies, this is an absolute requirement (e.g., hiring a person who speaks the language of an immigrant sample). The greater the sensitivity of the research questions, the greater the desirability of matching characteristics. For example, in a study of the sexual behavior of pregnant African American teenagers, the data collectors would ideally be African American women.

- *Unremarkable appearance.* Extremes of appearance should generally be avoided because participants may react to extremes and may alter their behavior or responses accordingly. For example, data collectors should generally not be very old or very young. They should not dress extremely casually (e.g., in shorts and tee shirts), nor very formally (e.g., with elaborate jewelry). While on the job, data collectors should never wear any article that would convey their political or social views (e.g., political buttons, jewelry with peace symbols, and so on).
- *Personality.* Data collectors should be pleasant (but not effusive), sociable (but not overly talkative or overbearing), and nonjudgmental (but not apathetic or unfeeling about the participants' lives). The goal is to have nonthreatening data collectors who can encourage candor and put participants at ease without interjecting their own values and biases.
- *Availability.* Data collectors should ideally be available for the entire data collection period to avoid having to recruit and train new staff. If the study is longitudinal, it is advantageous to hire data collectors who could potentially be available for subsequent rounds of data collection.

In some situations, researchers will not be able to select research personnel. For example, the data collectors may be the staff nurses employed at a hospital or graduate students in a school of nursing. Particularly in such situations, training of the data collection staff is important.

Training Data Collectors

Depending on the prior experience of the research personnel, training will need to cover both general procedures (e.g., how to conduct an interview) and procedures specific to the study (e.g., how to administer a particular set of questions or make certain observations). Training can often be accomplished in a single day, but in complex projects, it may require more time. The lead researcher is usually the best person to conduct the training and to develop training materials.

The data collection protocols, as discussed in the previous section, are usually a good foundation for the development of a **training manual**. The manual normally includes background materials, general instructions, specific instructions, and copies of all the data collection and administrative forms. Table 13-1 presents an example of a table of contents for a training manual for a quantitative interview study.

The heart of a training manual is the detailed instructions relating to the administration of the specific data collection instruments (in Table 13-1, these appear in section IV.C). These instructions are usually intended to provide complete information about exactly what the researcher is looking for so that there is no ambiguity about the nature of the data to be obtained. As an example, Table 13-2 provides **Q-by-Qs (question-by-question instructions)** for two structured questions.

The agenda for the training should generally cover the content of the training manual, elaborating on any portion that is especially difficult or complex. The training often includes demonstrations by the research team of fictitious data collection episodes, performed either live or on videotape. Finally, the training usually involves having the trainees do trial runs of data collection in front of the trainers to demonstrate their understanding of the instructions.

TIPS FOR DEVELOPING AND IMPLEMENTING DATA COLLECTION PLANS

Much of this chapter was devoted to guidance on how to develop and implement a data col-

TABLE 13-1	Example of a Table of Contents: Training Manual for an Interview Study

I. Introduction
   A. Background and Purpose of the Study
   B. The Research Team/Organizational Structure
II. Initial Study Procedures
   A. Tracing and Locating Respondents
   B. Initial Contact with Respondents and Arranging Appointments
   C. Answering Respondents' Questions
   D. Privacy and the Research Setting
   E. Avoiding Refusals and Nonresponse
   F. Informed Consent
III. The Role of the Interviewer
   A. Establishing an Appropriate Interviewing Relationship
   B. Knowing the Interview
   C. Avoiding Bias
   D. Obtaining Full Responses
   E. Recording Information
IV. Instructions for Conducting the Study Interview
   A. Guide to the Use of the Study Instruments
   B. Conventions and Abbreviations Used in the Instruments
   C. Question-by-Question Specifications
   D. Concluding the Interview
V. Administrative Forms and Procedures
   A. Obtaining Interviewing Assignments
   B. Pledge of Confidentiality
   C. Editing Completed Interviews
   D. Submitting Completed Interviews to the Project Director
   E. Errors and Missing Information
   F. Time Forms and Payment
Appendices: Data Collection and Administrative Forms

lection plan. We offer here a few additional tips.

- Although the flow chart in Figure 13-1 suggests a fairly linear process, the development of a data collection plan is often an iterative one. Be prepared to backtrack and make adjustments, recognizing that the ultimate goal is not to get to the bottom of the list of steps but rather to ensure that the process yields conceptually relevant data of the highest possible quality.
- In developing an instrument package, it may be necessary to evaluate tradeoffs between data quality and data quantity. If compromises have to be made, it is usually preferable to forego quantity. For example, it is better to have an excellent measure of the dependent variable with no supplementary measures to help in interpreting outcomes than to have mediocre measures of all desired variables. When data quality for key variables is poor, the results cannot be trusted, so additional information cannot possibly help to clarify the findings.
- Try to avoid, to the fullest extent possible, reinventing the wheel. It is inefficient and unnecessary to start from scratch—not only in developing an instrument but also in developing specific forms, protocols, training materials, and so on. Ask seasoned researchers if they have any materials that you may borrow or adapt for your study. Much of the material relating to data collection plans will *not* be available in published research articles (although it may be available in dissertations or research reports to federal funding agencies).
- Document what you are doing as you develop and implement your data collection plan—and save your documentation. You may need the information later in writing your research report, in requesting funding for a follow-up study, or in helping another researcher.

RESEARCH EXAMPLES

Data collection procedures are often not described in detail in research reports owing to space constraints in journals. However, a

TABLE 13-2	Examples of Question-by-Question Specifications
Question:	During the past year, did your child have an injury, poisoning, or other accident that required medical attention?
Q-by-Q:	This question asks whether the respondent's child had an injury, poisoning, or other type of accident that required *medical* attention. Included would be examination or treatment by a doctor, nurse, emergency medical technician, or other trained person—not simply application of a bandage at home or something else the respondent might do herself or himself. The response should be "yes" *only* if the injury, poisoning, or accident occurred within the 12 months before the date of the interview.
Question:	During your current pregnancy, have you made any visits to a doctor or nurse for prenatal care, that is, to be examined or talk about your pregnancy?
Q-by-Q:	This question asks if the respondent obtained prenatal care during this pregnancy. Being tested for pregnancy does *not* by itself constitute prenatal care, nor does obtaining pregnancy or abortion counseling. Prenatal care is concerned with the health and well-being of the mother and fetus and with a successful birth outcome. Prenatal care can be provided by a doctor, nurse, or midwife.

few examples of exemplary data collection procedures that were described in research journals are presented in Table 13-3. The examples represent efforts the researchers made to achieve high-quality data. More detailed information about the data collection plan for a quantitative and a qualitative study follow.

Data Collection in a Quantitative Study

Mercer, Ferketich, and DeJoseph (1993) examined partner relationships among 371 pregnant women. They tested a conceptual model of the influence of antepartal stress on partner relationships during pregnancy and early parenthood among those in high-risk and low-risk pregnancies. The model was based on earlier research by the study team.

Data were collected longitudinally through interviews and self-administered questionnaires with the pregnant women and, when possible, with their partners. Data were collected at five points in time: before delivery, during postpartal hospitalization, and at 1, 4, and 8 months after delivery.

The authors indicated that six criteria were used to select their battery of instruments: (1) evidence from prior studies that the instrument yielded high-quality data, (2) conceptual congruence with the theoretical underpinnings of the researchers' model, (3) standardization of the instruments for both men and women, (4) previous use in studies of childbearing families, (5) the clarity of individual questions in the instruments, and (6) instrument brevity. As an example of an instrument they selected, the dependent variable (partner relationships) was operationalized by the Locke-Wallace Marital Adjustment Test, a relatively brief measure of dyadic adjustment that had previously demonstrated adequate data quality. The investigators conducted a pilot study to test the clarity and acceptability of the instrument package to participants.

The interviewers for this study were primarily graduate nursing students, all of whom were trained and supervised by the project director. Team meetings were frequently held during the data collection period to ensure that consistent approaches to interviewing were maintained.

TABLE 13-3 Examples of Exemplary Data Collection Procedures	
RESEARCH QUESTION	**DATA COLLECTION PROCEDURE**
Quantitative Studies	
What are the risky drug and sexual behaviors and the mental health characteristics of homeless and drug-recovering women? (Nyamathi, Flaskerud, & Leake, 1997)	Participants were recruited by African American or Latina nurses who were trained in working with the homeless and drug-addicted women. Data were collected in face-to-face interviews with survey instruments administered in English and Spanish by nurses and outreach workers of the same ethnicity as the participant.
What factors influence the behavior of institutional caregivers when they interact with institutionalized, cognitively impaired elders? (Burgener & Shimer, 1993)	Observations were made as unobtrusively as possible. To decrease sensitivity of participants to the research team's presence, researchers spent time in the units before data collection. Every week during data collection, observers simultaneously observed the same episode and compared their observations to ensure a continuing level of consistency and objectivity.
Qualitative Studies	
What is the lived experience of parents after admission of their child to a pediatric intensive care unit? (Mu & Tomlinson, 1997)	Family interviews were conducted in private and in a comfortable area. Interviewers were advanced nurse clinicians who were trained in interviewing methods by the researcher. Interviews were tape recorded to ensure verbatim text, and transcriptions were done by an expert transcriber.
What are the ways in which primary caregivers to older relatives manage the caregiving experience? (Langner, 1993)	In-depth interview guides were developed based on a literature review and the researcher's clinical experience. A pilot study was used to refine the guide for clarity, content, and length. As the data collection progressed, new questions evolved and were added to the interview.

Data Collection in a Qualitative Study

Chalmers and Thomson (1996) conducted an in-depth study to explore and describe the meaning of the risk experience among women who had primary relatives with breast cancer. The study involved semi-structured interviews with 55 women. All interviews, which took place in the respondents' homes, were tape recorded.

The initial interview guide included questions that were developed from the research literature. The interview guide and the data collection process were pilot tested with two women. As the study evolved, new interview guides were developed as the questioning became more focused. Probing questions were used to clarify the meaning of responses and to pursue sensitively all topics until no additional information was elicited.

The researchers' report noted that they made every attempt to use effective interviewing techniques and to collect the highest possible quality data. Their techniques included the provision of privacy and a quiet environment, clarification of participants' comments, and showing acceptance of their comments.

The tape-recorded interviews were transcribed verbatim to maintain data integrity and to minimize interviewer biases. The analysis of qualitative data involves categorizing the narrative information (see Chapter 22). Most of the categorization was completed by the researcher who conducted the interview, but segments of transcribed data were categorized by the second researcher to ensure that there was agreement about how the data should be classified before analysis.

SUMMARY

Some researchers use existing data in their studies, which includes use of existing **records** or performance of a secondary analysis. However, most researchers collect new data and often develop a detailed **data collection plan** before they actually begin to collect their data—especially if the study is gathering quantitative data. Nurse researchers have available to them a wide variety of data collection approaches. Data collection methods vary along four important dimensions: structure, quantifiability, researcher obtrusiveness, and objectivity. Qualitative studies tend to be low on these dimensions, whereas quantitative studies tend to be high on them, but the researcher often has latitude in customizing a strategy. When research is highly structured, the researcher often uses formal data collection **instruments** or **tools**.

The three principal data collection approaches are self-report, observation, and biophysiologic measures. Most nursing research studies involve the use of **self-reports**, that is, data obtained by directly questioning participants regarding the phenomena of interest. The self-report method is strong with respect to its directness and versatility, but the major drawback is the potential for deliberate or unconscious distortions on the part of respondents. **Observational methods** are techniques for obtaining data through the direct observation of phenomena. A wide variety of human activity and traits are amenable to observation, including phenomena that may otherwise be impossible to measure in any other fashion. However, observation is subject to a variety of **observer biases** and may also result in distorted behavior on the part of participants. **Biophysiologic measures**, which are being used with greater frequency in clinical studies, tend to yield data that are objective and valid, although they are not immune to a variety of technical problems.

Qualitative studies often adopt data collection plans that are flexible and that evolve as the study progresses. Most quantitative studies, however, require considerable advance planning and progress through a series of specific steps—the first of which is a thorough identification and prioritization of all data needs. In addition to data for answering research questions, data may be needed to describe the sample, control extraneous variables, analyze biases, understand **subgroup effects,** interpret results, perform **manipulation checks**, and obtain administrative information.

Once the researcher has made decisions about data needs and data collection methods, existing measures of the variables should be sought for use or adaptation. The construction of new instruments requires considerable time and skill and should be undertaken only as a last resort. The selection of existing instruments should be based on such considerations as conceptual appropriateness, expected data quality, cost, population appropriateness, and reputation. Even when existing instruments are used, the instrument package should usually be pretested to determine its length, clarity, and overall suitability.

Before implementing the data collection plan, the researcher in a quantitative study usually develops data collection protocols, data collection forms, and data management procedures. In a qualitative study, data collection decisions usually evolve in the field—although qualitative researchers must still make a number of advance decisions, such as how to record research data. When the researcher cannot collect the data without assistance, he or she should carefully select and train the data collection staff.

STUDY ACTIVITIES

Chapter 13 of the *Study Guide to Accompany Nursing Research, Principles and Methods, 6th ed.*, offers various exercises and study suggestions for reinforcing the concepts presented in this chapter. Additionally, the following study questions can be addressed:

1. Indicate which method of data collection (self-report, observation, and so forth) you would use to operationalize the following variables, and why you have made that choice:
   a. Stress in hospitalized children
   b. Activity level among the noninstitutionalized elderly
   c. Pain in cancer patients
   d. Body image among obese individuals
2. Read a recent research report in a nursing journal, paying especially close attention to the data collection plan. What information about procedures that may affect data quality is missing from the report? How, if at all, does this absence affect your acceptance of the researchers' conclusions?
3. Read the following article and indicate which types of data (according to those listed under Identifying Data Needs) were collected: Maloni, J. A., Chance, B., Zhang, C., Cohen, A. W., Betts, D., & Gange, S. J. (1993). Physical and psychosocial side effects of antepartum hospital bed rest. *Nursing Research, 42,* 297–303.

SUGGESTED READINGS

Methodologic References

Collins, C., Given, B., Given, C. W., & King, S. (1988). Interviewer training and supervision. *Nursing Research, 37,* 122–124.

Davis, L. L. (1992). Instrument review: Getting the most from a panel of experts. *Applied Nursing Research, 5,* 194–197.

Fry, E. (1968). A readability formula that saves time. *Journal of Reading, 11,* 513–515.

Gunning, R. (1968). *The technique of clear writing* (rev. ed.). New York: McGraw Hill.

Jacobson, S. F. (1988). Evaluating instruments for use in clinical nursing research. In M. Frank-Stromberg (Ed.), *Instruments for clinical nursing research.* Norwalk, CT: Appleton & Lange.

Marlowe, D. P., & Crowne, D. (1960). A new scale of social desirability independent of psychopathology. *Journal of Consulting Psychology, 24,* 349–354.

Martin, P. A. (1993). Data management for surveys. *Applied Nursing Research, 6,* 142–144.

Reineck, C. (1991). Nursing research instruments: Pathway to resources. *Applied Nursing Research, 4,* 34–45.

Rew, L., Bechtel, D., & Sapp, A. (1993). Self-as-instrument in qualitative research. *Nursing Research, 42,* 300–301.

Substantive References

Burgener, S. C., & Shimer, R. (1993). Variables related to caregiver behaviors with cognitively impaired elders in institutional settings. *Research in Nursing & Health, 16,* 193–202.

Chalmers, K., & Thomson, K. (1996). Coming to terms with the risk of breast cancer. *Qualitative Health Research, 6,* 256–282.

Langner, S. R. (1993). Ways of managing the experience of caregiving to elderly relatives. *Western Journal of Nursing Research, 15,* 582–594.

Logan, J., & Jenny, J. (1990). Deriving a new nursing diagnosis through qualitative research: Dysfunctional ventilatory warning response. *Nursing Diagnosis, 1,* 37–43.

Mercer, R. T., Ferketich, S. L., & DeJoseph, J. F. (1993). Predictors of partner relationships during pregnancy and infancy. *Research in Nursing & Health, 16,* 45–56.

Mu, P., & Tomlinson, P. (1997). Parental experience and meaning construction during a pediatric health crisis. *Western Journal of Nursing Research*, 19, 608–636.

Nyamathi, A., Flaskerud, J., & Leake, B. (1997). HIV-risk behaviors and mental health characteristics among homeless or drug-recovering women and their closest sources of social support. *Nursing Research, 46*, 133–137.

Rajan, L. (1994). The impact of obstetric procedures and analgesia/anaesthesia during labour and delivery on breast feeding. *Midwifery, 10*, 87–103.

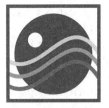

CHAPTER **14**

Self-Reports

Self-report data can be gathered either by oral interview or by written questionnaire. Interviews (and, to a lesser extent, questionnaires) can vary considerably with respect to their degree of structure and their question type. We begin by reviewing various approaches to collecting qualitative self-report data.

UNSTRUCTURED AND SEMI-STRUCTURED SELF-REPORT TECHNIQUES

Unstructured or loosely structured self-report methods offer the researcher flexibility in gathering information from study participants. When these methods are used, the researcher generally does not have a specific set of questions that must be asked in a specific order and worded in a given way. Instead, the researcher starts with some general questions or topics and allows the respondents (or **informants,** as they are often called in such studies) to tell their stories in a narrative fashion. Unstructured or semi-structured interviews, in other words, tend to be conversational and interactive in nature.

Investigations in almost all the qualitative traditions use unstructured approaches to gathering self-report data. Unstructured interviews encourage respondents to define the important dimensions of a phenomenon and to elaborate on what is relevant to them, rather than being guided by the investigator's a priori notions of relevance. Unstructured interviews should be the mode of choice when the researcher does not have a clear idea of what it is he or she does not know.

Types of Unstructured Self-Reports

Researchers use various approaches in collecting unstructured or semi-structured self-report data. The main methods are briefly described next.

1. **Completely unstructured interview.** When a researcher proceeds with no preconceived view of the content or flow of information to be gathered, he or she may conduct unstructured interviews with respondents. Unstructured interviews are conversational and typically are conducted in naturalistic settings. Their aim is to elucidate the respondents' perceptions of the world without imposing any of the researcher's views on them. A researcher using a completely unstructured approach may informally ask a broad question (sometimes called a **grand tour**

331

question) relating to the topic under investigation, such as, "Tell me about what happened when you first learned you had AIDS?" Subsequent questions are more focused and are guided by responses to the broad question. Ethnographic and phenomenologic studies generally rely heavily on unstructured interviews.

2. **Focused interview.** A researcher often wants to be sure that a given set of topics is covered in interviews with participants. In a focused or **semi-structured interview**, the interviewer uses a list of areas or questions to be covered with each respondent; the list is referred to as a **topic guide**. The interviewer's function is to encourage participants to talk freely about all the topics on the list and to record the responses, usually by tape recorder. Focused interviews are the most widely used method of collecting unstructured self-report data.

3. **Focus group interview.** A variant of the focused interview is the focus group interview, a technique that is becoming increasingly popular in the study of some health problems. In a focus group interview, a group of usually 5 to 15 people is assembled for a group discussion. Typically, the people selected are a fairly homogeneous group to promote a comfortable group dynamic. The interviewer (often called a **moderator**) guides the discussion according to a written set of questions or topics to be covered. A major advantage of a group format is that it is efficient—the researcher obtains the viewpoints of many individuals in a short time. One disadvantage is that some people are uncomfortable about expressing their views in front of a group.

4. **Life histories.** Life histories are narrative self-disclosures about a person's life experiences. Anthropologists and ethnographers frequently use the life history approach to learn about cultural patterns.

With this approach, the researcher asks the respondents to provide, in chronologic sequence, a narration of their ideas and experiences regarding some theme, either orally or in writing. Leininger (1985) noted that comparative life histories are especially valuable for the study of the patterns and meanings of health and health care, especially among elderly people. Her highly regarded essay provides a protocol for obtaining a life health care history.

5. **Critical incidents.** The critical incidents technique is a method of gathering information about people's behaviors by examining specific incidents relating to the behavior under investigation. The technique, as the name suggests, focuses on a factual incident, which may be defined as an observable and integral episode of human behavior. The word critical means that the incident must have a discernible impact on some outcome; it must make either a positive or negative contribution to the accomplishment of some activity of interest. For example, if we were interested in understanding why patients do not always follow their medication regimen, we might ask a sample of patients the following questions: "Think of the last time you failed to take your medications as prescribed. What led up to the situation? Exactly what did you do? Why did you feel it would be all right to miss taking the medicine?" The technique differs from other self-report approaches in that it focuses on something specific about which the respondent can be expected to testify as an expert witness. As an example, Janson-Bjerklie, Ferketich, and Benner (1993) used the critical incidents technique to examine asthmatic episodes in a sample of asthmatic adults.

6. **Diaries.** Personal diaries have long been used as a source of data in historical research. It is also possible to generate new

data for a nonhistorical study by asking study participants to maintain a diary over a specified period. The diaries may be completely unstructured; for example, individuals who have undergone an organ transplantation could be asked simply to spend 10 minutes a day jotting down their thoughts and feelings. Frequently, however, subjects are requested to make entries into a diary regarding some specific aspect of their experience, sometimes in a semi-structured format. For example, studies of the effect of nutrition during pregnancy on fetal outcomes frequently require subjects to maintain a complete diary of everything they ate over a 1- to 2-week period. Nurse researchers have used health diaries to collect information about how people prevent illness, maintain health, experience morbidity, and treat health problems.

Gathering Unstructured Self-Report Data

In most cases, the primary purpose of gathering unstructured self-report data is to enable the researcher to construct reality in ways that are consistent with the constructions of the people being studied. This goal requires the researcher to take steps to overcome communication barriers and to enhance the flow of meaning. An important issue is that the researcher and the respondents should have a common vocabulary. If the researcher is studying a different culture or a subgroup that uses distinctive terms or slang, efforts should be made even before data collection to understand those terms and their nuances.

Although unstructured interviews are conversational in nature, this does not mean that they should be entered into casually. The conversations are purposeful ones that require advance thought and preparation. For example, careful thought should be given to the wording of questions. To the extent possible, the word-

ing should make sense to the respondent and reflect his or her world view.

In addition to being a good questioner, the interviewer must be a good listener. Only by attending carefully to what the respondent is saying can the in-depth interviewer develop appropriate follow-up questions. Even when a topic guide is used, the interviewer must not let the flow of dialogue be bound by those questions. In unstructured interviews on a particular theme, many questions that appear on a topic guide are answered spontaneously over the course of the interview, usually out of sequence.

The researcher generally prepares for the interview by developing (mentally or in writing) the broad questions to be asked, and often by practicing the interview with a stand-in respondent. The researcher must also prepare respondents for the interview by putting them at ease insofar as is possible. Part of this process involves sharing pertinent information about the study (e.g., about the study aims and protection of confidentiality). Another part of this process is using the first few minutes for pleasantries and ice-breaking exchanges of conversation before the actual questioning begins.

Unstructured interviews are typically long—sometimes lasting up to several hours. Researchers often find that the respondents' construction of their experience only begins to emerge after lengthy, in-depth dialogues. Recording such abundant information can be handled in various ways. Some researchers take sketchy notes as the interview progresses, filling in the details as soon as is practical after the interview is completed. However, the generally preferred method is to tape record the interviews for later full transcription. Although some respondents balk or are overly self-conscious when their conversation is recorded, respondents typically forget about the presence of recording equipment after a few minutes. It is often useful to both tape record the interview and take notes during its progress (or immediately after its completion) to ensure the highest possible reliability of data.

The interviewer should also strive for a positive closure to the interview. In many cases, this involves providing the respondents with a summary of the important features of the interview, giving them ample opportunity to clarify, refine, or correct the interviewer's summary.

Evaluation of Unstructured Approaches

Unstructured interviews are an extremely flexible approach to gathering data and, in many research contexts, offer distinct advantages. In clinical situations, for example, it may be appropriate to let individuals talk freely about their problems and concerns, allowing them to take much of the initiative in directing the flow of information. In general, unstructured interviews are of greatest utility when a new area of research is being explored. In such situations, an unstructured approach may allow the investigator to ascertain what the basic issues or problems are, how sensitive or controversial the topic is, how easy it is to secure respondents' cooperation in discussing the issues, how individuals conceptualize and talk about the problems, and what range of opinions or behaviors exist that are relevant to the topic. Unstructured methods may also help elucidate the underlying meaning of a pattern or relationship repeatedly observed in more structured research.

On the other hand, unstructured methods are extremely time-consuming and demanding of the researcher's skill in analyzing and interpreting the resulting qualitative data. Samples tend to be small because of the quantity of information produced, so it may be difficult to know whether findings are reliable and could be generalized. Unstructured methods do not usually lend themselves to the rigorous testing of hypotheses concerning cause-and-effect relationships.

STRUCTURED SELF-REPORT INSTRUMENTS

A researcher using a structured approach always operates with a formal, written instrument, known as an **interview schedule**, when the questions are asked orally in either a face-to-face or telephone format. The instrument is called a **questionnaire** or sometimes an **SAQ** (**self-administered questionnaire**) when the respondents complete the instrument themselves, usually in a paper-and-pencil format but occasionally directly onto a computer. Some studies embed an SAQ into an interview schedule, with interviewers asking some questions orally but relying on respondents to answer others in writing.

Structured instruments consist of a set of questions (also known as **items**) in which the wording of both the question and, in most cases, the response alternatives is predetermined. When structured interviews or questionnaires are used, subjects are asked to respond to the same questions, in the same order, and they have the same set of options for their responses. Most nurse researchers who collect self-report data use instruments with a moderate to high degree of structure. In developing structured instruments, a great deal of effort is usually devoted to the content, form, and wording of the questions.

Question Form

Structured instruments themselves vary in their degree of structure through their combination of open-ended and closed-ended questions. **Open-ended questions** allow respondents to respond in their own words. The question, "What was the biggest problem you faced after your open-heart surgery?" is an example of an open-ended question. In questionnaires, the respondent is asked to give a written reply to open-ended items and, therefore, adequate space must be provided to permit a full response. In interviews, the interviewer is normally expected to quote the response verbatim or as closely as possible.

Closed-ended (or **fixed-alternative**) **questions** offer respondents a number of alternative replies, from which the subjects must choose the one that most closely matches the appropriate answer. The alternatives may range from the simple yes or no variety ("Have you smoked a cigarette within the past 24 hours?") to complex expressions of opinion or behavior.

Both open- and closed-ended questions have certain strengths and weaknesses. Good closed-ended items are often difficult to construct but easy to administer and, especially, to analyze. With closed-ended questions, the researcher needs only to tabulate the number of responses to each alternative to gain some understanding about what the sample as a whole thinks about an issue. The analysis of open-ended items, on the other hand, is often difficult and time-consuming. The procedure that is normally followed is the development of categories and the assignment of the open-ended responses to those categories. That is, the researcher essentially transforms the open-ended responses to fixed categories in a post hoc fashion so that tabulations can be made. This classification process takes considerable time and skill.

Closed-ended items are generally more efficient than open-ended questions in the sense that a respondent is normally able to complete more closed- than open-ended questions in a given amount of time. In questionnaires, subjects may be less willing to compose a written response than to check off or circle the appropriate alternative. With respondents who are unable to express themselves well verbally, closed-ended items have a distinct advantage. Furthermore, there are some types of questions that may seem less objectionable in closed form than in open form. Take the following example:

1. What was the gross annual income of your family last year?

2. In what range was your family's gross annual income last year?
   ( ) 1. under $25,000
   ( ) 2. $25,000 to $49,999
   ( ) 3. $50,000 to $74,999
   ( ) 4. $75,000 to $99,999
   ( ) 5. $100,000 or over

The second question is more likely to be answered by respondents because the range of options allows them a greater measure of privacy than the blunter open-ended question.

These various advantages of the fixed-alternative question are offset by some corresponding shortcomings. The major drawback of closed-ended questions lies in the possibility of the researcher neglecting or overlooking some potentially important responses. It is often difficult to see an issue from multiple points of view. The omission of possible alternatives can lead to inadequate understanding of the issues and to outright bias if respondents choose an alternative that misrepresents their position. When the area of research is relatively new, open-ended questions may be more suitable than closed-ended items for avoiding bias.

Another objection to closed-ended items is that they may be superficial. Open-ended questions allow for a richer and fuller perspective on the topic of interest, if the respondents are verbally expressive and cooperative. Some of this richness may be lost when the researcher later tabulates answers by developing a system of classification, but excerpts taken directly from the open-ended responses can be extremely valuable in a research report in imparting the flavor of the replies.

Finally, some respondents may object to being forced into choosing from among responses that do not reflect their opinions precisely. Open-ended questions give a lot of freedom to the respondent and, therefore, offer the possibility of spontaneity, which is unattainable when a set of responses is provided.

The decision to use open- and closed-ended questions is based on a number of important considerations, such as the sensitivity of the topic, the verbal ability of the respondents, the amount of time available, and so forth. Combinations of both types are highly recommended to offset the strengths and weaknesses of each. Questionnaires typically use fixed-alternative questions predominantly, to minimize the respondent's writing burden. Interview schedules, on the other hand, are more variable in their mixture of these two question types.

Specific Types of Closed-Ended Questions

It is often difficult to create good-quality closed-ended questions because the researcher must pay careful attention to the wording of the question and to the content, wording, and formatting of the response options. Nevertheless, the analytic advantages of closed-ended questions make it compelling to include them on structured instruments. Various types of closed-ended questions, many of which are illustrated in Table 14–1, are discussed below.

1. **Dichotomous questions** require the respondent to make a choice between two response alternatives, such as yes/no or male/female. Dichotomous questions are considered most appropriate for gathering factual information.

2. **Multiple-choice questions** offer more than two response alternatives. Dichotomous items often are considered too restrictive by respondents, who may resent being forced to see an issue as either yes or no. Graded alternatives are preferable for opinion or attitude questions because they give the researcher more information (intensity as well as direction of opinion) and because they give the respondent the opportunity to express a range of views. Multiple-choice questions most commonly offer three to seven alternatives.

3. **Cafeteria questions** are a special type of multiple-choice question that asks respondents to select a response that most closely corresponds to their view. The response options are generally full expressions of a position on the topic of interest.

4. **Rank-order questions** ask respondents to rank target concepts along some continuum, such as most favorable to least favorable or most to least important. Respondents are asked to assign a 1 to the concept that is most important, a 2 to the concept that is second in importance, and so on. Rank-order questions can be useful but need to be handled carefully because they are often misunderstood by respondents. Rank-order questions should not ask respondents to rank more than about 10 alternatives.

5. **Forced-choice questions** require respondents to choose between two alternative statements that represent polar positions or characteristics. Several personality tests use a forced-choice format.

6. **Rating questions** ask respondents to judge something along an ordered dimension. Rating questions are typically bipolar in nature, with the end points specifying the opposite extremes of a continuum. Rating questions require labeling of the end points, but sometimes intermediary points along the scale are also labeled. The number of gradations or points along the scale can vary but should always be an odd number, such as 7, 9, or 11, to allow for a neutral midpoint. (In the example in Table 14-1, the rating question has 11 points, numbered 0 to 10).

7. **Checklists** are items that encompass several questions on a topic and require the same response format. A checklist is often a two-dimensional arrangement in which a series of questions is listed along one dimension (usually vertically) and

TABLE 14-1   Examples of Closed-Ended Question Types

1. Dichotomous Question
   Have you ever been hospitalized?
   ( ) 1. Yes
   ( ) 2. No
2. Multiple-Choice Question
   How important is it to you to avoid a pregnancy at this time?
   ( ) 1. Extremely important
   ( ) 2. Very important
   ( ) 3. Somewhat important
   ( ) 4. Not at all important
3. Cafeteria Question
   People have different opinions about the use of estrogen-replacement therapy for women in menopause. Which of the following statements best represents your point of view?
   ( ) 1. Estrogen replacement is dangerous and should be totally banned.
   ( ) 2. Estrogen replacement may have some undesirable side effects that suggest the need for caution in its use.
   ( ) 3. I am undecided about my views on estrogen-replacement therapy.
   ( ) 4. Estrogen replacement has many beneficial effects that merit its promotion.
   ( ) 5. Estrogen replacement is a wonder cure that should be administered routinely to menopausal women.
4. Rank-Order Question
   People value different things about life. Below is a list of principles or ideas that are often cited when people are asked to name things they value most. Please indicate the order of importance of these values to you by placing a 1 beside the most important, 2 beside the next most important, and so forth.
   ( ) Achievement and success
   ( ) Family relationships
   ( ) Friendships and social interaction
   ( ) Health
   ( ) Money
   ( ) Religion
5. Forced-Choice Question
   Which statement most closely represents your point of view?
   ( ) 1. What happens to me is my own doing.
   ( ) 2. Sometimes I feel I don't have enough control over my life.
6. Rating Question
   On a scale from 0 to 10, where 0 means extremely dissatisfied and 10 means extremely satisfied, how satisfied are you with the nursing care you received during your hospitalization?
   Extremely dissatisfied   Extremely satisfied
           0   1   2   3   4   5   6   7   8   9   10

response alternatives are listed along the other. This two-dimensional character of checklists has led some people to call these **matrix questions**. Checklists are relatively efficient and easy for respondents to understand, but because they are difficult for an interviewer to read, they are used more frequently in self-administered questionnaires than in interviews. Figure 14-1 presents an example of a checklist.

8. **Calendar questions** are being used increasingly when researchers want to obtain retrospective information about the

Here are some characteristics of birth-control devices that are of varying importance to different people. How important a consideration has each of these been for you in choosing a birth-control method?

		Of Very Great Importance	Of Great Importance	Of Some Importance	Of No Importance
1.	Comfort				
2.	Cost				
3.	Ease of use				
4.	Effectiveness				
5.	Noninterference with spontaneity				
6.	Safety to you				
7.	Safety to partner				

Figure 14-1. Example of a checklist.

chronology of different events and activities in people's lives. Questions about start dates and stop dates of events are asked and recorded on a calendar grid, such as the one shown in Figure 14-2. Calendars are useful to respondents because they can often better reconstruct the dates of events when several events are recorded in juxtaposition.

9. **Visual analogue scales** (VASes) have come into increased use to measure subjective experiences, such as pain, fatigue, nausea, and dyspnea. The VAS is a straight line, the end anchors of which are labeled as the extreme limits of the sensation or feeling being measured. Subjects are asked to mark a point on the line corresponding to the amount of sensation experienced. Traditionally, the VAS line is 100 mm in length, which facilitates the derivation of a score from 0 to 100 through simple measurement of the distance from one end of the scale to the subject's mark on the line. An example of a VAS is presented in Figure 14-3.

Composite Scales

A **scale** is a device designed to assign a numeric score to people to place them on a continuum with respect to attributes being measured, like

a scale for measuring people's weight. Many studies that collect data through self-report use a composite psychosocial scale, the purpose of which is to discriminate quantitatively among people with different attitudes, fears, motives, perceptions, personality traits, and needs. Scales are generally created by combining several closed-ended items (such as those described in the previous section) into a single composite score. Scales are often incorporated into questionnaires and interview schedules, but they may be used independently. Many sophisticated scaling techniques have been developed, only two of which are discussed here.*

LIKERT SCALES

The most widely used scaling technique is the **Likert scale**, named after the psychologist Rensis Likert. A Likert scale consists of several declarative items that express a viewpoint on a

---

*Among the earliest types of attitude scale were the **Thurstone scales**, named after the psychologist L. L. Thurstone. The Thurstone approach to scaling is elaborate and time-consuming and has fallen into relative disuse. Another scaling method, developed by Louis Guttman in the 1940s, is known as the **Guttman** or **cumulative scales**. Advanced scaling procedures include ratio scaling, multidimensional scaling, and multiple scalogram analysis. Textbooks on psychological scaling and psychometric procedures should be consulted for more information about these alternative scaling strategies.

Pregnancy
(Code no. is Pregnancy no.)

Employment

1 = Employed

(Write in name of each employer)

Child Care

1 = Kindergarten / elementary school
2 = After/before school program
3 = Summer program/day camp
4 = Head Start
5 = Day care center/nursery school/ preschool
6 = Family day care/baby-sitter
7 = Grandparent
8 = Other relative
9 = Boyfriend/husband

(For each period, enter code in beginning month and end month, and connect with solid line)

Case # _____

	1999												2000												2001											
	JAN	FEB	MAR	APR	MAY	JUN	JUL	AUG	SEP	OCT	NOV	DEC	JAN	FEB	MAR	APR	MAY	JUN	JUL	AUG	SEP	OCT	NOV	DEC	JAN	FEB	MAR	APR	MAY	JUN	JUL	AUG	SEP	OCT	NOV	DEC
Pregnancy							1								1														2							2
Employment	1								1													1			Acme Insurance					1						
Employment (name)	Central Bank																																			
Child Care																						6	6		6											
Child Care																									7					7						

Figure 14-2. Example of a calendar grid (completed).

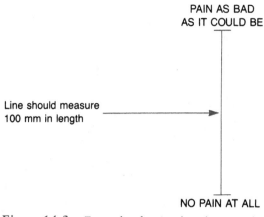

PAIN AS BAD
AS IT COULD BE

Line should measure
100 mm in length

NO PAIN AT ALL

Figure 14-3. Example of a visual analogue scale.

topic. Respondents are asked to indicate the degree to which they agree or disagree with the opinion expressed by the statement. Table 14-2 presents an illustrative six-item Likert scale for measuring attitudes toward the mentally ill. Ten to 15 statements are generally recommended for a good Likert scale; the example in Table 14-2 is shown only to illustrate key features. First, let us briefly discuss the procedure for constructing a Likert scale.

The first step is to develop a large pool of items or statements that clearly state different positions regarding the issue under consideration. Neutral statements or statements so extreme that virtually everyone would agree or disagree with them should be avoided. The aim is to spread out people with various attitudes or traits along a continuum. About equal numbers of positively and negatively worded statements should be chosen to avoid biasing the responses.*

There are differences of opinion concerning the appropriate number of response alternatives to use. Likert used five categories of agreement/disagreement responses, such as are shown in

---

*The advanced student who is developing a Likert scale for general use should consult a reference on psychometric procedures, such as *Psychometric Theory* by Nunnally and Bernstein (1994).

Table 14-2. Some investigators prefer a seven-point scale, adding the alternatives "slightly agree" and "slightly disagree." There is also a diversity of opinion about the advisability of including an explicit category labeled "uncertain." Some researchers argue that the inclusion of this option makes the task less objectionable to people who cannot make up their minds or have no strong feelings about an issue. Others, however, feel that the use of this undecided category encourages fence-sitting, or the tendency to not take sides. Investigators who do not give respondents an explicit alternative for indecision or uncertainty proceed in principle as though they were working with a five- or seven-point scale, even though only four or six alternatives are given: Nonresponse to a given statement is *scored* as though the neutral response were there and had been chosen.

After the Likert scale is administered to subjects, the responses must be scored. Typically, the responses are scored in such a way that endorsement of positively worded statements and nonendorsement of negatively worded statements are assigned a higher score. Table 14-2 illustrates what this procedure involves. The first statement is positively phrased so that agreement indicates a favorable attitude toward the mentally ill. The researcher, therefore, would assign a higher score to a person agreeing with this statement than to someone disagreeing with it. Because the item has five response alternatives, a score of 5 would be given to someone strongly agreeing, 4 to someone agreeing, and so forth. The responses of two hypothetical respondents are shown by a check or an X, and their scores for each item are shown in the right-hand columns of the table. Person 1, who agreed with the first statement, is given a score of 4, whereas person 2, who strongly disagreed, is given a score of 1. The second statement is negatively worded, and so the scoring is reversed—a 1 is assigned to those who strongly agree, and so forth. This reversal is necessary so that a high score will consistently reflect positive attitudes toward the mentally ill. When each item has been handled in

TABLE 14-2 Example of a Likert Scale to Measure Attitudes Toward the Mentally Ill

DIRECTION OF SCORING*	ITEM	RESPONSES†					SCORE	
		SA	A	?	D	SD	Person 1 (✓)	Person 2 (X)
+	1. People who have had a mental illness can become normal, productive citizens after treatment.		✓			X	4	1
−	2. People who have been patients in mental hospitals should not be allowed to have children.		X		✓		5	3
−	3. The best way to handle patients in mental hospitals is to restrict their activity as much as possible.		X		✓		4	2
+	4. Many patients in mental hospitals develop normal, healthy relationships with staff members and other patients.			✓	X		3	2
+	5. There should be an expanded effort to get the mentally ill out of institutional settings and back into their communities.	✓				X	5	1
−	6. Because the mentally ill cannot be trusted, they should be kept under constant guard.		X			✓	5	2
	TOTAL SCORE						26	11

*Researchers would not indicate the direction of scoring on a Likert scale administered to subjects. The scoring direction is indicated in this table for illustrative purposes only.
†SA, strongly agree; A, agree; ?, uncertain; D, disagree; SD, strongly disagree.

this manner, a person's total score can be determined by adding together individual item scores. Because total scores are computed in this manner, the term **summated rating scale** is sometimes used for such scales. The total scores of the two hypothetical respondents to the items in Table 14-2 are shown at the bottom of that table. These scores reflect a considerably more positive attitude toward the mentally ill on the part of person 1 than person 2.

The summation feature of Likert scales makes it possible to make fine discriminations among people with different points of view. A single Likert question allows people to be put into only five categories. A six-item scale, such as the one in Table 14-2, permits much finer gradation—from a minimum possible score of 6 (6×1) to a maximum possible score of 30 (6×5).

Likert scales are popular among nurse researchers. Coates (1997), for example, developed a Likert-type scale to assess nurses' caring efficacy. Kidd and Huddleston (1994) developed a 10-item Driving Practices Scale to measure risky driving. The items in their scale were developed on the basis of unstructured interviews with hospitalized trauma patients who had sustained injuries while driving.

SEMANTIC DIFFERENTIAL SCALES

Another technique that can be encountered in the research literature is known as the **semantic differential (SD)**. With the SD, the respondent is asked to rate a given concept (e.g., primary nursing, team nursing) on a series of bipolar adjectives, such as effective/ineffective, good/bad, important/unimportant, or strong/weak. Respondents are asked to place a check at the appropriate point on 7-point rating scales that extend from one extreme of the dimension to the other. An example of the format for an SD is shown in Figure 14-4.

The semantic differential has the advantages of being highly flexible and easy to construct. The concept being rated can be virtually anything—a person, place, situation, abstract idea, controversial issue, and so forth. Typically, several concepts are included on the

same schedule so that comparisons can be made across concepts (e.g., male nurse, female nurse, male physician, and female physician).

The researcher also has considerable freedom in constructing the bipolar scales. However, two considerations should guide the selection of the adjectives. First, the adjectives should be appropriate for the concepts being used and for the information being sought. The addition of the adjective pair tall/short in Figure 14-4 would add little understanding of how people react to the role of nurse practitioners.

The second consideration in the selection of adjective pairs is the extent to which the adjectives are measuring the same dimension or aspect of the concept. Osgood, Suci, and Tannenbaum (1957), through extensive research with SD scales, found that adjective pairs tend to cluster along three principal and independent dimensions that these authors labeled evaluation, potency, and activity. The most important group of adjectives includes those that are evaluative, such as effective/ineffective, valuable/worthless, good/bad, fair/unfair, and so forth. Potency adjectives include strong/weak and large/small, and examples of activity adjectives are active/passive and fast/slow. The reason these three dimensions need to be considered

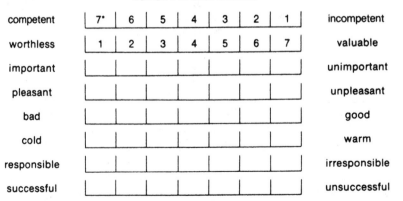

*The score values would not be printed on the form administered to actual subjects. The numbers are presented here solely for the purpose of illustrating how semantic differentials are scored.

Figure 14-4. Example of a semantic differential.

separately is that a person's evaluative rating of a concept is independent of the activity or potency ratings of that concept. For example, two people who associate high levels of activity with the concept of nurse practitioner might have divergent views with regard to how valuable they perceive the concept of nurse practitioner. The researcher must decide whether to represent all three of these dimensions or whether only one or two are needed. Each dimension or aspect must be scored separately.

The scoring procedure for SD responses is essentially the same as for Likert scales. Scores from 1 to 7 are assigned to each bipolar scale response, with higher scores generally associated with the positively worded adjective. Responses are then summed across the bipolar scales to yield a total score.

Semantic differentials have been used in a number of nursing studies. For example, Preski and Walker (1997) examined maternal identity in relation to the behavioral problems of 2- to 3-year-old children, and they developed an 11-item SD scale to measure maternal identity. Ganong (1993) developed a 40-item SD instrument called the First Impression Questionnaire, which was designed to measure attitudes toward an individual. He used the instrument to study whether nurses stereotype pregnant patients on the basis of their marital status.

EXISTING SELF-REPORT SCALES AND PSYCHOLOGICAL MEASURES

Many social psychological states and traits are of interest to those engaged in clinical nursing research, and many self-report scales have been developed to measure them, often using a Likert-type format. Table 14-3 illustrates a number of important constructs that have been measured with an existing composite scale by nurse researchers.

A special suggested readings section at the end of this chapter provides references for locating existing self-report scales. Additionally, both the nursing and nonnursing indexes and

abstracting services should be consulted for references to studies that have developed scales. The Cumulative Index to Nursing and Allied Health Literature (CINAHL) database includes information on the scales used in research studies. Information on standardized tests and psychological measures can be retrieved through a computerized literature search of the database called *Mental Measurement Yearbook*, produced by the Buros Institute of Mental Measurements, or through *Health and Psychosocial Instruments Online*.

Developing Structured Instruments

A careful, well-developed interview schedule or questionnaire cannot be prepared in minutes or even in hours. A researcher interested in designing a useful and accurate instrument must devote considerable time to analyzing the research requirements and attending to minute details. The steps for developing a structured instrument follow closely the steps outlined in Chapter 13. However, a few additional considerations should be mentioned.

Once data needs have been identified, it is often useful to cluster related constructs together as a basis for separate **modules** or areas of questioning in the instrument. For example, an interview schedule may consist of a module on demographic information, another on health symptoms, a third on stressful life events, and a fourth on health-promoting activities.

Before actually developing questions or selecting existing scales, it is necessary to decide whether to collect the data by means of interview or questionnaire because questions must often be worded somewhat differently depending on the mode of administration. The advantages and disadvantages of each are described in a later section.

Some thought needs to be given to the sequencing of modules and questions within modules to arrive at an order that is psychologically meaningful to respondents and encourages candor and cooperation. For exam-

TABLE 14-3	Examples of Concepts Frequently Measured With Composite Scales in Nursing Studies	
CONCEPT	**RESEARCH EXAMPLE REFERENCE**	**INSTRUMENT USED**
Anxiety	Collins & Rice, 1997	State-Trait Anxiety Inventory (STAI)
Coping	Houston, Eagen, Freeborg, & Dougherty, 1997 Hahn, Brooks, & Hartsough, 1993	Coping Resources Inventory (CRI) Lazarus Ways of Coping Scale
Depression	Flynn, 1997 Buchanan, Cowan, Burr, Waldron, & Kogan, 1993	Center for Epidemiological Studies Depression Scale (CES-D) Beck Depression Inventory (BDI)
Family functioning	Ford-Gilboe, 1997	Family Adaptability & Cohesion Evaluation Scales (FACES III)
Fatigue	Neuberger, et al., 1997	Multidimensional Assessment of Fatigue
Health practices	Flynn, 1997	Personal Lifestyle Questionnaire (PLQ)
Hope	Zorn, 1997	Miller Hope Scale (MHS)
Life satisfaction	Friedman, 1997 Topp & Stevenson, 1994	Satisfaction with Life Scale (SWLS) Life Satisfaction Scale (LSS)
Mood states	Neuberger, et al., 1997 Houston, Eagen, Freeborg, & Dougherty, 1997	Profile of Mood States (POMS) Multiple Affect Adjective Checklist (MAACL)
Pain	Neill, 1993 White, LeFort, Amsel, & Jeans, 1997	McGill Pain Questionnaire (MPQ) McGill Pain Questionnaire-Short Form (SF-MPQ)
Quality of life	LoBiondo-Wood, Williams, Wood, & Shaw, 1997 Nickel, et al., 1996	Quality of Life Index (QLI) Quality of Well-Being Scale (QWB)
Self-esteem	Flynn, 1997 Draucker, 1997	Rosenberg Self-Esteem Scale (RSE) Coopersmith Self-Esteem Inventory
Social Support	Ford-Gilboe, 1997 Richmond, 1997	Personal Resources Questionnaire (PRQ85) Social Support Questionnaire (SSQ)

(continued)

TABLE 14-3	Examples of Concepts Frequently Measured With Composite Scales in Nursing Studies (Continued)		
CONCEPT	**RESEARCH EXAMPLE REFERENCE**		**INSTRUMENT USED**
Stress	Beaton, Murphy, Pike, & Corneil, 1997 Woods, Lentz, Mitchell, Heitkemper, & Shaver, 1997		Symptoms of Stress Inventory (SOS) Life Experiences Survey (LES)
Symptoms of Distress	Collins & Rice, 1997 Samarel, Fawcett, & Tulman, 1997		Symptom Checklist-90 (SCL-90) Symptom Distress Scale (SDS)

ple, the schedule should begin with questions that are interesting and motivating. The instrument also needs to be arranged in such a way that distortions and biases are minimized. The possibility that earlier questions might influence replies to the subsequent questions should be kept in mind. Whenever both general and specific questions about a topic are to be included, the general question should be placed first to avoid putting ideas into people's heads.

Every instrument should be prefaced by introductory comments about the nature and purpose of the study. In interviews, the introductory comments would normally be read to the respondents by the interviewer and often incorporated into an informed consent form. In questionnaires, the introduction usually takes the form of a **cover letter** that accompanies the instrument. The introduction should be given considerable care and attention because it represents the first point of contact between the researcher and potential respondents. An example of a cover letter accompanying a mailed questionnaire is presented in Figure 14–5.

When a first draft of the instrument is in reasonably good order, discuss it critically with individuals who are knowledgeable about the construction of questionnaires and

with people who are familiar with the substantive content of your schedule. The instrument also should be reviewed by someone who is capable of detecting technical difficulties, such as spelling mistakes, grammatical errors, and so forth. When these various people have provided feedback, a revised version of the instrument can be pretested. The pretest should be administered to individuals who are similar to those who will ultimately participate in the study. Ordinarily, 10 to 20 pretested schedules are sufficient.*

ADMINISTRATION OF SELF-REPORT INSTRUMENTS

Interview schedules and questionnaires require different skills and different considerations in their administration. Both the quantity and the quality of the data gathered are influenced by the data collection procedures and the competency of the research personnel. In this section,

---

*If a new composite scale is being developed, a much larger pretest sample is advisable.

Dear _____ :

    We are conducting a study to examine how women who are approaching retirement age (age 55 to 65) feel about various issues relating to health and health care. This study, which is sponsored by the State Department of Health, will enable health-care providers to better meet the needs of women in your age group. Would you please assist us in this study by completing the enclosed questionnaire? Your opinions and experiences are very important to us and are needed to give an accurate picture of the health-related needs of women in the greater Middletown area.

    Your name was selected at random from a list of residents in your community. The questionnaire is completely anonymous, so you are not asked to put your name on it or to identify yourself in any way. We therefore hope that you will feel comfortable about giving your honest opinions. If you prefer not to answer any particular question, please feel perfectly free to leave it blank. Please do answer the questions if you can, though, and if you have any comments or concerns about any question, just write your comments in the margin.

    A postage-paid return envelope has been provided for your convenience. We hope that you will take a few minutes to complete and return the questionnaire to us—it should take only about 15 minutes of your time. To analyze the information in a timely fashion, we ask that you return the questionnaire to us by May 12.

    Thank you very much for your cooperation and assistance in this endeavor. If you would like a copy of the summary of the results of this study, please check the box at the bottom of page 10.

Figure 14-5. Fictitious example of a cover letter for a mailed questionnaire.

we examine the problems involved in instrument administration and ways of handling those difficulties.

Collecting Interview Data

The quality of interview data depends to a great extent on the proficiency of the interviewers. Interviewers for large survey organizations receive extensive general training in addition to specific training for individual studies. Although this introductory book cannot adequately cover all the principles of good interviewing, it can identify some of the major issues.

A primary task of the interviewer is to put respondents at ease so that they will feel comfortable in expressing their honest opinions.

The respondents' personal reaction to the interviewer can seriously affect their willingness to participate. Interviewers, therefore, should always be punctual (if an appointment has been made), courteous, and friendly. The interviewer should strive to appear unbiased and to create a permissive atmosphere that encourages candor. All opinions of the respondents should be accepted as natural—the interviewer generally should not express surprise, disapproval, or even approval.

When a structured interview schedule is being used, interviewers should follow the wording of the questions in the schedule precisely. Similarly, interviewers should not offer spontaneous explanations of what the questions mean. Repetitions of the questions are usually adequate to dispel any misunderstanding, particularly if the instrument has been properly pretested. The interviewer should not read the questions from the schedule mechanically. A naturalistic, conversational tone is essential in building rapport with respondents, and this tone is impossible to achieve if the interviewer is not thoroughly familiar with the questions.

When closed-ended questions with lengthy or complicated response alternatives are asked, or when a series of questions using the same alternative is posed, the interviewer should hand the subjects a **show card** that lists the response options. Individuals cannot be expected to remember detailed unfamiliar material and are sometimes inclined to choose the last alternative if they cannot recall earlier ones. Closed-ended items can be recorded by checking or circling the appropriate alternative (or, with computer-assisted personal interviewing [CAPI], by entering a code onto a computer), but responses to open-ended questions need to be recorded in full or tape recorded for later transcription. The interviewer should not paraphrase or summarize the respondent's reply.

Interviewers typically find that obtaining complete and relevant responses to open-ended questions is not always an easy matter.

Respondents often reply to seemingly straightforward questions with irrelevant discussions or partial answers, or they may say, "I don't know" to avoid giving their opinions on sensitive topics or to stall while they think over the question. In such cases, the job of the interviewer is to probe. The purpose of a **probe** is to elicit more useful information from a respondent than was volunteered during the first reply. A probe can take many forms: sometimes it involves a repetition of the original question, and sometimes it is a long pause intended to communicate to respondents that they should continue. Frequently, it is necessary to encourage a more complete response by a nondirective supplementary question, such as, "How is that?" The interviewer must be careful to use only *neutral* probes that do not influence the content of the subject's response. Box 14-1 gives some examples of neutral, nondirective probes that are used by professional interviewers to get more complete responses to questions. The ability to probe well is perhaps the greatest test of an interviewer's skill. To know when to probe and how to select the best probes, the interviewer must comprehend fully the purpose of each question and the type of information being

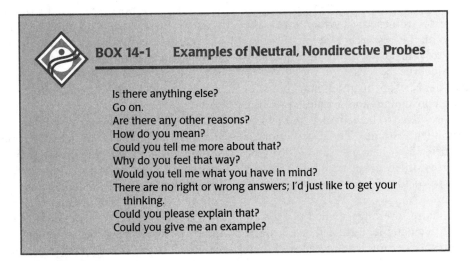

BOX 14-1   Examples of Neutral, Nondirective Probes

Is there anything else?
Go on.
Are there any other reasons?
How do you mean?
Could you tell me more about that?
Why do you feel that way?
Would you tell me what you have in mind?
There are no right or wrong answers; I'd just like to get your thinking.
Could you please explain that?
Could you give me an example?

sought, as spelled out in the question-by-question instructions (Q-by-Qs).

The guidelines for handling telephone interviews are essentially the same as those for face-to-face interviews, although additional effort usually is required to build rapport over the telephone. In both cases, the interviewer should strive to make the interview a pleasant and satisfying experience in which respondents are made to feel as though the information they are providing is important.

Collecting Questionnaire Data

Self-administered questionnaires can be distributed in a number of ways. The most convenient procedure is to distribute the questionnaires to a group of respondents who complete the instrument together at the same time. This approach has the obvious advantages of maximizing the number of completed questionnaires and allowing the researcher to clarify any possible misunderstandings about the instrument. Group administrations are often possible in educational settings and might also be feasible in some hospital or community situations.

Personal presentation of questionnaires to individual respondents is another alternative. Personal contact with respondents has been found to have a positive effect on the rate of questionnaires returned. Furthermore, the availability of the researcher or an assistant can be an advantage in terms of explaining and clarifying the purposes of the study or particular items. This method may be relatively time-consuming and expensive if the questionnaires have to be delivered and picked up at respondents' homes. The distribution of questionnaires in a clinical setting, on the other hand, is often inexpensive and efficient and likely to yield a high rate of completed questionnaires.

Questionnaires are often mailed to respondents. A problematic feature of this approach is that the **response rates** tend to be low. When only a small subsample of respondents return

their questionnaires, it may be unreasonable to assume that those who did respond were somehow typical of the sample as a whole. In other words, the researcher is faced with the possibility that those individuals who did not complete a questionnaire would, as a group, have answered the questions differently from those who did return it.

If the response rate is high, the risk of serious response bias may be negligible. A response rate greater than 60% is probably sufficient for most purposes, but lower response rates are common. The researcher generally should attempt to discover how representative the respondents are, relative to the target population, in terms of basic demographic characteristics, such as age, gender, marital status, and the like. This comparison may lead the researcher to conclude that respondents and nonrespondents are similar enough to assume the absence of serious biases. If demographic differences are found, the investigator will at least be in a position to make some inferences about the direction of the biases.

The response rate can be affected by the manner in which the questionnaires are designed and mailed. The physical appearance of the questionnaire can influence its appeal, so some thought should be given to the layout, quality and color of paper, method of reproduction, and typographic quality of the instrument. The standard procedure for distributing the questionnaire is to include with the instrument a cover letter and a stamped, addressed return envelope. Failure to enclose a return envelope could have a serious effect on the response rate.

The use of **follow-up reminders** has been found to be effective in achieving higher response rates for mailed questionnaires. This procedure involves the mailing of additional letters urging nonrespondents to complete and return their forms. Follow-up letters or notices are typically sent 2 to 3 weeks after the initial mailing. Sometimes, the reminder simply involves a letter of encouragement to nonrespondents. It is preferable, however, to enclose a second copy of the questionnaire with the reminder letter because many nonrespondents will have misplaced the original copy. Telephone follow-ups can be successful, but they are costly and involve a considerable amount of time. With anonymous questionnaires, the investigator may be unable to distinguish between respondents and nonrespondents for the purpose of sending follow-up letters. In such a situation, the simplest procedure is to send out a follow-up letter to the entire sample, thanking those individuals who have already answered and asking others to cooperate.

As questionnaires are returned, the investigator should keep a log of the incoming receipts on a daily basis. Each questionnaire should be opened, checked for usability, and assigned an identification number. Such record-keeping will assist the researcher in assembling the results, monitoring the response rate, and making decisions about the timing of follow-up mailings and cutoff dates.

The problems associated with mailed questionnaires cannot be handled using interpersonal skills. Building rapport in a questionnaire situation to enhance the response rate is difficult and often depends on attention to details. Even though these procedural matters may seem trivial, the success of the project may depend on their careful execution.

QUESTIONNAIRES VERSUS INTERVIEWS: AN ASSESSMENT

Self-administered questionnaires offer a number of advantages over personal interviews, but they have some drawbacks as well. Let us consider some of the following strong points of questionnaires:

1. *Cost.* Questionnaires, relative to interviews, are generally much less costly and require less time and energy to administer. Group-administered questionnaires are clearly the least expensive and time-consuming of any procedure. With a fixed amount of funds or time, a larger and more geographically diverse sample can usually be obtained with mailed questionnaires than with interviews.

2. *Anonymity.* Questionnaires, unlike interview schedules, offer the possibility of complete anonymity. Sometimes, a guarantee of anonymity is crucial in obtaining candid responses, particularly if the questions are of a highly personal or sensitive nature. Anonymous questionnaires often result in a higher proportion of socially unacceptable responses (i.e., responses that place the respondent in an unfavorable light) than face-to-face interviews.

3. *Interviewer bias.* The absence of an interviewer ensures that there will be no interviewer bias. Ideally, an interviewer is a neutral agent through whom questions and answers are passed. Studies have shown, however, that this ideal is difficult to achieve. Respondents and interviewers interact as humans, and this interaction can affect the subject's responses. This problem clearly is not present for questionnaires.

Despite these advantages, the strengths of interviews far outweigh those of questionnaires. It is true that interviews are costly, prevent respondent anonymity, and are subject to interviewer biases. Nevertheless, the numerous advantages described as follows have led many researchers to conclude that interviews are superior to questionnaires for most research purposes:

1. *Response rates.* The response rate tends to be high in face-to-face interviews. People are apparently more reluctant to refuse to talk to an interviewer who is directly in front of them than to discard or ignore a questionnaire. A well-designed and properly conducted interview study normally achieves a response rate in the vicinity of 80% to 90%. Because

nonresponse is not a random process, low response rates may introduce serious biases.

2. *Audience.* Many individuals simply cannot fill out a questionnaire. Examples include young children and blind, elderly, illiterate, or uneducated individuals. Interviews, on the other hand, are normally feasible with most people.

3. *Clarity.* Interviews offer some protection against ambiguous or confusing questions. The interviewer can determine whether questions have been misunderstood and can clarify matters. In questionnaires, items that are misinterpreted may go undetected by the researchers, and thus the responses may lead to erroneous conclusions.

4. *Depth of questioning.* The information obtained from questionnaires tends to be somewhat more superficial than interview data, partly because questionnaires ordinarily contain a preponderance of closed-ended items. Open-ended questions often engender resentment among questionnaire respondents, who dislike having to compose and write out a reply. Much of the richness and complexity of the human experience can be lost if closed-ended items are used exclusively. Furthermore, interviewers can enhance the quality of the self-report data through probing.

5. *Missing information.* Respondents are less likely to give "I don't know" responses or to leave a question unanswered in an interview situation than on questionnaires.

6. *Order of questions.* In an interview, the researcher has strict control over the order of presentation of the questions. Questionnaire respondents are at liberty to skip around from one section of the instrument to another. It is possible that a different ordering of questions from the one originally intended could bias the responses.

7. *Sample control.* Interviews permit greater control over the sample in the sense that the interviewer knows whether the person being interviewed is the intended respondent. It is not unusual to have individuals who receive questionnaires pass the instrument on to a friend, relative, secretary, and so forth. This kind of activity can change the characteristics of the sample.

8. *Supplementary data.* Finally, face-to-face interviews have an advantage in their ability to produce additional data through observation. The interviewer is in a position to observe or judge the respondents' level of understanding, degree of cooperativeness, social class, lifestyle, and so forth. These kinds of information can be useful in interpreting the responses.

Many of the advantages of face-to-face interviews also apply to telephone interviews. Complicated or detailed schedules or ones with sensitive questions are not well suited for telephone interviewing, but for relatively brief instruments, the telephone interview is more economical than personal interviews and tends to yield a higher response rate than mailed questionnaires.

RESPONSE BIASES

Although self-reports represent a powerful mechanism for obtaining data, researchers who use this approach should always be aware of the risk of **response biases**—that is, the tendency of some respondents to distort their responses. Perhaps the most pervasive problem is a person's tendency to present a favorable image of himself or herself. The **social desirability response bias** refers to the tendency of some individuals to misrepresent their responses consistently by giving answers that are congruent with prevailing social mores. This problem is often difficult to combat. Subtle, indirect, and delicately worded questioning sometimes can help to alleviate this response bias. The creation of a permissive atmosphere and provisions for respondent anonymity also encourage frankness.

Some response biases are most commonly observed in connection with composite scales. These biases are sometimes referred to as **response sets**. Scale scores are seldom entirely accurate and pure measures of the critical variable. A number of irrelevant factors are also being measured at the same time. Because these response-set factors can sometimes influence or bias responses to a considerable degree, investigators who construct scales must attempt to eliminate them or reduce their impact.

Extreme responses are an example of such a response set. This biasing factor results from the fact that some individuals consistently express their attitudes in terms of extreme response alternatives (e.g., "strongly agree"), and others characteristically endorse middle-range alternatives. This response style is a distorting influence in that extreme responses may not necessarily signify the most intense attitude toward the phenomenon under investigation. There appears to be little that a researcher can do to counteract this bias, although there are procedures for detecting its existence.

Some people have been found to agree with statements regardless of the content. In the research literature, these people are sometimes referred to as **yea-sayers**, and the bias is known as the **acquiescence response set**. A less common problem is the opposite tendency for other individuals, called **nay-sayers**, to disagree with statements independently of the question content. Although there apparently are some people for whom such tendencies are stable and enduring personality characteristics, acquiescence and its opposite counterpart can often be avoided or minimized by the simple strategy of **counterbalancing** positively and negatively worded statements.

The effects of response biases should not be exaggerated, but it is important that researchers who are using self-reports give these issues some thought. If an instrument or scale is being developed for general use by other researchers, it is recommended that evidence be gathered demonstrating that the scale is sufficiently free from the influence of response biases to measure the critical variable.

TIPS FOR DEVELOPING SELF-REPORT INSTRUMENTS

Although we all are accustomed to asking questions, the proper phrasing of questions in a research study is a delicate task. In this section, we provide some tips on the wording of questions and response options for self-report instruments. Although some of the advice is specific to structured self-reports, many of the suggestions are equally appropriate for unstructured interviews.

Tips for Wording the Questions

In wording questions for research purposes, the researcher must keep four important considerations in mind.

1. *Clarity.* Questions should be worded clearly and unambiguously—often a difficult task because respondents do not necessarily understand what information is needed and do not always have the same mind-set as the researcher.
2. *Ability of respondents to give information.* The researcher needs to consider whether the respondents can be expected to understand the question or are qualified to provide meaningful information.
3. *Bias.* Questions should be worded in a manner that will minimize the risk of response biases.
4. *Sensitive information.* In developing questions, the researcher should strive to be courteous, considerate, and sensitive to the needs and rights of respondents,

especially when asking questions of a highly private nature.

Here are some specific suggestions to keep in mind with regard to these four considerations:

- Clarify in your own mind the information that you are trying to obtain. The question, "When do you usually eat your evening meal?" might elicit such responses as "around 6 p.m." or "when my son gets home from soccer practice," or "when I feel like cooking." The question itself contains no words that are difficult, but the question is unclear because the intent of the researcher is not apparent.
- Try to state your questions in the affirmative rather than the negative, and particularly avoid sentences with double negatives.
- Avoid long sentences or phrases, and avoid technical terms if more common terms are equally appropriate. Try to use words that are simple enough for the *least* educated respondents in your sample. Do not assume that even members of your own profession will have extensive knowledge on all aspects of nursing and medical terminology.
- Avoid "double-barreled" questions that contain two distinct ideas or concepts. The statement, "The mentally ill are essentially incapable of caring for themselves and should, therefore, be denied any responsibilities or rights," might lead to conflicts of opinion in a single person, who might only agree with one part of the statement.
- Do not assume that respondents will be aware of or informed about issues or questions in which you are interested. Furthermore, avoid giving the impression that respondents *ought* to have the information. Questions on complex or specialized issues can be worded in such a way that a respondent will be comfortable admitting ignorance (e.g., "Many people

have not had an opportunity to learn much about the physiologic side-effects of oral contraceptives, but some people have picked up information on this subject. Do you happen to know of any such side effects?"). Another approach is to preface a question by a short statement of explanation about terminology or issues.

- Avoid leading questions that suggest a particular kind of answer. A question such as, "Do you agree that nurse–midwives play an indispensable role in the health team?" is not neutral.
- State a range of alternatives within the question itself when possible. For instance, the question, "Do you normally prefer to get up early in the morning on weekends?" is more suggestive of the "right" answer than "Do you normally prefer to get up early in the morning or to sleep late on weekends?"
- For questions that deal with socially unacceptable behavior or attitudes (e.g., excessive drinking habits, noncompliance with physician's instructions, and the like), closed-ended questions are often useful because it is easier to check off having engaged in socially disapproved actions than to verbalize those actions in response to an open-ended question. Furthermore, when the unacceptable behavior is actually presented to respondents as an option, they are more likely to realize that they are not alone in their behaviors or attitudes, and admissions of nonstandard behavior becomes less difficult.
- Impersonal wording of a question is sometimes useful in minimizing embarrassment and encouraging honesty. To illustrate this point, compare these two statements with which respondents would be asked to agree or disagree: (1) "I am personally dissatisfied with the nursing care I received during my hospitalization," (2) "The quality of nursing care in this hospital is unsatisfactory." A respondent might feel more comfortable about

admitting dissatisfaction with nursing care in the less personally worded second question.

- Researchers who are concerned about respondents' possible confusion or misinterpretation sometimes conduct **cognitive questioning** during the pretest phase of instrument development. Cognitive questioning invites respondents to think aloud about the meaning of the question and what comes to mind when they hear a question. For example, if we wanted to ask a question such as, "Are you exempt from this facility's age restrictions?" but we weren't sure if the respondent understood the concept of an exemption, we might in the pretest ask, "Please tell me in your own words what an exemption is. What did you have in mind when we asked you if you were exempt from the age restrictions?"

Tips for Preparing Response Alternatives

If closed-ended questions are used, the researcher also needs to make decisions about the form that the response alternatives will take. Below are some suggestions for preparing alternatives to closed-ended items.

- The responses options should adequately cover all the significant alternatives. If respondents are forced to choose a response from among options provided by the researcher, they should feel reasonably comfortable with the available options. As a safety measure, the researcher can have as one response option a phrase such as "other—please specify."
- The alternatives should be mutually exclusive (e.g., the following categories for a question on a person's age are *not* mutually exclusive: 30 years or younger, 30–40 years, 40–50 years, 50 years or older).
- There should be some underlying rationale for the order in which the alterna-

tives are presented to the respondent. Often, the options can be placed in order of decreasing or increasing favorability, agreement, or intensity. When the respondent is asked to choose from options that have no natural sequence or order, alphabetic ordering of the alternatives is less likely to lead the respondent to a particular response (e.g., see question 4 in Table 14-1).

- The response alternatives should not be too lengthy. One sentence or phrase for each alternative should almost always be sufficient to express a concept. In general, the response alternatives should be about equal in length.

Tips for Formatting an Instrument

The appearance and layout of the schedule may seem a matter of minor administrative importance. However, a poorly designed format can have substantive consequences if respondents (or interviewers) become confused, miss questions, or answer questions that they should have omitted. The format is especially important in questionnaires because respondents who are unfamiliar with the researcher's intent will not usually have an opportunity to ask questions. The following suggestions may be helpful in laying out an instrument:

- Try not to compress too many questions into too small a space. An extra page of questions is better than a schedule that appears cluttered and confusing and that provides inadequate space for responses to open-ended questions.
- Set off the response options from the question or stem itself in formatting alternative responses. These options are usually aligned vertically (Box 14-2). In a questionnaire, respondents can be asked either to circle the appropriate answer or to place a check mark in the appropriate box.
- Give special care to formatting **filter questions**, which are designed to route respondents through different sets of questions

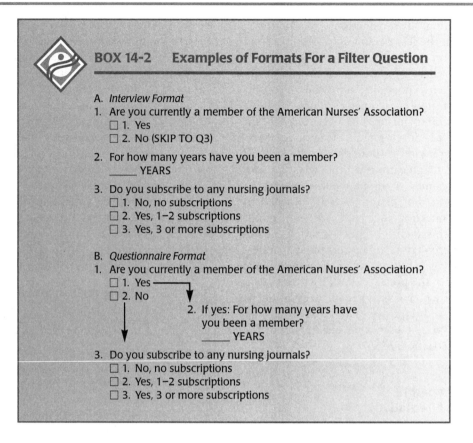

BOX 14-2   Examples of Formats For a Filter Question

A. *Interview Format*
1. Are you currently a member of the American Nurses' Association?
   ☐ 1. Yes
   ☐ 2. No (SKIP TO Q3)

2. For how many years have you been a member?
   _____ YEARS

3. Do you subscribe to any nursing journals?
   ☐ 1. No, no subscriptions
   ☐ 2. Yes, 1–2 subscriptions
   ☐ 3. Yes, 3 or more subscriptions

B. *Questionnaire Format*
1. Are you currently a member of the American Nurses' Association?
   ☐ 1. Yes
   ☐ 2. No

   2. If yes: For how many years have
      you been a member?
      _____ YEARS

3. Do you subscribe to any nursing journals?
   ☐ 1. No, no subscriptions
   ☐ 2. Yes, 1–2 subscriptions
   ☐ 3. Yes, 3 or more subscriptions

depending on their responses to earlier items. In interview schedules, the most typical procedure is to use **skip patterns** that instruct the interviewers to skip to a specific place in the schedule (e.g., SKIP TO Q3). In self-administered questionnaires, such skip patterns may be confusing, and it may be better to set off questions appropriate to only a subset of respondents apart from the main series of questions, as illustrated in Box 14-2, part B. A very important advantage of CAPI and computer-assisted telephone interviewing (CATI) is that the computer is programmed with the skip instructions, leaving no room for human error.
• Avoid forcing all readers to go through inapplicable questions in a questionnaire.

That is, question 2 in Box 14-2 could have been worded as follows: "If you are a member of the American Nurses' Association, for how long have you been a member?" The person who is not a member may not be sure how to handle this question and may be annoyed at having to read through material that is irrelevant.

RESEARCH EXAMPLES

Self-reports are the most commonly used method of collecting data for nursing research studies. This section provides some examples of both qualitative and quantitative studies that relied on self-reports.

Research Examples of Unstructured and Semi-Structured Self-Reports

An increasing number of published nursing studies are based on unstructured or semi-structured self-report methods. Table 14-4 briefly describes the research problems and data collection approaches used in six such studies. A more detailed description of a study using semi-structured interviews follows.

Gloersen, Kendall, Gray, McConnell, Turner, and Lewkowicz (1993) undertook a 2-year investigation into the phenomenon of "doing well" in people with AIDS. Their study sought to identify the processes that enhance AIDS patients' states of well-being. An in-depth focused interview approach was used "to generate an understanding of the concept of doing well because of its focus on exploring percep-

tions of well-being rather than on quantitative measures that would verify and define wellness a priori" (p. 47).

Five investigators conducted the interviews with a sample of 16 AIDS victims, who were selected based on their ability to articulate and discuss their experience of doing well with AIDS. The interviews averaged about 90 minutes in length. Among the questions posed to the respondents were the following: What is your experience of doing well with AIDS? What kinds of things have helped you to do well? What things have you done to help yourself do well? How is the experience of doing well changing over time? What helps you to continue to do well? Respondents were asked to elaborate on any aspect that was considered relevant to the general topic. Follow-up interviews were conducted with 8 of the 16 informants. All interviews were tape recorded and later transcribed. The interview-

TABLE 14-4 Examples of Studies That Collected Unstructured Self-Report Data

RESEARCH QUESTION	DATA COLLECTION METHOD
What is the process of healing among adult male survivors of childhood sexual abuse? (Draucker & Petrovic, 1996)	Unstructured interviews
What is the experience of suffering among people with multiple sclerosis? (Pollock & Sands, 1997)	Semi-structured interviews
What are patients' responses to the angioplasty experience? (Gulanick, Bliley, Perino, & Keough, 1997)	Focus group interviews
What are the factors that contribute to successful aging in a rural setting? (Laferriere & Hamel-Bissell, 1994)	Life histories
What are the beliefs of nurses and consumers about the nature of nursing's contribution in aged and extended care? (Cheek, O'Brien, Ballantyne, & Pincombe, 1997)	Critical incidents technique
What are the strategies or situations that stimulate or relieve nausea or vomiting during pregnancy? (O'Brien, Relyea, & Lidstone, 1997)	Diaries

ers supplemented the transcripts with their own notes, based on their observations during the interviews.

The researchers found that the AIDS victims used several dynamic processes to develop a sense of well-being. For example, every study participant identified *accepting* as an important concept. Other important processes included being active, mastering life, relating mind and body, being positive, participating in health care, and experiencing support.

Research Examples of Structured Self-Reports

Structured self-report instruments are used in most nursing research studies. Table 14-5 presents some examples of studies that have used structured interviews or questionnaires, together with information on response rates. A more detailed description of a questionnaire study follows.

Vortherms, Ryan, and Ward (1992) conducted a survey of nurses to determine their knowledge of, attitudes toward, and perceived barriers to pharmacologic management of pain in cancer patients. Using a number of questions from other instruments, the researchers developed an 82-item questionnaire. The questionnaire consisted of four modules, including a module on background and demographic questions, knowledge of the pharmacologic management of cancer pain, liberalness in pain management, and perceived barriers to pain management in the nurses' practice settings.

The researchers developed a 32-item knowledge test, comprising three subtests: knowledge of opioids, of pain, and of medication scheduling regimens. Test scores were computed in terms of percentage of correct re-

---

TABLE 14-5 Examples of Nursing Studies Using Structured Self-Reports

RESEARCH QUESTION	SAMPLE	ADMINISTRATION METHOD	RESPONSE RATE
How do college women perceive their risk for sexually transmitted disease (STD) infection, and what factors are related to STD risk prevention behaviors? (Hale & Trumbetta, 1996)	308 college women	Distributed questionnaires	90%
What are the current practices of nurse practitioners in assessing, preventing, and treating metabolic bone disease in low-birthweight infants? (Smith & Kirchhoff, 1997)	112 neonatal nurse practitioners	Mailed questionnaires	64%
How satisfied are patients with day-surgery services for eye surgery? (Law, 1997)	38 day-surgery eye patients	Telephone interviews	84%
What are the levels of satisfaction with and perceived barriers to health care among women in a Medicaid prepaid plan versus regular fee-for-service Medicaid program? (Reis, 1990)	98 Medicaid clients	Personal interviews	89%

sponses. Five items (with response options ranging from 1 to 5) were used to measure liberalness of nurses' attitudes in pain management. This summated rating scale (scores ranged from 0 to 24) was adapted from a scale previously used to measure physicians' liberalness in pain management. The questions on perceived barriers were all rating questions, in which respondents were asked to rate nine factors in terms of whether each was a barrier to pain management in their setting and also to rate other nurses and physicians in their settings on adequacy of pain management. Five pain management experts reviewed a draft of the questionnaire for clarity and appropriateness of the content, and survey experts reviewed it with respect to format and style. The questionnaire was pretested with a sample of nurses who had oncology experience.

The questionnaire, a cover letter, a stamped addressed return envelope, and a stamped addressed postcard were mailed to a systematic sample of 1173 nurses holding active licensure in Wisconsin. To encourage cooperation, the cover letter was printed on Pain Research Group/World Health Organization Collaborating Center letterhead. Anonymity was maintained by the use of a separate return postcard by which respondents indicated that they had sent in their questionnaires. Second and third mailings (with duplicate questionnaires and postcards) were sent at 6-week intervals to those who had not yet returned the postcards. A total of 790 nurses (68%) returned a completed questionnaire.

The researchers found that 59% of the nurses had worked with cancer patients in the prior 6 months, although only 7% worked in oncology settings. The scores on the knowledge test ranged from 11% to 93% correct. In general, nurses believed that a substantial minority of patients overreported pain, although they had fairly liberal attitudes toward pain management.

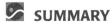 **SUMMARY**

Self-report data are collected by means of an oral **interview** or written **questionnaire**. Self-

reports vary widely in terms of their degree of structure or standardization. Unstructured methods provide both respondent and interviewer latitude in the formulation of questions and answers. Methods of collecting unstructured or loosely structured self-report data include the following: (1) **unstructured interviews**, which are conversational discussions on the topic of interest; (2) **semi-structured** or **focused interviews**, in which the interviewer is guided by a broad **topic guide** of questions to be asked; (3) **focus group interviews**, which involve discussions with small groups about topics covered in a topic guide; (4) **life histories**, which encourage respondents to narrate, in chronologic sequence, their life experiences regarding some theme; (5) the **critical incidents technique**, which involves probes about the circumstances surrounding a behavior or incident that is critical to some outcome of interest; and (6) **diaries**, in which respondents are asked to maintain daily records about some aspects of their lives. Unstructured methods tend to yield data of considerable depth and are useful in gaining an understanding about little-researched phenomena, but they are time-consuming and yield data that are challenging to analyze.

Most self-report data in nursing studies are collected through structured interview schedules or questionnaires. Questions in the instrument also vary in their degree of structure. **Open-ended questions** permit respondents to reply to questions in their own words. **Closed-ended** (or **fixed-alternative**) **questions** offer a number of alternative responses from which respondents are instructed to choose.

Closed-ended questions can take a number of different forms. The simplest type of fixed alternative (**dichotomous questions**) requires a choice between two options, such as yes or no. **Multiple-choice questions** provide respondents with a range of alternatives. **Cafeteria questions** are a special type of multiple-choice item in which respondents are asked to select a statement that best represents their view. Respondents are sometimes requested to **rank-**

order a list of alternatives along a continuum, usually from most favorable to least favorable. **Forced-choice questions** require respondents to choose between two competing positions. **Rating questions** ask respondents to judge something along an ordered, bipolar dimension. A **checklist** groups together several questions that require the same response format and that can be answered by placing a check in the appropriate space on a **matrix**. **Calendar questions** ask for information about the stop and start dates of various events, recorded on a calendar grid. A **visual analogue scale (VAS**es) is often used for the measurement of subjective experiences, such as pain and nausea.

Composite psychosocial **scales** are multiple-item self-report tools for quantitatively measuring the degree to which individuals possess or are characterized by target traits or attributes. The most common type of composite scale is the **Likert scale,** or **summated rating scale.** Likert scales present the respondent with a series of statements that are worded either favorably or unfavorably toward some phenomenon. Respondents are asked to indicate their degree of agreement or disagreement with each statement. A total score is derived by the summation of scores assigned to all items, which in turn are scored according to the direction of favorability expressed. The **semantic differential (SD)** is a second scaling procedure used for measuring the meaning of concepts to individuals. The technique consists of a series of bipolar rating scales on which respondents are asked to indicate their reaction toward some phenomenon. The scales may be measuring an evaluation (e.g., good/bad); activity (e.g., active/passive); or potency (e.g., strong/weak) dimension. Scoring of the SD proceeds in a fashion similar to that of Likert scales.

The quality of interview data depends heavily on the interpersonal skills of the interviewer. The interviewer must endeavor to put respondents at ease and build rapport with them. When respondents give incomplete or irrelevant replies to a question, the interviewer

must use a technique known as **probing** to solicit additional information.

Self-administered questionnaires can be distributed in various ways. Group administration to an intact group is the most convenient and economical procedure. Another approach is to mail questionnaires to individuals. The main problem with mailed questionnaires is that many people fail to respond to them, leading to the risk of a biased sample. A number of techniques, such as the use of **follow-up reminders** and good **cover letters**, are designed to increase the **response rate.**

On the whole, interviews suffer from fewer weaknesses than questionnaires. Questionnaires are less costly and time-consuming than interviews, offer the possibility of anonymity, and do not run a risk of interviewer bias. However, interviews yield a higher response rate, are suitable for a wider variety of individuals, are less likely to lead to misinterpretations of questions, and tend to provide richer data than questionnaires.

The researcher interested in using self-reports must contend with the possibility of reporting biases, which are often called **response-set biases** in the context of scales. This problem concerns the tendency of certain individuals to respond to items in characteristic ways, independently of the item's content. The **social desirability response bias** stems from a person's desire to appear in a favorable light. The **extreme response set** results when a person characteristically endorses extreme response alternatives. Another type of response bias is known as **acquiescence,** which designates an individual's tendency to agree with statements regardless of their content. A converse problem arises less frequently when a person disagrees with most statements.

STUDY ACTIVITIES

Chapter 14 of the *Study Guide to Accompany Nursing Research: Principles and Methods, 6th ed.,* offers various exercises for reinforcing the concepts presented in this chapter. Additionally, the following study questions can be addressed:

1. Identify which unstructured methods of self-report might be appropriate for the following research problems:
   a. What are the coping strategies of parents who have lost a child through sudden infant death syndrome?
   b. How do nurses in emergency rooms make decisions about their activities?
   c. What are the health beliefs and practices of Haitian immigrants in the United States?
2. The underutilization of nursing skills because of voluntary nonemployment is sometimes the cause of some concern. Suppose that you were planning to conduct a statewide study concerning the plans and intentions of nonemployed registered nurses in your state. Would you adopt an interview or questionnaire approach? How structured would your schedule be? Why?
3. Suppose that the investigation of nonemployed nurses were to be accomplished by means of a mailed questionnaire. Draft a cover letter to accompany the schedule.
4. Suppose that you were interested in studying the attitudes of men toward witnessing the births of their children in a hospital delivery room. Develop five positively worded and five negatively worded statements that could be used in constructing a Likert scale for such a study.
5. List 10 pairs of bipolar adjectives that would be appropriate for rating *all* the following concepts for an SD scale: cigarettes, alcohol, marijuana, heroin, cocaine.
6. Suggest ways of improving the following questions:
   a. When do you usually administer your injection of insulin?
   b. Would you disagree with the statement that nurses should not unionize?
   c. Do you agree or disagree with the following statement? Alcoholics deserve more pity than scorn and should be encouraged to seek medical rather than spiritual assistance.
   d. What is your opinion about the new health reform bill?
   e. Don't you think that the role of nurses ought to be expanded?

SUGGESTED READINGS

Methodologic References

General References on Self-Reports

Bradburn, N. M., & Sudman, S. (1979). *Improving interview method and questionnaire design.* San Francisco: Jossey-Bass.

Collins, C., Given, B., Given, C. W., & King, S. (1988). Interviewer training and supervision. *Nursing Research, 37,* 122–124.

Denzin, N. K. (1989). *The research act* (3rd ed.). New York: McGraw-Hill.

DeVellis, R. F. (1991). *Scale development: Theory and applications.* Newbury Park, CA: Sage.

Dillman, D. (1978). *Mail and telephone surveys: The total design method.* New York: John Wiley.

Flanagan, J. C. (1954). The critical-incident technique. *Psychological Bulletin, 51,* 327–358.

Gift, A. G. (1989). Visual analogue scales: Measurement of subjective phenomena. *Nursing Research, 38,* 286–288.

Goldman, A. E., & McDonald, S. S. (1987). *The group depth interview: Principles and practice.* Englewood Cliffs, NJ: Prentice-Hall.

Gordon, R. L. (1980). *Interviewing: Strategy, techniques and tactics* (3rd ed.). Homewood, IL: Dorsey Press.

Institute for Social Research. (1976). *Interviewer's manual, Survey Research Center* (rev. ed.). Ann Arbor: University of Michigan.

Kingry, M. J., Fiedje, L. B., & Friedman, L. L. (1990). Focus groups: A research technique for nursing. *Nursing Research, 39,* 124–125.

Krueger, R. A. (1988). *Focus groups: A practical guide for applied research.* San Mateo, CA: Sage.

Lee, K. A., & Kieckhefer, G. M. (1989). Measuring human responses using visual analogue scales. *Western Journal of Nursing Research, 11,* 128–132.

Leininger, M. M. (1985). Life-health-care history: Purposes, methods and techniques. In M. M. Leininger (Ed.), *Qualitative research methods in nursing.* New York: Grune & Stratton.

McCracken, G. (1988). *The long interview.* Newbury Park, CA: Sage.

Morgan, D. L. (1988). *Focus groups as qualitative research.* Newbury Park, CA: Sage.

Nunnally, J. C., & Bernstein, I. H. (1994). *Psychometric theory* (3rd ed.). New York: McGraw-Hill.

Osgood, C. E., Suci, G. J., & Tannenbaum, P. H. (1957). *The measurements of meaning.* Urbana, IL: University of Illinois Press.

Paterson, B., & Bramadat, I. J. (1992). Use of the preinterview in oral history. *Qualitative Health Research, 2,* 99–115.

Payne, S. (1951). *The art of asking questions.* Princeton, NJ: Princeton University Press.

Reiskin, H. (1992). Focus groups: A useful technique for research and practice in nursing. *Applied Nursing Research, 5,* 197–201.

Schuman, H., & Presser, S. (1996). *Questions and answers in attitude surveys: Experiments in questions form, wording and context.* Thousand Oaks, CA: Sage.

Spradley, J. (1979). *The ethnographic interview.* New York: Holt Rinehart & Winston.

Waltz, C. F., Strickland, O. L., & Lenz, E. R. (1991). *Measurement in nursing research* (2nd ed.). Philadelphia: F. A. Davis.

Woods, N. F. (1981). The health diary as an instrument for nursing research. *Western Journal of Nursing Research, 3,* 76–92.

Wykle, M. L., & Morris, D. L. (1988). The health diary. *Applied Nursing Research, 1,* 47–48.

References for Locating Scales and Psychological Measures

Anastasi, A. (1997). *Psychological testing* (7th ed.). Englewood Cliffs, NJ: Prentice Hall.

Buros, O. K. (1994). *Tests in print II.* Highland Park, NJ: Gryphon Press.

Cattell, J. B., & Warburton, F. W. (1967). *Objective personality and motivation tests.* Chicago: University of Illinois Press.

Chun, K. T., Cobb, S., & French, J. R. P., Jr. (1975). *Measures for psychological assessment.* Ann Arbor: Survey Research Center.

Corcoran, K., & Fischer, J. (1994). *Measures for clinical practice: A sourcebook.* New York: Macmillan.

Frank-Stromborg, M. (Ed.). (1988). *Instruments for clinical nursing research.* Norwalk, CT: Appleton and Lange.

Frank-Stromberg, M., & Olsen, S. (1997). *Instruments for clinical health care research.* Boston: Jones and Bartlett.

Keyser, D. J., & Sweetland, R. C. (Eds.) (1988). *Test critiques.* (Vol. 7). Kansas City, MO: Test Corporation of America.

McDowell, I., & Newell, C. (1987). *Measuring health: A guide to rating scales and questionnaires.* New York: Oxford University Press.

Mitchell, J. V., Jr. (Ed.). (1985). *The ninth mental measurements yearbook.* Lincoln, NE: University of Nebraska Press.

Reineck, C. (1991). Nursing research instruments: Pathway to resources. *Applied Nursing Research, 4,* 34–38.

Robinson, J. P., & Shaver, P. R. (1973). *Measures of social psychological attitudes* (rev. ed.). Ann Arbor: University of Michigan.

Shaw, M. E., & Wright, J. M. (1967). *Scales for the measurement of attitudes.* New York: McGraw-Hill.

Strickland, O. L., & Waltz, C. (1988). *Measurement of nursing outcomes: Vol. II. Measuring nursing performance.* New York: Springer.

Touliatos, J., Perlmutter, B. F., & Straus, M. A. (Eds.). (1990). *Handbook of family measurement techniques.* Newbury Park, CA: Sage.

Waltz, C. F., & Strickland, O. L. (1988). *Measurement of nursing outcomes: Vol. I. Measuring client outcomes.* New York: Springer.

Ward, M. J., & Felter, M. E. (1979). *Instruments for use in nursing education research.* Boulder, CO: Western Interstate Commission for Higher Education.

Ward, M. J., & Lindeman, C. A. (Eds.). (1978). *Instruments for measuring nursing practice and other health variables.* Washington, DC: U.S. Government Printing Office.

Substantive References

Beaton, R. D., Murphy, S. A., Pike, K. C., & Corneil, W. (1997). Social support and network conflict in firefighters and paramedics. *Western Journal of Nursing Research, 19*, 297–313.

Buchanan, L. M., Cowan, M., Burr, R., Waldron, C., & Kogan, H. (1993). Measurement of recovery from myocardial infarction using heart rate variability and psychological outcomes. *Nursing Research, 42*, 74–78.

Cheek, J., O'Brien, B., Ballantyne, A., & Pincombe, J. (1997). Using critical incidents technique to inform aged and extended care nursing. *Western Journal of Nursing Research, 19*, 667–682.

Coates, C. J. (1997). The caring efficacy scale: Nurses' self-reports of caring in practice settings. *Advanced Practice Nursing Quarterly, 3*, 53–59.

Collins, J. A., & Rice, V. H. (1997). Effects of relaxation intervention in phase II cardiac rehabilitation. *Heart & Lung, 26*, 31–44.

Draucker, C. B. (1997). Early family life and victimization in the lives of women. *Research in Nursing & Health, 20*, 399–412.

Draucker, C. B., & Petrovic, K. (1996). Healing of adult male survivors of childhood sexual abuse. *Image—The Journal of Nursing Scholarship, 28*, 325–330.

Flynn, L. (1997). The health practices of homeless women. *Nursing Research, 46*, 72–77.

Ford-Gilboe, M. (1997). Family strengths, motivation, and resources as predictors of health promotion behavior in single-parent and two-parent families. *Research in Nursing & Health, 20*, 205–217.

Friedman, M. M. (1997). Social support sources among older women with heart failure. *Research in Nursing & Health, 20*, 319–327.

Ganong, L. (1993). Nurses' perceptions of married and unmarried pregnant patients. *Western Journal of Nursing Research, 15*, 352–362.

Gloersen, B., Kendall, J., Gray, P., McConnell, S., Turner, J., & Lewkowicz, J. W. (1993). The phenomena of doing well in people with AIDS. *Western Journal of Nursing Research, 15*, 44–54.

Gulanick, M., Bliley, A., Perino, B., & Keough, V. (1997). Patients' responses to the angioplasty experience. *American Journal of Critical Care, 6*, 25–32.

Hahn, W. K., Brooks, J. A., & Hartsough, D. M. (1993). Self-disclosure and coping styles in men with cardiovascular reactivity. *Research in Nursing & Health, 16*, 275–282.

Hale, P. J., & Trumbetta, S. L. (1996). Women's self-efficacy and sexually transmitted disease prevention behaviors. *Research in Nursing & Health, 19*, 101–110.

Houston, S., Eagen, M., Freeborg, S., & Dougherty, D. (1997). A comparison of structured versus guided preheart catheterization information on mood states and coping resources. *Applied Nursing Research, 9*, 189–194.

Janson-Bjerklie, S., Ferketich, S., & Benner, P. (1993). Predicting the outcomes of living with asthma. *Research in Nursing & Health, 16*, 241–250.

Kidd, P., & Huddleston, S. (1994). Psychometric properties of the Driving Practices Questionnaire: Assessment of risky driving. *Research in Nursing & Health, 17*, 51–58.

Laferriere, R. H., & Hamel-Bissell, B. P. (1994). Successful aging of oldest old women in the Northeast Kingdom of Vermont. *Image—The Journal of Nursing Scholarship, 26*, 19–23.

Law, M. (1997). A telephone survey of day-surgery eye patients. *Journal of Advanced Nursing, 25*, 355–363.

LoBiondo-Wood, G., Williams, L., Wood, R. P., & Shaw, B. W. (1997). Impact of liver transplantation on quality of life. *Applied Nursing Research, 10*, 27–32.

Neill, K. M. (1993). Ethnic pain styles in acute myocardial infarction. *Western Journal of Nursing Research, 15*, 531–543.

Neuberger, G. B., Press, A. N., Lindsley, H. B., Hinton, R., Cagle, P. E., Carlson, K., Scott, S., Dahl, J., & Kramer, B. (1997). Effects of exercise on fatigue, aerobic fitness, and disease activity measures in persons with rheumatoid arthritis. *Research in Nursing & Health, 20*, 195–204.

Nickel, J. T., Salsberry, P. J., Caswell, R. J., Keller, M. D., Long, T., & O'Connell, M. (1996). Quality of life in nurse case management of persons with AIDS receiving home care. *Research in Nursing & Health, 19*, 91–99.

O'Brien, B., Relyea, J., & Lidstone, T. (1997). Diary reports of nausea and vomiting during pregnancy. *Clinical Nursing Research, 6*, 239–252.

Pollock, S. E., & Sands, D. (1997). Adaptation to suffering: Meaning and implications for nursing. *Clinical Nursing Research, 6,* 171–185.

Preski, S., & Walker, L. O. (1997). Contributions of maternal identity and lifestyle to young children's adjustment. *Research in Nursing & Health, 20,* 107–117.

Reis, J. (1990). Medicaid maternal and child health care: Prepaid plans vs. private fee-for-service. *Research in Nursing & Health, 13,* 163–171.

Richmond, T. S. (1997). An explanatory model of variables influencing postinjury disability. *Nursing Research, 46,* 262–269.

Samarel, N., Fawcett, J., & Tulman, L. (1997). Effect of support groups with coaching on adaptation to early stage brest cancer. *Research in Nursing & Health, 20,* 15–26.

Smith, S. L., & Kirchhoff, K. T. (1997). *Journal of Obstetric, Gynecologic, and Neonatal Nursing, 26,* 297–302.

Topp, R., & Stevenson, J. S. (1994). The effects of attendance and effort on outcomes among older adults in a long-term exercise program. *Research in Nursing & Health, 17,* 15–24.

Vortherms, R., Ryan, P., & Ward, S. (1992). Knowledge of, attitudes toward, and barriers to pharmacologic management of cancer pain in a statewide random sample of nurses. *Research in Nursing & Health, 15,* 459–466.

White, C. L., LeFort, S. M., Amsel, R., & Jeans, M. (1997). Predictors of the development of chronic pain. *Research in Nursing & Health, 20,* 309–318.

Woods, N. F., Lentz, M., Mitchell, E. S., Heitkemper, M., & Shaver, J. (1997). PMS after 40: Persistence of a stress-related symptom pattern. *Research in Nursing & Health, 20,* 329–340.

Zorn, C. R. (1997). Factors contributing to hope among noninstitutionalized elderly. *Applied Nursing Research, 10,* 94–100.

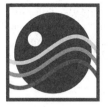

CHAPTER **15**

Observational Methods

Scientific observation involves the systematic selection, observation, and recording of behaviors,
events, and settings relevant to a problem under
investigation. Like self-report methods, observational methods can vary in terms of structure,
from unstructured methods that usually result
in qualitative data to structured approaches that
yield quantitative data. Both structured and unstructured methods are discussed in this chapter.
First, however, we present an overview of some
general issues.

OBSERVATIONAL ISSUES

When a nurse researcher observes an event—
such as a nurse administering an injection
to a patient—he or she typically has a clear
idea about what is to be observed and under
what circumstances it will take place. The researcher cannot absorb and record an infinite number of details and must, therefore,
have some guidelines specifying the manner in
which the observations are to be focused and
recorded. In this section, we indicate the versatility of observational methods and point
out some considerations for observing phenomena in a research context.

Phenomena Amenable to Observations

Nurse researchers usually make observational
records of either human behaviors or the characteristics of individuals, events, environments,
or objects. The following list of observable phenomena is meant to be suggestive rather than
exhaustive:

1. *Characteristics and conditions of individuals.* A broad variety of information
   about people's attributes and states can
   be gathered by direct observation. We
   refer not only to relatively enduring
   traits of individuals, such as their physical appearance, but also to more temporary conditions, such as physiologic
   symptoms that are amenable to observation. We include here physiologic conditions that can be observed either directly
   through the senses, or with the aid of
   observational apparatus, such as a radio-
   graph. To illustrate this class of observable phenomena, the following could be
   used as dependent or independent variables in a nursing research investigation:
   the sleep or wake state of patients, the
   presence of edema in congestive heart

failure, turgor of the skin in dehydration, the manifestation of decubitus ulcers, alopecia during cancer chemotherapy, or symptoms of infusion phlebitis in hospitalized patients. For example, Cureton-Lane and Fontaine (1997) observed the sleep patterns of children in a pediatric intensive care unit in relation to such factors as noise and light levels, contact with caregivers, and parental presence.

2. *Activities.* Many actions are amenable to observation and constitute valuable data for nurse researchers. Activities that serve as an index of health status or physical and emotional functioning are particularly important. As illustrations, the following kinds of activities lend themselves to an observational study: patients' eating habits and trends, bowel movements in postsurgical patients, length and number of visits by friends and relatives to hospitalized patients, and aggressive actions among children in the hospital playroom. For example, Beck, Heacock, Mercer, Walls, Rapp, and Vogelpohl (1997) studied the dressing behavior of cognitively impaired nursing home residents who were exposed to an intervention to promote dressing independence.

3. *Skill attainment and performance.* Nurses and nurse educators are routinely called on to develop skills among clients and students. The attainment of these skills is often manifested behaviorally, and in such cases, an observational assessment is appropriate. For example, a nurse researcher might want to observe the following kinds of behavior: the ability of nursing students to insert a urinary catheter properly, the ability of stroke patients to scan a food tray if homonymous hemianopia is present, the ability of diabetic patients to test their urine for sugar and acetone, or the ability of a newborn to exhibit sucking behavior when positioned for breastfeeding. Nurses' on-the-job per-

formance and decision-making behaviors are also of interest to researchers in terms of understanding how to make improvements to the practice of nursing. Larson, Bryan, Adler, and Blane (1997), for example, observed more than 2500 episodes of staff handwashing in an intensive care unit, focusing on handwashing frequency and practices.

4. *Verbal communication behaviors.* The content and structure of people's conversations are readily observable, easy to record, and, thus, an obvious source of data. Among the kinds of verbal communications that a nurse researcher may be interested in observing are information giving by nurses to patients, nurses' conversations with grieving relatives, exchange of information among nurses at change-of-shift report, dialogue of residents in a nursing home, and conversations in a rural public health clinic. For example, Hall (1996) studied the effectiveness of communication between nurses and ventilated patients using observational methods.

5. *Nonverbal communication behaviors.* People communicate their fears, wants, and emotions in many ways other than just with words. For nurse researchers, nonverbal communication represents an extremely fruitful area for research because nurses are often called on to be sensitive to nonverbal cues. The kinds of nonverbal behavior amenable to observational methods include facial expressions, touch, posture, gestures and other body movements, and extralinguistic behavior (i.e., the manner in which people speak, aside from the content, such as the intonation, loudness, and continuity of the speech). As an example, Routasalo (1996) studied nurses' and elderly patients' use of nonnecessary touch; verbal communication that occurred in connection with the touching was also recorded

to understand better the situations in which nonnecessary touching was used.

6. *Environmental characteristics.* An individual's surroundings may have a profound effect on his or her behavior, and a number of studies have explored the relationship between certain observable attributes of the environment on the one hand and human beliefs, actions, and needs on the other. Examples of observable environmental attributes include the following: the noise levels in different areas of a hospital, the decor in a nursing home, the safety hazards in an elementary school classroom, or the cleanliness of the homes in a community. For example, Russell and Champion (1996) observed safety hazards in the homes of low-income mothers with preschool children in relation to the mothers' health beliefs and the children's previous injury histories.

Units of Observation

In selecting behaviors, attributes, or situations to be observed, the investigator must decide what constitutes a unit. There are two basic approaches, which are best considered as the end points of a continuum. The **molar approach** entails observing large units of behavior and treating them as a whole. For example, psychiatric nurse researchers might engage in a study of patient mood swings. An entire constellation of verbal and nonverbal behaviors might be construed as signaling aggressive behaviors, and another set might constitute passive behaviors. Most in-depth, unstructured observational studies use a molar approach. At the other extreme, the **molecular approach** uses small and highly specific behaviors as the unit of observation. Each movement, action, gesture, or phrase is treated as a separate entity, or perhaps is broken down into even smaller units. The choice of approaches depends to a large degree on the nature of the problem and the preferences of the investigator. The molar

approach is more susceptible to observer errors and distortions because of greater ambiguity in what is being observed. On the other hand, in reducing the observations to more concrete and specific elements, the investigator may lose sight of the activities that are at the heart of the inquiry.

The Observer–Observed Relationship

The researcher can interact with individuals in the observational setting to varying degrees. The issue of the relationship between the observer and those observed is important and has stirred much controversy. Two important aspects of this issue concern intervention and concealment. The decisions a researcher makes in establishing a strategy for handling these considerations should be based on an understanding of the ethical and methodologic implications.

In observational studies, intervention may involve an experimental intervention of the type described in Chapter 8 on experimental designs. For example, a nurse researcher may observe patients' postoperative behaviors after an intervention designed to improve the patients' ability to cough and breathe after surgery. In observational studies, however, the researcher sometimes intervenes to structure the research setting without necessarily introducing an experimental treatment, that is, without manipulating the independent variable. This approach is sometimes referred to as the use of **directed settings**. For instance, researchers sometimes stage a situation to provoke specific behavioral patterns. Certain events or activities are rare in naturalistic settings, and therefore, it is inexpedient to await their manifestation. For example, a number of social psychological investigations have studied the behavior of bystanders in crisis situations. Because crises are unpredictable and infrequent, investigators have staged emergencies to observe helping behavior (or lack of it) among onlookers. Such studies are considered high on the intervention dimension. Studies in which the researcher intervenes to elicit behaviors of interest may be practical when there is little opportunity to observe activities or events as they unfold naturalistically. However, such studies are sometimes criticized on the grounds of artificiality and may suffer from serious problems of external validity.

The second dimension that concerns the relationship between the observer and the observed is the degree to which subjects are aware of the observation and their status as study participants. In naturalistic settings, researchers are sometimes concerned that their presence, if known, would alter the behaviors under observation. In some situations, therefore, observers may adopt a completely passive role, attempting insofar as possible to become unobtrusive bystanders. The problem of behavioral distortions that result from the known presence of an observer has been called a **reactive measurement effect** or, more simply, **reactivity**. One approach to minimizing the problem of reactivity is to make the observations without people's knowledge, through some type of concealment. For example, a nurse could monitor patients' conversations surreptitiously by means of the call system located at the nurses' station. In laboratory environments or in some directed settings, concealed observations can be accomplished through the use of one-way mirrors.

Concealment offers the researcher a number of distinct advantages, even beyond the reduction of reactivity. Some individuals might deny a researcher the privilege of observing them altogether, so that the alternative to concealed observation might be no observation at all. Total concealment, however, may be difficult to attain except in formal or highly active observational settings. Furthermore, concealed observation, without the knowledge and consent of those observed, is ethically problematic (see Chapter 6).

A second situation is one in which the subjects are aware of the researcher's presence but may not be aware of the investigator's underlying motives. This approach offers the researcher the opportunity of getting more in-depth information than is usually possible with total concealment. Also, because the researcher is not totally concealed, there may be fewer ethical problems. Nevertheless, the issues of subject deception and failure to obtain informed voluntary consent remain thorny ones. Furthermore, a serious drawback of this second approach is the possibility that the interaction between the observer and the observed will alter the subjects' behavior. Even when the observed individuals are unaware of being participants in a research study, there is always a risk that the researcher's presence will alter their normal activities, mannerisms, or conversations.

The researcher will be confronted with methodologic, substantive, or ethical issues at every point along the concealment and intervention dimensions. Some of these problems will be irrelevant in particular projects, but the investigator should assess carefully the relative weaknesses of an approach against the possible advantages it might offer.

OBSERVATIONAL METHODS: UNSTRUCTURED OBSERVATIONS

Qualitative studies sometimes involve the collection of unstructured or loosely structured observational data, often as an important supplement to self-report data. The aim of qualitative research is typically to understand the behaviors and experiences of people as they actually occur in naturalistic settings. Therefore, the qualitative researcher's aim is to observe and record information about people and their environments with a minimum of structure and researcher-imposed interference.

Unstructured observational data are often gathered in field settings through a process referred to as **participant observation**. In participant observation research, the investigator participates in the functioning of the social group under investigation and strives to observe and record information within the contexts, structures, and symbols that are relevant to the group members. Although it is beyond the scope of this book to describe in detail the methods used in participant observation research, we describe some of the salient issues.

The Observer–Participant Role

The role that an observer plays in the social group under investigation is important because the social position of the observer determines what he or she is likely to see. That is, the behaviors that are likely to be available for observation depend on the observer's position in a network of relations.

Leininger (1985) noted that the observer's role typically evolves through a sequence of four phases:

1. Primarily observation
2. Primarily observation with some participation
3. Primarily participation with some observation
4. Reflective observation

In the initial phase, the researcher observes and listens to those under study to obtain a broad view of the situation. This phase allows both the observer and the observed to "size up" each other, to become acquainted, and to become more comfortable in interacting. In phase 2, observation is enhanced by a modest degree of participation. As the researcher participates more actively in the activities of the social group, the reactions of people to specific researcher behaviors can be more systematically studied. In phase 3, the researcher strives to become a more active participant, learning by the actual experience of doing rather than just by watching and listening. In phase 4, the researcher reflects on the total process of what transpired and how people interacted with and reacted to the researcher.

The observer must overcome at least two major hurdles in assuming a satisfactory role regarding subject-informants. The first is to gain entrée into the social group under investigation; the second is to establish rapport and develop trust within the social group. Without

gaining entrée, the study cannot proceed; but without the trust of the group, the researcher will typically be restricted to what Leininger (1985) refers to as "front stage" knowledge, that is, information that is distorted by the group's protective facades. The goal of the participant observer is to "get back stage"—to learn about the true realities of the group's experiences and behaviors. On the other hand, being a fully participating member does not *necessarily* offer the best perspective for studying a phenomenon—just as being an actor in a play does not offer the most advantageous view of the performance.

Interpersonal skills play an important part in developing the appropriate role in participant observation research. Wilson (1985) noted that successful participant observation research may require researchers to "go through channels, cultivate relationships, contour [their] appearances, withhold evaluative judgments, and be as unobtrusive and charming as possible" (p. 376).

Gathering Unstructured Observational Data

During the initial phase of a naturalistic observational inquiry, it is often useful to gather some written or pictorial descriptive information that provides an overview of the environment. In an institutional setting, for example, it may be helpful to obtain a floor plan, an organizational chart, an annual report, and so on. Then, a preliminary personal tour of the site should be undertaken to gain familiarity with the ambience of the site and to note major activities, social groupings, transactions, and events. In community studies, it is usually useful to "map" key aspects of the community environment, such as community resources (e.g., churches, businesses, public transportation, community centers), community liabilities (e.g., vacant lots, empty stores, public housing units), and social and environmental characteristics (e.g., condition of streets and buildings, traffic patterns, types of signs, children playing in public places.). Researchers sometimes conduct what is referred to as a **windshield survey**, which involves an intensive tour in an automobile to map important features of the community under study.

The next step is to identify a meaningful way to sample observations and to select observational locations. Sampling by time and by event are common strategies for observational sampling (these strategies are discussed later in this chapter). It is generally useful to use a combination of positioning approaches in selecting observational locations. **Single positioning** means staying in a single location for a period to observe behaviors and transactions in that location. **Multiple positioning** involves moving around the site to observe behaviors from different locations. **Mobile positioning** involves following a person throughout a given activity or period.

Because participant observers cannot spend a lifetime in one site and because they cannot be in more than one place at a time, observation is almost always supplemented with information obtained in unstructured interviews or conversations. For example, an informant may be asked to describe what went on in a meeting that the observer was unable to attend, or informants may be asked to describe an event that occurred before the observer entered the field. In such a case, the informant functions as the observer's observer.

The participant observer typically places few restrictions on the nature of the data collected, in keeping with the goal of minimizing observer-imposed meanings and structure. Nevertheless, participant observers often have a broad plan for the types of information to be gathered. Among the aspects likely to be considered relevant are the following:

1. *The physical setting.* What are the main features of the physical setting? What is the context within which human behavior unfolds? What types of behaviors and characteristics are promoted (or constrained) by the physical environment?

2. *The participants.* What are the characteristics of the people being observed? How many people are there? What are their roles? Who is given free access to the setting—who "belongs"? What brings these people together?

3. *Activities and interactions.* What is going on—what are the participants doing? Is there a discernible progression of activities? How do the participants interact with one another? What methods do they use to communicate, and how frequently do they do so? What type of affect is manifested during their interactions? How are the participants interconnected to one another or to the activities underway?

4. *Frequency and duration.* When did the activity or event begin, and when is it scheduled to end? How much time has elapsed? Is the activity a recurring one, and if so, how regularly does it recur? How typical of such activities is the one that is under observation?

5. *Intangible factors.* What did *not* happen (especially if it ought to have happened)? Are the participants saying one thing verbally but communicating other messages nonverbally? What types of things were disruptive to the activity or situation?

Recording Unstructured Observations

The most common forms of record keeping in participant observation and other unstructured observational studies are logs and field notes. A **log** is a daily record of events and conversations that transpire in the observational setting. **Field notes** may include the daily log but tend to be much broader, more analytic, and more interpretive than a simple listing of occurrences. Field notes represent the participant observer's efforts to record information and also to synthesize and understand the data.

Field notes are sometimes categorized according to the purpose they will serve during the analysis and integration of information. **Observational notes** are objective descriptions of events and conversations; information such as time, place, activity, and dialogue are recorded as completely and objectively as possible. **Theoretical notes** are interpretive attempts to attach meaning to observations. **Methodologic notes** are instructions or reminders about how subsequent observations will be made. **Personal notes** are comments about the researcher's own feelings during the research process. Table 15-1 presents some examples of all four types of field notes from a fictitious observational study of an in vitro fertilization clinic.

The success of any participant observation study depends heavily on the quality of the logs and field notes. It is essential to record observations while still in the process of collecting information because memory is bound to fail if there is too long a delay. On the other hand, the participant observer cannot usually perform the recording function by openly carrying a clipboard, pens, and paper because this action would undermine the observer's role as an ordinary participant of the group. The researcher, therefore, must develop the skill of making detailed mental notes that can later be committed to a permanent record. Alternatively, the observer can try to jot down unobtrusively a phrase or sentence that will later serve as a reminder of an event, conversation, or impression. At a later point—preferably as soon as possible—the observer can use the brief notes and mental recordings to develop

TABLE 15-1 Example of Field Notes: Study of an In Vitro Fertilization Facility	
Observational notes	Couple A entered the center for the first time at about 7:00 PM on a Tuesday evening. Mrs. A sat very stiffly on the chair next to the receptionist's desk, and Mr. A sat beside her. Both parties looked uncomfortable and tense. There was little interaction between them until they were called in for the initial consultation. While in the waiting area, Mrs. A picked up several magazines, thumbed through them absently, and then put them down again. Mr. A spent most of the time smoking cigarettes, staring at the ceiling or at the entrance to the office. Couple A spent about 15 minutes in the waiting area. When their names were called, Mrs. A jumped as though startled and then moved quickly toward the door. She turned back once to make sure Mr. A was following, and when she saw that he was just rising, motioned for him to follow her.
Theoretical notes	Tension is a common feature among couples waiting for their initial consultation. However, the tension seems to stem from different sources and manifests itself in different ways. Some couples seem not to be persuaded that in vitro fertilization (IVF) is right for them; these couples seem embarrassed and tend not to communicate with one another. The source of tension seems to stem less from conflict about whether to try IVF than from the fear of disappointment. These couples tend to engage in continuous *sotto voce* discussions about what they've heard about IVF while waiting for their intake.
Methodologic notes	I decided yesterday to make more systematic observations of couples immediately after they complete their initial interview. This decision was spurred by an incident yesterday in which both partners left the office in tears.
Personal notes	My progress in understanding what these couples seeking IVF treatment are going through is very uneven. Two days ago, I was confident that patterns were falling into place. But this afternoon, a little girl in the waiting room (an adopted daughter of a couple undergoing treatment) made me painfully aware of how much more complex the phenomenon of infertility and its social and psychological meanings really are.

the more extensive field notes. The use of portable computers with word processing capabilities can greatly facilitate the recording and organization of notes in the field.

Evaluation of Unstructured Observation

Unstructured observation is a method of collecting research data that has both opponents and proponents. Researchers who support the use of unstructured methods point out that these techniques usually provide a deeper and richer understanding of human behaviors and social situations than is possible with more standardized procedures. Participant observation is particularly valuable, according to this view, for its ability to "get inside" a particular situation and lead to a more complete understanding of its complexities. Furthermore, unstructured observational approaches are inherently flexible and, therefore, permit the observer greater freedom to reconceptualize the problem after becoming more familiar with the situation. Advocates of qualitative observational research also claim that structured, quantitatively oriented methods are too mechanistic and superficial to render a meaningful account of the intricate nature of human behavior.

Critics of the unstructured approach point out a number of methodologic shortcomings. Observer bias and observer influence are prominent difficulties. Not only is there a concern that the observer may lose objectivity in recording actual observations, there also is the possibility that the observer will inappropriately sample events and situations to be observed. Once the researcher begins to participate in a group's activities, the risk of emotional involvement becomes a salient issue. The researcher in the new member role may fail to attend to many scientifically relevant aspects of the situation or may develop a myopic view on issues of importance to the group. Participant observation techniques, thus, may be an unsuitable approach to study problems when one suspects that the risk of identification is strong. Finally, unstructured

observational methods depend more on the observational and interpersonal skills of the observer than do highly structured techniques—skills that may be difficult to cultivate.

On the whole, it appears that unstructured observational methods are extremely profitable for in-depth, exploratory research in which the investigator wishes to establish an adequate conceptualization of the important variables in a social setting or wants to develop hypotheses. The more structured observational methods discussed in the next section tend to be better suited to the formal testing of research hypotheses.

OBSERVATIONAL METHODS: STRUCTURED OBSERVATIONS

Structured observational methods differ from unstructured techniques in the specificity of behaviors or events selected for observation, in the advance preparation of record-keeping forms, and in the kinds of activities in which the observer engages. The observer using a structured observational procedure may still have room for making inferences and exercising judgment but is restrained with regard to the kinds of phenomena that will be watched and recorded. The creativity of structured observation lies not in the observation itself but rather in the formulation of a system for accurately categorizing, recording, and encoding the observations and for sampling the phenomena of interest. Because structured techniques depend on plans developed before the actual observation, they are not considered appropriate when the investigator has limited knowledge about the phenomena under investigation.

Categories and Checklists

The most common approach to making structured observations of ongoing events and behaviors consists of the construction of a category system to which the observed phenomena can be assigned. A **category system** represents an attempt to designate in a systematic or quantitative fashion the qualitative behaviors and events transpiring within the observational setting.

CONSIDERATIONS
IN USING CATEGORY SYSTEMS

One of the most important requirements of a category system is the careful and explicit definition of the behaviors and characteristics to be observed. Each category should be explained in detail with an operational definition so that observers will have relatively clearcut criteria for assessing the occurrence of the phenomenon in question. For example, Hurley, Volicer, Hanrahan, Houde, and Volicer (1992) developed an observational scale for measuring discomfort in noncommunicative patients with advanced Alzheimer's disease. An example of a behavioral indicator for the Discomfort Scale is "noisy breathing," which is defined as follows:

> Noisy breathing: negative sounding noise on inspiration or expiration; breathing looks strenuous, labored, or wearing; respirations sound loud, harsh, or gasping; difficulty breathing or trying hard at attempting to achieve good gas exchange; episodic bursts of rapid breaths or hyperventilation. (Hurley, Volicer, Hanrahan, Houde, & Volicer, 1992, p. 373)

In developing or selecting a categorization scheme, the researcher must make a number of important decisions. One decision concerns the exhaustiveness of the phenomena to be observed and the number of categories to be included. Some category systems are constructed such that *all* observed behaviors of a certain type (e.g., all body movements) can be classified into one, and only one, category.

A contrasting technique is to develop a nonexhaustive system in which only *particular* types of behavior are categorized. For example, if we were observing the aggressive behavior of autistic children, we might develop such categories as "strikes another child," "kicks or hits walls or floors," "calls other children names," "throws objects around the room," and so forth. In this restricted category system, many behaviors (all those that are nonaggressive) would not be classified. Such nonexhaustive systems are adequate for many research purposes. However, they run the risk of providing data that are difficult to interpret. When a large number of observed behaviors are unclassified, the investigator may have difficulty in placing the categorized behaviors into a proper context.

Virtually all category systems require that the observer make some inferences, but there is considerable variability on this dimension. Weiss's (1992) Tactile Interaction Index (TII) for observing patterns of interpersonal touch is an example of a system that requires a modest amount of inference. For example, one dimension of the TII concerns the location or part of an individual's body that is touched, classified in one of 19 relatively straightforward categories (e.g., abdomen, arm, back, and so on).

On the other hand, a category system such as the Abnormal Involuntary Movement Scale (AIMS) requires considerably more inference. The AIMS system, which was developed by the National Institute for Mental Health and frequently used to study tardive dyskinetic movements (e.g., Grace et al., 1996; Littrell and Magill, 1993) contains such broad categories as "incapacitation due to abnormal movements." Even when such categories are accompanied by detailed definitions and descriptions, there is a heavy inferential burden placed on the observer. The decision concerning how much observer inference is appropriate depends on a number of factors, including the research purposes and the skills of the observers. Beginning researchers are advised to construct or use category systems that require only a moderate degree of inference.

Once a category system has been developed or selected, the researcher can proceed to construct a **checklist,** which is the instrument used by the observer to record observed phenomena. Whether one constructs a new category system or uses an existing one, the system should be subjected to pilot runs to assess its suitability for the intended study.

CHECKLISTS FOR EXHAUSTIVE SYSTEMS

When an observer uses an exhaustive system (i.e., when all behaviors of a certain type—such as verbal interaction—are observed and recorded), the researcher must be especially careful to define the categories in such a way that the observers know when one behavior ends and a new one begins. Another essential feature of exhaustive systems is that the referent behaviors should be mutually exclusive. If overlapping categories are not eliminated, then the observer may have difficulty in deciding how to classify a particular observation. The underlying assumption in the use of such a category system is that behaviors, events, or attributes that are allocated to a particular category are equivalent to every other behavior, event, or attribute in that same category.

The checklist is generally formatted with the list of behaviors or events from the category system on the left and space for tallying the frequency or duration of occurrence of behaviors on the right. In complex social situations with multiple actors, the right-hand portion may be divided into panels according to characteristics of the actors (e.g., nurse/physician; male patients/female patients) or by individual subjects' names or identification numbers.

The task of the observer using this approach is to place all behaviors in only one category for each element. By **element,** we refer to either a unit of behavior, such as a sentence in a conversation, or to a time interval. To illustrate, suppose that we were interested in studying the problem-solving behavior of a group of public health workers developing a maternal–child health program in a rural area. We might construct a category system such as the following: (1) information seeking, (2) information giv-ing, (3) problem describing, (4) suggestion proposing, (5) suggestion opposing, (6) suggestion supporting, (7) summarizing, and (8) miscellaneous. The observer would be required to classify every group member's contribution—using, for example, each sentence as the element—to the problem-solving process in terms of one of these eight categories. By employing such a system, it would be possible to analyze, for example, the relationship between a group member's role, status, or characteristics on the one hand and the types of problem-solving behaviors engaged in on the other.

The second manner in which this approach can be used is to categorize the relevant behaviors at regular time intervals. For example, in an observational system for analyzing the motor activities of infants, the researcher might want to use 15-second time intervals as the basic recording unit. That is, the observer would be expected to record infant movements occurring within a 15-second period. Checklists based on exhaustive category systems are demanding of the observer because the recording task is continuous.

CHECKLISTS FOR NONEXHAUSTIVE SYSTEMS

The second approach, which is sometimes referred to as a **sign system,** begins with a listing of categories of behaviors that may or may not be manifested by the subjects. The observer's task is to watch for instances of the behaviors on the list. When a behavior occurs, the observer either places a check mark beside the appropriate behavior to designate its occurrence or makes a cumulative tally of the number of times the behavior was witnessed. The product of this type of endeavor is a kind of demography of events transpiring within the observational period. With this type of checklist, the observer does not classify *all* the behaviors or characteristics of the individuals being observed but rather identifies the occurrence and frequency of particular behaviors. A hypothetical example of a checklist using the sign system for describing patients' abilities to perform selected activities of daily living is presented in Table 15-2.

Rating Scales

Structured observations can be recorded in a number of ways other than through the use of category systems and checklists. The major alternative is to use **rating scales** that require the observer to rate some phenomenon in terms of points along a descriptive continuum. The ratings usually are quantified during the subsequent analysis of the observational data.

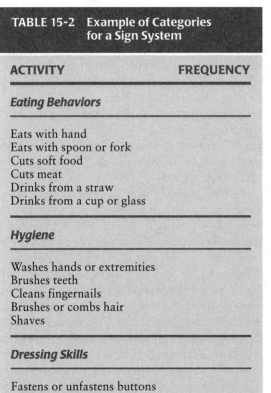

TABLE 15-2	Example of Categories for a Sign System

ACTIVITY	FREQUENCY
Eating Behaviors	
Eats with hand	
Eats with spoon or fork	
Cuts soft food	
Cuts meat	
Drinks from a straw	
Drinks from a cup or glass	
Hygiene	
Washes hands or extremities	
Brushes teeth	
Cleans fingernails	
Brushes or combs hair	
Shaves	
Dressing Skills	
Fastens or unfastens buttons	
Fastens or unfastens snaps	
Pulls zipper up or down	
Ties or unties shoelaces	
Puts on or takes off eyeglasses	
Fastens or unfastens buckle	
Puts in or takes out dentures	

Rating scales normally are used in one of two ways. The observer may be required to make ratings of behaviors or events at frequent intervals throughout the observational period in much the same way that a checklist would be used. Alternatively, the observer may use the rating scales to summarize an entire event or transaction after the observation is completed. Postobservation ratings require the observer to integrate a number of activities and to judge which point on a scale most closely fits the interpretation given to the overall situation. For example, suppose that we were interested in comparing the behaviors of nurses working in intensive care units with those of nurses in other units. After 15-minute observation sessions, the observer might be asked to rate the perceived anxiety level of the nursing staff in each unit as a whole, or that of individual members. The rating scale item might take the following form:

> According to your perceptions, how tense were the nurses in the observed unit?
> 1. Extremely relaxed
> 2. Rather relaxed
> 3. Somewhat relaxed
> 4. Neither relaxed nor tense
> 5. Somewhat tense
> 6. Rather tense
> 7. Extremely tense

The same information could be solicited using a graphic rating scale format:

```
       1    2    3    4    5    6    7
       |    |    |    |    |    |    |
    Extremely     Neither      Extremely
    relaxed       relaxed        tense
                  nor tense
```

Rating scales can also be used as an extension of checklists wherein the observer records not only the occurrence of some behavior but also some qualitative aspect of it, such as its magnitude or intensity. Weiss's (1992) TII once again provides a good example. Her category scheme comprises four dimensions: location (part of body touched); action (the specific gesture or movement used, such as grabbing, hitting, patting, and so on); duration (temporal length of the touch); and intensity. Observers using the index must both classify the nature and duration of the touch *and* rate the intensity on a four-point scale: light, moderate, strong, and deep. When rating scales are coupled with a category scheme in this fashion, considerably more information about the phenomena under investigation can be obtained. The disadvantage of this approach is that it places an immense burden on the observer, particularly if there is an extensive amount of activity.

Constructing Versus Borrowing Structured Observational Instruments

The development, testing, refining, and retesting of a new category scheme or rating scale may require weeks or even months of effort, particularly if the system is intended to be used in a variety of settings and with a variety of subjects. In some cases, a researcher may have no alternative but to design new observational instruments. For example, the researcher may be investigating a relatively new area or may be expanding an area of inquiry with a new population of subjects for whom existing tools may be inappropriate. As in the case of self-report instruments, however, we encourage researchers to explore the literature fully for potentially usable observational instruments.

Many observational systems have been constructed with the intent of being applied to a variety of research situations. Generalized systems, such as the AIMS system described earlier, should be scrutinized before proceeding to design a new system. The use of an existing system not only saves a considerable amount of work but also facilitates comparisons among investigations.

A few sourcebooks describe available observational checklists for certain research applications. For example, the reference books by Frank-Stromborg (1988) and Strickland and Waltz (1988), which describe instruments for measuring variables of relevance to nursing, include some observational instruments. Perhaps the best source for such tools, however, is the current research literature on the topic of interest. For example, if you wanted to conduct an observational study of maternal–infant bonding behavior, a good place to begin would be to review recently completed research on this or similar topics to obtain clues about how maternal bonding was operationalized. Table 15-3 provides examples of some concepts of interest to nurse researchers for which observational instruments have been developed and lists a recent study that used these instruments.

Observational Sampling

Structured observational methods rarely involve the recording of all behaviors or activities that occur in a given situation. The investigator must often decide how and when the system will be applied. Observational sampling methods represent a mechanism for obtaining representative examples of the behavior being observed without having to observe for prolonged periods. Note that observational sampling concerns the selection of behaviors to be observed, not the selection of study participants.

One frequently used system is the **time-sampling method**. This procedure involves the selection of periods during which the observations will occur. The timeframes may be systematically selected (e.g., every 30 seconds at 2-minute intervals) or may be selected at random. As a hypothetical example, suppose we were studying the interaction patterns of mothers and their handicapped children. Some of the mothers have received specific preparation from a community health nurse for dealing with their conflict over the child's dependence–independence needs, and a control group of mothers has not received this intervention. To examine the effects of this special program, the behavior of the mothers and children are observed in a playground setting. During a 1-hour observation period, we decide to sample behaviors rather than to observe the entire ses-

TABLE 15-3	Examples of Observational Instruments Used by Nurse Researchers	
CONCEPT	**RESEARCH EXAMPLE REFERENCE**	**INSTRUMENT**
Caregiver behaviors	Burgener & Shimer, 1993	Interaction Behavior Measure (IBM)
Confusion	Miller, Neelon, Dalton, Ng'andu, Bailey, Layman, & Hosfeld, 1996	NEECHAM Confusion Scale
Functional ability	Sisson, 1995	Barthel Functional Index
Home environment quality for children	Tesh & Holditch-Davis, 1997	Home Observation for Measurement of the Environment (HOME)
Infant development	Pickler, Frankel, Walsh, & Thompson, 1996 Becker, Engelhardt, Steinmann, & Kane, 1997	Anderson Behavioral State Scale (ABSS) Bayley Scales of Infant Development
Infant feeding performance	Pickler, Frankel, Walsh, & Thompson, 1996	Complex Feeding Scale
Mother–infant interaction	Becker, Englehardt, Steinmann, & Kane, 1997	Nursing Child Assessment Teaching Scales (NCATS)
Pain in children	Pederson, 1996 Maikler, 1991	Observational Scale of Behavioral Distress Maximally Discriminative Facial Movement Coding System
Pressure ulceration	Lewicki, Mion, Splane, Samstag, & Secic, 1997	Braden Scale for Predicting Pressure Sore Risk
Quality of nursing care	Norman & Redfern, 1996	Quality of Patient Care Scale (QualPacs)

sion. For the sake of simplicity, let us say that 3-minute observations will be made. If we use a systematic sampling approach, we would observe for 3-minutes, then cease observing for a prespecified period, say 3 minutes. Using this scheme, a total of 10 3-minute observations would be made. A second approach is to sample randomly 3-minute periods from the total of 20 such periods in an hour. The decision with regard to the length and number of periods for

creating a suitable sample must be influenced by the aims of the research. In establishing time units, one of the most important considerations is determining a psychologically meaningful timeframe. A good deal of pretesting and experimentation with different sampling plans is essential in developing or adapting observational strategies. Algase, Kupferschmid, Beel-Bates, and Beattie (1997) used time sampling in their study of the stability of daily wandering behavior among cognitively impaired nursing home residents.

Event sampling is a second system for obtaining a set of observations. This approach selects integral behaviors or events of a prespecified type for observation. Event sampling requires that the investigator either have some knowledge concerning the occurrence of events or be in a position to await their occurrence. Examples of integral events that may be suitable for event sampling include shift changes of nurses in a hospital, cast removals of pediatric patients, epileptic seizures, and cardiac arrests in the emergency room. This sampling approach is preferable to time sampling when the events of principal interest are infrequent throughout the day and are at risk of being missed if specific time sampling frames are established. In addition, event sampling has the advantage that the observation treats situations in their entirety rather than fragmenting them into discontinuous segments. Still, when behaviors and events are relatively frequent, time sampling does have the virtue of enhancing the representativeness of the observed behaviors. Time sampling and event sampling can sometimes be profitably combined. As an example of a study that used event sampling, Roach, Larson, and Bartlett (1996) studied the extent to which critical care nurses practice intravascular site care according to written protocols, using site care episodes as the events to sample.

Structured Observations by Nonresearch Personnel

The research we have discussed thus far involves situations in which the researcher (or an observer assistant) observes ongoing events or behaviors of relevance to the research problem and then codes information relating to what has been seen in some specified period. Other forms of observational data-gathering methods provide more global information about the characteristics, activities, and behaviors of individuals. Such methods often involve asking nonresearch personnel to record information about another person or a group on structured scales, based on their own observations. This method has much in common (in terms of format and scoring procedures) with the self-report scales described in Chapter 13; the primary difference is that the person completing the scale describes the attributes and behaviors of people other than himself or herself, based on observation. For example, a mother might be asked to describe the temperament of her infant, staff nurses might be asked to evaluate the functional capacity of nursing home residents, or a nursing supervisor might be asked to assess the nursing competency of nurses on the unit. As with self-report instruments, researchers might decide to construct their own behavior-rating scale for a specific research purpose, or they might choose to use or adapt an existing scale. Some of the references cited in Chapter 13 and at the end of this chapter identify such observational instruments.

The use of nonresearch personnel to provide observational data has a number of practical advantages. It is an economical method compared with using trained observers. For example, an observer might have to watch children for hours or days to describe fully the nature and intensity of certain behavior problems when a parent or teacher could readily do this. In some situations, the behaviors of interest might never be capable of observation by an outsider because of reactivity problems, because they occur in private situations, or because they constitute rare events (e.g., sleepwalking).

On the other hand, such methods may have all the same problems as self-report scales (such as response-set biases) in addition to the problem of observer bias. Observer bias may in some cases be extreme, such as often happens when parents are asked to provide information about their children. Nonresearch observers are typically not trained, and inter-observer agreement usually cannot be determined. Thus, this approach has a number of problems but will inevitably continue to find many research applications because, in many cases, there are no alternatives.

Several nurse researchers have used third-party observers to collect research data. For example, Bournaki (1997) asked parents to rate the temperaments of their children using the Middle Childhood Temperament Questionnaire in a study of children's pain-related responses to venipunctures (observations by the researcher were used to measure the children's behavioral responses). Winslow (1997) asked the caregivers of Alzheimer's patients to rate the problematic behavior of the patients in a study of stress outcomes among family caregivers. Swanson, Maas, and Buckwalter (1994) asked Alzheimer's disease patients' primary nurses to rate the patients' functional abilities using the Geriatric Rating Scale and the Functional Abilities Checklist.

MECHANICAL AIDS IN OBSERVATIONS

Our discussion has focused on those types of observations that are made by observers directly through the use of their sensory organs. In this section, we look at mechanical devices or other equipment that can be used either as an extension of the human senses or as a means of securing permanent records of observational data.

The health care field has a rich store of devices and equipment designed to make available to observers conditions or attributes that are ordinarily imperceptible. Nasal specula, stethoscopes, bronchoscopes, radiographic and imaging equipment, ultrasound technology, and a myriad of other medical instruments make it possible for health care personnel to gather observational information concerning the health status and bodily functioning of patients.

In addition to equipment for enhancing physiologic observations, several mechanical devices are available for recording behaviors and events. These techniques make possible categorization at a later time. When the behav-

ior of interest is primarily auditory, tape recordings can be obtained and used as a permanent observational record. Transcripts from such recordings can then be prepared to facilitate the coding or classification process. Other technologic instruments to aid auditory observation have been developed, such as laser devices that are capable of recording sounds by being directed on a window to a room, and voice tremor detectors that are sensitive to stress.

When a visual record is desired, videotapes are likely to be the most suitable media. In addition to being permanent, videotapes offer the possibility of capturing complex behaviors that would elude categorization by an on-the-spot observer. Visual records are also more capable of capturing fine units of behavior, such as micromomentary facial expressions, than is the naked eye. Videotapes offer the possibility of checking the accuracy of the coders and, thus, are useful as an aid to training. Finally, it is often easier to conceal a camera than a human observer, and in some situations, this feature would constitute a major advantage. Video records also have a number of drawbacks, some of which are fairly technical, such as lighting requirements, lens limitations, and so forth. Other serious problems result from the fact that the camera angle adopted could present a lopsided view of an event or situation. Also, some study participants may be more self-conscious in front of a video camera than they would otherwise be. Still, for many applications, permanent visual records offer unparalleled opportunities to expand the range and scope of observational studies.

Also of interest is the growing technology for assisting with the encoding and recording of observations made directly by on-the-spot observers. For example, there is equipment that permits the observer to enter observational data directly into a computer as the observation occurs, and in some cases, the equipment can be used to record physiologic data concurrently. Such a system was used in an interesting nursing study by White, Williams,

Alexander, Powell-Cope, and Conlon (1990), who tested whether a taped bedtime story read to hospitalized children by their parents would help to ease separation anxiety.

OBSERVER BIASES

Although observation is an extremely important method of data collection, it must be acknowledged that both unstructured and structured observational data are vulnerable to a number of distortions and biases. Human perceptual errors and inadequacies are a continuous threat to the quality of obtained information. Observation and interpretation are demanding tasks, requiring attention, sensation, perception, and conception. To accomplish these activities in a completely objective fashion is probably impossible, although structured category systems are designed to reduce observer subjectivity.

Several types of observational biases are especially common. One bias is referred to as the **enhancement of contrast effect**. The observer may tend to distort the observation in the direction of dividing the content into clearcut entities. The converse effect—a bias toward **central tendency**—occurs when extreme events are distorted toward a middle ground. A series of biases are in a category described as **assimilatory**. The observer may tend to distort observations in the direction of identity with previous inputs. This bias would have the effect of miscategorizing information in the direction of regularity and orderliness. Assimilation to the expectations and attitudes of the observer also occurs.

Rating scales and other evaluative observations are susceptible to several distinct types of bias. The **halo effect** refers to the tendency of the observer to be influenced by one characteristic in judging other unrelated characteristics. For example, if we formed a positive general impression of a person, we would probably be likely to rate that person as intelligent, loyal, and dependable simply because these traits are positively valued. Rating scales may reflect the personality traits of the observer. The **error of leniency** is the tendency for the observer to rate everything positively, and the **error of severity** is the contrasting tendency to rate too harshly.

Needless to say, these biases are much more likely to operate when a high degree of observer inference is required by the observational tasks. The careful construction and pretesting of checklists and rating scales (with structured observation) and the proper training of observers are techniques that can play an important role in minimizing or estimating these problematic biases. Although the degree of observer bias is not necessarily a function of the degree of structure imposed on the observation, it is generally more difficult to assess the extent of bias when using unstructured methods.

TIPS FOR GATHERING OBSERVATIONAL DATA

By the time we reach adulthood, many of us have lost some of our native ability to learn through careful observation. We may even have to "unlearn" habits of filtering out details of the world around us. Below are some suggestions for how to proceed in an observational study.

- Observers ideally should view the behaviors and events under observation in a neutral and nonjudgmental fashion. The people being observed are more likely to mask their emotions or behave in an atypical fashion if they think they are being critically appraised. Even positive cues (such as nodding approval) often should be withheld because approval may induce repetition of a behavior that might not otherwise have occurred.

- The adequate training and preparation of observers is essential to the collection of high-quality observational data. If people are to become good instruments for collecting observational data, then they must be trained to observe in such a way that accuracy is maximized and biases are minimized. Even when the investigator who designed the study does most or all of the observing, self-training and dry runs are essential. The setting during the trial period should resemble as closely as possible the settings that will be the focus of the actual observations.
- Ideally, training should include practice sessions during which the comparability of the observers' recordings is assessed. That is, two or more observers should watch a trial event or situation, and observations should then be compared. Procedures for establishing the **interrater reliability** of structured observational instruments are described in Chapter 17.

- With both structured and unstructured methods of observation, it is usually useful to spend a period of time with study participants before the actual observations and recording of data. Having a warm-up period helps to relax people (especially if audio or video equipment is being used) and can be extremely helpful to observers (e.g., if the participants have a linguistic style to which the observer must adjust, such as a strong regional accent).

RESEARCH EXAMPLES

Table 15-4 presents several examples of observational studies conducted by nurse researchers. Two other examples that illustrate observational research in greater detail follow. The first is an example of an ethnographic study in which participant observation was used, and the second is a quantitative study that used structured instruments.

TABLE 15-4 Examples of Studies Using Observation

RESEARCH QUESTION	TYPE OF OBSERVATION	PHENOMENON OBSERVED
What is the context within which heavy use of the emergency department occurs, and what is its meaning to patients and clinicians? (Malone, 1996)	Participant observation	Interactions between emergency nurses and "frequent fliers" (repeat users of emergency services)
What are the experiences and needs of patients with brain tumors? (Leavitt, Lamb, & Voss, 1996)	Unstructured observation	Verbal communications of brain tumor patients in support groups
What is the effectiveness of a special program to teach children with disabilities about handwashing? (Day, Arnaud, & Monsma, 1993)	Structured checklist	Children's handwashing
What are the structure, process, and outcomes of nurse practitioner–patient encounters? (Courtney & Rice, 1997)	Structured ratings	Nurse practitioners' care of clients in a primary care setting

Research Example of an Unstructured Observation

Chase (1995) conducted an ethnographic study of the "culture" of the critical care unit to examine the social context within which nurses' critical care clinical judgment occurs. Field work was done over a 2-year period, primarily in an 11-bed open heart surgical intensive care unit.

Participant observations were conducted about twice weekly during the 2 years of the study. Nurse managers granted access to the nursing unit under study, and individual nurses agreed to be observed. Although initially the observations were fairly general, more focused observations were undertaken later in the field work in response to initial observations about communication patterns. The early observations also led the researcher to conduct observations for several months in a 10-bed general surgical intensive care unit, for comparison purposes. Extensive field notes were recorded at each observational session. In addition, frequent methodologic and analytic memos were written to capture emerging patterns or to develop new understandings of observations. As is typical in participant observation, the unstructured observations were supplemented with in-depth interviews with 10 nurses who were followed extensively.

Chase concluded that parallel hierarchies for nurses and physicians allowed for checks on clinical judgment both within and across professional lines. Such rituals as the nursing report and physician rounds provided a context for a critique of judgment processes. Communication of judgment, which was frequently an open and casual conversation, was viewed as contributing to better patient outcomes.

Research Example of a Structured Observation

Miller and Holditch-Davis (1992) compared the interactions of preterm infants and their parents with the infants' interactions with nurses. A sample of 29 high-risk preterm infants were observed weekly from 7:00 PM to 11:00 PM. All infants received at least 2 minutes of parental care and 2 minutes of nursing care during the observational session. During the observations, occurrences of infant and caregiver behaviors were recorded every 10 seconds, according to a behavioral scoring system that had been developed by other researchers. There was an audible signal at the end of each 10-second epoch, at which time the observer recorded the behaviors on a computer used as an event recorder. Each observation was conducted by one of two observers.

The researchers measured various dimensions of behavior. One dimension was caregiver involvement. For this variable, infant time spent with parents and nurses was divided into four mutually exclusive levels of involvement: contact (touching, holding); routine care (feeding, changing diaper); low-level nursing care (e.g., taking vital signs); and high-level nursing care (e.g., respiratory care). Contact was scored only if no other type of involvement occurred in the 10-second epoch; if one of the other three levels occurred in the same epoch, the one that occupied the greatest amount of time was scored. Other dimensions scored included the infant's behavior, the infant's sleep–wake state, and caregiver stimulation.

The researchers found that nurses and parents provided different types of stimulation to the infants. Nurses were more likely to engage in procedural care, and parents were more likely to hold, talk to, move, and touch the infants affectionately. The infants demonstrated more large body movements and jitters when they were with the nurses and more active sleep and smiles when they were with the parents.

SUMMARY

Observational methods are techniques for acquiring information for research purposes through the direct observation and recording of phenomena. In any observational setting—whether it be in a natural field situation or laboratory setup—the observer must have a plan regarding the nature of the phenomena to be observed. The researcher usually selects an appropriate **unit of observation**. The **molar approach** entails the observation of large segments of behaviors and events as integral units. The **molecular approach**, on the other hand, treats small, specific actions as separate entities.

The investigator must make decisions concerning the relationship between the observer and the people observed. The decisions relate primarily to the dimensions of concealment and intervention. **Concealment** refers to the degree to which the observed people are aware that they are being observed or that they are the subjects of a research study. The problem of behavioral distortions stemming from the presence of an observer (known as **reactivity**) is a major reason for making concealed observations. **Intervention** refers to the degree to which the investigator structures the observational setting in line with research demands as opposed to being a passive observer.

Like self-reports, observational methods vary in terms of structure. Qualitative studies generally collect unstructured observational data, often using a procedure known as participant observation. **Participant observation** is a method that has been used by anthropologists and sociologists as a means of understanding cultures, institutions, and social groups. The participant observer endeavors to obtain information about the dynamics of the social group within the subject's own frame of reference, without imposing a preconceived structure based on the researcher's world view.

In the initial phase of a participant observation study, the researcher is primarily an observer and gathers a preliminary understanding of the site. As time passes, the researcher typically becomes a more active participant and also develops a plan for sampling events and selecting observational positions. The observer usually samples events to be observed through a combination of **single positioning**, **multiple positioning**, and **mobile positioning**. The final phase of the research involves reflective observation about the activities that transpired.

Participant observers typically collect information about the setting, participants, activities and interactions, frequency and duration of events, and intangible factors. **Logs** of daily events and **field notes** are the major methods of recording data. Field notes have multiple purposes and may be categorized as **observational notes, theoretical notes, methodologic notes**, and **personal notes**.

Structured observational methods impose a number of constraints on the observer for the purpose of maximizing observer accuracy and objectivity and for obtaining an adequate representation of the phenomena of interest. Two types of data collection forms are used most commonly by observers in structured situations. **Checklists** are tools for recording the appearance or frequency of prespecified behaviors, events, or characteristics. Checklists are based on the development of **category systems** for encoding the observed phenomena. The researcher constructing a category system must make a number of decisions concerning its exhaustiveness, generality, inference requirements, and training demands. One type of checklist is based on the **sign system** and is used as a demographic record of the types of behavior that occurred during the observational session. A second format is used to analyze exhaustively ongoing events and activities.

Rating scales are the second most common record-keeping tool for structured observations. The observer using a rating scale is required to rate some phenomenon according to points along a dimension that is typically bipolar (e.g., passive/aggressive or excellent health/poor health). Ratings are generally made either during the observational setting at specific intervals (e.g., every 5 minutes) or after the observation is completed.

Most structured observations make use of some form of sampling plan for selecting the behaviors, events, and conditions to be observed. One frequently used approach is **time sampling**, which involves the specification of the duration and frequency of both the observational periods and the intersession intervals.

Event sampling selects integral behaviors or events of a special type for observation.

Technologic advances have greatly augmented the researcher's capacity to collect, record, and preserve observational data. Such devices as tape recorders, movie cameras, videotape cameras, and laser devices permit behaviors and events to be categorized after their occurrence.

Observational methods, although extremely valuable to nurse researchers, are subject to a variety of biasing effects. The greater the degree of observer inference and judgment, the more likely it is that perceptual errors and distortions will occur. Among the most prevalent observer biases are the **enhancement of contrast effect**, **central tendency bias**, the **halo effect**, **assimilatory biases**, **errors of leniency**, and **errors of severity**.

STUDY ACTIVITIES

Chapter 15 of the *Study Guide to Accompany Nursing Research: Principles and Methods, 6th ed.*, offers various exercises and study suggestions for reinforcing the concepts presented in this chapter. Additionally, the following study questions can be addressed:

1. Suppose you were interested in observing the behavior of fathers in the delivery room during the birth of their first child. Identify the observer–observed relationship on the concealment and intervention dimensions that you would recommend adopting for such a study, and defend your recommendation. What are the possible drawbacks of your approach, and how might you deal with them?

2. Would a psychiatric nurse researcher be well suited to conduct a participant observation study of the behavior of psychiatric nurses and their interactions with clients? Why or why not?

3. A nurse researcher is planning to study temper tantrums displayed by hospitalized children. Would you recommend using a time sampling approach? Why or why not?

4. Below is a list of problem statements. Indicate which of these problems could be studied by using some form of observational method. For each problem that is amenable to observation, specify whether you think a structured or unstructured approach would be preferable.
   a. Does team nursing versus primary nursing affect the type of communication patterns between nurses and patients?
   b. Is there a relationship between prenatal instruction and delivery room behaviors of primiparas?
   c. Is the number of hours of direct clinical practice for student nurses related to their performance on the licensure examination?
   d. Do the attitudes of nurses toward abortion affect the quality of care given to abortion patients?
   e. Do industrial alcohol programs have a positive impact on on-the-job accident rates?
   f. Is the touching behavior of nurses related to their ethnic or cultural background?

SUGGESTED READINGS

Methodologic References

Dowrick, P., & Biggs, S. J. (Eds.). (1983). *Using video: Psychological and social applications*. New York: John Wiley and Sons.

Frank-Stromberg, M. (Ed.). (1988). *Instruments for clinical nursing research*. Norwalk, CT: Appleton & Lange.

Kerlinger, F. (1986). *Foundations of behavioral research* (3rd ed.). New York: Holt, Rinehart & Winston.

Leininger, M. (1985). Ethnography and ethnonursing: Models and modes of qualitative data analysis. In M. Leininger (Ed.), *Qualitative research methods in nursing.* New York: Grune & Stratton.

Lobo, M. L. (1992). Observation: A valuable data collection strategy for research with children. *Journal of Pediatric Nursing, 7,* 320–328.

Lofland, J., & Lofland, L. (1984). *Analyzing social settings: A guide to qualitative observation and analysis.* Belmont, CA: Wadsworth.

McCall, G. J., & Simmons H. L. (Eds.). (1969). *Issues in participant observation: A text and reader.* Reading, MA: Addison-Wesley.

Morrison, E. F., Phillips, L. R., & Chal, Y. M. (1990). The development and use of observational measurement scales. *Applied Nursing Research, 3,* 73–86.

Schatzman, L., & Strauss, A. (1982). *Field research: Strategies for a natural sociology* (2nd ed.). Englewood Cliffs, NJ: Prentice-Hall.

Strickland, O. L., & Waltz, C. (Eds.). (1988). *Measurement of nursing outcomes.* New York: Springer.

Ward, M. J., & Lindemann, C. (Eds.). (1979). *Instruments for measuring nursing practice and other health care variables.* Hyattsville, MD: Department of Health, Education and Welfare.

Wilson, H. S. (1985). *Research in nursing.* Menlo Park, CA: Addison-Wesley.

Substantive References

Algase, D. L., Kupferschmid, B., Beel-Bates, C. A., & Beattie, E. (1997). Estimates of the stability of daily wandering behavior among cognitively impaired long-term care residents. *Nursing Research, 46,* 172–178.

Beck, C., Heacock, P., Mercer, S. O., Walls, R. C., Rapp, C. G., & Vogelpohl, T. S. (1997). Improving dressing behavior in cognitively impaired nursing home residents. *Nursing Research, 46,* 126–132.

Becker, P. T., Engelhardt, K. F., Steinmann, M. F., & Kane, J. (1997). Infant age, context, and family system influences on the interactive behavior of mothers of infants with mental delay. *Research in Nursing & Health, 20,* 39–50.

Bournaki, M. C. (1997). Correlates of pain-related responses to venipunctions in school-aged children. *Nursing Research, 46,* 147–154.

Burgener, S. C., & Shimer, R. (1993). Variables related to caregiver behaviors with cognitively impaired elders in institutional settings. *Research in Nursing & Health, 16,* 193–202.

Chase, S. K. (1995). The social context of critical care clinical judgment. *Heart and Lung, 24,* 154–162.

Courtney, R., & Rice, C. (1997). Investigation of nurse-practitioner-patient interactions. *Nurse Practitioner, 22,* 46–48.

Cureton-Lane, R. A., & Fontaine, D. K. (1997). Sleep in the pediatric ICU. *American Journal of Critical Care, 6,* 56–63.

Day, R. A., Arnaud, S. S., & Monsma, M. (1993). Effectiveness of a handwashing program. *Clinical Nursing Research, 2,* 24–40.

Grace, J., Bellus, S. B., Raulin, M. L, Herz, M. I., Priest, B. L., Brenner, V., Donnelly, K., Smith, P. & Gunn, S. (1996). Long-term impact of clozapine and psychosocial treatment on psychiatric symptoms and cognitive functioning. *Psychiatric Services, 47,* 41–45.

Hall, D. S. (1996). Interactions between nurses and patients on ventilators. *American Journal of Critical Care, 5,* 293–297.

Hurley, A. C., Volicer, B. J., Hanrahan, P. A., Houde, S., & Volicer, L. (1992). Assessment of discomfort in advanced Alzheimer patients. *Research in Nursing & Health, 15,* 369–377.

Larson, E. L., Bryan, J. L., Adler, L. M., & Blane, C. (1997). A multifaceted approach to changing handwashing behavior. *American Journal of Infection Control, 25,* 3–10.

Leavitt, M. B., Lamb, S. A., & Voss, B. S. (1996). Brain tumor support group: Content themes and mechanisms of support. *Oncology Nursing Forum, 23,* 1247–1256.

Lewicki, L. J., Mion, L., Splane, K. G., Samstag, D., & Secic, M. (1997). Patient risk factors for pressure ulcers during cardiac surgery. *AORN Journal, 65,* 938–942.

Littrell, K., & Magill, A. M. (1993). The effect of clozapine on preexisting tardive dyskinesia. *Journal of Psychosocial Nursing and Mental Health Services, 31,* 14–18.

Maikler, V. E. (1991). Effects of a skin refrigerant/anesthetic and age on the pain responses of infants receiving immunizations. *Research in Nursing & Health, 14,* 397–402.

Malone, R. E. (1996). Almost "like family": Emergency nurses and "frequent flyers." *Journal of Emergency Nursing, 22,* 176–183.

Miller, D. B., & Holditch-Davis, D. (1992). Interaction patterns of parents and nurses with high-risk preterm infants. *Research in Nursing & Health, 15*, 187–197.

Miller, J., Neelon, V., Dalton, J., Ng'andu, N., Bailey, D., Layman, E., & Hosfeld, A. (1996). The assessment of discomfort in elderly confused patients. *Journal of Neuroscience Nursing, 28*, 175–182.

Norman, I. J., & Redfern, S. J. (1996). The validity of two quality assessment instruments. *International Journal of Nursing Studies, 33*, 660–668.

Pederson, C. (1996). Promoting parental use of nonpharmacologic techniques with children during lumbar punctures. *Journal of Pediatric Oncology Nursing, 13*, 21–30.

Pickler, R. H., Frankel, H. B., Walsh, K. M., & Thompson, N. M. (1996). Effects of nonnutritive sucking on behavioral organization and feeding performance in preterm infants. *Nursing Research, 45*, 132–135.

Roach, H., Larson, E., & Bartlett, D. B. (1996). Intravascular site care: Are critical care nurses practicing according to written protocols? *Heart & Lung, 25*, 401–408.

Routasalo, P. (1996). Non-necessary touch in the nursing care of elderly people. *Journal of Advanced Nursing, 23*, 904–911.

Russell, K. M., & Champion, V. L. (1996). Health beliefs and social influence in home safety practices of mothers with preschool children. *Image—The Journal of Nursing Scholarship, 28*, 59–64.

Sisson, R. A. (1995). Cognitive status as a predictor of right hemisphere stroke outcomes. *Journal of Neuroscience Nursing, 27*, 152–156.

Swanson, E. A., Maas, M. L., & Buckwalter, K. C. (1994). Alzheimer's residents' cognitive and functional measures. *Clinical Nursing Research, 3*, 27–41.

Tesh, E. M., & Holditch-Davis, D. (1997). HOME inventory and NCATS: Relation to mother and child behavior during naturalistic observations. *Research in Nursing & Health, 20*, 295–307.

Weiss, S. J. (1992). Measurement of the sensory qualities in tactile interaction. *Nursing Research, 41*, 82–86.

White, M. A., Williams, P. D., Alexander, D. J., Powell-Cope, G. M., & Conlon, M. (1990). Sleep onset latency and distress in hospitalized children. *Nursing Research, 39*, 134–139.

Winslow, B. W. (1997). Effects of formal supports on stress outcomes in family caregivers of Alzheimer's patients. *Research in Nursing & Health, 20*, 27–37.

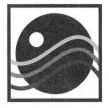

CHAPTER **16**

Biophysiologic and Other Data Collection Methods

Most nursing research studies involve the collection of data through self-reports and observations. However, other methods of collecting data are available, and several of these are reviewed in this chapter. The most important alternative method is the use of biophysiologic measures.

BIOPHYSIOLOGIC MEASURES

The trend in nursing research has been toward increased clinical, patient-centered investigations and an expanded use of measures to assess the physiologic status of study participants. Indeed, the National Institute for Nursing Research has emphasized the need for more physiologically based nursing research.

Many variables that are of interest in clinical research do not require biophysiologic instrumentation for their measurement. Data on physiologic activity or dysfunction can often be gathered through direct observation. For example, phenomena such as vomiting, cyanosis, postcardiotomy delirium, edema, and wound status can be observed for presence and intensity. Other biophysiologic data can be gathered by asking people directly. Examples of possible self-report measures include assessment of pain, ratings of fatigue, and reports of nausea. This section focuses on biophysiologic phenomena that require the use of specialized technical apparatus that yield quantitative measures.

Settings in which nurses operate are typically filled with a wide variety of technical instruments for measuring physiologic functions. It is beyond the scope of this book to describe in any detail the many kinds of biophysiologic measures available to nurse researchers. Our objectives are to present an overview of potential measures for clinical nursing studies, to illustrate their use in a research context, and to direct the interested reader to supplementary sources for further information.

Purposes of Biophysiologic Measures

Clinical nursing studies often involve specialized equipment and instruments both for creating independent variables (e.g., an intervention using biofeedback equipment) and for measuring dependent variables. For the most part, our discussion focuses on the use of biophysiologic measures as outcome or dependent variables.

Most nursing studies in which biophysiologic measures have been used fall into one of five classes.

1. *Studies of basic physiologic processes that are relevant to nursing care.* Such studies often involve subjects who are healthy and normal or some subhuman animal species. For example, McCarthy, Lo, Nguyen, and Ney (1997) studied the effect of the protein density of food on the food intake and nutritional status of tumor-bearing rats. Liehr, Meininger, Mueller, Chandler, and Chan (1997) studied blood pressure reactivity in a sample of healthy adolescents during angry and normal talk.

2. *Explorations of the ways in which nursing actions or medical interventions affect the health outcomes of patients.* For example, Penny-MacGillivray (1996) studied the effects of bathing newborns at two different times (after the admission assessment examination and 4 hours after birth) in terms of infant body temperature. Banasik and Emerson (1996) studied the effects of three different positions (supine, right lateral, and left lateral) on arterial and venous blood gases in postoperative cardiac surgery patients.

3. *Evaluations of a specific nursing procedure or intervention.* These studies differ from the studies in the second category in that they involve a new intervention that is being tested, usually in comparison with standard methods of care. Typically, these studies involve a hypothesis stating that the innovative nursing procedure will result in improved biophysiologic outcomes among patients. For example, Byers and Smyth (1997) studied the effect of a music intervention on the noise annoyance, heart rate, and blood pressure in cardiac surgery patients. Collins and Rice (1997) studied the effects of

a relaxation intervention and guided imagery on psychological and physiologic outcomes in adults with cardiovascular disease.

4. *Studies to improve the measurement and recording of biophysiologic information regularly gathered by nurses.* For example, Moniaci and Kraus (1997) did a study to determine if blood pressure values obtained from the calves of neonates correlated with measurements obtained from the umbilical arterial catheter. Krenzischek and Tanseco (1996) compared the results of hemoglobin measured at the bedside with measurements done in the laboratory and found that the two were comparable.

5. *Studies of the correlates of physiologic functioning in patients with health problems.* For example, Lewicki, Mion, Splane, Samstag, and Secic (1997) studied various biophysiologic measures (e.g., hemoglobin, hematocrit, and serum albumin levels) in cardiac patients in relation to their risk for developing pressure ulcers. Caudell and Gallucci (1995) explored the relationship between physiologic (e.g., heart rate, skin conductance) and selected psychosocial (e.g., mood state, coping) variables among women undergoing a cognitive stress test.

The physiologic phenomena that interest nurse researchers run the full gamut of available measures. Some of these measures are discussed in the next section.

Types of Biophysiologic Measures

Physiologic measurements can be classified in one of two major categories. **In vivo measurements** are those that are performed directly within or on living organisms themselves. One example of an in vivo measure is oxygen saturation measurement through a pulse oximeter. An **in vitro measurement**, by contrast, is performed outside the organism's body, as in the case of measuring serum potassium concentration in the blood drawn from a patient.

IN VIVO MEASURES

In vivo measures often involve the use of highly complex instrumentation systems. An **instrumentation system** is the apparatus and equipment used to measure one or more attributes of a subject and the presentation of that measurement data in a manner that humans can interpret. Organism–instrument systems involve up to six major components: (1) stimulus, (2) subject, (3) sensing equipment, (4) signal-conditioning equipment, (5) display equipment, and (6) recording, data processing, and transmission equipment. These components and their interrelationships are presented in Figure 16–1. The role of each component is briefly described as follows:

1. *Stimulus.* Many physiologic measurements require some type of external stimulus. The stimulation may be engendered by another human, as in the case of requests for deep and rapid breathing by the patient when recording electrical activity from the brain. The stimulus

may also be produced by electrical or mechanical equipment, such as an external pacemaker and cardiac defibrillator.

2. *Subject.* Human bodies consist of chemical, electrical, mechanical, thermal, hydraulic, pneumatic, and other systems interacting with each other and with the outside world. Communication of the human organism with the external environment consists of various inputs (e.g., sensory inputs, inspired air, or liquid and food intake) and outputs (e.g., speech, body movements, expired air, or wastes). Most of these inputs and outputs are easily amenable to measurements. The major bodily systems—circulatory, respiratory, and so forth—also communicate with each other internally, as do smaller subsystems, such as organs and cells. Biomedical instrumentation constitutes the tools for measuring the information communicated by these diverse elements.

3. *Sensing equipment.* Sensing equipment normally consists of one or more transducers. Generally defined, a *transducer* is a device that converts one form of energy into another. Transducers are used

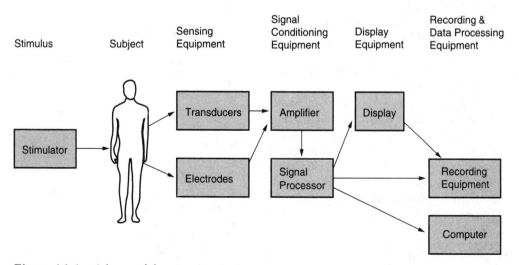

Figure 16-1. Schema of the organism–instrument system.

in organism–instrument systems to measure physical phenomena by producing an electrical signal proportional to these phenomena. Electrical signals permit presentations of the desired physiologic information in a highly useful form. With an electrical analogue of the critical physiologic event, the scientist can store the event on a computer file for later inspection and analysis.

4. *Signal-conditioning equipment.* In virtually all physiologic measures, two signals are produced by the subject: the key physiologic signal—such as the electrocardiographic signal—and an interference signal. An important function of signal-conditioning equipment is to reject the interference signal and to amplify the desired physiologic signal from the transducer.

5. *Display equipment.* Display devices convert the modified electrical signals into visual or auditory output. For example, an oscilloscope is a device that allows for the visual observation of the waveform of a signal. It is used to display and measure the time, phase, voltage, or frequency of a physiologic signal. With sophisticated equipment, a television monitor that shows interpretation of the various physiologic functions under scrutiny is often available.

6. *Recording, data processing, and transmission equipment.* For research purposes, it is usually necessary to obtain a permanent record of the physiologic measurements for subsequent scrutiny and analysis. The recording equipment can be a unit that is either separate from the display device or integrated with it. The use of computer-linked equipment has the advantage of permitting information to be transmitted and replayed for convenient and detailed analysis.

Not all instrumentation systems involve all six components. Some systems, such as an electronic thermometer, are simple; other systems are extremely complex. For example, there are some electronic monitors that, although they are miniaturized and can be put into place during ambulation, yield simultaneous measures of such physiologic variables as cardiac responsivity, respiratory rate and rhythm, core temperature, and muscular activity.

In vivo instruments have been developed to measure all bodily functions, and technologic improvements continue to advance our ability to measure biophysiologic phenomena more accurately, more conveniently, and more rapidly than ever before. The uses to which such instruments have been put by nurse researchers is richly diverse and impressive. Table 16-1 presents examples of research questions that have been posed by nurse researchers relating to the various physiologic systems, together with a list of the physiologic variables measured. Of course, most nurse researchers who have gathered physiologic data have used data from two or more physiologic systems. For example, it is common for nurses to use data on vital signs (e.g., temperature, heart rate, or blood pressure) in their investigations. It is also common for nurses to combine information from in vivo measures with that from in vitro measures.

IN VITRO MEASURES

With in vitro measures, data are gathered by extracting some physiologic material from subjects and submitting it for laboratory analysis. Nurse researchers may or may not be involved in the extraction of the material; however, the analysis is normally done by highly specialized laboratory technicians. Generally, each laboratory establishes a range of normal values for each measure, and this information is critical for interpreting the results of laboratory tests.

Several classes of laboratory analysis have been used in studies by nurse researchers, including the following:

TABLE 16-1 Examples of Nursing Studies Using In Vivo Measures	
RESEARCH QUESTION	**MEASUREMENTS**
What are the responses to circumcision among unanesthetized newborn males and those having dorsal penile nerve block? (Williamson, 1997)	Circulatory function: blood pressure, heart rate, cardiac rhythm
Does lung volume reduction improve pulmonary function and quality of life in patients with bullous emphysema? (Vaca, Osterloh, Daake, & Noedel, 1996)	Respiratory function: forced expiratory volume in 1 second; residual volume; forced vital capacity; minute volume ventilation
What is the effect of facial cooling on tympanic temperature? (Thomas, Savage, & Brengelmann, 1997)	Neurologic function: tympanic and esophageal body temperature
What is the effect of muscle-strength training on the functional status of patients with osteoarthritis at the knee joint? (Schilke, Johnson, Housh, & O'Dell, 1996)	Musculoskeletal function: extension and flexion strength of the legs; range of motion at the knee
What are the effects of ovarian hormones on gastric mobility in rats with varying ovarian hormone status? (Heitkemper & Bond, 1995)	Gastrointestinal function: gastric contractile activity through a gastric tension transducer
What is the relationship between the frequency of urinary incontinence in older women and various functional, urologic, and environmental characteristics? (Wyman, Elswick, Ory, Wilson, & Fantl, 1993)	Genitourinary function: maximal cystometric bladder capacity, using saline infusion cystometry

- *Chemical measures,* such as measures of hormone levels, sugar levels, or potassium levels
- *Microbiologic measures,* such as bacterial counts and identification
- *Cytologic or histologic measures,* such as tissue biopsies

Because nurse researchers as a rule are not responsible for the analysis of in vitro extractions, it is unnecessary to explain relevant instrumentation or procedures, and it is impossible to catalog the thousands of laboratory tests available. To give students a sense of how in vitro measures have been used by nurse researchers, we present some examples in Table 16-2. Laboratory analyses of blood and urine samples are the most frequently used in vitro measures in nursing investigations.

Selecting a Biophysiologic Measure

For nurses unfamiliar with the hundreds of biophysiologic measures available in institutional settings, the selection of one or more appropriate measures of important research variables may pose a real challenge. There are, unfortunately, no comprehensive handbooks to guide interested researchers to the measures, instruments, and interpretations that may be required in collecting physiologic data. Probably the best approach is to consult a knowledgeable colleague or an expert at a local institution. It also may be possible to obtain useful information

TABLE 16-2	Examples of Nursing Studies Using In Vitro Measures

RESEARCH QUESTION	MEASUREMENTS
What is the extent to which gender, age, height, and weight predict selected physiologic outcomes? (Brown, Knapp, & Radke, 1997)	Blood tests: hemoglobin concentration; serum glucose concentration; serum cholesterol concentration
What is the relationship between psychological distress, sleep quality, and physiologic stress among women diagnosed with fibromyalgia? (Shaver, Lentz, Landis, Heitkemper, Buchwald, & Woods, 1997)	Urine tests: urinary catecholamines and cortisol
What are the effects of a nurse-delivered smoking cessation intervention on short-term smoking abstinence among hospitalized postoperative patients? (Wewers, Bowen, Stanislaw, & Desimone, 1994)	Saliva test: saliva cotinine level
What is the difference between the use of a scrub brush and use of soap alone in reducing bacteria? (Loeb, Wilcox, Smaill, Walter, & Duff, 1997)	Bacterial cultures: hand bacterial counts
What are the effects of 72 hours of sleep deprivation on wound healing in rats? (Landis & Whitney, 1997)	Cell histology: extent of polymorphonuclear cells, macrophages, fibroblasts, and connective tissue in tissue samples

on biophysiologic measures from original research articles on a problem similar to your own, a review article on the central phenomenon under investigation, manufacturers' catalogs, and exhibits of manufacturers at professional conferences.

Obviously, the most basic issue to address in selecting a physiologic measure is whether the measure will yield good information about the research variable under investigation. In some cases, the researcher will need to consider whether the variable should be measured by observation or self-report instead of (or in addition to) using biophysiologic equipment or apparatus. For example, stress could be measured by asking people questions (e.g., using the State–Trait Anxiety Inventory); by observing their behavior during exposure to stressful stimuli; or by measuring heart rate, blood pressure, or levels of adrenocorticotropic hormone in urine samples.

Several other considerations should be kept in mind in selecting a biophysiologic measure, several of which have been noted by Lindsey and Stotts (1989). These include the following:

- Is the equipment or laboratory analysis you will need readily available to you? If not, can it be borrowed, rented, or purchased?
- If equipment must be purchased, is it affordable? Can funding be acquired to cover the purchase (or rental) price?
- Can you operate the required equipment and interpret its results, or will you need training? Are there resources available to help you with operation and interpretation?
- Will you encounter any difficulties in obtaining permission to use the necessary equipment from an Institutional Review Board or other institutional authority?
- Does the measure need to be direct (e.g., a direct measure of blood pressure by way

of an arterial line), or is an indirect measure (e.g., blood pressure measurement by way of a sphygmomanometer) sufficient?

- Will continuous monitoring be necessary (e.g., electrocardiogram readings), or is a point-in-time measure adequate?
- Will your activities during data collection permit you to record data simultaneously, or will you need an instrument system with recording equipment (or a research assistant)?
- Will a mechanical stimulus be needed to get appropriate or meaningful measurements? Does available equipment include the required stimulus?
- Will a single measure of your dependent variable be sufficient, or is it preferable to operationalize your research variable using multiple measures? If multiple measures are better, what burden does this place on you as a researcher and on patients as research subjects?
- Are your measures likely to be influenced by reactivity (i.e., the subjects' awareness of their subject status)? If so, can alternative or supplementary nonreactive measures be identified, or can the extent of reactivity bias be assessed?
- Can your research variable be measured using a noninvasive procedure, or is an invasive procedure required?
- Is the measure you plan to use sufficiently accurate and sensitive to variation?
- Are you thoroughly familiar with rules and safety precautions, such as grounding procedures, especially when using electrical equipment?

The difficulty in choosing biophysiologic measures for nursing research investigations lies not in their shortage, nor in their questionable utility, nor in their inferiority to other methods. Indeed, they are plentiful, often highly reliable and valid, and extremely useful in clinical nursing studies. However, great care must be exercised in selecting appropriate instruments or laboratory analyses with regard to practical, ethical, medical, and technical considerations.

Research Example of a Study Using Biophysiologic Measures

Topf (1992) used an experimental design to test whether sleep was affected by a person's ability to control hospital noises. Subjects were randomly assigned to three groups: (1) those who received instruction in control over critical care unit (CCU) sounds and were subjected to a noisy condition, (2) those who received no instruction and were subjected to a noisy condition, or (3) those who were subjected to a quiet condition. Data were collected in a sleep laboratory that simulated a CCU environment so that actual noise levels could be controlled.

Twenty different measures of sleep were used in this study, one of which was a self-reported rating of sleep quality and 19 of which were physiologic. The physiologic measures included sleep efficiency; minutes in bed, asleep, and awake in various sleep stages; and number of stage shifts, intrasleep awakenings, and rapid-eye-movement periods. The physiologic data were obtained through polysomnograph equipment, which included electroencephalogram (EEG), electromyogram (EMG), and electrooculogram (EOG) recordings. The recordings yielded 1000-page sleep records. The unit of analysis for coding the sleep records was each page of the record. The stage of sleep of each page was recorded on a sleep summary sheet using well-established sleep stage criteria.

Subjects in all three groups changed into sleepwear at about 9:30 PM, and then the polysomnograph technician taped EEG, EOG, and EMG electrodes in place. At 10:25 PM, subjects were instructed to retire for the night, and the polysomnograph wires were connected to wall outlets in the subjects' rooms. The polysomnograph equipment was calibrated by the technician, who then recorded sleep according to standardized procedures. The technician also turned on an amplifier and audiotape recorder with CCU nighttime sounds for subjects in the two noise conditions.

The actual measures were derived through scoring by a doctorally prepared polysomnograph specialist. A second doctorally prepared polysomnographer scored some records (one sleep record randomly selected out of every five) to establish interscorer agreement. Agreement between the two scorers ranged between 78% and 94%.

The findings indicated that subjects' sleep patterns were strongly related to whether there was noise in the laboratory but were not a function of the instruction.

RECORDS AND AVAILABLE DATA

Thus far, we have examined a number of data collection strategies for which it was assumed that the researcher would be responsible for actually collecting the data and, in some cases, developing the data collection instruments. However, data that are routinely gathered for nonresearch purposes are often used to answer research questions.

Data Sources

The places where a nurse researcher is likely to find useful records are too numerous to list here, but a few suggestions may be helpful. Within a hospital or other health care setting, excellent records are kept routinely and systematically. For example, patient charts, physicians' order sheets, care plan statements, printouts of recordings of biophysiologic measures, and so forth all constitute rich data sources. In addition to medical and nursing records, hospitals maintain financial records, personnel records, nutritional records, and so forth. Educational institutions maintain various records. For example, most schools of nursing have permanent files on their students. Public school systems also keep records, including both academic and health-related information. Indus-

tries and businesses normally maintain a variety of records that may interest industrial nurse researchers, such as information on employees' absenteeism, health status, on-the-job accidents, job performance ratings, alcoholism or drug problems, and so forth. In addition to institutional records, personal documents such as diaries and letters should be considered as possible data sources. Table 16-3 illustrates some of the data sources and types of variables measured in nursing studies that have used existing records.

Advantages and Disadvantages of Using Records

The use of information from records is advantageous to the researcher for several reasons. The most salient advantage of existing records is that they are an economical source of information; the collection of original data is often time-consuming and costly. The use of preexisting records also permits an examination of trends over time, if the information is of the type that is collected repeatedly. Problems of reactivity and response biases may be completely absent when the researcher obtains information from records. Furthermore, the investigator does not have to be concerned with obtaining cooperation from participants.

On the other hand, because the researcher has not been responsible for the collection and recording of information, he or she may be unaware of the limitations, biases, or incompleteness of the records. Two of the major sources of bias in records are **selective deposit** and **selective survival**. If the records available for use do not constitute the entire set of all possible such records, the investigator must somehow deal with the question of how representative the existing records are. Many record keepers intend to maintain an entire universe or set of records rather than a sample but may fail to adhere to this ideal. The lapses from the ideal may be the result of some systematic biases, and the careful researcher should attempt to learn just what those biases may be.

TABLE 16-3   Examples of Nursing Studies Using Existing Records

RESEARCH QUESTION	DATA SOURCE	RESEARCH VARIABLES
What are the changes in continence status after hip fracture repair? (Palmer, Myers, & Fedenko, 1997)	Medical records	Incidence of incontinence; preoperatively and postoperatively; cognitive impairment; gender
Is there a relationship between the presence of apnea and the number of days it takes a premature infant to attain full oral feeding? (Mandich, Ritchie, & Mullett, 1996)	Daily nursing notes; medical records	Number of days between first attempted oral feeding and full oral feeding; number of apnea instances; receipt of aminophylline
What is the difference in the incidence of diarrhea among patients given one of three formulas with varying fiber concentrations administered through nasogastric tube? (Reese, Means, Hanrahan, Clearman, Colwill, & Dawson, 1996)	Medical records; bedside flow sheet	Medications; prior food aversions; fiber concentration; incidence of diarrhea and other gastrointestinal discomforts
How effective is the Creighton model ovulation method of natural family planning in avoiding and achieving a pregnancy? (Fehring, Lawrence, & Philpot, 1994)	Clinic logbooks	Number of clinic sessions attended; reason for program withdrawal; pregnancies; pregnancy outcomes; referral codes
Do falls among older nursing home residents predict subsequent disease onset? (Miceli, Waxman, Cavalieri, & Lage, 1994)	Physician progress notes; medical records; physician order sheets; nursing assessment records	Onset of new medical conditions; incidence of falling; circumstance of any fall; cognitive and functional status; medication use; fatality

An additional problem with which researchers must contend is the increasing reluctance of institutions to make their records available for scientific studies. The Privacy Act, a federal regulation enacted to protect individuals against possible misuse of records, has made hospitals, agencies, schools, and industrial organizations sensitive to the possibility of legal action from individuals who think that their right to privacy has been violated. The major issue here is the divulgence of an individual's identity. If records are maintained with an identifying number rather than a name, permission to use the records may be readily granted. However, most institutions *do* maintain records by their clients' names. In such a situation, the researcher may need the assistance of personnel at the institution to maintain client anonymity, and some organizations may be unwilling to use their personnel for such purposes.

A number of other difficulties in the use of records for research purposes may be relevant. Sometimes, the records have to be verified in terms of their authenticity, authorship, or accuracy, a task that may be difficult to execute if the records are old. The researcher using records must be prepared to deal with forms and file systems that he or she does not understand. Codes and symbols that had meaning to the record keeper may have to be translated to be usable. In using records to study trends, the researcher should always be alert to the possibility of changes in record-keeping procedures. For example, does a dramatic increase or decrease in the incidence of sudden infant death syndrome reflect changes in the causes or cures of this problem, or does it reflect a change in diagnosis or record keeping?

These considerations suggest that, although existing records may be plentiful, inexpensive, and accessible, they should not be used without paying attention to potential problems and weaknesses.

Research Example of a Study Using Available Data

Davis and Nomura (1990) were concerned about the appropriate frequency of assessing patients' vital signs after surgery. They noted that hospitals typically have protocols governing the frequency of this monitoring but that the frequencies specified vary considerably from hospital to hospital, and such variations appear to be based on tradition rather than on scientific data. The purpose of their investigation was to determine whether the protocol in effect in one specific hospital (a 450-bed acute care hospital in a large urban area) was appropriate for class I surgical patients. The protocol in effect was q 15 minutes × 4, q ½ hour × 2, q 1 hour × 1, and q 4 hours × 4.

Various hospital records were obtained for 250 surgical patients who were determined to be class I by an anesthesiologist. Charts of patients over a 1-year period for those undergoing five different types of surgical procedures were randomly selected. Data were gathered from the admit/discharge sheet; surgical permit; anesthesia record; recovery room record; unit record of temperature, pulse, respiration, and blood pressure; intake/output sheet; medication record; doctor's progress notes; and nurses' notes.

The investigators' analysis focused primarily on the timing of vital signs outside abnormal parameters and the occurrence of abnormal signs and symptoms such as nausea and vomiting and urinary retention. The pattern of findings revealed a dramatic reduction in vital signs outside normal parameters between the first and second hours after surgery, with few signs occurring at hour 4 or beyond. Newly occurring abnormal vital signs appeared in only 2% of the sample in hour 3 on the unit, and none of these patients had recurrences in the following hour. Based on this analysis, the protocol in the hospital in which the study was conducted was changed. Unless otherwise ordered by the physician, the new frequency is q 15 minutes × 1, q 30 minutes × 2, q 1 hour × 1, q 4 hours × 4.

Q METHODOLOGY

Q methodology is the term used by Stephenson (1975) to refer to a constellation of substantive, statistical, and psychometric concepts relating to research on individuals. Q methodology utilizes a procedure known as the **Q sort**, which involves the sorting of a deck of cards according to specified criteria.

Q-Sort Procedures

In a Q sort, study participants are presented with a set of cards on which words, phrases, statements, or other messages are written. Participants are then asked to sort the cards according to a particular dimension, such as approval/disapproval, most like me/least like me, or highest priority/lowest priority. The number of cards to be sorted is typically between 60 and 100. Usually, the cards are sorted into 9 or 11 piles, with the number of cards placed in each pile determined by the researcher. A common practice is to have the subjects distribute the cards such that fewer cards are placed at either of the two extremes and more cards are placed toward the middle. Table 16-4 shows a hypothetical distribution of 60 cards, with the specification of the number of cards to be placed in each of the nine piles.

The sorting instructions and the objects to be sorted in a Q-sort investigation vary according to the requirements of the research. Attitudes can be studied by asking people to sort statements in terms of agreement/disagreement or approval/disapproval. The researcher can study personality by developing cards on which personality characteristics are described. People can then be requested to sort items on a "very much like me" to "not at all like me" continuum. Self-concept can be explored by comparing responses to this "like me" dimension to people's responses elicited when the instructions are to sort cards according to what they consider ideal personality traits. Q sorts can be used to great advantage in studying individuals in depth. For example, participants could be asked to sort traits as they apply to themselves in different roles, such as employee, parent, spouse, friend, and so forth. The technique can also be used to gain information concerning how individuals see themselves, how they perceive others seeing them, how they believe others would like them to be, and so forth. Other applications include asking patients to rate nursing behaviors on a continuum of most helpful to least helpful; asking nursing students to rate aspects of their educational preparation along a most useful to least useful continuum; and asking cancer patients to rate various aspects of their treatment in terms of a most distressing to least distressing dimension.

The number of cards in a Q sort varies according to the research problem. However, it is unwise to use fewer than 50 or 60 items because it is difficult to achieve stable and reliable results with a smaller number. On the other hand, 100 to 150 cards are normally considered the upper limit because the task becomes tedious and difficult with larger numbers.

The analysis of data obtained through Q sorts is a somewhat controversial matter. The options range from the most elementary, descriptive statistical procedures, such as rank ordering, averages, and percentages, to highly complex procedures, such as factor analysis. Factor analysis, a procedure designed to reveal the underlying dimensions or common elements in a set of items, is described in Chapter 20. Some researchers insist that factor analysis is essential in the analysis of Q-sort data.

Q sorts can be constructed by researchers and tailored to the needs of specific studies. However, there are also existing Q sorts that can be used. The advantages of using a previously developed Q sort are that it is time-saving, provides opportunities for comparisons with other studies, and generally includes established information about the quality of data yielded by the procedure. One example of a widely used Q sort is the Child-Rearing Practices Report (CRPR), a 91-item Q sort that provides information about parenting behavior. Hillman (1997) used the CRPR to compare the

TABLE 16-4	Example of a Distribution of Q-Sort Cards							
	APPROVE OF LEAST							**APPROVE OF MOST**
Category	1	2	3	4	5	6	7	8	9
Number of cards	2	4	7	10	14	10	7	4	2

child-rearing practices of parents of children with cancer and parents of healthy children.

Evaluation of Q Methodology

Q methodology can be a powerful methodologic tool, but like other data collection techniques, it has a number of drawbacks as well. On the plus side, we have seen that Q sorts are extremely versatile and can be applied to a wide variety of problems. Unlike many other clinical approaches, Q methodology can be an objective and (usually) reliable procedure for the intensive study of an individual. Q sorts have been used effectively to study the progress of people during different phases of therapy, particularly psychotherapy. The requirement that individuals place a predetermined number of cards in each pile virtually eliminates response-set biases that often characterize responses to written scale items. Furthermore, the task of sorting cards may be more agreeable to some people than completing a paper-and-pencil instrument.

On the other hand, it is difficult and time-consuming to administer Q sorts to a large sample of individuals. The sampling problem is further compounded by the fact that Q sorts cannot normally be administered through the mail, thereby resulting in difficulties in obtaining a geographically diverse sample of participants. Some critics have argued that the forced procedure of distributing cards according to the researcher's specifications is artificial and actually excludes information concerning how people would ordinarily distribute their opinions.

Another criticism of Q-sort data relates to permissible statistical operations. Most statistical tests and procedures assume that responses to items are independent of one another. Likert-type scales exemplify items that are totally independent: a person's response of agree/disagree to one item does not in any way restrict responses to other items. Techniques of this type are known as **normative measures**. Normative measures can be interpreted by comparing individual scores with the average score for a group. The Q-sort technique is a forced-choice procedure, wherein a person's response to one item depends on, and is restricted by, responses to other items. Referring to Table 16-4, a respondent who has already placed two cards in category 1 ("approve of least") is not free to place another item in this same category.* Such an approach produces what are known as **ipsative** measures. With ipsative measures, the average of a group is an irrelevant point of comparison because the average is identical for all individuals. With a nine-category Q sort such as is shown in Table 16-4, the average value of the sorted cards will always be five. (The average value of a *particular item* can be meaningfully computed and compared among individuals or groups, however.) Strictly speaking, ordinary statistical tests of significance are inappropriate for use with nonindependent ipsative measures. In practice, many researchers feel that the violation of assumptions in applying standard statistical procedures to Q-sort data is not a serious transgression, particularly if the number of items is large.

Research Example of a Study Using Q Methodology

Von Essen and Sjödén (1993) compared the perceptions of psychiatric inpatients and nursing staff regarding the importance of various nurse caring behaviors. A total of 61 patients and 63 nurses in four psychiatric short-term hospital wards in Sweden were the subjects in this study.

Data were collected by means of a Q-sort instrument called the Caring Assessment Instrument (CARE-Q), modified for this study and translated into Swedish. The CARE-Q consists of 50 caring behaviors that subjects were asked

---

*People are usually told, however, that they can move cards from one pile to another until the desired distribution is obtained.

to place on a seven-point continuum from most important to least important. The cards had to be placed to conform to a symmetric distribution with 1, 4, 10, 20, 10, 4, and 1 cards in the respective piles. The patients were asked: "In order to make you feel cared for, how important is it that the staff . . . ?"

The CARE-Q items designated nursing behaviors conceptualized as comprising six subscales: Accessible, Explains and Facilitates, Comforts, Anticipates, Monitors, and Trusting Relationship. For example, the Comfort subscale consists of nine items, such as "touches the patient when he/she needs comfort" and "sits down with the patient." In the version used by the inpatients, the word *patient* was replaced by the word *you.* Each behavior was given a value from 1 to 7, corresponding to the subject's placement of it in the distribution.

The findings indicated that patients assigned a higher average value to the Explains and Facilitates subscale than nurses did. Nursing behaviors in this category were ranked as number 1 by patients and as number 6 by staff. By contrast, staff gave a higher average value to the Comforts subscale than did the patients.

PROJECTIVE TECHNIQUES

Questionnaires, interview schedules, and psychological tests and scales normally depend on the respondents' capacity for self-insight or willingness to share personal information with the researcher. **Projective techniques** include a variety of methods for obtaining psychological measures with only a minimum of cooperation required of the person. Projective methods give free play to study participants' imagination and fantasies by providing them with a task that permits an almost unlimited number and variety of responses. The rationale underlying the use of projective techniques is that the manner in which a person organizes and reacts to unstructured stimuli is a reflection of the person's needs, motives, attitudes, values, or personality characteristics. A stimulus of low structure is sufficiently ambiguous that respondents can read-in their own interpretations and in this way provide the researcher with information about their perception of the world. In other words, people project part of themselves into their interactions with phenomena, and projective techniques represent a means of taking advantage of this fact.

Types of Projective Techniques

Projective techniques are highly flexible because virtually any unstructured stimuli or situation can be used to induce projective behaviors. One class of projective methods uses pictorial materials. The **Rorschach ink blot test** is one example of a **pictorial projective device.** Another example is the Thematic Apperception Test (TAT). The TAT materials consist of 20 cards that contain pictures. People are requested to make up a story for each picture, inventing an explanation of what led up to the event shown, what is happening at the moment, what the characters are feeling and thinking, and what kind of outcome will result. The responses are then scored according to some scheme for the variables of interest to the researchers. Variables that have been measured by TAT-type pictures are achievement motivation, need for affiliation, parent–child relationships, attitude toward minority groups, creativity, attitude toward authority, and fear of success. Randell (1993) used the TAT to study the changes experienced by older primiparous women during pregnancy.

Verbal projective techniques present participants with an ambiguous verbal stimulus rather than a pictorial one. There are two classes of verbal methods: association techniques and completion techniques. An example of an association technique is the **word-association method,** which presents participants with a series of words, to which they respond with the first thing that comes to mind. The word list often combines both neutral and emotionally tinged words, which are included for the purpose of detecting impaired thought processes or internal conflicts. The word-association technique has also been used to study creativity, interests, and attitudes. The most common completion technique is **sentence completion**. The person is supplied with a set of incomplete sentences and is asked to complete them in any desired manner. This approach is frequently used as a method of measuring attitudes or some aspect of personality. Some examples of incomplete sentences include the following:

> When I think of a nurse, I feel. . . .
> The thing I most admire about nurses is. . . .
> A good nurse should always. . . .

The sentence stems are designed to elicit responses toward some attitudinal object or event in which the investigator is interested. Responses are typically categorized or rated according to a prespecified plan.

A third class of projective measures falls into a category known as **expressive methods**. These techniques encourage self-expression, in most cases, through the construction of some product out of raw materials. The major expressive methods are play techniques, drawing and painting, and role playing. The assumption is that people express their feelings, needs, motives, and emotions by working with or manipulating various materials.

Evaluation of Projective Measures

Projective measures are among the most controversial in the behavioral sciences. Critics point out that it is difficult to score projective techniques objectively. A high degree of inference is required in gleaning information from projective tests, and the quality of the data depends heavily on the sensitivity and interpretive skill of the investigator or analyst. It has been pointed out that the interpretation of the responses by the researcher is almost as projective as the participants' reactions to original stimuli.

Another problem with projective techniques is that there have been difficulties in demonstrating that they are, in fact, measuring the variables that they purport to measure. If a pictorial device is used to score aggressive expressions, can the researcher be confident that individual differences in aggressive responses really reflect underlying differences in aggressiveness?

Projective techniques have supporters as well as critics in the research community. People have advocated using projective devices, arguing that they probe the unconscious mind, encompass the whole personality, and provide data of a breadth and depth unattainable by more traditional methods. One useful feature of projective instruments is that they are less susceptible to faking than self-report measures. Another strength is that it is often easier to build rapport and gain people's interest with a projective measure than with a questionnaire or scale. Finally, some projective techniques are particularly useful with special groups, especially with children.

Research Example of a Study Using a Projective Measure

Janelli (1993) undertook a study to determine whether there is a difference between how older men and older women perceive their body image. The sample consisted of 89 older men and women from several long-term care facilities.

One of the measures that Janelli used to measure body image perception was the Draw-A-Person (DAP) Technique, a paper-and-pencil projective test. Each older person was instructed as follows: "Draw a person: You may make it any way you wish, but draw a whole person, not just the face" (p. 332). Based on the drawings, three variables were created: (1) area, considered to reflect self-assessment in relation to the environment; (2) height, interpreted as an indication of feelings of self-significance; and (3) centeredness, considered to reflect the person's general security level and orientation to reality. The area measure was obtained by placing a transparency of graphic paper measured in quarter-inch squares over the drawing. Height was measured from top to bottom of the figure with a ruler, to the nearest quarter of an inch. Centeredness was measured by how far the center of the drawing was from the center of the page. Janelli, who acknowledged that "no consensus exists among researchers that the DAP Technique represents a projection of a person's own body image" (p. 332) also administered the self-report Body Cathexis Scale (BCS) as a supplementary measure of body image.

The findings indicated that men and women had comparable scores on the BCS. However, on the DAP measures, the men drew figures that were larger in area, taller, and more centered than the drawings of the women. Janelli concluded that the women had a poorer body image perception than the men, as measured by the DAP Technique.

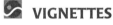 ## VIGNETTES

Another data collection alternative we examine is called vignettes. Vignettes rely on self-reports by study participants but involve a stimulus.

Uses of Vignettes

Vignettes are brief descriptions of an event or situation to which respondents are asked to react. The descriptions can either be fictitious or based on fact, but they are always structured to elicit information about respondents' perceptions, opinions, or knowledge about some phenomenon under study. The vignettes are often written, narrative descriptions, but researchers have also begun to use videotaped vignettes that portray a specific situation. The questions posed to respondents after the presentation of the vignettes typically are closed-ended (e.g., "On the nine-point scale below, rate how well you believe the nurse in this story handled the situation"). Normally, the number of vignettes included in a study ranges from 4 to 10.

The purpose of the study in which vignettes are used is sometimes not revealed to study participants. This technique has sometimes been used as an indirect measure of attitudes, prejudices, and stereotypes through the use of embedded or hidden descriptors. For example, a researcher interested in exploring attitudes toward, or stereotypes of, male nurses could present people with a series of vignettes describing fictitious nurses in terms of, say, their education, family background, nursing experience, and so forth. For each vignette, the nurse would be described as a male half the time (at random) and as a female the other half. The participants could then be asked to describe the fictitious nurses in terms of likableness, friendliness, cheerfulness, effectiveness, and so forth. Any differences in the participants descriptions presumably result from attitudes toward appropriate sex-role behavior.

Evaluation of Vignettes

Vignettes are often an economical means of eliciting information about how people might behave in situations that would be difficult to observe in daily life. For example, we might want to assess how patients would react to or feel about nurses with different types of personalities and personal styles of interaction. In clinical settings, it would be difficult to expose patients to many different nurses, all of whom have been evaluated as having different personalities. Another advantage of vignettes is that it is possible to manipulate the stimuli (the vignettes) experimentally by randomly assigning vignettes to groups, as in the example about male nurses. Furthermore, vignettes often represent an interesting task for subjects. Finally, vignettes can be incorporated into mailed questionnaires and are therefore an inexpensive data collection strategy.

Vignettes are handicapped by some of the same problems as other self-report techniques. The principal problem is that of response biases. If a respondent describes how he or she would react in a situation portrayed in the vignette, how accurate is that description of the respondent's actual behavior? However, there is some evidence from a recent study by nurse researchers (Lanza, Carifio, Pattison, & Hicks, 1997) that validates the use of vignettes to explore certain phenomena.

Research Example of a Study Using Vignettes

McDonald and Bridge (1991) were interested in examining the effect of gender stereotyping on nursing care. Using a factorial design, they created an experimental manipulation that involved the use of a written vignette.

The vignette, which described a 3-day postoperative colostomy patient, simulated a typical shift report for a medical-surgical patient. Eight separate packets, corresponding to eight different experimental conditions, were created. The vignettes in the packet appeared to be identical but differed in three ways: gender of the patient (male versus female); patient health status (described as stable or unstable); and memory load (high versus low). With respect to the latter, subjects in the low memory load condition read only the colostomy vignette, whereas those in the high memory load condition read several other vignettes. Box 16–1 presents a sample vignette from this study, for the unstable female condition.

The sample of 160 female medical-surgical nurses was randomly assigned to one of the eight conditions (2 × 2 × 2). After reading their vignette package, nurses were instructed to estimate to the nearest minute the time they would plan for each of 16 nursing actions (e.g, patient ambulation, patient chair time, emotional support). The results indicated that nurses planned significantly more ambulation, analgesic administration, and emotional support for the patient described as male than for the same patient described as female.

COGNITIVE AND NEUROPSYCHOLOGICAL TESTS

Nurse researchers sometimes are interested in assessing the cognitive skills of study participants. There are several different types of **cognitive tests**.

Types of Cognitive Tests

Intelligence tests represent attempts to evaluate the general, global ability of individuals to perceive relationships and solve problems. Aptitude tests are designed to measure a person's potential for achievement, usually achievement of an academic nature. In practice, the terms aptitude, intelligence, and general mental ability are often used interchangeably. Of the many such tests available, some have been developed for indi-

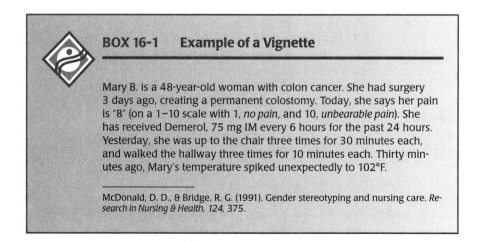

BOX 16-1   Example of a Vignette

Mary B. is a 48-year-old woman with colon cancer. She had surgery 3 days ago, creating a permanent colostomy. Today, she says her pain is "8" (on a 1–10 scale with 1, *no pain*, and 10, *unbearable pain*). She has received Demerol, 75 mg IM every 6 hours for the past 24 hours. Yesterday, she was up to the chair three times for 30 minutes each, and walked the hallway three times for 10 minutes each. Thirty minutes ago, Mary's temperature spiked unexpectedly to 102°F.

McDonald, D. D., & Bridge, R. G. (1991). Gender stereotyping and nursing care. *Research in Nursing & Health, 124,* 375.

vidual (one-on-one) administration, whereas others have been developed for group use. Individual tests, such as the Stanford-Binet or Wechsler I.Q. tests, must be given to a participant by a person who has received training as a tester. Group tests of ability, such as the Scholastic Assessment Test (SAT), can be administered with little training. Intelligence or aptitude tests give either scores for global ability or subscores for several different areas, such as quantitative, verbal, and spatial ability. Nurse researchers have been particularly likely to use ability tests in studies of high-risk groups, such as children who had a low birthweight. Good sources for learning more about ability tests are the books by Anastasi (1997) and Walsh and Betz (1995).

Some cognitive tests are specially designed to assess neuropsychological functioning among those with potential cognitive impairments, such as the Mini-Mental Status Examination (MMSE). These tests capture varying types of competence, such as the ability to concentrate and the ability to remember. Nurses have used such tests extensively in studies of elderly patients and patients with Alzheimer's disease.

Nurse researchers are also sometimes interested in achievement tests, which are designed to measure a person's present level of proficiency or mastery of a given area of knowledge. Because both practicing nurses and nurse educators are involved, to differing degrees, in teaching, the measurement of instructional effectiveness is an area in which some nurse researchers are understandably interested. Achievement tests may be standardized to be used by thousands of test users or specially constructed to assess specific knowledge. Standardized tests are instruments that have been carefully developed and tested and that normally cover broad achievement objectives. The constructors of such tests establish **norms**, which make possible the comparison of study participants with a reference group. The NLN Achievement Test is an example of a standardized test. For specific learning objectives, the researcher may be required to construct a new test. The development of an achievement test that is objective, accurate, and valid is a challenging task. Ebel's (1991) book entitled *Essentials of Educational Measurement* (5th ed.) is a useful reference for those readers interested in achievement test construction.

Research Example of a Study Using Cognitive Testing

Sauvé, Walker, Massa, Winkle, and Sheinman (1996) conducted a longitudinal study of the prevalence, type, severity, and natural evolution of cognitive impairments among patients who survived sudden cardiac arrest. Their aim was to understand patterns of cognitive recovery in these survivors. A sample of 25 patients underwent extensive neuropsychological testing during their hospitalization (within 3 weeks of their initial cardiac arrest), with additional testing 6 to 9 weeks, 12 to 15 weeks, and 22 to 25 weeks after the event.

The battery of tests used in this study assessed orientation, attention, concentration, memory (both short-term and delayed recall), reasoning, and motor performance. Several of the tasks, such as the test that measured motor speed, were computer-based, allowing millisecond reaction time measurements. The researchers also administered the Neurobehavior Cognitive Status Examination (NCSE), a screening test designed to assess intellectual function in several ability areas (e.g., orientation, language, memory, construction, calculation, and reasoning). Another test used was the Symbol-Digit Modalities Test, which assesses the ability to direct focus to a stimulus. The Controlled Oral Word Association Test is a task that requires people to generate as many words as possible in three 60-second trials, in response to an initial letter supplied by the tester.

The researchers found that, during hospitalization, most patients had mild to severe impairments in one or more areas of cognitive functioning. Six months after the arrest event, nearly one third of the patients continued to be impaired, particularly in terms of memory deficits.

TIPS FOR COLLECTING DATA WITH ALTERNATIVE METHODS

The methods described in this chapter represent important data collection alternatives to self-report and observations. Below are a few suggestions regarding the use of these alternative methods.

- Sometimes, the methods used in this chapter are attractive because they are unusual and may therefore seem like a more creative approach to collecting data than self-report and observational methods. However, the prime considerations in selecting a data collection method should always be the conceptual congruence between the constructs of interest and the method and the quality of data that the method yields.
- If you decide to use an alternative method such as a projective technique or a Q sort, a good strategy might be to supplement it with a more traditional measure of the construct as a means of assessing the validity of the alternative approach.
- Most of the techniques described in this chapter yield quantitative data. However, several can also be used to collect qualitative data. Records, for example, may be narrative accounts, such as nurses' notes. Projective techniques are often scored quantitatively but almost always yield narrative data that can be analyzed qualitatively. The questions asked of study participants after they read a vignette could also be open-ended questions amenable to qualitative analysis (e.g., "How would you recommend handling the situation described here?").
- As in other methods of data collection, the importance of adequate training of the data collectors cannot be overemphasized. Even when using existing records, the data collectors need to be trained with respect to the extraction of relevant information and the recording of that information on appropriate forms.

SUMMARY

This chapter reviewed several data collection strategies that are used less frequently than those described in Chapters 14 and 15. For certain research problems, these alternative techniques—and especially **biophysiologic measures**—may be strong candidates as methods of collecting data.

The trend in nursing research is toward increasing numbers of clinical, patient-centered investigations in which biophysiologic indicators of patients' health status are used as dependent variables. Many examples of instruments and laboratory tests used in nursing studies were described. Particular attention was paid to the **instrumentation systems** used for **in vivo measures** (those performed within or on living organisms). The components of an organism–instrument system are the stimulus, subject, sensing equipment, signal-conditioning equipment, display equipment, and recording equipment. Blood tests and urine tests are the most frequently used **in vitro measures** (those performed outside the organism's body). Despite the clearcut utility of biophysiologic measures for nursing science, great care must be taken in selecting such measures with regard to practical, technical, and ethical considerations.

Existing **records** are often used by researchers in the conduct of scientific investigations. Such records provide an economical source of information. In using records, the researcher should try to determine how representative and accurate they are. Two major sources of bias in records are **selective deposit** and **selective survival**.

Q sorts involve having people sort a set of statements into piles according to specified criteria. Attitudes, personality, and self-concept are some of the traits that may be measured by Q methodology. One limitation in the use of

Q sorts is that they produce **ipsative measures,** wherein the average across cards is an irrelevant basis of comparison inasmuch as the forced-choice approach produces the same average for all subjects. This differs from other techniques that produce **normative measures** because each choice is independent of other choices.

Projective techniques encompass a variety of data collection methods that rely on people's projection of psychological traits or states in response to vaguely structured stimuli. **Pictorial methods** present a picture or cartoon and ask the participant to describe what is happening, what led up to the event, or what kind of action is needed. **Verbal methods** present people with an ambiguous verbal stimulus rather than a picture. Two types of verbal methods are **word association** and **sentence completion. Expressive methods** take the form of play, drawing, or role playing.

Vignettes are brief descriptions of some event, person, or situation to which respondents are asked to react. Vignettes are often incorporated into questionnaires or interview schedules. They may be used to assess respondents' hypothetical behaviors, opinions, and perceptions.

Cognitive tests are sometimes used by nurse researchers. Various aspects of cognitive functioning can be measured by such tests, including intelligence or aptitude tests, tests of neuropsychological functioning, and achievement tests.

STUDY ACTIVITIES

Chapter 16 of the *Study Guide to Accompany Nursing Research: Principles and Methods, 6th ed.*, offers various exercises and study suggestions for reinforcing the concepts presented in this chapter. Additionally, the following study questions can be addressed:

1. Formulate a research problem in which each of the following could be used as the measurements for the dependent variable:
   a. Blood pressure
   b. EMGs
   c. Thermograms
   d. Blood sugar levels
2. Identify some of the in vivo or in vitro measures you might use to address the following research questions:
   a. Does clapping the lungs before suctioning result in better patient outcomes than suctioning without clapping?
   b. What is the effect of various bed positions on the development of respiratory acidosis or alkalosis?
   c. What are the cardiovascular effects of administering liquid potassium chloride in three different solutions (orange juice, fruit punch, cranberry juice)?
   d. What is the rate of respiratory increase for designated decreases in the pH level of cerebrospinal fluid?
3. Suppose that you were interested in studying the following variables: professionalism in nurses, fear of death in patients, achievement motivation in nursing students, job satisfaction among industrial nurses, fathers' reactions to their newborn infants, and patients' needs for affiliation. Describe at least two ways of collecting data relating to these concepts, using the following approaches:
   a. Vignettes
   b. Verbal projective techniques
   c. Pictorial projective techniques
   d. Records
   e. Q sorts

SUGGESTED READINGS

Methodologic References

Biophysiologic References

Abbey, J. (Guest Ed.). (1978). Symposium on bio-instrumentation for nurses. *Nursing Clinics of North America, 13,* 561–640.

Bauer, J. D., Ackermann, P. G., & Toro, G. (1982). *Clinical laboratory methods* (9th ed.). St. Louis: C. V. Mosby.

Cromwell, L., Weibell, F. J., & Pfeiffer, E. A. (1980). *Biomedical instrumentation and measurements* (2nd ed.). Englewood Cliffs, NJ: Prentice-Hall.

Ferris, C. D. (1980). *Guide to medical laboratory instruments*. Boston: Little, Brown.

Fischbach, F. (1995). *A manual of laboratory and diagnostic tests* (5th ed.). Philadelphia: Lippincott-Raven.

Kraemer, H. C. (1992). *Evaluating medical tests*. Newbury Park, CA: Sage.

Lindsey, A. M. (1984). Research for clinical practice: Physiological phenomena. *Heart & Lung, 13,* 496–507.

Lindsey, A. M., & Stotts, N. A. (1989). Collecting data on biophysiologic variables. In H. S. Wilson, *Research in nursing* (2nd ed.). Menlo Park, CA: Addison-Wesley.

Pagana, K. D., & Pagana, T. J. (1993). *Diagnostic testing and nursing implications: A case study approach* (4th ed.). St. Louis: C. V. Mosby.

Pugh, L. C., & DeKeyser, F. G. (1995). Use of physiologic variables in nursing research. *Image—The Journal of Nursing Scholarship, 27,* 273–276.

Weiss, M. D. (1973). *Biomedical instrumentation*. Philadelphia: Chilton Book Company.

Widmann, F. K. (1983). *Clinical interpretation of laboratory tests* (9th ed.). Philadelphia: F. A. Davis.

Other Data Collection Methods

Aaronson, L. S., & Burman, M. E. (1994). Use of health records in research: Reliability and validity issues. *Research in Nursing & Health, 17,* 67–74.

Anastasi, A. (1997). *Psychological testing.* (7th ed.). Englewood Cliffs, NJ: Prentice Hall.

Angell, R. C., & Freedman, R. (1953). The use of documents, records, census materials, and indices. In L. Festinger & D. Katz (Eds.), *Research methods in the behavioral sciences* (pp. 300–326). New York: Holt, Rinehart & Winston.

Block, J. (1978). *The Q-Sort method in personality assessment and psychiatric research.* (2nd ed.). Springfield, IL: Charles C. Thomas.

Ebel, R. (1991). *Essentials of educational measurement* (5th ed.) Englewood Cliffs, NJ: Prentice Hall.

Flaskerud, J. H. (1979). Use of vignettes to elicit responses toward broad concepts. *Nursing Research, 28,* 210–212.

Kerlinger, F. N. (1986). *Foundations of behavioral research* (3rd ed.). New York: Holt, Rinehart & Winston.

Lanza, M. L. (1988). Development of a vignette. *Western Journal of Nursing Research, 10,* 346–351.

Semeomoff, B. (1976). *Projective techniques.* New York: John Wiley and Sons.

Simpson, S. H. (1989). Use of Q-sort methodology in cross-cultural nutrition and health research. *Nursing Research, 38,* 289–290.

Stephenson, W. (1975). *The study of behavior: Q technique and its methodology.* Chicago: University of Chicago Press.

Tetting, D. W. (1988). Q-sort update. *Western Journal of Nursing Research, 10,* 757–765.

Walsh, W. B., & Betz, N. E. (1995). *Tests and assessment* (3rd ed.) Englewood Cliffs, NJ: Prentice Hall.

Waltz, C. F., Strickland, O. L., & Lenz, E. R. (1991). *Measurement in nursing research* (2nd ed.). Philadelphia: F. A. Davis.

Substantive References

Biophysiologic Studies

Banasik, J. L., & Emerson, R. J. (1996). Effect of lateral position on arterial and venous blood gases in postoperative cardiac surgery patients. *American Journal of Critical Care, 5,* 121–126.

Brown, J. K., Knapp, T. R., & Radke, K. J. (1997). Sex, age, height, and weight as predictors of selected physiologic outcomes. *Nursing Research, 46,* 101–104.

Byers, J. F., & Smyth, K. A. (1997). Effect of a music intervention on noise annoyance, heart rate, and blood pressure in cardiac surgery patients. *American Journal of Critical Care, 6,* 183–191.

Caudell, K. S., & Gallucci, B. B. (1995). Neuroendocrine and immunological responses of women to stress. *Western Journal of Nursing Research, 17,* 672–692.

Collins, J. A., & Rice, V. H. (1997). Effects of relaxation intervention in phase II cardiac rehabilitation. *Heart & Lung, 26,* 31–44.

Heitkemper, M. M., & Bond, E. F. (1995). Gastric motility in rats with varying ovarian hormone status. *Western Journal of Nursing Research, 17,* 9–19.

Krenzischek, D. A., & Tanseco, F. V. (1996). Comparative study of bedside and laboratory measurements of hemoglobin. *American Journal of Critical Care, 5,* 427–432.

Landis, C. A., & Whitney, J. D. (1997). Effects of 72 hour sleep deprivation on wound healing in the rat. *Research in Nursing & Health, 20,* 259–267.

Lewicki, L. J., Mion, L., Splane, K. G., Samstag, D., & Secic, M. (1997). Patient risk factors for pressure ulcers during cardiac surgery. *AORN Journal, 65,* 933–942.

Liehr, P., Meininger, J. C., Mueller, W., Chandler, S. P., & Chan, W. (1997). Blood pressure reactivity in urban youth during angry and normal talking. *Journal of Cardiovascular Nursing, 11,* 85–94.

Loeb, M. B., Wilcox, L., Smaill, F., Walter, S., & Duff, Z. (1997). A randomized trial of surgical scrubbing with a brush compared to antiseptic soap alone. *American Journal of Infection Control, 25,* 11–15.

McCarthy, D. O., Lo, C., Nguyen, H., & Ney, D. M. (1997). The effect of protein density of food on food intake and nutritional status of tumor-bearing rats. *Research in Nursing & Health, 20,* 131–138.

Moniaci, V., & Kraus, M. (1997). Determining the relationship between invasive and noninvasive blood pressure values. *Neonatal Network: Journal of Neonatal Nursing, 16,* 51–56.

Penny-MacGillivray, T. (1996). A newborn's first bath: When? *Journal of Obstetric, Gynecologic, and Neonatal Nursing, 25,* 481–487.

Schilke, J. M., Johnson, G. O., Housh, T. J., & O'Dell, J. R. (1996). Effects of muscle-strength training on the functional status of patients with osteoarthritis of the knee joint. *Nursing Research, 45,* 68–72.

Shaver, J., Lentz, M., Landis, C, Heitkemper, M. M., Buchwald, D. S., & Woods, N. F. (1997). Sleep, psychological distress, and stress arousal in women with fibromyalgia. *Research in Nursing & Health, 20,* 247–257.

Thomas, K. A., Savage, M. V., & Brengelmann, G. L. (1997). *American Journal of Critical Care, 6,* 46–51.

Topf, M. (1992). Effects of personal control over hospital noise on sleep. *Research in Nursing & Health, 15,* 19–28.

Vaca, K. J., Osterloh, J. F., Daake, C. J., & Noedel, N. R. (1996). *American Journal of Critical Care, 5,* 412–419.

Wewers, M. E., Bowen, J. M., Stanislaw, A. E., & Desimone, V. B. (1994). A nurse-delivered smoking cessation intervention among hospitalized postoperative patients. *Heart & Lung, 23,* 151–156.

Williamson, M. L. (1997). Circumcision anesthesia: A study of nursing implications for dorsal penal nerve block. *Pediatric Nursing, 23,* 59–63.

Wyman, J. F., Elswick, R. K., Ory, M. G., Wilson, M. S., & Fantl, J. A. (1993). Influence of functional, urological, and environmental characteristics on urinary incontinence in community dwelling older women. *Nursing Research, 42,* 270–275.

Studies Using Other Data Collection Methods

Davis, M. J., & Nomura, L. A. (1990). Vital signs of class I surgical patients. *Western Journal of Nursing Research, 12,* 28–41.

Fehring, R. J., Lawrence, D., & Philpot, C. (1994). Use effectiveness of the Creighton model ovulation method of family planning. *Journal of Obstetric, Gynecologic, and Neonatal Nursing, 23,* 303–309.

Hillman, K. A. (1997). Comparing child-rearing practices in parents of children with cancer and parents of healthy children. *Journal of Pediatric Oncology Nursing, 14,* 53–67.

Janelli, L. M. (1993). Are there body image differences between older men and women? *Western Journal of Nursing Research, 15,* 327–339.

Lanza, M. L., Carifio, J., Pattison, I., & Hicks, C. (1997). Validation of a vignette simulation of assault on nurses by patients. *Image—The Journal of Nursing Scholarship, 29,* 151–154.

Mandich, M., Ritchie, S. K., & Mullett, M. (1996). Transition time to oral feeding in premature infants with and without apnea. *Journal of Obstetric, Gynecologic, and Neonatal Nursing, 25,* 771–776.

McDonald, D. D., & Bridge, R. G. (1991). Gender stereotyping and nursing care. *Research in Nursing & Health, 14,* 373–378.

Miceli, D. L., Waxman, H., Cavalieri, T., & Lage, S. (1994). Prodromal falls among older nursing home residents. *Applied Nursing Research, 7,* 18–27.

Palmer, M. H., Myers, A. H., & Fedenko, K. M. (1997). Urinary continence changes after hip-fracture repair. *Clinical Nursing Research, 6,* 8–24.

Randell, B. P. (1993). Growth versus stability: Older primiparous women as a paradigmatic case for persistence. *Journal of Advanced Nursing, 18,* 518–525.

Reese, J. L., Means, M. E., Hanrahan, K., Clearman, B., Colwill, M., & Dawson, C. (1996). Diarrhea associated with nasogastric feedings. *Oncology Nursing Forum, 23,* 59–68.

Sauvé, M. J., Walker, J. A., Massa, S. M., Winkle, R. A., & Sheinman, M. M. (1996). Patterns of cognitive recovery in sudden cardiac arrest survivors. *Heart & Lung, 25,* 172–181.

von Essen, L., & Sjödén, P. (1993). Perceived importance of caring behaviors to Swedish psychiatric inpatients and staff, with comparisons to somatically-ill samples. *Research in Nursing & Health, 16,* 293–303.

CHAPTER **17**

Assessing Data Quality

Data collection methods vary considerably in their ability to capture adequately the phenomena in which nurse researchers are interested. An ideal data collection procedure is one that measures or captures the constructs in a way that is relevant, credible, accurate, unbiased, and sensitive. For most concepts of interest to nurse researchers, there are few data collection procedures that match this ideal. Biophysiologic methods have a much higher chance of success in attaining these goals than self-report or observational methods, but no method is perfect. In this chapter, we discuss criteria for evaluating the quality of data obtained in a research project. We begin with a discussion of the principles of measurement and the assessment of quantitative data. Later in this chapter, we discuss the assessment of qualitative data.

MEASUREMENT

Quantitative studies derive data through the measurement of research variables. **Measurement** may be defined as follows: "Measurement consists of rules for assigning numbers to objects to represent quantities of attributes" (Nunnally, 1978, p. 2). As this definition implies, quantification is intimately associated

with measurement. An often-quoted statement by early American psychologist L. L. Thurstone advances a position assumed by many quantitative researchers: "Whatever exists, exists in some amount and can be measured." The notion underlying this statement is that attributes of objects are not constant: they vary from day to day, from situation to situation, or from one object to another. This variability is capable of a numeric expression that signifies *how much* of an attribute is present in the object. Quantification is used to communicate that amount. The purpose of assigning numbers, then, is to differentiate between people or objects that possess varying degrees of the critical attribute.

Rules and Measurement

The definition of measurement indicates that numbers must be assigned to objects according to specified rules rather than haphazardly. Quantification in the absence of rules would be meaningless. The rules for measuring temperature, weight, blood pressure, and other physical attributes are familiar to us. Rules for measuring many variables for nursing research studies, however, have to be invented. Whether the data are collected by way of observation, self-report, or some other method, the researcher must specify under what conditions and according to what criteria the numeric values are to be assigned to the characteristic of interest.

As an example, suppose we were studying attitudes toward the distribution of condoms in school-based clinics and asked parents to express their extent of agreement with the following statement:

> Teenagers should be taught to "say no" rather than having contraceptives available to them in schools.
> ( ) Strongly agree
> ( ) Agree
> ( ) Slightly agree
> ( ) Undecided
> ( ) Slightly disagree
> ( ) Disagree
> ( ) Strongly disagree

The responses to this question can be quantified by developing a system for assigning numbers to them. Note that *any* rule would satisfy the definition of measurement. We could assign the value of 30 to "strongly agree," 27 to "agree," 20 to "slightly agree," and so on, but there is no apparent justification for doing so. Therefore, in measuring attributes, we must strive not only to develop rules but also to develop good, meaningful rules. Without any *a priori* information about the "distance" between the seven options, the most defensible procedure is to adopt a simplified scheme of assigning a 1 to "strongly agree" and a 7 to "strongly disagree." This rule would quantitatively differentiate, in increments of one point, among people who have seven different reactions to the statement. In developing a new set of rules for measuring attributes, the researcher seldom knows in advance if his or her rules really are the best possible. In essence, a new set of measurement rules constitutes a researcher's hypothesis concerning how an attribute functions and varies. The adequacy of the hypothesis—that is, the worth of the measuring tool—needs to be assessed empirically.

In developing rules, the researcher must strive to link the numeric values to reality. To state this requirement somewhat more technically, the measurement procedures must be isomorphic to reality. The term **isomorphism** signifies equivalence or similarity between two phenomena. A measurement tool cannot be useful unless the measures resulting from it have some correspondence with the real world.

To illustrate the concept of isomorphism, suppose the Scholastic Assessment Test (SAT) were administered to 10 people, who obtained the following scores: 345, 395, 430, 435, 490, 505, 550, 570, 620, and 640. These values are shown at the top of Figure 17–1. Let us further suppose that in reality the true scores of these same 10 people on a hypothetically perfect test were as follows: 360, 375, 430, 465, 470, 500, 550, 610, 590, and 670. These values are shown at the bottom of Figure 17–1. This figure shows that, although not perfect, the test came fairly close to representing the true scores of the 10 subjects. Only two individuals (H and I) were improperly ordered as a result of the actual test. This example illustrates a measure whose isomorphism with reality is fairly high, but improvable.

The researcher almost always works with fallible measures. Instruments that measure psychological phenomena are less likely to correspond to reality than physical measures, but few instruments are totally immune from error. Techniques for evaluating how much error is present in a measuring instrument are discussed later in this chapter.

Advantages of Measurement

What exactly does measurement accomplish? Consider how handicapped nurses and doctors—and researchers—would be in the absence of measurement. What would happen, for example, if there were no measures of weight, temperature, or blood pressure? Only intuition, guesses, personal judgments, and subjective evaluations would remain.

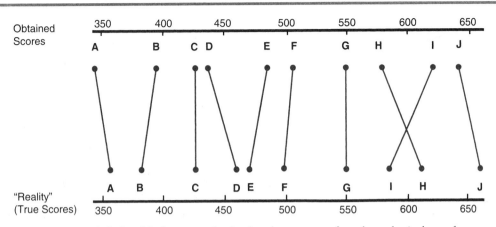

Figure 17-1. Relationship between obtained and true scores for a hypothetical set of test scores.

One of the principle strengths of measurement is that it removes much of the guesswork in gathering information. Because measurement is based on explicit rules, the information tends to be objective. An objective measure is one that can be independently verified by others. Two people measuring the weight of a person using the same scale would be likely to get identical results. Two people scoring a standardized self-report stress scale would be likely to arrive at identical scores. Not all scientific measures are completely objective, but most are likely to incorporate rules for minimizing subjectivity.

An additional advantage is that measurement makes it possible to obtain reasonably precise information. Instead of describing Nathan as "rather tall," we can depict him as a man who is 6 feet 2 inches tall. If we chose, or if the research requirements demanded it, we could obtain even more precise height measurements. Because of the possibility for precision, the researcher's task of differentiating among people who possess different degrees of an attribute becomes considerably easier.

Finally, measurement constitutes a language of communication. Numbers are much less vague than words and therefore are capable of communicating information to a broad audience. If a researcher reported that the average oral temperature of a sample of postoperative patients was somewhat high, different readers might develop different conceptions about the physiologic state of the sample. However, if the researcher reported an average temperature of 99.6°F, there is no possibility of ambiguity or misinterpretation.

Errors of Measurement

The measurement of attributes does not occur in a vacuum. Both the procedures involved in applying the measurement and the object being measured are susceptible to numerous influences that could alter the resulting information. Some of the factors that impinge on the measurement process can be controlled to a certain degree, and attempts should always be made to do so, but such efforts are rarely completely successful.

If an instrument is not perfectly accurate, then the measures it yields can be said to contain a certain degree of error. Conceptually, an **observed** (or **obtained**) **score** can be decomposed into two parts—an error component and a true component. This can be written symbolically as follows:

$$\text{Obtained score} = \text{True score} \pm \text{Error}$$

or

$$X_O = X_T \pm X_E$$

The first term in this equation represents the actual, observed score for some measurement. For example, it could represent a patient's systolic blood pressure or a score on a scale of anxiety. The X_T stands for the true value that would be obtained if it were possible to arrive at an infallible measure. The **true score** is a hypothetical entity—it can never be known because measures are *not* infallible. The final term in the equation is the **error of measurement**. The difference between true and obtained scores is the result of factors that affect the measurement and result in distortions.

Decomposing obtained scores in this fashion brings to light an important point. When a researcher measures an attribute of interest, he or she is also *measuring* attributes that are not of interest. The true score component is what one hopes to isolate; the error component is a composite of other factors that are also being measured, contrary to the researcher's wishes. This concept can be illustrated with an exaggerated example. Suppose a researcher were measuring the weight of 10 people on a spring scale. As each subject steps on the scale, our fictitious researcher places a hand on the subject's shoulder and applies some pressure. The resulting measures (the X_Os) will all be biased in an upward direction because the scores reflect the influence of both the subject's actual weight (X_T) and the researcher's pressure (X_E). Errors of measurement are problematic because they represent an unknown quantity and also because they are variable. In this example, the amount of pressure applied would undoubtedly vary from one subject to the next. In other words, the proportion of true score component in an obtained score varies from one person to the next.

Many factors contribute to errors of measurement. Among the most common are the following seven factors:

1. *Situational contaminants.* Scores can be affected by the conditions under which they are produced. A study participant's awareness of an observer's presence (the reactivity problem) is one source of bias. The anonymity of the response situation, the friendliness of the researchers, or the location of the data gathering can all affect a subject's responses. Other environmental factors, such as the temperature, humidity, lighting, time of day, and so forth, can represent sources of measurement error.

2. *Transitory personal factors.* The scores of an individual may be influenced by a variety of temporary personal states such as fatigue, hunger, anxiety, mood, and so forth. In some cases, these factors can affect a measurement directly, as in the case of anxiety affecting a measurement of pulse rate. In other cases, temporary personal factors can alter individuals' scores by influencing their motivation to cooperate, act naturally, or do their best.

3. *Response-set biases.* A number of relatively enduring characteristics of the respondents can interfere with accurate measures of the target attribute. Response sets such as social desirability, extreme responses, and acquiescence are potential problems in self-report measures, particularly in psychological scales (see Chapter 13).

4. *Administration variations.* Alterations in the methods of collecting data from one subject to the next could result in variations in obtained scores that have little to do with variations in the target attribute. If observers alter their coding categories or definitions, if interviewers improvise the wording of a question, if test administrators change the test instructions, or if some physiologic measures are taken before a feeding and others are taken after a feeding, then measurement errors can potentially occur.

5. *Instrument clarity.* If the directions for obtaining measures are vague or poorly understood, then scores may be affected by this ambiguity and misunderstanding.

For example, questions in a self-report instrument may be interpreted differently by different respondents, leading to a distorted measure of the critical variable. Observers may miscategorize observations if the classification scheme is unclear.

6. *Item sampling.* Errors are sometimes introduced as a result of the sampling of items used to measure an attribute. For example, a nursing student's score on a 100-item test of general nursing knowledge will be influenced to a certain extent by *which* 100 questions are included on the examination. A person might get 95 questions correct on one test but only 90 right on another similar test.

7. *Instrument format.* Several technical characteristics of an instrument can influence the obtained measurements. Open-ended questions may yield different information than closed-ended questions. Oral responses to a specific question may be at odds with responses to a written form of the same question. The ordering of questions within an instrument may also influence responses.

This list represents a sampling of the sources of measurement error with which a researcher must deal. Other common problems will come to light in other sections of this chapter.

RELIABILITY OF MEASURING INSTRUMENTS

The reliability* of an instrument that yields quantitative data is a major criterion for assessing its quality and adequacy. Essentially, the **reliability** of an instrument is the degree of consistency with which it measures the at-

tribute it is supposed to be measuring. If a scale gave a reading of 120 pounds for a person's weight one minute, and a reading of 150 pounds in the next minute, we would naturally be wary of using that scale because the information would be unreliable. The less variation an instrument produces in repeated measurements of an attribute, the higher its reliability. Thus, reliability can be equated with the stability, consistency, or dependability of a measuring tool.

Another way of defining reliability is in terms of accuracy. An instrument can be said to be reliable if its measures accurately reflect the true scores of the attribute under investigation. This definition links reliability to the issues raised in the discussion of measurement error. We can make this relationship clearer by stating that an instrument is reliable to the extent that errors of measurement are absent from obtained scores. A reliable measure is one that maximizes the true score component and minimizes the error component. The greater the error, the lower the reliability.

These two ways of approaching the concept of reliability (consistency and accuracy) are not so different as they might at first appear. The errors of measurement that impinge on an instrument's accuracy also affect its consistency. The example of the scale that produced variable weight readings should clarify this point. Suppose that the true weight of a person is 125 pounds, but that two independent measurements yielded 120 and 150 pounds. In terms of the equation presented in the previous section, we could express the measurements as follows:

$$120 = 125 - 5$$
$$150 = 125 + 25$$

The values of the errors of measurement for the two trials are -5 and $+25$, respectively. These errors produced scores that are both inconsistent *and* inaccurate. We must conclude that our fictitious spring scale is highly unreliable.

The reliability of a measuring tool can be assessed in several different ways. The method

---

*The discussion of reliability presented here is based entirely on classic measurement theory. Readers concerned with assessing the reliability of instructional measures that can be classified as mastery type or criterion referenced should consult Thorndike and Hagen (1990).

chosen depends to a certain extent on the nature of the instrument but also on the aspect of the reliability concept that is of greatest interest. The aspects that have received major attention are stability, internal consistency, and equivalence.

Stability

The **stability** of a measure refers to the extent to which the same results are obtained on repeated administrations of the instrument. The estimation of reliability here focuses on the instrument's susceptibility to extraneous factors from one administration to the next.

Assessments of the stability of a measuring tool are derived through procedures that evaluate **test–retest reliability**. The researcher administers the same test to a sample of individuals on two occasions and then compares the scores obtained. The comparison procedure is performed objectively by computing a **reliability coefficient,** which is a numeric index of the magnitude of the test's reliability.

To explain a reliability coefficient, we must first briefly discuss the concepts underlying the statistic known as the **correlation coefficient.*** We have pointed out repeatedly that a scientist often strives to detect and explain the relationships among phenomena: Is there a relationship between patients' gastric acidity levels and incidents of emotional upset? Is there a relationship between body temperature and perceptions of the passage of time? The correlation coefficient is an important tool for quantitatively describing the magnitude and direction of a relationship. The computation of this index does not concern us here. It is more important to understand how to read a correlation coefficient.

Two variables that are obviously related to one another are people's height and weight. Tall people tend, on average, to be heavier than short people. We would say that there was a

perfect relationship if the tallest person in a population were the heaviest, the second tallest person were the second heaviest, and so forth. The correlation coefficient summarizes how perfect a relationship is. The possible values for a correlation coefficient range from -1.00 through .00 to $+1.00$. If height and weight were perfectly correlated, then the correlation coefficient expressing this relationship would be 1.00. Because the relationship does exist but is not perfect, the correlation coefficient is probably in the vicinity of .50 or .60. The relationship between height and weight can be described as a **positive relationship** because increases in height tend to be associated with increases in weight.

When two variables are totally unrelated, the correlation coefficient is equal to zero. One might expect that women's dress sizes are unrelated to their intelligence. Large women are as likely to perform well on tests of ability as small women. The correlation coefficient summarizing such a relationship would presumably be in the vicinity of .00.

Correlation coefficients running from .00 to -1.00 express what is known as **inverse** or **negative relationships**. When two variables are inversely related, increases in one variable are associated with *decreases* in the second variable. Suppose that there is an inverse relationship between a nurse's age and attitude toward abortion. This means that, on the average, the greater the age of the nurse, the *less* favorable the attitude. If the relationship were perfect (i.e., if the oldest nurse had the least favorable attitude and so on), then the correlation coefficient would be equal to -1.00. In actuality, the relationship between age and abortion attitudes is probably modest—in the vicinity of $-.20$ or $-.30$. A correlation coefficient of this magnitude describes a weak relationship wherein older nurses tend to be unfavorable and younger nurses tend to be favorable toward abortion, but a "crossing of lines" is not unusual. That is, a number of younger nurses oppose abortion, and a number of older nurses are not opposed.

---

*Computational procedures and additional information concerning correlation coefficients (Pearson's *r*) are presented in Chapter 18.

Now we are prepared to discuss the use of correlation coefficients to compute reliability estimates. In the case of test–retest reliability, a sample would be administered the instrument twice. Suppose, for example, we were interested in the stability of a scale to measure self-esteem in adolescents. Because self-esteem is presumably a fairly stable attribute that does not change markedly from one day to the next, we would expect a measure of it to yield consistent scores on two separate administrations. As a check on the instrument's stability, we might arrange to administer the scale 3 weeks apart to a sample of teenagers. Fictitious data for this example are presented in Table 17-1. It can be seen that, generally, the differences in the scores on the two testings are not large. The reliability coefficient for test–retest estimates is the correlation coefficient between the two sets of scores. In this example, the computed reliability coefficient is .95, which is high.

The value of the reliability coefficient theoretically can range between −1.00 and +1.00, just as in the case of other correlation coefficients. A negative coefficient would have been obtained in the self-esteem example if teenagers who had high self-esteem scores at time 1 had low scores at time 2. In practice, reliability coefficients normally range between .00 and 1.00. The higher the coefficient, the more stable the measure. For most purposes, reliability coefficients above .70 are considered satisfactory. In some situations, a higher coefficient may be required, or a lower one may be considered acceptable.

The test–retest method is a relatively easy and straightforward approach to estimating reliability. It is a method that can be used with self-report, observational, and physiologic measures. However, the test–retest approach has certain disadvantages. One problem is that many traits of interest *do* change over time, independently of the stability of the measure. Attitudes, behaviors, moods, knowledge, physical condition, and so forth can be modified by intervening experiences between the two testings. The procedures used to estimate stability confound changes resulting from random fluctuations and those resulting from true modifications in the attribute being measured. Still, there are many attributes (such as self-esteem) that are relatively enduring characteristics for which a test–retest approach is suitable.

Stability estimates suffer from other problems, however. One possibility is that the subjects' responses or observer's coding on the second administration will be influenced by the memory of their responses or coding on the first administration, regardless of the actual values on the second day. This memory interference will result in a spuriously high reliability coefficient. Another difficulty is that subjects may actually change as a result of the first administration. Finally, people may not be as careful using the same instrument a second time. If they find the procedure boring on the second occasion, then the responses could be haphazard, resulting in a spuriously low estimate of stability.

In summary, the test–retest approach is a procedure for estimating the stability of a measure over time. On the whole, reliability coefficients tend to be higher for short-term retests than for long-term retests (i.e., those greater than 1 or 2 months) because of actual changes in the

TABLE 17-1	Fictitious Data for Test–Retest Reliability of Self-Esteem Scale		
SUBJECT NUMBER	**TIME 1**	**TIME 2**	
1	55	57	
2	49	46	
3	78	74	
4	37	35	
5	44	46	
6	50	56	
7	58	55	
8	62	66	
9	48	50	
10	67	63	$r = .95$

attribute being measured. Stability indexes are most appropriate for relatively enduring characteristics such as personality, abilities, or certain physical attributes such as height.

Internal Consistency

Composite scales and tests that involve a summation of items are often evaluated in terms of their internal consistency. Ideally, scales designed to measure an attribute are composed of a set of items, all of which are measuring the critical attribute and nothing else. On a scale to measure empathy in nurses, it would be inappropriate to include an item that is a better measure of diagnostic competence than empathy. An instrument may be said to be **internally consistent** or **homogeneous** to the extent that all of its subparts are measuring the same characteristic.

The internal consistency approach to estimating an instrument's reliability is probably the most widely used method among researchers today. These procedures are popular not only because they are economical (they require only one test administration) but also because they are the best means of assessing one of the most important sources of measurement error in psychosocial instruments, the sampling of items.

One of the oldest methods for assessing internal consistency is the **split-half technique**. In this approach, the items composing a test are split into two groups and scored independently, and the scores on the two half-tests are used to compute a correlation coefficient. To illustrate this procedure, the fictitious scores from the first administration of the self-esteem scale are reproduced in the second column of Table 17-2. For the sake of simplicity, we will say that the total instrument consists of 20 questions. To compute a split-half reliability coefficient, the items must be divided into two groups of 10. Although a large number of possible splits is possible, the usual procedure is to use odd items versus even items. One half-test, therefore, consists of items 1, 3, 5, 7, 9, 11, 13, 15, 17, and 19, and the even-numbered items compose the second half-test. The scores on the two halves for our example are shown in the third and fourth columns of Table 17-2. The correlation coefficient describing the relationship between the two half-tests is an estimate of the internal consistency of the self-esteem scale. If the odd items are measuring the same attribute as the even items, then the reliability coefficient should be high. The correlation coefficient computed on the fictitious data is .67.

The correlation coefficient computed on split halves of a measure tends to underesti-

---

TABLE 17-2   Fictitious Data for Split-Half Reliability of the Self-Esteem Scale

SUBJECT NUMBER	TOTAL SCORE	ODD-NUMBERS SCORE	EVEN-NUMBERS SCORE	
1	55	28	27	
2	49	26	23	
3	78	36	42	
4	37	18	19	
5	44	23	21	
6	50	30	20	
7	58	30	28	
8	62	33	29	
9	48	23	25	
10	67	28	39	$r = .80$

mate systematically the reliability of the entire scale. Other things being equal, longer scales are more reliable than shorter ones. The correlation coefficient computed on the data in Table 17-2 is an estimate of reliability for a 10-item instrument, not a 20-item instrument. To overcome this difficulty, a formula has been developed for adjusting the correlation coefficient to give an estimate of reliability for the entire test. The correction equation, which is known as the **Spearman-Brown prophecy formula,** is as follows:

$$r^1 = \frac{2r}{1 + r}$$

where r = the correlation coefficient computed on the split halves

r^1 = the estimated reliability of the entire test

Using the formula, the reliability for our hypothetical 20-item measure of self-esteem would be as follows:

$$r^1 = \frac{(2)\,(.67)}{1 + .67} = .80$$

The split-half technique is easy to use and eliminates most of the problems associated with the test–retest approach. However, the split-half technique is handicapped by the fact that different reliability estimates can be obtained by using different splits; that is, it makes a difference whether one uses an odd–even split, a first-half–second-half split, or some other method of dividing the items into two groups. For this reason, the split-half approach is increasingly being replaced by formulas that compensate for this deficiency.

The two most widely used methods are **coefficient alpha** (or **Cronbach's alpha**) and the **Kuder-Richardson formula 20** (abbreviated KR-20). KR-20 is a specialized version of coefficient alpha, used with tests that are scored dichotomously for a right or wrong answer. It is beyond the scope of this text to explain in detail the application of these methods. However, because coefficient alpha is a widely used index of reliability, the reader may wish to consult an advanced text on psychometrics, such as Cronbach (1990) or Nunnally and Bernstein (1994).[*]

Both the coefficient alpha and KR-20 produce a reliability coefficient that can be interpreted in the same fashion as other reliability coefficients described here. That is, the normal range of values is between .00 and +1.00, and higher values reflect a higher degree of internal consistency. Coefficient alpha is preferable to the split-half procedure because it gives an estimate of the split-half correlation for *all possible* ways of dividing the measure into two halves.

In summary, indices of homogeneity or internal consistency estimate the extent to which different subparts of an instrument are equivalent in terms of measuring the critical attribute. The split-half technique has been used to estimate homogeneity, but the coefficient alpha is a preferable method. None of these approaches considers fluctuations over time as a source of unreliability.

Equivalence

A researcher may be interested in estimating the reliability of a measure by way of the **equivalence** approach under one of two circumstances: (1) when different observers or researchers are using an instrument to measure the same phenomena at the same time, or (2) when two presumably parallel instruments are administered to individuals at about the same time. In both

---

[*]The coefficient alpha equation, for the advanced student, is as follows:

$$r = \frac{k}{k - 1}\left[1 - \frac{\Sigma\sigma_i^2}{\sigma v^2}\right]$$

where r = the estimated reliability

k = the total number of items in the test

σ_i^2 = the variance of each individual item

σy^2 = the variance of the total test scores

Σ = the sum of

situations, the aim is to determine the consistency or equivalence of the instruments in yielding measurements of the same traits in the same people.

In Chapter 15, we pointed out that a potential weakness of observational methods is the fallibility of the observer. The greater the interpretive burden on the observer, the higher is the risk of observer error or bias. The accuracy of observer ratings and classifications can be enhanced by careful training, the development of clearly defined and nonoverlapping categories, the use of a small number of categories, and the use of behaviors that tend to be molecular rather than molar. Even when care is taken to design an observational system that minimizes the possibility of error, the researcher should assess the reliability of the instrument. In this case, the "instrument" includes both the category or rating system developed by the researcher and the observer making the measurements.

Interrater (or **interobserver**) **reliability** is estimated by having two or more trained observers watching some event simultaneously and independently recording the relevant variables according to a predetermined plan or coding system. The resulting records can then be used to compute an index of equivalence or agreement. Several procedures for arriving at such an index are possible. For certain types of observational data (e.g., ratings and frequency counts within a category system), correlation techniques are often suitable. That is, a correlation coefficient may be computed to demonstrate the strength of the relationship between one observer's ratings or frequencies and another's.

Another procedure is to compute reliability as a function of agreements, using the following equation:

$$\frac{\text{Number of agreements}}{\text{Number of agreements + disagreements}}$$

This simple formula unfortunately tends to overestimate observer agreements. If the be-

havior under investigation is one that observers code for absence or presence every, say, 10 seconds, then by chance alone, the observers will agree 50% of the time. Other approaches to estimating interrater reliability may be of interest to advanced students. Techniques such as Cohen's kappa, analysis of variance, intraclass correlations, and rank-order correlations have been used to assess the reliability of observational measures.

The second situation in which the equivalence of measures is evaluated is when two alternative, parallel forms of a single instrument are available. This type of research problem is unlikely to present itself frequently in nursing research, except in methodologic studies or in an educational context. For example, alternate forms of a test of nursing knowledge might be needed. In such a case, the two forms should be administered to a sample of individuals in immediate succession, randomly alternating the order of presentation of the forms. The correlation coefficient between the two sets of scores would be an index of reliability of equivalence. This procedure is adopted to determine whether the two instruments are, in fact, measuring the same attribute. The researcher uses this technique to assess the errors of measurement resulting from errors in item sampling.

Interpretation of Reliability Coefficients

The reliability coefficients computed according to the procedures just described can be used as an important indicator of the quality of a quantitative measure. A measure that is unreliable interferes with an adequate testing of a researcher's hypotheses. If data fail to confirm a research prediction, one possibility is that the measuring tools were unreliable—not necessarily that the expected relationships do not exist. There is no standard for what an acceptable reliability coefficient should be. If a researcher is interested only in making group-level comparisons, then coefficients in the vicinity of .70 might be sufficient (although coefficients of .80 or greater are highly desirable). By group-level comparisons, we mean that the investigator is interested in comparing the scores of such groups as male versus female, smoker versus nonsmoker, experimental versus control, and so forth. However, if measures are to be used as a basis for making decisions about individuals, then the reliability coefficient ideally should be .90 or better. For instance, if a score on a test were to be used as a criterion for admission to a graduate nursing program, then the accuracy of the test would be of critical importance to both individual applicants and the school of nursing.

The reliability coefficient has a special interpretation that should be briefly explained without elaborating on technical details. This interpretation relates to the earlier discussion of decomposing an observed score into an error component and a true component. Suppose that we have just administered a scale that measures empathy to 50 nurses. It would be expected that the scores would vary from one nurse to another because some nurses are more empathic than others. Some of the variability in scores is true variability, reflecting real individual differences in the attribute being measured; some of the variability, however, is error. Thus,

$$V_O = V_T + V_E$$

where V_O = observed total variability in scores

V_T = true variability

V_E = variability owing to random errors

A reliability coefficient is directly associated with this equation. *Reliability is the proportion of true variability to the total obtained variability,* or

$$r = \frac{V_T}{V_O}$$

If, for example, the reliability coefficient were .85, then 85% of the variability in obtained scores could be said to represent true individual differences, and 15% of the variability would reflect random, extraneous fluctuations. Looked at in this way, it should be clearer why instruments with reliability lower than .70 are risky to use.

Table 17-3 illustrates different forms of reliability evaluations that nurse researchers have

TABLE 17-3 Examples of Reliability Assessments by Nurse Researchers

INSTRUMENT	TYPE OF RELIABILITY	RELIABILITY COEFFICIENT	REFERENCE
Index of Professional Nursing Governance	Internal consistency Test–retest	.97 .77	Hess, 1998
NEECHAM Confusion Scale	Internal consistency Interrater reliability	.90 .91	Neelon, Champagne, Carlson, & Funk, 1996
Smoking and Women Questionnaire	Test–retest (1–3 weeks) Cronbach's alpha	.84 .83	Gulick & Escobar-Florez, 1995

used to assess instruments that they or others developed.

VALIDITY

The second important criterion by which a quantitative instrument's adequacy is evaluated is its validity. **Validity** refers to the degree to which an instrument measures what it is supposed to be measuring. When a researcher develops an instrument to measure patients' hopelessness, how can its developer really know that the resulting scores validly reflect this construct and not something else, such as depression? Problems of validity relate to the question, Are we really measuring the attribute we think we are measuring?

Like reliability, validity has a number of different aspects and assessment approaches. Unlike reliability, however, the validity of an instrument is extremely difficult to establish. There are no formulas or equations that can easily be applied to the scores of the hypothetical hopelessness scale to estimate how good a job the scale is doing in measuring the critical variable.

The reliability and validity of an instrument are not totally independent qualities of an instrument. *A measuring device that is unreliable cannot possibly be valid.* An instrument cannot be validly measuring the attribute of interest if it is erratic, inconsistent, and inaccurate. An unreliable tool would be measuring too many other factors associated with random error to be considered a valid indicator of the target variable. However, an instrument can be reliable without being valid. Suppose we had the idea to assess anxiety in patients by measuring the circumference of their wrists. We could obtain highly accurate, consistent, and precise measurements of the wrist circumferences, but such measures would not be valid indicators of anxiety. Thus, the high reliability of an instrument provides no evidence of its

validity for an intended purpose; the low reliability of a measure *is* evidence of low validity.

The methodologic literature abounds with terms relating to different facets of the validity question. One aspect is known as face validity. **Face validity** refers to whether the instrument *looks* as though it is measuring the appropriate construct. Although face validity should not be considered as primary evidence for the quality of an instrument, it may be helpful for a measure to have face validity if other types of validity have also been demonstrated. For example, it might be easier to persuade people to participate in an evaluation if the evaluation instruments have face validity. Three other aspects of validity are of greater importance in assessments of an instrument: content validity, criterion-related validity, and construct validity.

Content Validity

Content validity is concerned with the sampling adequacy of items for the construct that is being measured. Content validity is relevant for both affective measures (i.e., measures relating to feelings, emotions, and psychological traits) and cognitive measures.

For cognitive measures, the validity question being asked is, How representative are the questions on this test of the universe of all questions that might be asked on this topic? Suppose we were interested in testing the knowledge of a group of lay people concerning the seven danger signals of cancer identified by the American Cancer Society. To be representative, or content valid, the questions on the test would have to include items from each of the seven danger signals, or "CAUTION":

Change in bowel or bladder habits
A sore that does not heal
Unusual bleeding or discharge
Thickening or lump in breast or elsewhere
Indigestion or difficulty in swallowing
Obvious change in wart or mole
Nagging cough or hoarseness

Content validity is also relevant in the development of affective measures. The person who wanted to develop a new instrument would begin by developing a thorough conceptualization of the construct of interest so that the measure would adequately capture the entire domain. Such a conceptualization might come from rich first-hand knowledge but is more likely to come from an exhaustive literature review or from a qualitative inquiry. For example, Frank-Stromborg (1989) made efforts to enhance the content validity of her Reaction to the Diagnosis of Cancer Questionnaire. She began by asking 340 cancer patients the following open-ended question: "What do you remember of your feelings when first told you had cancer?" Prevalent themes that emerged in the responses to this question were then incorporated into items in the scale, thus reflecting the major content areas experienced by cancer patients.

The content validity of an instrument is necessarily based on judgment. There are no completely objective methods of ensuring the adequate content coverage of an instrument. However, it is becoming increasingly common to use a panel of experts in the content area to evaluate and document the content validity of new instruments. The panel typically consists of at least three experts, but a larger number may be advisable if the construct is complex. The experts are asked to evaluate individual items on the new measure as well as the entire instrument. Two key issues in such an evaluation are whether individual items are relevant and appropriate in terms of the construct and whether the items adequately measure all dimensions of the construct. With regard to assessing the relevance of items, some researchers compute interrater agreement indexes and a formal **content validity index** (CVI) across the experts' ratings of each item's relevance. One widely used procedure is to have experts rate items on a 4-point scale (from 1 = not relevant to 4 = very relevant). The CVI for the total instrument is the percentage of total items rated by the experts as either 3 or 4. A CVI score of .80 or better is generally considered to have good content validity.

Criterion-Related Validity

Criterion-related validity involves a pragmatic approach to validity assessment. The researcher attempting to establish the criterion-related validity of an instrument is not seeking to ascertain how well the tool is measuring a particular theoretical trait. The emphasis is on establishing the relationship between the instrument and some other criterion. The instrument, whatever abstract attribute it is measuring, is said to be valid if its scores correlate highly with the criterion. For example, if a measure of birth control use among sexually active teenage girls correlates highly with subsequent premarital pregnancies, then the birth control measure could be described as having good validity. In terms of the criterion-related validation approach, the key issue is whether the instrument is a useful predictor of subsequent behaviors, experiences, or conditions.

One requirement of the criterion-related approach to validation is the availability of a reasonably reliable and valid criterion with which the measures on the target instrument can be compared. This is, unfortunately, seldom easy. If we were developing an instrument to predict the nursing effectiveness of nursing students, we might use subsequent supervisory ratings as our criterion. However, how can we be sure that these ratings are valid and reliable? In fact, the supervisory ratings might themselves be in need of validation. Thus, the criterion-related validity is particularly appropriate when there is a concrete and easily measured criterion. For example, a measure to predict whether a smoker will or will not be successful at quitting smoking 4 weeks after a cessation intervention has available a very clearcut and objective criterion.

Once the criterion is selected, the validity can be assessed easily and straightforwardly. The scores on the predictor instrument are correlated with the criterion variable. The magnitude of the correlation coefficient is a direct estimate of how valid the instrument is, according to this method of validation. To illustrate, suppose a team of nurse researchers developed a scale to measure professionalism among nurses. They administer the instrument to a sample of nurses and at the same time ask the nurses to indicate how many articles they have published. The publications variable was chosen as one of many potential objective criteria of professionalism. Fictitious data are presented in Table 17-4. The correlation coefficient of .83 indicates that the professionalism scale correlates reasonably well with the number of articles a nurse has published. Whether the scale is really measuring professionalism is a somewhat different issue—an issue that is the concern of construct validation discussed in the next section.

A distinction is sometimes made between two types of criterion-related validity. The distinction is not usually an important one, but the terms are used frequently enough to warrant their mention. **Predictive validity** refers to the adequacy of an instrument in differentiating between the performance or behaviors of individuals on some future criterion. When a school of nursing correlates the incoming SAT scores of students with subsequent grade-point averages, the predictive validity of the SATs for nursing school performance is being evaluated. **Concurrent validity** refers to the ability of an instrument to distinguish individuals who differ in their present status on some criterion. For example, a psychological test to differentiate between those patients in a mental institution who can and cannot be released could be correlated with current behavioral ratings of health care personnel. The difference between predictive and concurrent validity, then, is the difference in the timing of obtaining measurements on a criterion.

Validation by means of the criterion-related approach is most often used in applied or practically oriented research. Criterion-related validity is helpful in assisting decision makers by giving them some assurance that their decisions will be effective, fair, and, in short, valid.

Construct Validity

Validating an instrument in terms of **construct validity** is a difficult and challenging task. The instrument designer adopting this approach is concerned with the questions: What is this measuring device really measuring? Is the abstract concept under investigation being ade-

TABLE 17-4 Fictitious Data for Criterion-Related Validity Example		
SUBJECT	**SCORE ON PROFESSIONALISM SCALE**	**NUMBER OF PUBLICATIONS**
1	25	2
2	30	4
3	17	0
4	20	1
5	22	0
6	27	2
7	29	5
8	19	1
9	28	3
10	15	1

$r = .83$

quately measured with this instrument? Unlike criterion-related validity, construct validity is more concerned with the underlying attribute than with the scores that the instrument produces. The scores are of interest only insofar as they constitute a valid basis for inferring the degree to which a subject possesses some characteristic. Unfortunately, the more abstract the concept, the more difficult it is to establish the construct validity of the measure; at the same time, the more abstract the concept, the less suitable it is to validate a measure by the criterion-related approach. Actually, it is really not just a question of suitability but also of feasibility. What objective criterion is there for such concepts as empathy, grief, role conflict, or separation anxiety?

Despite the obstacles and difficulties encountered in assessing the construct validity of instruments, this activity is a vital component of scientific progress. The constructs in which scientists are interested must be reliably and validly measured. The significance of construct validity is in its linkage with theory and theoretical conceptualization. In validating a measure of death anxiety, we would probably be less concerned with the adequate sampling of items or with relating the resultant scores to a criterion than with the extent to which the measure corresponds to a theory of death anxiety that is acceptable to us.

Construct validation can be approached in several ways, but there is always an emphasis on logical analysis and the testing of relationships predicated on the basis of theoretical considerations. Constructs are usually explicated in terms of other concepts; therefore, the researcher should be in a position to make predictions about the manner in which the construct will function in relation to other constructs.

One approach to construct validation is the **known-groups technique**. In this procedure, groups that are expected to differ on the critical attribute because of some known characteristic are administered the instrument. For instance, in validating a measure of fear of the labor experience, one might contrast the scores of primiparas and multiparas. Because one would expect that women who had never given birth would experience more anxiety than women who had already had children, one might question the validity of the instrument if such differences did not emerge. There is not necessarily an expectation that the differences would be great. It would be expected that some primiparas would feel little anxiety, and some multiparas would express some fears. On the whole, however, it would be anticipated that some group differences would be reflected in the average scores. As another example of the known-groups technique, consider the example of validating a measure concerning limitations in functional ability. One might choose people with emphysema and people without emphysema to validate the instrument. The validity of the instrument might be questioned if differences in scores between the two groups did not occur because one would expect that people with emphysema would have experienced limitations in functional ability.

Another method of construct validation consists of an examination of relationships based on theoretical predictions, which is really a variant of the known-groups approach. A researcher might reason as follows:

- According to theory, construct X is positively related to construct Y.
- Instrument A is a measure of construct X; instrument B is a measure of construct Y.
- Scores on A and B are correlated positively, as predicted by the theory.
- Therefore, it is inferred that A and B are valid measures of X and Y.

This logical analysis is fallible and does not constitute proof of construct validity but is important as a type of evidence, nevertheless.

A significant advance in the area of construct validation is the procedure developed by Campbell and Fiske (1959) known as the **multitrait–multimethod matrix method** (**MTMM**). This procedure makes use of the concepts of convergence and discriminability. **Convergence** refers to evidence that different methods of measuring a construct yield similar results. Different approaches to measurement should converge on the construct. **Discriminability** refers to the ability to differentiate the construct being measured from other similar constructs. Campbell and Fiske argued that evidence of both convergence and discriminability should be brought to bear in the construct validity question.

To help explain the MTMM approach, fictitious data from a study to validate a "need for autonomy" measure are presented in Table 17-5. In using this approach, the researcher must measure the critical concept by two or more methods. Suppose we measured need for autonomy in a sample of nursing home residents by having the residents respond to a self-report summated rating scale (the measure we are attempting to validate); having nurses rate each person after observing him or her in a task designed to elicit different degrees of autonomy; and having the residents respond to a pictorial (projective) stimulus depicting an autonomy-relevant situation. A second requirement of the MTMM approach is that we must also measure constructs from which we wish to differentiate the key construct, using the same measuring methods. In the current example, suppose that

we decided to differentiate "need for autonomy" from "need for affiliation." One requirement for the MTMM is that the discriminant concept must be similar to the focal concept. In our example, the two traits meet this criterion: one would expect, on the average, that people who exhibited a high degree of need for autonomy would be relatively low in terms of need for affiliation. The point of including both concepts in a single validation study is to gather evidence that the two concepts are, in fact, distinct rather than two different labels for the same underlying attribute.

The numbers in Table 17-5 represent the correlation coefficients between the scores on the six different measures (two traits $\times$ three methods). For instance, the coefficient of $-.38$ at the intersection of A1–B1 expresses the relationship between the self-report scores on the need for autonomy and need for affiliation measures. Recall that a minus sign before the correlation coefficient signifies an inverse relationship. In this case, the $-.38$ tells us that there was a slight tendency for people scoring high on the need for autonomy scale to score low on the need for affiliation scale. (The numbers in parentheses along the diagonal of this matrix are the reliability coefficients.)

TABLE 17-5 Multitrait–Multimethod Matrix

METHOD*	TRAITS†	METHOD 1		METHOD 2		METHOD 3	
		A_1	B_1	A_2	B_2	A_3	B_3
Method 1	A_1	(.88)					
	B_1	$-.38$	(.86)				
Method 2	A_2	.60	$-.19$	(.79)			
	B_2	$-.21$	.58	$-.39$	(.80)		
Method 3	A_3	.51	$-.18$	.55	$-.12$	(.74)	
	B_3	$-.14$	.49	$-.17$	.54	$-.32$	(.72)

*Methods: 1, self-report summated scale; 2, observational rating; 3, projective test.

†Traits: A, need for autonomy trait; B, need for affiliation trait.

Various aspects of the MTMM matrix have a bearing on the construct validity question. The most direct evidence (convergence) comes from the correlations between two different methods for measuring the same trait. In the case of A1–A2, the coefficient is .60, which is reasonably substantial. Convergent validity should be sufficiently large to encourage further scrutiny of the matrix. Second, the convergent validity entries should be higher (in terms of absolute magnitude*) than those correlations between measures that have neither method nor trait in common. That is, A1–A2 should be greater than A2–B1 or A1–B2. Inspection of the table reveals that, indeed, .60 surpasses the "heterotrait–heteromethod" values of −.21 and −.19. This requirement is a minimum one, which, if failed, should cause the researcher to have serious doubts about the measures. Third, the convergent validity coefficients should be greater than the coefficients between measures of different traits by a single method. Once again, the matrix in Table 17-5 fulfills this criterion: A1–A2 (.60) and A2–A3 (.55) are higher than A1–B1 (−.38), A2–B2 (−.39) and A3–B3 (−.32). The last two requirements provide some evidence for discriminant validity.

The MTMM approach can be extended to include more traits and more methods. The difficulty is in administering a large number of measures to a sample of subjects. Also, the evidence is seldom as clearcut as in this contrived example, and therefore, additional measures may create undesirable confusion. Indeed, a common problem with the MTMM method is that of interpretation of the pattern of coefficients. Another issue is that there is no clearcut criterion for determining whether the requirements of the MTMM method have been met—that is, there are no objective mechanisms for assessing the magnitude of similarities and differences within the matrix. On the other hand, the MTMM method continues to be a valuable

tool for exploring the validity of instruments. The researcher may decide to utilize the concepts underlying the procedure even when the full model is not feasible. Perhaps in some cases only an A1–B1 type of combination is possible, whereas in others, A1–A2–A3 would be manageable. The execution of any portion of the model is better than no effort to estimate construct validity and generally is preferable to a content validity approach alone for most concepts of interest to nurse researchers.

Another approach to construct validation employs a statistical procedure known as factor analysis. Although factor analysis, which will be discussed in Chapter 20, is computationally complex, it is conceptually rather simple. **Factor analysis** is essentially a method for identifying clusters of related variables. Each cluster, called a **factor**, represents a relatively unitary attribute. The procedure is used to identify and group together different measures of some underlying attribute. In effect, factor analysis constitutes another means of looking at the convergent and discriminant validity of a large set of measures. Indeed, a procedure known as **confirmatory factor analysis** is sometimes used as a method for analyzing MTMM data (Ferketich, Figueredo, & Knapp, 1991; Lowe & Ryan-Wenger, 1992).

In summary, construct validation uses both logical and empirical procedures. Like content validity, construct validity requires a judgment pertaining to what the instrument is measuring. Unlike content validity, however, the logical operations required by construct validation are typically linked to a theory or conceptual framework. Construct and criterion-related validity share an empirical component, but in criterion-related validity, there is usually a pragmatic, objective criterion with which to compare a measure rather than a second measure of an abstract theoretical construct.

Interpretation of Validity

Like reliability, validity is not an all-or-nothing characteristic of an instrument. An instrument

---

*The **absolute magnitude** refers to the value without a plus or minus sign. A value of −.50 is of a higher absolute magnitude than +.40.

cannot really be said to possess or lack validity; it is a question of degree. Furthermore, although we have referred to the process of testing the validity of an instrument as validation, it is inappropriate to speak of the process as yielding proof of validity. Like all tests of hypotheses, the testing of an instrument's validity is not proved, established, or verified but rather is supported to a greater or lesser degree by evidence.

Strictly speaking, a researcher does not validate the instrument itself but rather some application of the instrument. A measure of anxiety may be valid for presurgical patients on the day before an operation but may not be valid for nursing students on the morning of a final examination. Of course, some instruments may be valid for a wide range of uses with different types of samples, but each use requires new supporting evidence. In a sense, validation is a never-ending process. The more evidence that can be gathered that an instrument is measuring what it is supposed to be measuring, the more confidence researchers will have in its validity.

Nurse researchers have become increasingly sophisticated in assessing the validity of measures. Table 17-6 presents some examples of measures that have been subjected to a validation process by nurse researchers.

OTHER CRITERIA FOR ASSESSING QUANTITATIVE MEASURES

Reliability and validity are the two most important aspects to consider in evaluating a quantitative measure. If an instrument can be shown to be reasonably reliable and valid for a specific purpose, then the researcher can have some assurance that the results of a study will be meaningful. High reliability and validity are a necessary, though insufficient, condition for good scientific research.

A researcher sometimes needs to consider other qualities of an instrument in addition to its validity and reliability. These additional criteria are by no means a substitute for reliability and validity but may in some cases be

TABLE 17-6	Examples of Validity Assessments by Nurse Researchers	
INSTRUMENT	**TYPE OF VALIDITY**	**PROCEDURE**
Cardiac Event Threat Questionnaire, a measure of threat related to cardiac events (Bennett, Puntenney, Walker, & Ashley, 1996)	Content Construct	Review by panel of experts Confirmatory factor analysis; correlation with Profile of Mood States
H & H Lactation Scale, a measure of insufficient milk supply (Hill & Humenick, 1996)	Content Predictive Construct	Review by three experts in lactation Correlation with level of breastfeeding 8 weeks postpartum Correlation with a similar breastfeeding tool (convergence); factor analysis
Sense of Belonging Scale, a self-report measure of a person's sense of belonging and well-being (Hagerty & Patusky, 1995)	Content Construct	Review by a panel of 7 experts Known groups (contrasting scores of students, depressed patients and nuns); factor analysis; correlation with other similar measures

equally important. Indeed, several of these qualities are directly related to the issues raised in the preceding two sections.

Efficiency

Instruments of comparable reliability and validity may still differ in their efficiency. An instrument that requires 10 minutes of a subject's time to measure his or her social support is efficient in comparison with an instrument to measure the same attribute that requires 30 minutes to complete. One aspect of efficiency is the number of items incorporated in an instrument. Long instruments tend to be more reliable than shorter ones. There is, however, a point of diminishing returns. As an example, consider a 40-item scale to measure feelings of guilt among parents of handicapped children. Let us say that we find a reliability of .94 for the scale, using coefficient alpha as our index of internal consistency. Using the Spearman-Brown formula, we can estimate how reliable the scale would be with only 30 items:

$$r^1 = \frac{kr}{1 + [(1 - k)r]} = \frac{.75\,(.94)}{1 - [.25\,(.94)]} = .92$$

where k = the factor by which the instrument is being incremented or decreased; in this case, $k = 30 \div 40 = .75$

As this calculation shows, a 25% reduction in the length of the instrument resulted in this case in a negligible decrease in reliability, from .94 to .92. Most researchers probably would be willing to sacrifice a modest amount of reliability in exchange for the opportunity to substantially reduce the subjects' response burden and data collection costs.

Efficiency is more characteristic of certain types of data collection procedures than others. In a questionnaire or interview, closed-ended questions are more efficient than open-ended items. Self-report scales tend to be less time-consuming than projective instruments for a comparable amount of information. Of course, a researcher may decide that other ad-

vantages (such as depth of information) offset a certain degree of inefficiency. Other things being equal, however, it is desirable to select as efficient an instrument as possible.

Sensitivity

The sensitivity of an instrument affects how small a variation in an attribute can be reliably detected and measured. A yardstick marked off with only three divisions for feet would result in a highly insensitive measure of a person's height. The yardstick could be made more sensitive to variations in height by subdividing each foot into 12 equal sections for inches, and the process could be continued until a sufficiently sensitive measuring tool was obtained for the purposes needed. Unfortunately, it is not this easy to increase the sensitivity of most instruments.

The sensitivity of an instrument determines how discriminating its measurements will be between individuals with differing amounts of an attribute. Using the yardstick marked off in feet only, it would be impossible to discriminate between a person who is 5 feet 8 inches tall and one who is 6 feet 3 inches tall: both would be measured as 6 feet, measuring to the nearest foot. There are statistical procedures that permit a researcher to enhance the sensitivity of paper-and-pencil measures by assessing the degree to which each item is contributing to the instrument's power to make discriminations. These **item analysis techniques** are described in detail in texts on measurement and psychometric theory. Several references are noted at the end of this chapter.

The sensitivity of an instrument is most likely to become an issue in certain kinds of situations. When changes in the level of an attribute are being closely monitored, as in the case of many physiologic measurements, then it is important to use a sensitive device. If important decisions are to be based on the measures resulting from an instrument, then its sensitivity is highly relevant. Experimenters must also be concerned with the sensitivity of measuring tools whenever the treatments they are introducing are not markedly different from their control conditions. In the nursing research literature, there are many examples of studies in which differences between conditions were not detected. Part of the difficulty in many nursing intervention studies is that new interventions are compared with older interventions rather than with no intervention at all. When experimental and control conditions are not maximally different—as must often be the case in nursing research—then highly sensitive instruments may be required to detect differences in the effects of the treatments.

Other Criteria

A few remaining qualities that should be considered in assessing a quantitative instrument can be noted. Most of the following 10 criteria are actually aspects of the reliability and validity issues:

1. *Objectivity.* There should be as little room as possible for disagreements between two or more independent researchers applying the instrument to measure the same phenomenon.
2. *Comprehensibility.* The subject or the researcher should be able to comprehend the behaviors required to secure accurate and valid measures.
3. *Balance.* The instrument designer should strive for a balanced measure to minimize response-set biases and to facilitate content validity.
4. *Speededness.* For most types of instruments, the researcher should be sure that adequate time is allowed to obtain complete measurements without rushing the measuring process.
5. *Unidimensionality.* A measuring tool should be designed to produce separate scores for unitary concepts that can be isolated.
6. *Range.* The instrument should be capable of achieving a meaningful measure from the smallest expected value of the variable to the largest.
7. *Linearity.* A researcher normally strives to construct measures that are equally accurate and sensitive over the entire range of values.
8. *Signal-to-noise ratio.* In physiologic measures, it is important to use instruments and procedures that maximize the signal reading and minimize the interference noise.
9. *Reactivity.* The instrument should, insofar as possible, avoid affecting the attribute that is being measured.
10. *Simplicity.* Other things being equal, a simple instrument is more desirable than a complex instrument inasmuch as complicated measures run a greater risk of having errors.

ASSESSMENT OF QUALITATIVE DATA

The methods of assessment described in this chapter apply to structured data collection instruments that yield quantitative scores. For the most part, these procedures cannot be meaningfully applied to such qualitative materials as unstructured interview responses or narrative descriptions from a participant observer's field notes. However, this does not imply that qualitative researchers are unconcerned with the quality of their data collection techniques. The central question underlying the concepts of reliability and validity is: Do the data collected by the researcher reflect the truth? Certainly, qualitative researchers are as eager as quantitative researchers to have their findings reflect the true state of human experience.

Many qualitative nurse researchers seek to evaluate the quality of their data and their findings through procedures that have been outlined by Lincoln and Guba (1985), two proponents of the naturalistic paradigm of inquiry. These researchers have suggested four criteria for establishing the **trustworthiness** of qualitative data: credibility, dependability, confirmability, and transferability. Table 17-7 presents some examples of qualitative nursing studies that have used various techniques to establish the trustworthiness of the data.

Credibility

Careful qualitative researchers take steps to improve and evaluate the **credibility** of their data and conclusions, which refers to confidence in the truth of the data. Lincoln and Guba (1985) point out that the credibility of an inquiry involves two aspects: first, carrying out the investigation in such a way that the believability of the findings is enhanced, and second, taking steps to *demonstrate* credibility. Credibility of qualitative data and the resulting findings is the aspect of data quality on which most methodologic attention has fo-

cused. Lincoln and Guba suggest a variety of techniques for improving and documenting the credibility of qualitative research, several of which are discussed next.

PROLONGED ENGAGEMENT AND PERSISTENT OBSERVATION

Lincoln and Guba recommend several activities that make it more likely that credible data and interpretations will be produced. A first and very important step is **prolonged engagement**—the investment of sufficient time in the data collection activities to have an in-depth understanding of the culture, language, or views of the group under study and to test for misinformation and distortions. Prolonged engagement is also essential for building trust and rapport with informants.

TABLE 17-7   **Examples of Assessments of Data Quality in Qualitative Nursing Studies**

RESEARCH QUESTION	ASSESSMENT PROCEDURE
What are the social and cultural constructions of "nerves" in two fishing communities? (Davis & Joakimsen, 1997)	Method triangulation (participant observation, interviews) Investigator triangulation Time triangulation Space triangulation Person triangulation
What is the essential structure of spiritual care as viewed by Christian patients? (Conco, 1995)	Member checks Peer debriefings Thick description Method triangulation (interviews, field notes) Time triangulation
What is the personal or subjective experience of forgetfulness among elders? (Cromwell, 1994)	Member checks Peer debriefing Partial audit Thick description
What is the experience of therapeutic reading offered through bibliotherapy? (Cohen, 1994)	Member checks Peer debriefing Negative case analysis Independent audit Time triangulation

Credible data collection in naturalistic inquiries also involves **persistent observation**, which concerns the salience of the data being gathered and recorded. Persistent observation refers to the researchers' focus on the characteristics or aspects of a situation or a conversation that are relevant to the phenomena being studied. As Lincoln and Guba (1985) note, "If prolonged engagement provides scope, persistent observation provides depth" (p. 304).

TRIANGULATION

The technique known as triangulation is also used to improve the likelihood that qualitative findings will be found credible. **Triangulation** refers to the use of multiple referents to draw conclusions about what constitutes the truth. Denzin (1989) identified four types of triangulation: data triangulation, investigator triangulation, theory triangulation, and method triangulation.

Data triangulation involves the use of multiple data sources in a study to obtain diverse views for the purpose of validating conclusions. There are three basic types of data triangulation—time, space, and person. **Time triangulation** involves collecting data on the same phenomenon at different points in time. This concept is similar to test–retest reliability assessment; that is, the point is not to study the phenomenon longitudinally but rather to determine the congruence of the phenomenon across time. **Space triangulation** involves collecting data on the same phenomenon in multiple sites. The aim is to validate the data by testing for consistency across sites. Finally, **person triangulation** involves collecting data from different levels of persons: individuals, groups (e.g., dyads, triads, families), and collectives (e.g., organizations, communities, institutions), with the aim of validating data through multiple perspectives on the phenomenon.

The second major type of triangulation is **investigator triangulation**, which refers to the use of two or more trained researchers to analyze and interpret a set of data. Through collaboration, investigators can reduce the possibility of a biased or one-sided interpretation of the data. Moreover, if the investigators bring to the analysis task a complementary blend of skills and expertise, the analysis and interpretation can benefit from divergent perspectives. The concept of investigator triangulation is conceptually similar to the use of interrater reliability in quantitative studies.

With **theory triangulation**, the researcher uses competing theories or hypotheses in the analysis and interpretation of a single set of data. A qualitative researcher who develops competing hypotheses while still in the field is an a good position to test the validity of each because the flexible design of qualitative studies provides ongoing opportunities to direct the inquiry and to sample relevant informants. Theory triangulation can help the researcher to rule out rival hypotheses and to prevent premature conceptualizations. The quantitative analogue for theory triangulation is construct validation, especially through a convergent validity approach.

Method triangulation involves the use of multiple methods in collecting data about the same phenomenon. In purely qualitative studies*, the researcher may use a combination of unstructured data collection methods, such as interviews, observations, and diaries. Indeed, many qualitative studies use a rich blend of methods to develop a comprehensive understanding of a phenomenon. Multiple data collection methods provide an opportunity for evaluating the extent to which an internally consistent picture of the phenomenon emerges.

Although Denzin's (1989) seminal work discussed these four types of triangulation as a method of converging on valid understandings about a phenomenon, other types have been suggested. For example, Kimchi, Polivka, and

---

*We have already discussed method triangulation involving a combination of qualitative and quantitative approaches (see Chapter 11).

Stevenson (1991) have described **analysis triangulation**, which is the use of two or more analytic techniques to analyze the same set of data. Divergent analytic strategies offer another opportunity to validate the meanings inherent in a qualitative data set. Finally, the term **multiple triangulation** has been used to describe the process used by researchers when more than one of these types of triangulation is used in the collection and analysis of the same data set.

In summary, the purpose of using triangulation is to provide a basis for convergence on the truth. By using multiple methods and perspectives, researchers strive to sort out "true" information from "error" information.

EXTERNAL CHECKS: PEER DEBRIEFING AND MEMBER CHECKS

Two other techniques that Lincoln and Guba (1985) recommend for establishing credibility involve activities that provide an external validation of the inquiry process. **Peer debriefing** is a session held with one or more objective peers to review and explore various aspects of the inquiry. Peer debriefing is a process that exposes the researcher to the searching questions of others who are experienced in the methods of naturalistic inquiry, the phenomenon being studied, or both. These sessions can also be useful to the researcher interested in testing some working hypotheses or in exploring avenues to pursue in the emerging research design.

A **member check** refers to the provision of feedback to the study participants regarding the data and the researcher's emerging findings and interpretations, including securing the participants' reactions. Member checking with study participants can be carried out both informally in an ongoing way as data are being collected and more formally after the data have been collected and fully analyzed. Lincoln and Guba consider member checking the most important technique for establishing the credibility of qualitative data.

SEARCHING FOR DISCONFIRMING EVIDENCE

The credibility of a data set can be enhanced by the researcher's systematic search for data that will challenge an emerging categorization or descriptive theory. The search for disconfirming evidence occurs through purposive sampling methods but is facilitated through other processes already described here, such as prolonged engagement and peer debriefings. As noted in Chapter 12, the purposive sampling of individuals who can offer conflicting accounts or points of view can greatly strengthen a comprehensive description of a phenomenon.

Lincoln and Guba (1985) refer to a similar activity of **negative case analysis**—a process by which the researcher revises his or her hypotheses through the inclusion of cases that appear to disconfirm earlier hypotheses. The goal of this procedure is to refine a hypothesis or theory continually until it accounts for *all* cases without exception.

RESEARCHER CREDIBILITY

Another aspect of credibility discussed by Patton (1990) is **researcher credibility**, that is, the faith that can be put in the researcher. In qualitative studies, the researcher *is* the data collecting instrument as well as the creator of the analytic process; therefore, the researcher's training, qualifications, and experience are important in establishing confidence in the data.

It is sometimes argued that, for readers to have confidence in the validity of a qualitative study's findings, the research report should contain information about the researcher, including information about credentials. In addition, the report may need to make clear the personal connections the researcher had to the people, topic, or community under study. For example, it is relevant for a reader of a report on AIDS patients' coping mechanisms to know that the researcher is HIV positive. Patton argues that the researcher should report "any personal and professional information that may have affected data collection, analysis and interpretation—negatively or positively. . ." (p. 472).

Dependability

The **dependability** of qualitative data refers to the stability of data over time and over conditions. This is similar conceptually to the stability aspect of reliability assessments in quantitative studies (and similar also to time triangulation).

One approach to assessing the dependability of data is to undertake a procedure referred to as **stepwise replication**. This approach, which is analogous to the conventional split-half technique, involves having a research group of two or more people who can be divided into two teams. These teams deal with data sources separately and conduct, essentially, independent inquiries through which data can be compared. Ongoing, regular communication between the teams is essential for the success of this procedure.

Another technique relating to dependability is the **inquiry audit**. An inquiry audit involves a scrutiny of the data and relevant supporting documents by an external reviewer, an approach that also has a bearing on the confirmability of the data, as we discuss next.

Confirmability

Confirmability refers to the objectivity or neutrality of the data, such that there would be agreement between two or more independent people about the data's relevance or meaning. In qualitative studies, the issue of confirmability does not focus on the characteristics of the researcher (is he or she objective and unbiased?) but rather on the characteristics of the data (are the data confirmable?).

Inquiry audits can be used to establish both the dependability and confirmability of the data. In an inquiry audit, the investigator must develop an **audit trail**, that is, a systematic collection of materials and documenta-

tion that will allow an independent auditor to come to conclusions about the data. There are six classes of records that are of special interest in creating an adequate audit trail: (1) the raw data (e.g., field notes, interview transcripts); (2) data reduction and analysis products (e.g., theoretical notes, documentation on working hypotheses); (3) process notes (e.g., methodologic notes, notes from member check sessions); (4) materials relating to intentions and dispositions (e.g., personal notes on intentions); (5) instrument development information (e.g., pilot forms); and (6) data reconstruction products (e.g., drafts of the final report).

Once the audit trail materials are assembled, the inquiry auditor proceeds to audit, in a fashion analogous to a financial audit, the trustworthiness of the data and the meanings attached to them. Although the auditing task is complex, it can serve as an invaluable tool for persuading others that qualitative data are worthy of confidence.

Transferability

In Lincoln and Guba's (1985) framework, **transferability** refers essentially to the generalizability of the data, that is, the extent to which the findings from the data can be transferred to other settings or groups. This is, to some extent, a sampling and design issue rather than an issue relating to the soundness of the data. However, as Lincoln and Guba note, the responsibility of the investigator is to provide sufficient descriptive data in the research report so that consumers can evaluate the applicability of the data to other contexts: "Thus the naturalist cannot specify the external validity of an inquiry; he or she can provide only the thick description necessary to enable someone interested in making a transfer to reach a conclusion about whether transfer can be contemplated as a possibility" (p. 316). **Thick description**, a widely used term among qualitative researchers, refers to a rich and thorough description of the research setting or context and of the transactions and processes observed during the inquiry. Thus, if there is to be transferability, the burden of proof rests with the investigator to provide sufficient information to permit judgments about contextual similarity.

TIPS FOR ASSESSING DATA QUALITY

Researchers can place little confidence in their findings if their data collection instruments and procedures yield data that are of poor quality. With quantitative instruments, it has become a customary procedure for the developers to estimate the validity and reliability of their tools before making them available for general use. Such an evaluation is often referred to as a **psychometric assessment** of an instrument. However, it is the responsibility of all researchers—not just the researchers who develop instruments—to ensure high-quality data. In this section, we provide some additional guidance relating to data quality.

- If you are using an existing quantitative instrument, you should always choose a measure with demonstrated high reliability and validity. If you are considering an instrument for which you can find no published psychometric information, it is wise to contact the developer of the instrument and ask about evidence of validity and reliability.
- As Table 17-3 illustrates, reliability estimates vary according to the procedures used to obtain them. In selecting an instrument, the researcher needs to determine which aspect of reliability (stability, internal consistency, or equivalence) is most relevant to the attribute and instrument under consideration.
- Even if you choose an instrument that previously was demonstrated to be reliable, this is no guarantee of its high quality for your study. An instrument's relia-

bility is not a fixed entity. *The reliability of an instrument is a property not of the instrument but rather of the instrument when administered to a certain sample under certain conditions.* A scale developed to measure dependence in hospitalized adults may be unreliable for use with hospitalized adolescents, or for the elderly in nursing homes, and so forth. This means that you should always learn about the characteristics of the group with whom or for whom the instrument was developed. If the original group was similar to your target group, then the reliability estimate provided by the scale developer is probably a reasonably good index of the instrument's accuracy and consistency for your study.

- The prudent researcher should not be satisfied with an instrument that will *probably* be reliable in his or her study. The recommended procedure is to compute estimates of reliability whenever data are collected for a scientific investigation. For physiologic measures that are relatively impervious to random fluctuations stemming from personal or situational factors, this procedure may be unnecessary. However, observational tools, self-report measures, tests of knowledge or ability, and projective tests—all of which are highly susceptible to errors of measurement—should be subjected to a reliability check as a routine step in the research process.
- If you are developing a new composite self-report or observational scale (or modifying an existing one), you should be aware that the reliability of such scales is partly a function of their length or number of items. To improve the reliability, more items tapping the same concept should be added.
- The reliability of an instrument is related in part to the heterogeneity of the sample with which it is used. The more homogeneous the sample (i.e., the more similar their scores), the lower the reliability coefficient

will be. This is because instruments are designed to measure differences among those being measured. If the sample is homogeneous, then it is more difficult for the instrument to discriminate reliably among those who possess varying degrees of the attribute being measured.

- It is generally easy to glean information about the psychometric properties of quantitative instruments—a reliability coefficient or validity coefficient can be briefly and readily communicated. However, many qualitative researchers fail to include information on data quality in their research reports. When information on data quality is totally absent in qualitative reports, readers have no way of knowing how trustworthy the data are, and this makes the utilization of the knowledge more problematic. It is important for researchers within both paradigms to take steps to enhance and document data quality and to summarize in a research report what the results of those steps were.

 ## RESEARCH EXAMPLES

In this section, we describe the efforts of a team of researchers to develop and evaluate a structured observational instrument, and of another researcher to evaluate her qualitative data.

Research Example Involving Assessment of a Structured Scale

Prescott, Ryan, Soeken, Castorr, Thompson, and Phillips (1991) undertook several activities to develop and refine the Patient Intensity for Nursing Index (PINI). The PINI is a 10-item scale for nurses to use in evaluating the intensity of nursing care and the nursing skill level needed by individual patients. The PINI includes items relating to severity of illness, dependency, complexity of care, and time.

After an initial development study, the research team performed an extensive psychometric evaluation. Interrater reliability was assessed by having day and evening RNs from one unit in each of five hospitals use the PINI on the same 150 patients as closely in time as possible (i.e., late in the shift for day nurses, early in the shift for night nurses). The overall interrater reliability was .62. Internal consistency of the PINI was also assessed. The reliability coefficient, based on the Cronbach alpha method, was .85.

Four substudies were undertaken for the validity testing, using data on 6445 patients collected by 487 RNs. The nurses worked in various clinical units of five hospitals in several states. The first study involved a factor analysis, which revealed that the PINI measures three underlying constructs: severity of illness, dependency, and complexity. The second substudy involved the testing of six hypotheses that predicted the relationship of PINI scores to other existing measures, such as length of hospital stay and scores on the hospital patient classification. All the hypotheses were supported. The third substudy involved comparing PINI scores for two groups of patients with different requirements, based on diagnostic-related group ratings. The low and high nursing intensity groups had substantially different PINI scores, as expected. Finally, the fourth substudy involved comparing nurses' ratings of one item on the PINI—hours of care—with observer-recorded time data. Although nurses completing the PINI tended to overestimate time requirements, agreement between the nurses and the observers was reasonably high. The researchers concluded that "the psychometric evaluation of the PINI as a measure of nursing intensity has been very positive" (p. 219).

Research Example Involving Assessment of Qualitative Data

Gagliardi (1991) conducted an in-depth inquiry to better understand the experiences of families living with a child with Duchenne muscular dystrophy. Three families that had a young boy (aged 7 to 9 years) with Duchenne were included in the study. The researcher visited each family weekly over a 10-week period and engaged in participant observation, including involvement in play activities, trips to summer camps, watching television with family members, and participation in family conversations. Logs of the observations were maintained the same day. Periodically, the researcher wrote analytic memoranda that were used to examine the researcher's emotions, biases, and conflicts.

In-depth unstructured interviews with family members were also conducted; the interviews were taped and later transcribed. Interviews were conducted twice over the 10-week period and then a third time 1 year later.

Gagliardi used several procedures to evaluate and document data quality. First, triangulation was used: data triangulation was achieved by interviewing multiple members of the family, and method triangulation was achieved by collecting both observational and self-report data. Member checks were undertaken by having family members verify themes emerging in the data during the second and third interviews. The grouping of narrative materials into themes was also verified by having two external auditors and several colleagues independently categorize a sample of the data, resulting in a 90% rate of agreement. The researcher met with her colleagues every 3 weeks to explore areas of disagreement and to help further reduce bias.

SUMMARY

Measurement involves a set of rules according to which numeric values are assigned to objects to represent varying degrees of some attribute. Measurement is advantageous to quantitative researchers because it offers objectivity, precision, and a tool for communication. However, researchers must strive to develop or use measurements whose rules are **isomorphic** with reality.

Few, if any, measuring instruments used by researchers are pure or infallible. **Obtained scores**—that is, the actual measurements obtained through the administration of the instruments—can be decomposed into a true score and an error component. **True scores** are hypothetical entities that represent the values that would be obtained if it were possible to construct a perfect measure. The error component, or **error of measurement**, represents the inaccuracies present in the measurement process. Sources of measurement error include situational contaminants, response-set biases, transitory personal factors, and several others.

One important characteristic of a measuring tool is its **reliability**, which refers to the degree of consistency or accuracy with which an instrument measures an attribute. The higher the reliability of an instrument, the lower the amount of error present in the obtained scores. Several empirical methods assess various aspects of an instrument's reliability. The **stability** aspect, which concerns the extent to which the instrument yields the same results on repeated administrations, is evaluated by **test–retest procedures**. The **internal consistency** or **homogeneity** aspect of reliability refers to the extent to which all the instrument's subparts or items are measuring the same attribute. Internal consistency may be evaluated using either the **split-half reliability** technique or **Cronbach's alpha** method. When the focus of a reliability assessment is on establishing **equivalence** between observers in rating behaviors, estimates of **interrater** or **interobserver reliability** may be obtained. Most of the methods of estimating reliability rely on the calculation of a **reliability coefficient**, an index that reflects the proportion of true variability in a set of scores to the total obtained variability. Reliability coefficients generally range in value from a low of .00 to 1.00, with higher values reflecting increased reliability.

Validity refers to the degree to which an instrument measures what it is supposed to be measuring. **Face validity** refers to whether the instrument appears, on the face of it, to be measuring the appropriate construct. **Content validity** is concerned with the sampling adequacy of the content being measured. **Criterion-related validity** focuses on the relationship or correlation between the instrument and some outside criterion. **Construct validity** refers to the adequacy of an instrument in measuring the abstract construct of interest. Approaches to assessing the construct validity of a measuring tool include **factor analysis** and the **known-groups technique,** which contrasts the scores of groups that are presumed to differ on the attribute. Another construct validity approach is the **multitrait–multimethod matrix technique,** which is based on the concepts of convergence and discriminability. **Convergence** refers to evidence that different methods of measuring the same attribute yield similar results. **Discriminability** refers to the ability to differentiate the construct being measured from other similar concepts.

Although high reliability and validity are essential criteria for assessing the quality of an instrument, other characteristics of the tool may also be important. Other criteria for evaluating a measuring tool include its efficiency, sensitivity, objectivity, comprehensibility, balance, speededness, unidimensionality, range, linearity, signal-to-noise ratio, frequency response, reactivity, and simplicity.

Data quality is equally important in qualitative and quantitative research. In both, the fundamental issue is whether one can have confidence that the data represent the true state of the phenomena under study. The criteria often used to assess the **trustworthiness** of qualitative data are credibility, dependability, confirmability, and transferability. **Credibility,** roughly analogous to validity in a quantitative study, refers to the believability of the data. Various techniques and activities can be used to improve and document the credibility of qualitative data, including **prolonged engagement,** which strives for adequate scope of data coverage, and **persistent observation,** which is aimed at achieving adequate depth. **Triangulation** is

the process of using multiple referents to draw conclusions about what constitutes the truth, and is therefore an important tool for validating qualitative data and its subsequent analysis. The five major forms include **data triangulation, investigator triangulation, theory triangulation, method triangulation,** and **analysis triangulation.** Two especially important tools for establishing credibility are **peer debriefings,** wherein the researcher obtains feedback about data quality and interpretive issues from peers, and **member checks,** wherein informants are asked to comment on the data and on the researcher's interpretations. Credibility can also be enhanced through a systematic search for disconfirming evidence (such as through a **negative case analysis**) or by having an investigator or team of investigators whose credibility is evident through their training and experience.

Dependability of qualitative data refers to the stability of data over time and over conditions. **Confirmability** refers to the objectivity or neutrality of the data. Independent **inquiry audits** by external auditors can be used to assess and document dependability and confirmability. **Transferability** refers to the extent to which findings from the data can be transferred to other settings or groups. Transferability can be enhanced by the use of **thick descriptions** of the context of the data collection.

🔁 STUDY ACTIVITIES

Chapter 17 of the *Study Guide to Accompany Nursing Research: Principles and Methods, 6th ed.,* offers various exercises and study suggestions for reinforcing the concepts presented in this chapter. Additionally, the following study questions can be addressed:

1. Explain in your own words the meaning of the following correlation coefficients:
   a. The relationship between intelligence and grade-point average was found to be .72.

b. The correlation coefficient between age and gregariousness was −.20.

c. It was revealed that patients' compliance with nursing instructions was related to their length of stay in the hospital ($r = -.50$).

2. Suppose the split-half reliability of an instrument to measure attitudes toward contraception was .70. Calculate the reliability of the full scale using the Spearman-Brown formula.

3. If a researcher had a 20-item scale whose reliability was .60, about how many items would have to be added to achieve a reliability of .80?

4. An instructor has developed an instrument to measure knowledge of research terminology. Would you say that more reliable measurements would be yielded before or after a year of instruction on research methodology, using the exact same test, or would there be no difference? Why?

5. What types of groups do you feel might be useful for a known-groups approach to validating measures of the following: emotional maturity, attitudes toward alcoholics, territorial aggressiveness, job motivation, and subjective pain?

6. Suppose you were interested in doing an in-depth study of people's struggles with obesity. Outline a data collection plan that would include opportunities for various types of triangulation.

▶ SUGGESTED READINGS

Methodologic References

Armstrong, G. D. (1981). The intraclass correlation as a measure of interrater reliability of subjective judgments. *Nursing Research, 30,* 314–315.

Banik, B. J. (1993). Applying triangulation in nursing research. *Applied Nursing Research, 6,* 47–52.

Berk, R. A. (1990). Importance of expert judgment in content-related validity evidence. *Western Journal of Nursing Research, 12,* 659–670.

Brink, P. J. (1991). Issues of reliability and validity. In J. M. Morse (Ed.), *Qualitative nursing research: A contemporary dialogue.* Newbury Park, CA: Sage.

Campbell, D. T., & Fiske, D. W. (1959). Convergent and discriminant validation by the multitrait-multimethod matrix. *Psychological Bulletin, 56,* 81–105.

Cronbach, L. J. (1990). *Essentials of psychological testing* (5th ed.). New York: Harper & Row.

Davis, L. L., & Grant, J. S. (1993). Guidelines for using psychometric consultants in nursing studies. *Research in Nursing & Health, 16,* 151–155.

DeKeyser, F. G., & Pugh, L. C. (1990). Assessment of the reliability and validity of biochemical measures. *Nursing Research, 39,* 314–317.

Denzin, N. K. (1989). *The research act* (3rd ed.). New York: McGraw-Hill.

Ferketich, S. L., Figueredo, A., & Knapp, T. R. (1991). The multitrait-multimethod approach to construct validity. *Research in Nursing & Health, 14,* 315–319.

Goodwin, L. D., & Goodwin, W. L. (1991). Estimating construct validity. *Research in Nursing & Health, 14,* 235–243.

Grant, J. S., & Davis, L. L. (1997). Selection and use of content experts for instrument development. *Research in Nursing & Health, 20,* 269–274.

Guilford, J. P. (1964). *Psychometric methods* (2nd ed.). New York: McGraw-Hill.

Hoffart, N. (1991). A member check procedure to enhance rigor in naturalistic research. *Western Journal of Nursing Research, 13,* 522–534.

Hutchinson, S., & Wilson, H. S. (1992). Validity threats in scheduled semistructured research interviews. *Nursing Research, 41,* 117–119.

Kimchi, J., Polivka, B., & Stevenson, J. S. (1991). Triangulation: Operational definitions. *Nursing Research, 40,* 364–366.

Kirk, J., & Miller, M. L. (1985). *Reliability and validity in qualitative research.* Beverly Hills, CA: Sage.

Laschinger, H. K. S. (1992). Intraclass correlations as estimates of interrater reliability in nursing research. *Western Journal of Nursing Research, 14,* 246–251.

Lincoln, Y. S., & Guba, E. G. (1985). *Naturalistic inquiry.* Newbury Park, CA: Sage.

Lowe, N. K., & Ryan-Wenger, N. M. (1992). Beyond Campbell and Fiske: Assessment of convergent and discriminant validity. *Research in Nursing & Health, 15,* 67–75.

Lynn, M. R. (1986). Determination and quantification of content validity. *Nursing Research, 35,* 382–385.

Nunnally, J. (1978). *Psychometric theory.* (2nd ed.) New York: McGraw-Hill.

Nunnally, J., & Bernstein, I. H. (1994). *Psychometric theory.* (3rd ed.). New York: McGraw-Hill.

Patton, M. Q. (1990). *Qualitative evaluation and research methods.* Newbury Park, CA: Sage.

Rodgers, B. L., & Cowles, K. V. (1993). The qualitative research audit trail: A complex collection of documentation. *Research in Nursing & Health, 16,* 219–226.

Slocumb, E. M., & Cole, F. L. (1991). A practical approach to content validation. *Applied Nursing Research, 4,* 192–195.

Thomas, S. D., Hathaway, D. K., & Arheart, K. L. (1992). Face validity. *Western Journal of Nursing Research, 14,* 109–112.

Thorndike, R. L., & Hagen, E. (1990). *Measurement and evaluation in psychology and education* (5th ed.). New York: John Wiley and Sons.

Tilden, V. P., Nelson, C. A., & May, B. A. (1990). Use of qualitative methods to enhance content validity. *Nursing Research, 39,* 172–175.

Waltz, C. F., Strickland, O. L., & Lenz, E. R. (1991). *Measurement in nursing research* (2nd ed.). Philadelphia: F. A. Davis.

Substantive References

Bennett, S. J., Puntenney, P. J., Walker, N. L., & Ashley, N. D. (1996). Development of an instrument to measure threat related to cardiac events. *Nursing Research, 45,* 266–270.

Cohen, L. J. (1994). What is the experience of therapeutic reading? *Western Journal of Nursing Research, 16,* 426–437.

Conco, D. (1995). Christian patients' views of spiritual care. *Western Journal of Nursing Research, 17,* 266–276.

Cromwell, S. L. (1994). The subjective experience of forgetfulness among elders. *Qualitative Health Research, 4,* 444–462.

Davis, D. L., & Joakimsen, L. M. (1997). Nerves as status and nerves as stigma: Idioms of distress and social action in Newfoundland and Northern Norway. *Qualitative Health Research, 7,* 370–390.

Frank-Stromborg, M. (1989). Reaction to the diagnosis of cancer questionnaire: Development and psychometric evaluation. *Nursing Research, 38,* 364–369.

Gagliardi, B. A. (1991). The family's experience of living with a child with Duchenne muscular dystrophy. *Applied Nursing Research, 4,* 159–164.

Gulick, E. E., & Escobar-Florez, L. (1995). Reliability and validity of the Smoking and Women Questionnaire among three ethnic groups. *Public Health Nursing, 12,* 117–126.

Hess, R. G. (1998). Measuring nursing governance. *Nursing Research, 47,* 35–42.

Hagerty, B. M., & Patusky, K. (1995). Developing a measure of sense of belonging. *Nursing Research, 44,* 9–13.

Hill, P. D., & Humenick, S. S. (1996). Development of the H & H Lactation Scale. *Nursing Research, 45,* 136–140.

Neelon, V. J., Champagne, M. T., Carlson, J. R., & Funk, S. G. (1996). *Nursing Research, 45,* 324–330.

Prescott, P. A., Ryan, J. W., Soeken, K. L., Castorr, A. H., Thompson, K. O., & Phillips, C. Y. (1991). The Patient Intensity for Nursing Index: A validity assessment. *Research in Nursing & Health, 14,* 213–221.

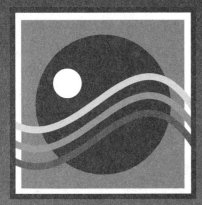

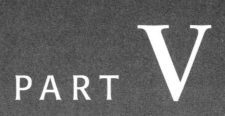

PART V

The Analysis
of Research Data

Quantitative Analysis: Descriptive Statistics

Statistical analysis is a method for rendering quantitative information meaningful and intelligible. Without the aid of statistics, the quantitative data collected in a research project would be little more than a chaotic mass of numbers. Statistical procedures enable the researcher to reduce, summarize, organize, evaluate, interpret, and communicate numeric information.

Some students are intimidated by statistics, but it may be of some comfort to know that mathematic talent is not required to use or understand statistical analysis. To apply and interpret most statistics, only logical thinking ability is needed. This textbook does not emphasize the theoretical rationale or mathematic derivation of statistical operations. In fact, even computation is underplayed because this is not a statistics textbook and because statistics are seldom calculated by hand in this era of computers. Our emphasis is on how to use statistics appropriately in different research situations and how to understand what they mean once they have been applied.

Statistics usually are classified as either descriptive or inferential. **Descriptive statistics** are used to describe and synthesize data. Averages and percentages are examples of descriptive statistics. Actually, when such indexes are calculated on data from a population, they are referred to as **parameters.** A descriptive index from a sample is called a **statistic.** Most scientific questions are about parameters, but researchers usually calculate statistics to estimate those parameters. When researchers use statistics to make inferences or draw conclusions about a population, **inferential statistics** are required. This chapter discusses descriptive statistics, and Chapter 19 focuses on inferential statistics. First, however, we must discuss the concept of levels of measurement.

LEVELS OF MEASUREMENT

Scientists have developed a system for categorizing different types of measures. This classification system is important because the analytic operations that can be performed on data depend on the measurement level used. Four major classes, or levels, of measurement have been identified: nominal, ordinal, interval, and ratio.

Nominal Measurement

The lowest level of measurement is referred to as nominal measurement. This level involves the assignment of numbers simply to classify characteristics into categories. Examples of variables amenable to nominal measurement include gender, blood type, and nursing specialty.

The numeric codes assigned in nominal measurement are not intended to convey any quantitative information. If we establish a rule to classify males as 1 and females as 2, the numbers in and of themselves have no meaning. The number 2 here clearly does not mean "more than" 1. It would be perfectly acceptable to reverse the code and use 1 for females and 2 for males. The numbers are merely symbols that represent two different values of the gender attribute. Indeed, instead of numeric codes, we could as easily have chosen alphabetical symbols, such as *M* and *F*. We recommend, however, thinking in terms of numeric codes if the subsequent analysis of data involves the use of a computer.

Nominal measurement provides no information about an attribute except that of equivalence and nonequivalence. If we were to "measure" the gender of Peter, Charles, Bob, Margot, and Sarah, we would—according to our rule—assign them the codes 1, 1, 1, 2, and 2, respectively. Peter, Charles, and Bob are considered equivalent with respect to the target attribute but are not equivalent to the other two subjects.

The basic requirements for measuring attributes on the nominal scale are that the classifications must be mutually exclusive and collectively exhaustive. For example, if we were measuring ethnicity, we might establish the following scheme: 1 = whites, 2 = African Americans, 3 = Hispanics. Each subject must be classifiable into one and only one of these categories. The requirement for collective exhaustiveness would not be met if, for example, there were several individuals of Asian descent in the sample.

The numbers used in nominal measurement cannot be treated mathematically. Although it might make perfectly good sense to determine the average weight of a sample of subjects, it is nonsensical to calculate the average gender of a sample. However, the elements assigned to each category can be enumerated, and statements can be made concerning the frequency of occurrence in each class. In a sample of 50 patients, we might find 30 males and 20 females. We could also say that 60% of the subjects are male and 40% are female. However, no further mathematic operations would be meaningful with data from nominal measures.

It may strike some readers as odd to think of the categorization procedure we have been describing as measurement. If the definition of measurement is recalled, however, it can be seen that nominal measurement does, in fact, involve the assignment of numbers to attributes according to rules. The rules are not sophisticated, to be sure, but they are rules nonetheless.

Ordinal Measurement

The next level in the measurement hierarchy is ordinal measurement. Ordinal measurement permits the sorting of objects on the basis of their standing on an attribute relative to each other. This level of measurement goes beyond a mere categorization: the attributes are *ordered* according to some criterion. If a researcher were to rank-order subjects from the heaviest to the lightest, then we would say that an ordinal level of measurement had been used.

The fundamental difference between nominal and ordinal measurement is that, with ordinal measurement, information concerning not only equivalence but also relative standing or ordering among objects is indicated. When we assign numbers to a person's religious affiliation, the numbers have no inherent meaning or significance. Now, consider this scheme for measuring a client's ability to perform activities of daily living: (1) completely dependent, (2) needs another person's assistance, (3) needs mechanical assistance, (4) completely independent. In this case, the measurement is ordinal. The numbers are not arbitrary—they signify incremental ability to perform the activities of daily living. The individuals assigned a value of four are equivalent to each other with regard to their ability to function *and*, relative to those in all the other categories, have more of that attribute.

Ordinal measurement does not, however, tell us anything about how much greater one level of an attribute is than another level. We do not know if being completely independent is twice as good as needing mechanical assistance, nor do we know if the difference between needing another person's assistance and needing mechanical assistance is the same as that between needing mechanical assistance and being completely independent. Ordinal measurement only tells us the relative ranking of the levels of an attribute.

As in the case of nominal scales, the types of mathematical operations permissible with ordinal-level data are rather restricted. Averages are generally meaningless with rank-order measures. Frequency counts, percentages, and several other statistical procedures to be discussed in Chapter 19 are appropriate for analyzing ordinal-level data.

Interval Measurement

Interval measurement occurs when the researcher can specify both the rank-ordering of objects on an attribute and the distance between those objects. The distances between the numeric values on an interval scale represent equal distances in the attribute being measured. Most psychological and educational tests are based on interval scales. The Scholastic Assessment Test (SAT) is an example of this level of measurement. A score of 550 on the SAT is higher than a score of 500, which in turn is higher than 450. Additionally, a difference between 550 and 500 on the test is presumably equivalent to the difference between 500 and 450.

Interval measures, then, are more informative than ordinal measures, but one piece of information that interval measures fail to provide is the absolute magnitude of the attribute. The Fahrenheit scale for measuring temperature illustrates this point. A temperature of 60°F is 10°F warmer than 50°F. A 10°F difference similarly separates 40°F and 30°F, and the two differences in temperature are equivalent. However, it cannot be said that 60°F is twice as hot as 30°F, or three times as hot as 20°F. The assignment of numbers to temperature on the Fahrenheit scale involves an arbitrary zero point. Zero on the thermometer does not signify a total absence of heat. In interval scales, there is no real or rational zero point.

The use of interval scales greatly expands the researcher's analytic possibilities. The intervals between numbers can be meaningfully added and subtracted: the interval between 10°F and 5°F is 5°F, or $10 - 5 = 5$. This same operation could not be performed with ordinal measures. Because of this capability, interval-level data can be averaged. It is perfectly reasonable, for example, to compute an average daily temperature for hospitalized patients from whom temperature readings are taken four times a day. Many widely used statistical procedures require that measurements be made on at least an interval scale.

Ratio Measurement

The highest level of measurement is **ratio measurement**. Ratio scales are distinguished from interval scales by virtue of having a rational, meaningful zero. Measures on a ratio scale provide information concerning the rank-ordering of objects on the critical attribute, the intervals between objects, and the absolute magnitude of the attribute for the object. Many physical measures provide ratio-level data. A person's weight, for example, is measured on a ratio scale because zero weight is an actual possibility. It is perfectly acceptable to say that someone who weighs 200 pounds is twice as heavy as someone who weighs 100 pounds.

Because ratio scales have an absolute zero, all arithmetic operations are permissible. One can meaningfully add, subtract, multiply, and divide numbers on a ratio scale. Consequently, all the statistical procedures suitable for interval-level data are also appropriate for ratio-level data. Ratio measurement constitutes the measurement ideal for scientists but is unattainable for most attributes of a psychological nature.

Comparison of the Levels

The four levels of measurement constitute a hierarchy, with ratio scales at the pinnacle and nominal measurement at the base. When one moves from a higher to a lower level of measurement, there is always an information loss. Let us demonstrate this using an example relating to data on the weight of a sample of individuals. Table 18-1 presents fictitious data for 10 subjects. The second column shows the ratio-level data, that is, their actual weight in

pounds. The ratio measure gives us complete information concerning the absolute weight of each subject and the differences in weights between all pairs of subjects.

In the third column, the original data have been converted to interval measures by assigning a score of 0 to the lightest individual (Katy), a score of 5 to the person 5 pounds heavier than the lightest person (Lindsay), and so forth. Note that the resulting scores are still amenable to addition and subtraction; the differences in pounds are equally far apart, even though they are at different parts of the scale. The data no longer tell us, however, anything about the absolute weights of the people in this sample. Katy, the lightest individual, might be a 10-pound infant or a 150-pound adult.

In the fourth column of Table 18-1, ordinal measurements were assigned by rank-ordering the sample from the lightest, who was assigned the score of 1, to the heaviest, who was assigned the score of 10. Now even more information is missing. The data provide no indication of how much heavier Nathan is than Katy. The difference separating them might be as little as 5 pounds or as much as 150 pounds.

Finally, the fifth column presents nominal measurements in which all subjects were classified as either heavy or light. The criterion applied in categorizing individuals was arbitrarily

TABLE 18-1 Fictitious Data for Four Levels of Measurement				
SUBJECTS	**RATIO-LEVEL**	**INTERVAL-LEVEL**	**ORDINAL-LEVEL**	**NOMINAL**
Nathan	180	70	10	2
Katy	110	0	1	1
Alex	165	55	8	2
Lauren	130	20	5	1
Kevin	175	65	9	2
Lindsay	115	5	2	1
Rosanna	125	15	4	1
Chad	150	40	7	1
Tom	145	35	6	1
Megan	120	10	3	1

TABLE 18-2 Research Examples of Variables Measured at Different Levels of Measurement		
RESEARCH QUESTION	**CONCEPT OR MEASURE**	**LEVEL OF MEASUREMENT**
What are the correlates of sleep patterns during hospitalization among patients with cardiac disease? (Redeker, Tamburri, & Howland, 1998)	Quantity of sleep in minutes	Ratio
	Duration of awakenings	Ratio
	Sleep Loss Scale	Interval
	NYHA Functional Classification	Ordinal
	Gender	Nominal
What are the multidimensional aspects of nicotine dependence and cigarette smoking among black and white women smokers? (Ahijevych & Gillespie, 1997)	Race	Nominal
	Perceived nicotine dependence	Interval
	Time to first cigarette in day	Ratio
	Plasma cotinine level	Ratio
What are adolescents' views and practices relating to tatooing? (Armstrong & Murphy, 1997)	Tattoo experience (yes/no)	Nominal
	Grades in school	Ordinal
	Purpose of tattooing (scale)	Interval
	Age at first tattoo	Ratio
What are the linkages among sexual risk taking, substance use, and AIDS knowledge among pregnant adolescents and young mothers? (Koniak-Griffin & Brecht, 1995)	Frequency of substance use	Ordinal
	AIDS knowledge	Ratio
	Number of sexual partners	Ratio
	Use versus nonuse of condoms	Nominal

set as a weight either greater than 150 pounds (2) or less than or equal to 150 pounds (1). The available information is very limited. Within any one category, there are no clues as to who is heavier than whom. With this level of measurement, Nathan, Alex, and Kevin are considered equivalent. They are equivalent with regard to the attribute heavy/light as defined by the classification criterion.

This example illustrates that at every successive level in the measurement hierarchy, there is a loss of information. It also illustrates another point: when one has information at one level, one can always manipulate the data to arrive at a lower level, but the converse is not true. If we were only given the nominal measurements, it would be impossible to reconstruct the actual weights.

It is not always a straightforward task to identify the level of measurement for a particular instrument. Usually, nominal measures and

ratio scales are discernible with little difficulty, but the distinction between ordinal and interval measures is more problematic. Some methodologists argue that most psychological measures that are treated as interval measures are really only ordinal measures. Most writers seem to believe that, although such instruments as Likert scales produce data that are, strictly speaking, ordinal level, the distortion introduced by treating them as interval measures is too small to warrant an abandonment of powerful statistical analyses. Table 18-2 presents examples of concepts that nurse researchers have operationalized at different levels of measurement.

FREQUENCY DISTRIBUTIONS

Raw quantitative data that are neither analyzed nor organized are overwhelming. It is not

TABLE 18-3		AIDS Knowledge Test Scores							
22	27	25	19	24	25	23	29	24	20
26	16	20	26	17	22	24	18	26	28
15	24	23	22	21	24	20	25	18	27
24	23	16	25	30	29	27	21	23	24
26	18	30	21	17	25	22	24	29	28
20	25	26	24	23	19	27	28	25	26

even possible to discern general trends until some order or structure is imposed on the data. Consider the 60 numbers presented in Table 18-3. Let us assume that these numbers represent the scores of 60 high school students on a 30-item test to measure knowledge about AIDS—scores that we will take to be measured on a ratio scale because there is a rational zero point (zero answers correct). Visual inspection of the numbers in this table does not really help us understand how the students performed.

A set of data can be completely described in terms of three characteristics: the shape of the distribution of values, central tendency, and variability. Central tendency and variability are dealt with in subsequent sections.

Constructing Frequency Distributions

Frequency distributions represent a method of imposing some order on a mass of numeric data. A **frequency distribution is** a systematic arrangement of numeric values from the lowest to the highest, together with a count of the number of times each value was obtained. The fictitious test scores of the 60 students are presented as a frequency distribution in Table 18-4. This organized arrangement makes it convenient to see at a glance what the highest and lowest scores were, what the most common score was, where the bulk of scores tended to cluster, and how many students were in the sample (total sample size is typically depicted as *N* in research reports). None of this was easily discernible before the data were organized.

The construction of a frequency distribution is simple. It consists basically of two parts: the observed values or measurements (the *X*s) and the frequency or count of the observations falling in each class (the *f*s). The values are listed in numeric order in one column, and the corresponding frequencies are listed in another. Table 18-4 shows the intermediary step in which the observations were actually tallied by the familiar method of four vertical bars and then a slash for the fifth observation. The only requirement for a frequency distribution is that the classes of observation must be mutually exclusive and collectively exhaustive. The sum of the numbers appearing in the frequency column must be equal to the size of the sample. In less verbal terms, $\Sigma f = N$, which translates as the sum of (signified by the Greek letter sigma, Σ) the frequencies (f) equals the sample size (N).

It is often useful to display not only the frequency counts for different values but also the percentages of the total, as shown in the fourth column of Table 18-4. The percentages are calculated by the simple formula: $\% = (f \div N) \times 100$. Just as the sum of all frequencies should equal N, the sum of all percentages should equal 100.

Rather than listing frequencies in tabular form, some researchers display their data graphically. Graphs have the advantage of being able to communicate a lot of information almost instantaneously. The most widely used types of graphs for displaying interval- and ratio-level data are **histograms and frequency polygons**. These two types are actually similar forms of presenting the same data.

Histograms and frequency polygons are constructed in much the same fashion. First, score classes are placed on a horizontal dimension, with the lowest value on the left, ascending to the highest value on the right. Next, the vertical dimension is used to designate the frequency count or, alternatively, percentages. The numbering of the vertical axis usually begins with zero. Using these dimensions as a base, a histogram is constructed by drawing bars above the score classes to the height corresponding to the frequency for that score class. An example is presented in Figure 18-1, using the same fictitious data on students' AIDS knowledge test scores.

Instead of vertical bars, the frequency polygon uses dots connected by straight lines to show frequencies for score classes. A dot corresponding to the frequency is placed above each score, as shown in Figure 18-2. It is con-

ventional to connect the figure to the base (zero line) at the score below the minimum value obtained and above the maximum value obtained. In this particular example, however, the graph is terminated at 30 and brought down to the base at that point with a dotted line because a score of 31 was not possible.

Shapes of Distributions

A distribution of numeric values such as those displayed in a frequency polygon can assume an almost infinite number of shapes. However, there are general aspects of the shape that can be described verbally. A distribution is said to be **symmetric** in shape if, when folded over, the two halves of the distribution would be superimposed on one another. In other words, symmetric distributions consist of two halves that are mirror images of one another. All the distributions shown in Figure 18-3 are symmetric. With real data sets, the distributions are rarely as perfectly symmetric as shown in this

TABLE 18-4	Frequency Distribution of Test Scores		
SCORE (X)	**TALLIES**	**FREQUENCY (f)**	**PERCENTAGE (%)**
15	I	1	1.7
16	II	2	3.3
17	II	2	3.3
18	III	3	5.0
19	II	2	3.3
20	IIII	4	6.7
21	III	3	5.0
22	IIII	4	6.7
23	LHT	5	8.3
24	LHT IIII	9	15.0
25	LHT II	7	11.7
26	LHT I	6	10.0
27	IIII	4	6.7
28	III	3	5.0
29	III	3	5.0
30	II	2	3.3
		$N = 60 = \Sigma f$	$\Sigma\% = 100.0\%$

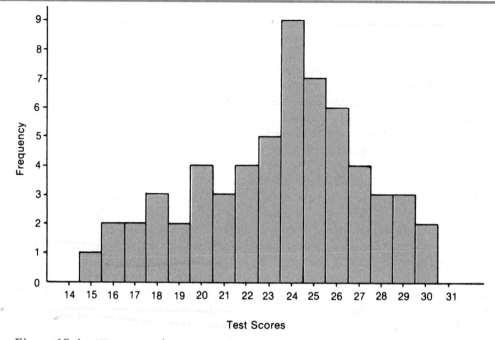

Figure 18-1.   Histogram of test scores.

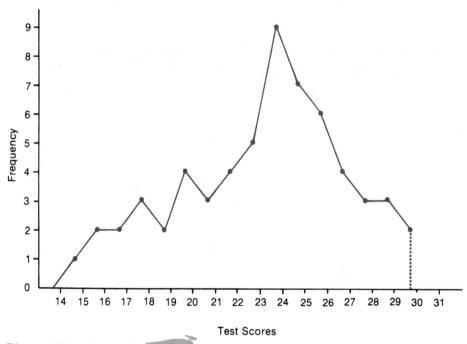

Figure 18-2.   Frequency polygon of test scores.

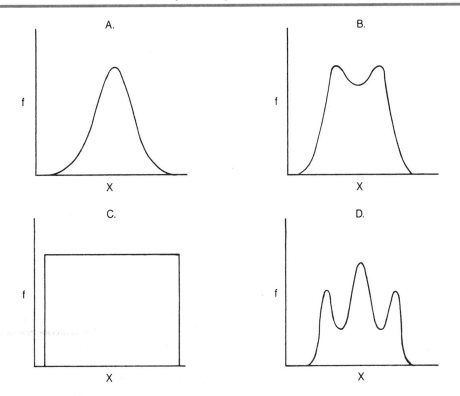

Figure 18-3.   Examples of symmetric distributions.

figure. However, minor discrepancies are often ignored in trying to characterize the shape of a distribution.

Asymmetric distributions usually are described as being skewed. In skewed distributions, the peak is off center, and one tail is longer than the other. Distributions that are skewed are usually described in terms of the direction of the skew. When the longer tail is pointing toward the right, the distribution is said to be **positively skewed.** Figure 18-4A depicts a positively skewed distribution. If, on the other hand, the tail points to the left, the skew is described as negative. A **negatively skewed** distribution is illustrated in Figure 18-4B. An example of an actual attribute that is positively skewed is personal income. The bulk of people have low to moderate incomes, with relatively

few people in high-income brackets in the right-hand tail of the distribution. An example of a negatively skewed attribute is age at death. Here, the bulk of people are at the upper end of the distribution, with relatively few people dying at an early age.

A second aspect of a distribution's shape is its modality. A **unimodal distribution** is one that has only one peak or high point (i.e., a value with high frequency), whereas a **multimodal distribution** has two or more peaks (i.e., two or more values of high frequency). The most common type of multimodal distribution is one with two peaks, which is called **bimodal**. Figure 18-3A is unimodal, as are both graphs in Figure 18-4. Multimodal distributions are illustrated in Figure 18-3B and D. Symmetry and modality are completely independent as-

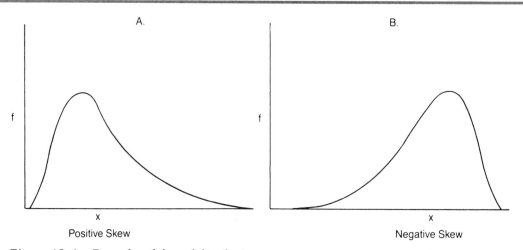

Figure 18-4. Examples of skewed distributions.

pects of a distribution. Knowledge of skewness does not tell you anything about how many peaks the distribution has.

Some distributions are encountered so frequently that special names are used to designate them. Of particular interest in statistical analysis is the distribution known as the **normal distribution** (sometimes called a **bell-shaped curve**). A normal distribution is one that is symmetric, unimodal, and not too peaked, as illustrated by the distribution in Figure 18-3A. Many physical and psychological attributes of humans have been found to approximate a normal distribution. Examples include height, intelligence, and grip strength. As we will see in Chapter 19, the normal distribution plays a central role in inferential statistics.

CENTRAL TENDENCY

Frequency distributions are an important means of imposing order on a set of raw data and of clarifying group patterns. For many purposes, however, a group pattern is of less interest to a researcher than an overall summary of a group's characteristics. The researcher usually asks such questions as, "What is the average oxygen con-

sumption of myocardial infarction patients during bathing?" "What is the average blood pressure reading of hypertensive patients during relaxation therapy?" "How knowledgeable is the average pregnant teenager about nutrition?" Such questions seek a single number that best represents a whole distribution of data values. Because an index of typicalness is more likely to be representative if it comes from the center of a distribution than if it comes from either extreme, such indexes are referred to as measures of **central tendency.** To lay people, the term *average* is normally used to designate central tendency. Researchers seldom use this term because it is ambiguous, inasmuch as there are three commonly used kinds of averages, or indexes of central tendency: the mode, the median, and the mean. Each can be used as an index to characterize a whole set of measurements.

The Mode

The **mode** is that numeric value in a distribution that occurs most frequently. The mode is the simplest to determine of the three measures of central tendency. Actually, the mode is not computed but rather is determined through inspection of a frequency distribution. In the following distribution of numbers, one can readily determine that the mode is 53:

50 51 51 52 53 53 53 53 54 55 56

The score of 53 was obtained four times, a higher frequency than for any other number. In the example presented earlier, the mode of the AIDS knowledge test scores is 24 (see Table 18-4). In multimodal distributions, of course, there is more than one score value that has high frequencies. The mode is seldom used in research reports as the only index of central tendency. Modes are a quick and easy method of determining the most popular score at a glance but are unsuitable for further computation and also are rather unstable. By unstable, we mean that modes tend to fluctuate widely from one sample drawn from a population to another sample drawn from the same population. The mode is infrequently used, except for describing typical values on nominal-level measures. For instance, researchers often characterize their samples by providing modal information on nominal-level demographic variables, as in the following example: "The typical (modal) subject was an unmarried white female, living in an urban area, with no prior history of sexually transmitted diseases."

The Median

The **median** is that point on a numeric scale above which and below which 50% of the cases fall. As an example, consider the following set of values:

2 2 3 3 4 5 6 7 8 9

The value that divides the cases exactly in half is 4.5, which is the median for this set of numbers. The point that has 50% of the cases above and below it is halfway between 4 and 5. An important characteristic of the median is that it does not take into account the quantitative values of individual scores. The median is an index of average *position* in a distribution of numbers. The median is insensitive to extreme values. Let us take the previous example to illustrate this point, making only one small change:

2 2 3 3 4 5 6 7 8 99

Despite the fact that the last value has been increased from 9 to 99, the median remains unchanged at 4.5. Because of this property, the median is often the preferred index of central tendency when the distribution is skewed and when one is interested in finding a typical value for variables measured on an ordinal scale or higher. In research reports, the median may be abbreviated as **Md** or **Mdn**.

The Mean

The **mean** is the point on the score scale that is equal to the sum of the scores divided by the total number of scores. The mean is the index of central tendency that is usually referred to as an average. The computational formula for a mean—which everyone knows, but whose symbols should be learned—is

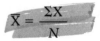

$$\overline{X} = \frac{\Sigma X}{N}$$

where $\overline{X}$ = the mean
Σ = the sum of
X = each individual raw score
N = the number of cases

Let us apply the above formula to calculate the mean weight of eight subjects whose individual weights are as follows:

85 109 120 135 158 177 181 195

$$\overline{X} = \frac{85 + 109 + 120 + 135 + 158 + 177 + 181 + 195}{8} = 145$$

Unlike the median, the mean is affected by the value of each and every score. If we were to exchange the 195-pound subject in this example for a subject weighing 275 pounds, the mean would increase from 145 to 155. A substitution of this kind would leave the median unchanged.

The mean is unquestionably the most widely used measure of central tendency. Many of the important tests of statistical significance, described in Chapter 19, are based on the mean. When researchers work with interval-level or ratio-level measurements, the mean, rather than the median or mode, is almost always the statistic reported. In research reports, the mean is often symbolized as M or $\overline{X}$.

Comparison of the Mode, Median, and Mean

Of the three indexes of central tendency, the mean is the most stable. If repeated samples were drawn from a given population, the means would vary or fluctuate less than the modes or medians. Because of its stability, the mean is the most reliable estimate of the central tendency of the population.

The arithmetic mean is the most appropriate index in situations in which the concern is for totals or combined performance of a group. If a school of nursing were comparing two graduating classes in terms of scores on a National League for Nursing Achievement Test, then the calculation of two means would be in order. Sometimes, however, the primary concern is learning what a typical value is, in which case a median might be preferred. In efforts to understand the economic well-being of United States citizens, for example, we would get a distorted impression of the financial status of the typical individual by considering the mean. The mean in this case would be inflated by the wealth of a small minority. The median, on the other hand, would reflect more realistically how the average person fared financially.

When a distribution of scores is symmetric and unimodal, the three indexes of central tendency coincide. In skewed distributions, the values of the mode, median, and mean differ. The mean is always pulled in the direction of the long tail, as shown in Figure 18-5.

The level of measurement plays a role in determining the appropriate index of central tendency that can be used to describe a variable. In general, the mode is appropriate for nominal measures, the median is appropriate for ordinal measures, and the mean is appropriate for interval and ratio measures. However, the

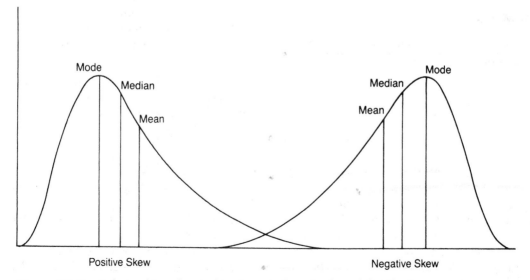

Positive Skew   Negative Skew

Figure 18-5. Relationships of central tendency indexes in skewed distributions.

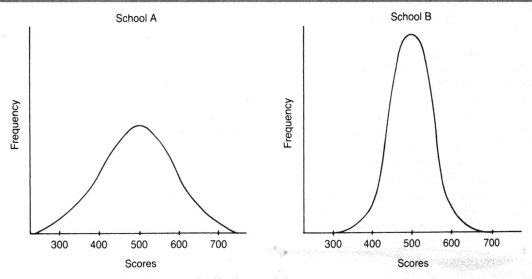

Figure 18-6. Two distributions of different variability.

higher the level of measurement, the greater the flexibility one has in choosing a descriptive statistic. Variables measured on an interval or ratio scale can use any of the three indexes of central tendency, although it is usually preferable to use the mean.

VARIABILITY

Measures of central tendency do not give a total picture of a distribution. Two sets of data with identical means could be different from one another in several respects. For one thing, two distributions with the same mean could be very different in shape: they could be skewed in opposite directions, for example. The characteristic of concern in this section is how spread out or dispersed the data are. The variability of two distributions can be different, even when the means are identical.

Consider the two distributions in Figure 18-6, which represent the hypothetical scores of freshman students from two schools of nursing on the SAT. Both distributions have an average of 500, but the patterns of scores are clearly different. In school A, there is a wide range of scores: from scores below 300 to some above 700. This school has many students who performed among the best possible but also has many students who scored well below the national average. In school B, on the other hand, there are few students at either extreme. School A is said to be more **heterogeneous** than school B, and school B is said to be more **homogeneous** than school A.

To describe a distribution adequately, there is a need for a measure of variability that expresses the extent to which scores deviate from one another. Several such indexes have been developed, the most common of which are the range, semiquartile range, and standard deviation.

The Range

The range is simply the highest score minus the lowest score in a given distribution. In the examples shown in Figure 18-6, the range for school A is about 500 (750 − 250), and the range for school B is about 300 (650 − 350). The range indicates the distance on the score scale between the lowest and highest values.

The chief virtue of the range is the ease with which it can be computed. As an index of variability, the shortcomings of the range outweigh this modest advantage. The range, being based on only two scores, is a highly unstable index. From sample to sample drawn from the same population, the range tends to fluctuate considerably. Another difficulty with the range is that it ignores completely variations in scores between the two extremes. In school B of Figure 18-6, suppose that only one student obtained a score of 250 and one other student obtained a score of 750. The range of both schools would then be 500, despite obvious differences in the heterogeneity of scores. For these reasons, the range is used largely as a gross descriptive index and is typically reported in conjunction with, not instead of, other measures of variability.

Semiquartile Range*

A previous section described the median as the point below which 50% of the cases fall. It is computationally possible to determine the point below which any percentage of the scores fall. For example, an admissions committee for a school of nursing might establish a minimum standard at the 40th percentile on the SAT for its entrants. The **semiquartile range** is calculated on the basis of quartiles within a distribution. The upper quartile (Q_3) is the point below which 75% of the cases fall, and the lower quartile (Q_1) is the point below which 25% of the scores lie.† The semiquartile range (SQR) is half the distance between Q_1 and Q_3, or

$$SQR = \frac{Q_3 - Q_1}{2}$$

_____

*Some statistical texts use the term *semiquartile range,* whereas others refer to this statistic as the *semiinterquartile range* or the *quartile deviation.*

†The computational formulas for percentiles are not presented here. Most standard statistics texts contain this information.

The semiquartile range indicates half the range of scores within which the middle 50% of scores lie. Because this index is a measure based on middle cases rather than extreme scores, it is considerably more stable than the range. In the case of the two nursing schools in Figure 18-6, school A would have a semiquartile range in the vicinity of 125, and the semiquartile range of school B would be about 75. The addition of one deviant case at either extreme for school B would leave the semiquartile range virtually untouched.

Standard Deviation

With interval- or ratio-level data, the most widely used measure of variability is the standard deviation. Like the mean, the standard deviation considers every score in a distribution. The standard deviation summarizes the average amount of deviation of values from the mean.

What is needed in a variability index is some way of capturing the degree to which scores deviate from one another. This concept of deviation is represented in both the range and the semiquartile range by the presence of a minus sign, which produces an index of deviation, or difference, between two score points. The standard deviation is similarly based on score differences. In fact, the first step in calculating a standard deviation is to compute deviation scores for each subject. A **deviation score** (usually symbolized with a small x) is the difference between an individual score and the mean. If a person weighed 150 pounds and the sample mean were 140, then the person's deviation score would be +10. Symbolically, the formula for a deviation score is

$$x = X - \overline{X}$$

Because what one is essentially looking for is an *average* deviation, one might think that a good variability index could be arrived at by summing the deviation scores and then dividing by the number of cases. This gets us close to a good solution, but the difficulty is that the sum

TABLE 18-5	Computation of a Standard Deviation	
X	$x = X - \overline{X}$	$x^2 = (X - \overline{X})^2$
4	−3	9
5	−2	4
6	−1	1
7	0	0
7	0	0
7	0	0
8	1	1
9	2	4
10	3	9
$\Sigma X = 63$	$\Sigma x = 0$	$\Sigma x^2 = 28$
$\Sigma X/N = \overline{X}$		
$= 63/9 = 7$		

$$SD = \sqrt{\frac{28}{9}} = \sqrt{3.11} = 1.76$$

of a set of deviation scores is always zero. Table 18-5 presents an example of deviation scores computed for nine numbers. As shown in the second column, the sum of the xs is equal to zero. The deviations above the mean always balance exactly those deviations below the mean.

The standard deviation overcomes this problem by squaring each deviation score before summing. After dividing by the number of cases, one takes the square root to bring the index back to the original unit of measurement. The formula for the standard deviation (often abbreviated as s or SD)* is

$$SD = \sqrt{\frac{\Sigma x^2}{N}}$$

---

*Some statistical texts indicate that the formula for an unbiased estimate of the population SD is

$$SD = \sqrt{\frac{\Sigma x^2}{N - 1}}$$

Knapp (1970) clarifies when N or $N - 1$ should be used in the denominator. He indicates that N is appropriate when the researcher is interested in *describing* variation in sample data.

A standard deviation has been completely worked out in the example in Table 18-5. First, a deviation score is calculated for each of the nine raw scores by subtracting the mean ($\overline{X} = 7$) from them. The third column shows that each deviation score is squared, thereby converting all values to positive numbers. The squared deviation scores are summed ($\Sigma x^2 = 28$), divided by 9 (N), and a square root taken to yield an SD of 1.76.

Most researchers routinely report the standard deviation of a variable along with the mean. Sometimes, however, one will find a reference to an index of variability known as the variance. The **variance** is simply the value of the standard deviation before a square root has been taken. In other words,

$$\text{Variance} = \frac{\Sigma x^2}{N} = SD^2$$

In the above example, the variance is 1.76^2, or 3.11. The variance is less widely reported because it is an index that is not in the same unit of measurement as the original data. The variance, however, is an important component in many inferential statistical tests that will be encountered later.

A standard deviation is typically more difficult for students to interpret than other statistics, such as the mean or range. In our previous example, we calculated an SD of 1.76. One might well ask, 1.76 *what*? What does the number mean? We will try to answer these questions from several vantage points. First, as we already know, the standard deviation is an index of the variability of scores in a data set. If two distributions had a mean of 25.0, but one had an SD of 7.0 and the other had an SD of 3.0, then we would immediately know that the second sample was more homogeneous.

A convenient way to conceptualize the standard deviation is to think of it as an average of the deviations from the mean. The mean tells us the single best point for summarizing an entire distribution, whereas a standard deviation tells us how much, on average, the scores deviate from that mean. A standard deviation might thus be interpreted as an indication of our degree of error when we use a mean to describe the entire sample.

The standard deviation can also be used in interpreting individual scores from within a distribution. Suppose we had a set of weight measures from a sample whose mean weight was 125 pounds and whose SD was 10 pounds. We can think of the standard deviation as actually providing a standard of variability. Weights greater than 1 SD away from the mean (i.e., greater than 135 or less than 115 pounds) are greater than the average variability for that distribution. Weights less than 1 SD from the mean, by consequence, are less than the average variability for that sample.

When the distribution of scores is normal or nearly normal, it is possible to say even more about the standard deviation. There are about 3 SDs above and 3 SDs below the mean with normally distributed data. To illustrate some further characteristics, suppose that we had a normal distribution of scores whose mean was 50 and whose SD was 10, as shown in Figure 18-7. In a normal distribution such as this, a fixed percentage of cases falls within certain

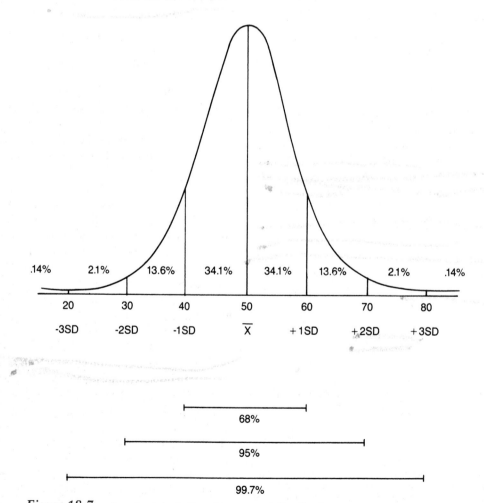

Figure 18-7. Standard deviations in a normal distribution.

distances from the mean. Sixty-eight percent of all cases fall within 1 SD of the mean (34% above and 34% below the mean). In this example, nearly 7 of every 10 scores fall between 40 and 60. Ninety-five percent of the scores in a normal distribution fall within 2 SDs from the mean. Only a handful of cases—about 2% at each extreme—lie more than 2 SDs from the mean. Using this figure, we can see that a person who obtained a score of 70 got a higher score than about 98% of the sample.

In summary, the standard deviation is a useful index of variability that can be used to describe an important characteristic of a distribution and that also can be used to interpret the score or performance of an individual in relation to others in the sample. Like the mean, the standard deviation is a stable estimate of a population parameter and also is used extensively in more advanced statistical procedures. The standard deviation is the preferred measure of a distribution's variability but is appropriate only for variables measured on the interval or ratio scale.

BIVARIATE DESCRIPTIVE STATISTICS: CONTINGENCY TABLES AND CORRELATION

The discussion has so far focused on a description of single variables. The mean, mode, standard deviation, and so forth are all used in describing data for one variable at a time. We have been examining what is referred to as **univariate** (one-variable) **descriptive statistics**. As indicated throughout this text, research is usually concerned with relationships between variables. What is needed, then, is some method of describing such relationships. In this section, we look at **bivariate** (two-variable) **descriptive statistics**.

Contingency Tables

A **contingency table** is essentially a two-dimensional frequency distribution in which the frequencies of two variables are cross-tabulated.

Suppose we had data on subjects' gender and responses to a question on whether they were nonsmokers, light smokers (less than one pack per day), or heavy smokers (one pack per day or more). We might be interested in learning if there is a tendency for men to smoke more heavily than women or vice versa. Some fictitious data on these two variables are presented in Table 18-6. It is difficult to make sense of these data in their present form. To describe the data, we need a method of organizing this mass of numbers. The best way to do so in a manner that highlights the research question is to construct a contingency table.

A contingency table for the data in Table 18-6 is presented in Table 18-7. Six cells are created by placing one variable (gender) along the horizontal dimension and the other variable (smoking status) along the vertical dimension at the left-hand side. The system of bars and crosshatches can then be used to tabulate the number of subjects belonging in each cell. The first subject, who has a code of 1 for gender and 1 for smoking status, would be marked in the upper left-hand cell, and so on. After all subjects have been assigned to the appropriate cells, the frequencies can be tabulated and percentages computed. This simple procedure allows us to see at a glance that, in this particular sample, women were more likely to be nonsmokers and less likely to be heavy smokers than men. Contingency tables, or cross-tabulations as they are sometimes called, are easy to construct and have the ability to communicate a lot of information. The use of contingency tables is usually restricted to nominal data or to ordinal data that have few values or ranks. In the gender–smoker relationship example, gender is a nominal measure, and smoking status, as operationally defined, is an ordinal measure. We will encounter contingency tables again in the discussion on inferential statistics in Chapter 19.

Correlation

The most common method of describing the relationship between two measures is through

TABLE 18-6	Fictitious Data for Gender–Smoking Relationship	
SUBJECT NUMBER	SUBJECT GENDER*	SMOKING STATUS†
01	1	1
02	2	3
03	2	1
04	1	2
05	1	1
06	2	2
07	2	1
08	2	3
09	1	1
10	2	3
11	1	2
12	1	3
13	1	1
14	2	3
15	2	1
16	2	2
17	2	3
18	1	1
19	2	2
20	1	2
21	1	1
22	1	3
23	1	2
24	2	2
25	2	1
26	1	3
27	2	3
28	1	1
29	1	3
30	1	2
31	2	1
32	1	1
33	2	2
34	1	2
35	1	1
36	2	2
37	2	3
38	2	3
39	2	2
40	1	2
41	1	1
42	2	1
43	1	2
44	2	2

*Gender: 1, female; 2, male.
†Smoking status: 1, nonsmoker; 2, light smoker; 3, heavy smoker.

correlation procedures. The computation of a correlation coefficient is normally performed when two variables are measured on either the ordinal, interval, or ratio scale. Correlation coefficients were briefly described in Chapter 17, and this section extends that discussion.

The correlation question asks, To what extent are two variables related to each other? For example: "To what extent are height and weight related?" "To what degree are anxiety test scores and blood pressure measures related?" These questions can be answered graphically or, more commonly, by the calculation of an index that describes the magnitude of the relationship.

The graphic representation of a correlation between two variables is called a **scatter plot** or **scatter diagram**. To construct a scatter plot, one first sets up a scale for the two variables constructed at right angles, making a rectangular coordinate graph. The range of values for one variable (X) is scaled off along the horizontal axis, and the same is done for the second variable (Y) along the vertical axis. One example is presented in Figure 18-8. To locate the position for subject A, one goes two units to the right along the X axis, and one unit up on the Y axis. The same procedure is followed for all subjects, resulting in the scatter plot shown. The letters shown on the plot in this figure have been included to help identify each point. Normally, only the dots appear on the diagram.

From a scatter plot, it is possible to determine both the direction and approximate magnitude of a correlation. The direction of the slope of points indicates the direction of the correlation. It may be recalled from Chapter 17 that correlations can be either positive or negative in direction. A positive correlation is obtained when high values on one variable are associated with high values on the second variable. If the slope of points begins at the lower left-hand corner and extends to the upper right-hand corner, then the relationship is positive. In the current example, we would say that X and Y are positively related. Inspection of the values shows that, indeed, people who

TABLE 18-7 Contingency Table for Gender–Smoking Relationship Data

| | GENDER | | | | | |
| SMOKING STATUS | Female | | Male | | Total | |
	N	%	N	%	N	%
Nonsmoker	10	45%	6	27%	16	36%
Light smoker	8	36%	8	35%	16	36%
Heavy smoker	4	18%	8	36%	12	27%
Total	22	50%	22	50%	44	100%

have a high score on variable X also tend to have a high score on variable Y, and low scorers on X tend to score low on Y.

A negative (or inverse) relationship is one in which high values on one variable are related to low values on the other. On a scatter plot, negative relationships are depicted by points that slope from the upper left-hand corner to the lower right-hand corner. A negative correlation is shown in Figure 18-9A and D.

Relationships are described as perfect when it is possible to predict perfectly the value of

Subject	X	Y
a	2	1
b	5	7
c	10	10
d	8	7
e	10	9
f	4	3
g	1	2
h	7	6
i	4	5
j	9	10

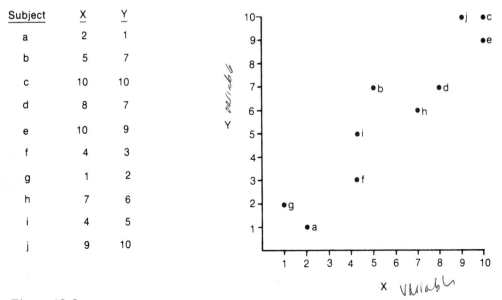

Figure 18-8. Construction of a scatter plot.

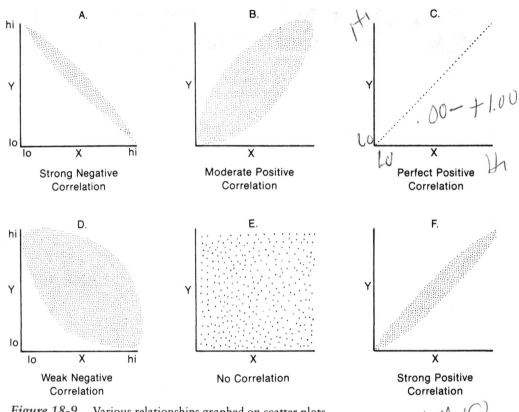

Figure 18-9. Various relationships graphed on scatter plots.

one variable by knowing the value of the second. For instance, if all people who were 6 feet 2 inches tall weighed 180 pounds, and all people who were 6 feet 1 inch tall weighed 175 pounds, and so on, then we could say that weight and height were perfectly, positively related. In such a situation, one would only need to be informed of a person's height to know his or her weight, or vice versa. On a scatter plot, a perfect relationship is represented by a sloped straight line, as shown in Figure 18-9C. When a relationship is not perfect, as is usually the case, one can interpret the degree of correlation from a scatter plot by seeing how closely the points cluster around a straight line. The more closely packed the points are around a diagonal slope, the higher the correlation. When the points are scattered all over the graph, the relationship is very low or

nonexistent. Various degrees and directions of relationships are presented in Figure 18-9.

Usually, it is more informative and efficient to express the direction and magnitude of a linear relationship by computing a correlation coefficient. As noted in Chapter 17, the correlation coefficient is an index whose values range from −1.00 for a perfect negative correlation, through zero for no relationship, to +1.00 for a perfect positive correlation. All correlations that fall between .00 and −1.00 are negative, and all correlations that fall between .00 and +1.00 are positive. The higher the absolute value of the coefficient (i.e., the value disregarding the sign), the stronger is the relationship. A correlation of −.80, for instance, is much stronger than a correlation of +.20.

The most commonly used correlation index is the **product–moment correlation coefficient,** also referred to as **Pearson's r.** This coefficient is computed when the variables being correlated have been measured on either an interval or ratio scale. (The correlation index generally used for ordinal-level measures is **Spearman's rho,** discussed in Chapter 19). The calculation of the *r* statistic is rather laborious and seldom performed by hand.*

Perfect correlations (+1.00 and −1.00) are extremely rare in research with humans. It is difficult to offer guidelines on what should be interpreted as strong or weak relationships. This determination depends, to a great extent, on the nature of the variables. If we were to measure patients' body temperatures both orally and rectally, a correlation of .70 between the two measurements would be considered low. For most variables of a social or psychological nature, however, an *r* of .70 is high; correlations between variables of a psychosocial nature are typically in the .10 to .40 range.

THE COMPUTER AND DESCRIPTIVE STATISTICS

In the previous sections, we introduced the basic concepts of statistics that are used to organize, summarize, and describe data. In this section, we work through a fictitious example of a study and illustrate these concepts through the use of computer printouts. This section aims to make the concepts less abstract by illustrating them with some data and to familiarize the reader with printouts from a standard computer pro-

gram called Statistical Package for the Social Sciences (SPSS).

Suppose that a nurse researcher were interested in improving the childbirth outcomes among a group of young, low-income pregnant women. A program of intensive health care, nutritional counseling, and contraceptive counseling is implemented, and an experiment is designed to test the effect of the program: half of a sample of pregnant women, assigned randomly, will receive the special treatment, and the other half will be assigned to a group receiving routine care. The two outcomes that the researcher is primarily interested in are the birthweight of the infant and whether the young woman becomes pregnant again within 18 months of delivery. Some fictitious data for this example, including data on various maternal characteristics, are presented in Table 18-8.

Figure 18-10 presents a frequency distribution printout for the birthweight variable. Under the term VALUE, each birthweight in the sample is listed in ascending order. In the next column, FREQUENCY, the number of occurrences of each birthweight is indicated. Thus, there was one 76-ounce baby, two 89-ounce babies, and so on. The next column, PERCENT, indicates the percentage of birthweights in each class: 3.3% of the babies weighed 76 ounces at birth, 6.7% weighed 89 ounces, and so on. The next column, VALID PERCENT, shows the percentage in each category after removing any missing data. In this example, birthweights were obtained for all 30 cases, but if one piece of data had been missing, the adjusted frequency for the 76-ounce baby would have been 3.4% (1 ÷ 29 rather than 30). The last column, CUM PERCENT, adds the percentage for a given birthweight value to the percentage for all preceding values. Thus, we can tell by looking at the row for 99 ounces that, cumulatively, 33.3% of the babies weighed *under* 100 ounces.

The bottom of this printout lists several of the descriptive statistics discussed in this chapter. The MEAN is equal to 104.7, whereas the MEDIAN is 102.5, and the MODE is 99. This

---

*For those who may wish to understand how a correlation coefficient is computed, we offer the following formula:

$$r_{xy} = \frac{\Sigma (X - \overline{X})(Y - \overline{Y})}{\sqrt{[\Sigma(X - \overline{X})^2][\Sigma(Y - \overline{Y})^2]}}$$

where r_{xy} = the correlation coefficient for variables X and Y
  X = an individual score for variable X
  $\overline{X}$ = the mean score for variable X
  Y = an individual score for variable Y
  $\overline{Y}$ = the mean score for variable Y
  Σ = the sum of

			TABLE 18-8 Fictitious Data on Low-Income Pregnant Women		
GROUP*	INFANT BIRTHWEIGHT	REPEAT PREGNANCY†	MOTHER'S AGE (YEARS)	NO. OF PRIOR PREGNANCIES	SMOKING STATUS‡
1	107	1	17	1	1
1	101	0	14	0	0
1	119	0	21	3	0
1	128	1	20	2	0
1	89	0	15	1	1
1	99	0	19	0	1
1	111	0	19	1	0
1	117	1	18	1	1
1	102	1	17	0	0
1	120	0	20	0	0
1	76	0	13	0	1
1	116	0	18	0	1
1	100	1	16	0	0
1	115	0	18	0	0
1	113	0	21	2	1
2	111	1	19	0	0
2	108	0	21	1	0
2	95	0	19	2	1
2	99	0	17	0	1
2	103	1	19	0	0
2	94	0	15	0	1
2	101	1	17	1	0
2	114	0	21	2	0
2	97	0	20	1	0
2	99	1	18	0	1
2	113	0	18	0	1
2	89	0	19	1	0
2	98	0	20	0	0
2	102	0	17	0	0
2	105	0	19	1	1

*Group: 1, experimental; 2, control.

†Repeat pregnancy: 1, yes; 0, no.

‡Smoking status: 1, smokes; 0, does not smoke.

suggests that the distribution is somewhat skewed. The RANGE is 52, which is equal to the MAXIMUM of 128 minus the MINIMUM of 76. The SD (STD DEV) is 10.955, and the VARIANCE is 120.010 (10.955²).

In addition to tabular information, such as that shown in Figure 18-10, many computer programs can produce graphic materials. Figure 18-11 presents a histogram for the variable, mother's age. In this case, all the values for age are shown on the vertical axis, and the frequency is shown on the horizontal axis. The histogram shows at a glance that the modal age is 19 ($f = 7$) and that this variable is negatively skewed (i.e., there are fewer younger than older girls). Descriptive statistics shown at the bottom of the printout indicate that the mean age for this group is 18.167, with an SD of 2.086.

If we were interested in comparing the repeat-pregnancy experience of the two groups of young women (experimental versus control), we would instruct the computer to cross-tabulate the two variables, as shown in the contingency table in Figure 18-12. This cross-tabulation resulted in four cells: (1) experimental subjects with no repeat pregnancy (upper left-hand cell); (2) control subjects with no repeat pregnancy (upper right-hand cell); (3) experimental subjects with a repeat pregnancy (lower left-hand cell); and (4) control subjects with a repeat pregnancy (lower right-hand cell). Each cell contains four pieces of information, which we will explain for the first cell. The first number is the number of subjects in that cell. Ten

```
--------------------------------------------------------------------------------
Page   2                        SPSS/PC+

WEIGHT    INFANT BIRTH WEIGHT


                                                   Valid      Cum
Value Label              Value  Frequency  Percent Percent    Percent

                           76       1       3.3     3.3       3.3
                           89.      2       6.7     6.7      10.0
                           94       1       3.3     3.3      13.3
                           95       1       3.3     3.3      16.7
                           97       1       3.3     3.3      20.0
                           98       1       3.3     3.3      23.3
                           99       3      10.0    10.0      33.3
                          100       1       3.3     3.3      36.7
                          101       2       6.7     6.7      43.3
                          102       2       6.7     6.7      50.0
                          103       1       3.3     3.3      53.3
                          105       1       3.3     3.3      56.7
                          107       1       3.3     3.3      60.0
                          108       1       3.3     3.3      63.3
                          111       2       6.7     6.7      70.0
                          113       2       6.7     6.7      76.7
                          114       1       3.3     3.3      80.0
                          115       1       3.3     3.3      83.3
                          116       1       3.3     3.3      86.7
                          117       1       3.3     3.3      90.0
                          119       1       3.3     3.3      93.3
                          120       1       3.3     3.3      96.7
                          128       1       3.3     3.3     100.0
                                 -------  -------  -------
                Total              30     100.0   100.0
--------------------------------------------------------------------------------
Page   3                        SPSS/PC+

WEIGHT    INFANT BIRTH WEIGHT


Mean       104.700    Std err      2.000    Median     102.500
Mode        99.000    Std dev     10.955    Variance   120.010
Kurtosis      .473    S E Kurt      .833    Skewness     -.254
S E Skew      .427    Range       52.000    Minimum     76.000
Maximum    128.000    Sum       3141.000

Valid cases    30    Missing cases      0
--------------------------------------------------------------------------------
```

Figure 18-10. SPSS Computer Printout: Frequency Distribution of Infant Birthweight.

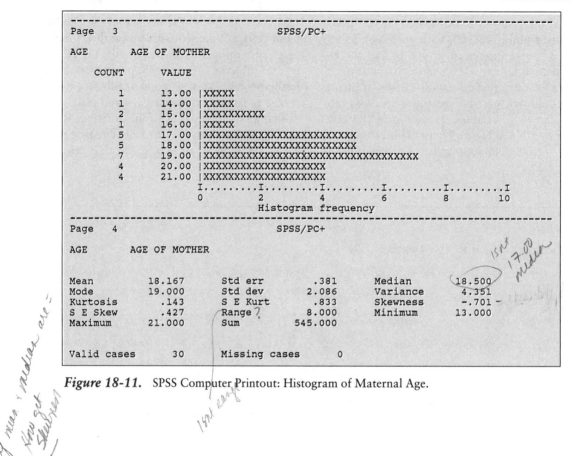

Figure 18-11. SPSS Computer Printout: Histogram of Maternal Age.

Figure 18-12. SPSS Computer Printout: Cross-Tabulation of Repeat Pregnancy, by Group.

experimental subjects did not have a repeat pregnancy within 18 months of their delivery. The next number is the *row* percentage: 47.6% of the women who did not become pregnant again were in the experimental group (10 ÷ 21). The next number represents the *column* percentage: 66.7% of those in the experimental group did not become pregnant (10 ÷ 15). The last number is the *overall* percentage of women in that cell (10 ÷ 30 = 33.3%). This order need not be memorized. It is shown in the upper left-hand corner of the table:

COUNT
ROW PCT
COL PCT
TOT PCT

Thus, Figure 18-12 indicates that a somewhat higher percentage of experimental subjects (33.3%) than controls (26.7%) experienced a repeat pregnancy. The row totals on the far right indicate that, overall, 30.0% of the sample ($N = 9$) had a subsequent pregnancy. The column total at the bottom indicates that, overall, 50.0% of the subjects were in the experimental group, and 50.0% were in the control group.

TIPS FOR APPLYING LEVELS OF MEASUREMENT AND DESCRIPTIVE STATISTICS

A knowledge of basic statistical methods is indispensable for those who want to keep abreast of research developments in their field—and for those undertaking a research project. Even researchers who conduct a basically qualitative study typically use some descriptive statistics for characterizing their sample. In this section, we provide some suggestions on the application of descriptive statistics.

- In operationalizing research variables, it is usually best to select or construct measures on as high a level of measurement as possible, especially for measures that will be used as dependent variables. This guideline is based on the fact that higher levels of measurement generally yield more information and are amenable to more powerful and sensitive analytic procedures than lower levels.

- Although it is generally preferable to use the highest possible level of measurement, there are exceptions to this guideline. For example, researchers sometimes use people's scores on interval- or ratio-level measures to create groups, and sometimes group membership is more meaningful or interpretable than continuous scores. For example, for some research and clinical purposes, it may be more relevant to designate infants as being of low birthweight or normal birthweight (nominal level) than to use actual birthweight values (ratio level).

- Descriptive statistics (percentages, means, standard deviations, and so on) are used for a variety of purposes in research reports. Sometimes—in purely descriptive studies—they are used directly to answer research questions, but inferential statistics (discussed in Chapter 19) are more likely to be used for this purpose. Descriptive statistics are most likely to be used to describe sample characteristics, to provide descriptive information about the distribution of key research variables in the study, and to document certain features of the research methods (e.g., the response rate or the attrition rate).

- When variables are measured on a nominal or ordinal scale, the nature of the measures limits the type of descriptive statistics that is appropriate. However, for variables measured on an interval or ratio scale, the researcher may wish to report multiple measures of central tendency or variability—particularly when the distribution is skewed. With asymmetric distributions, all three indexes of central tendency contain new information.

- In research reports, correlations are often reported in a **correlation matrix**, which is a two-dimensional display of the correlations among a set of variables. Every variable is displayed in both a row and a column, and the correlation coefficients among them are displayed at the intersection. An example of a correlation matrix is presented in the next section.

RESEARCH EXAMPLE

Bernhard and Sheppard (1993) conducted a study to examine the relationships among perceived health, menopausal symptoms, and self-care activities in perimenopausal and post-menopausal women. A total of 101 women in a large midwestern city responded to a newspaper advertisement for "menopausal women" and completed a self-administered questionnaire. The questionnaire included demographic information and four composite scales: the Health Perceptions Questionnaire (HPQ), the Menopause Symptom Checklist (MSC), the Self-Care Responses Questionnaire (SCR), and the Dyadic Adjustment Scale (DAS).

The research report for this study contained a variety of descriptive statistics, displayed in a number of tables. Table 18-9 shows a portion of their first table, which presented frequency information on sample characteristics. This table indicates that the typical woman who participated in the study was a married white woman with at least some college education.

The researchers then computed measures of central tendency and variability for their

---

TABLE 18-9 Demographic Characteristics of Study Participants

CHARACTERISTIC		PERCENTAGE (*N* = 101)
Race	White	96
	Other	4
Marital status	Married	64
	Divorced/separated	25
	Living together	4
	Widowed	4
	Single	3
Education	Some high school	1
	High school graduate	12
	Some college	49
	College graduate	26
	Graduate degree	12
Religion	Protestant	74
	Catholic	17
	Other	5
	None	4

Adapted from Bernhard, L. A., & Sheppard, L. (1993). Health, symptoms, self-care, and dyadic adjustment in menopausal women. *Journal of Obstetric, Gynecologic, and Neonatal Nursing, 22,* Table 1, with permission.

TABLE 18-10   Descriptive Statistics for Key Study Variables

VARIABLE	M	SD	RANGE	N
Health perceptions	124.84	10.01	91–144	59*
Menopause symptoms				
Total symptoms	12.99	5.49	0–26	90
Worrisome symptoms	2.49	3.15	0–20	90
Self-care responses	116.19	13.82	72–143	95
Dyadic adjustment	107.25	15.75	57–128	75

*Variations in numbers are due to missing data and to an administrative error with regard to an incorrect form of the Health Perceptions Questionnaire given to 39 women.

Adapted from Bernhard, L. A., & Sheppard, L. (1993). Health, symptoms, self-care, and dyadic adjustment in menopausal women. *Journal of Obstetric, Gynecologic, and Neonatal Nursing, 22,* Table 2, with permission.

---

primary study variables, as shown in Table 18-10. For each of the four scales included in the questionnaire, the table shows the mean, standard deviation, range, and number of sample members. Note that this last piece of information had to be included as a separate column in this table because varying numbers of respondents completed the four scales.

Information on the extent to which the various scales were intercorrelated is presented in Table 18-11, which is in the form of a **correlation matrix**. To read a correlation matrix, one finds the row for one of the variables and reads across until the row intersects with the column for a second variable. Table 18-11 lists, on the left, six variables: responses to a question on self-rated health and scores on the various scales (including total and subscale scores on the MSC). The numbers in the top row, from 1 to 6, correspond

---

TABLE 18-11   Intercorrelations Among Key Study Variables

VARIABLE	1	2	3	4	5	6
1. Self-rated health	1.00					
2. Health Perceptions Questionnaire	.44	1.00				
3. Menopause Symptom Checklist (total symptoms)	−.30	−.19	1.00			
4. Menopause Symptom Checklist (worrisome symptoms)	−.26	.30	.38	1.00		
5. Self-Care Responses Questionnaire	.12	.43	.03	−.16	1.00	
6. Dyadic Adjustment Scale	−.02	.19	.03	.15	−.14	1.00

Adapted from Bernhard, L. A., & Sheppard, L. (1993). Health, symptoms, self-care, and dyadic adjustment in menopausal women. *Journal of Obstetric, Gynecologic, and Neonatal Nursing, 22,* Table 3, with permission.

to the six variables: 1 is self-rated health, 2 is HPQ scores, and so forth. The correlation matrix shows, in the first column, the value of the correlation coefficient between self-rated health on the one hand and all six variables on the other. At the intersection of row 1 and column 1, we find the value 1.00, which simply indicates that self-rated health scores are perfectly correlated with themselves. The next entry in the first column represents the correlation between self-rated health and HPQ scores; the value of .44 (which can be read as +.44) indicates a moderate and positive relationship between these two variables: women who rated their health as excellent tended to have higher scores on the HPQ than women who said their health was fair or poor. By contrast, self-rated health was virtually unrelated to dyadic adjustment with a partner: women who had strong dyadic relationships were as likely to rate their health positively as women whose relationships were more troubled ($r = -.02$).

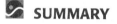

SUMMARY

There are four major **levels of measurement**. **Nominal measurement** classifies characteristics of attributes into mutually exclusive categories. **Ordinal measurement** involves the sorting of objects on the basis of their relative standing to each other on a specified attribute. **Interval measurement** indicates not only the rank-ordering of objects on an attribute but also the amount of distance between each object. Distances between numeric values on the interval scale represent equivalent distances in the attribute being measured. **Ratio measurement**, which constitutes the highest form of measurement, is distinguished from interval measurement by virtue of having a rational zero point.

Descriptive statistics enable the researcher to reduce, summarize, and describe quantitative data obtained from empirical observations and measurements. A **frequency distribution** is one of the easiest methods of imposing some

order on a mass of numbers. In a frequency distribution, numeric values are ordered from the lowest to the highest with a count of the number of times each value was obtained. **Histograms** and **frequency polygons** are two common methods of displaying frequency information graphically.

A set of data may be completely described in terms of the shape of the distribution, central tendency, and variability. The most important attributes of the distribution's shape are its symmetry and modality. A distribution is **symmetric** if its two halves are mirror images of each other. A **skewed distribution**, by contrast, is asymmetric, with one tail longer than the other. The modality of a distribution refers to the number of peaks present: a **unimodal distribution** has one peak, and a **multimodal distribution** has more than one peak.

Measures of **central tendency** are indexes, expressed as a single number, that represent the average or typical value of a set of scores. The **mode** is the numeric value that occurs most frequently in the distribution (or with greater frequency than other scores in its vicinity). The **median** is that point on a numeric scale above which and below which 50% of the cases fall. The **mean** is the arithmetic average of all the scores in the distribution. In general, the mean is the preferred measure of central tendency because of its stability and its usefulness in further statistical manipulations.

Variability refers to the spread or dispersion of the data. Measures of variability include the range, the semiquartile range, and the standard deviation. The **range** is the distance between the highest and lowest score values. The **semiquartile range** indicates one half of the range of scores within which the middle 50% of scores lie. The most commonly used measure of variability is the **standard deviation**. This index is calculated by first computing **deviation scores**, which represent the degree to which the scores of each person deviate from the mean. The standard deviation is designed to indicate how much, on average, the scores deviate from the mean. A related index, the **variance**, is equal to the standard deviation squared.

Bivariate descriptive statistics describe the existence and magnitude of relationships between two variables. A **contingency table** is a two-dimensional frequency distribution in which the frequencies of two variables are cross-tabulated. When the scores have been measured on an ordinal, interval, or ratio scale, it is more common to describe the relationship between two variables with correlational procedures. A **correlation coefficient** can be calculated to express in numeric terms the direction and magnitude of a linear relationship. The values of the correlation coefficient range from −1.00 for a perfect negative correlation, through .00 for no relationship, to +1.00 for a perfect positive correlation. The most frequently used correlation coefficient is the **product–moment correlation coefficient**, also referred to as **Pearson's** *r*. The graphic representation of a relationship between two variables is called a **scatter plot** or **scatter diagram**.

 STUDY ACTIVITIES

Chapter 18 of the *Study Guide to Accompany Nursing Research: Principles and Methods, 6th ed.*, offers various exercises and study suggestions for reinforcing the concepts presented in this chapter. Additionally, the following study questions can be addressed:

1. Construct a frequency distribution for the following set of scores obtained from a scale to measure attitudes toward primary nursing:

   32 20 33 22 16 19 25 26 25 18 22 30 24
   26 27 23 28 26 21 24 31 29 25 28 22 27
   26 30 17 24

2. Construct a frequency polygon or histogram with the data from above. Describe the resulting distribution of scores

in terms of symmetry and modality. How closely does the distribution approach a normal distribution?

3. What are the mean, median, and mode for the following set of data?

   13 12 9 15 7 10 16 8 6 1

   Compute the range and standard deviation.

4. Two hospitals are interested in comparing the tenure rates of their nursing staff. Hospital A finds that the current staff has been employed for a mean of 4.3 years, with an SD of 1.5. Hospital B, on the other hand, finds that the nurses have worked there for a mean of 6.4 years, with an SD of 4.2 years. Discuss what these results signify.

SUGGESTED READINGS

Methodologic References

Jaccard, J., & Becker, M. A. (1990). *Statistics for the behavioral sciences.* Belmont, CA: Wadsworth.

Judd, C. M., Smith, E. R., & Kidder, L. R. (1991). *Research methods in social relations* (6th ed.). Fort Worth, TX: Holt, Rinehart & Winston.

Knapp, T. R. (1970). N vs. N − 1. *American Educational Research Journal, 7,* 625–626.

McCall, R. B. (1997). *Fundamental statistics for behavioral sciences* (7th ed.). Pacific Grove, CA: Brooks-Cole.

Munro, B. H., & Page, E. N. (1997). *Statistical methods for health-care research* (3rd ed.). Philadelphia: Lippincott-Raven

Polit, D. F. (1996). *Data analysis and statistics for nursing research.* Stamford, CT: Appleton & Lange.

Triola, M. (1998). *Elementary statistics* (7th ed.). Menlo Park, CA: Addison-Wesley.

Substantive References

Ahijevych, K., & Gillespie, J. (1997). Nicotine dependence and smoking topography among black and white women. *Research in Nursing & Health, 20,* 505–514.

Armstrong, M. L., & Murphy, K. P. (1997). Tattooing: Another adolescent risk behavior warranting health education. *Applied Nursing Research, 10,* 181–189.

Bernhard, L. A., & Sheppard, L. (1993). Health, symptoms, self-care, and dyadic adjustment in menopausal women. *Journal of Obstetric, Gynecologic, and Neonatal Nursing, 22,* 456–461.

Koniak-Griffin, D., & Brecht, M. L. (1995). Linkages between sexual risk-taking, substance use, and IDS knowledge among pregnant adolescents and young mothers. *Nursing Research, 44,* 341–345.

Redeker, N. S., Tamburri, L., & Howland, C. L. (1998). Prehospital correlates of sleep in patients hospitalized with cardiac disease. *Research in Nursing & Health, 21,* 27–37.

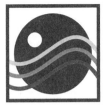

Inferential Statistics

Descriptive statistics are useful for summarizing empirical information, but usually the researcher wants to do more than simply describe data. **Inferential statistics,** which are based on the **laws of probability,** provide a means for drawing conclusions about a population, given the data obtained for the sample. Inferential statistics would help us with such questions as, "What do I know about the average 3-minute Apgar score of premature babies (the population) after having learned that a sample of 50 premature babies had a mean Apgar score of 7.5?" or "What can I conclude about the effectiveness of an intervention to promote breast self-examination among women older than 25 years of age (the population) after having found in a sample of 200 women that 50% of the experimental subjects but only 20% of the controls practiced breast self-examination 3 months later?" With the assistance of inferential statistics, researchers make judgments about or generalize to a large class of individuals based on information from a limited number of subjects.

With inferential statistics, the researcher estimates the parameters of a population from the sample statistics. These estimates are based on probability, and, as we shall see, probabilistic estimates involve a certain degree of error. The difference between estimates based on inferential statistics and estimates arrived at through the ordinary thinking process is that the statistical method provides a framework for making judgments in a systematic, objective fashion. Different researchers working with identical data would be likely to come to the same conclusion after applying inferential statistical procedures.

SAMPLING DISTRIBUTIONS

If a sample is to be used as a basis for making estimates of population characteristics, then it is clearly advisable to obtain as representative a sample as possible. As we saw in Chapter 12, random samples (i.e., probability samples) are the most effective means of securing representative samples. Inferential statistical procedures are based on the assumption of random sampling from populations—although this assumption is widely violated and ignored.

Even when random sampling is used, however, it cannot be expected that sample characteristics will be identical to population characteristics. Suppose we had a population of

10,000 freshmen nursing students who had taken the Scholastic Assessment Test (SAT). Let us say, for the sake of this example, that the mean SAT score for this population is 500 and the standard deviation (SD) is 100. Now, suppose that we do not know these parameters but that we must estimate them by using the scores from a random sample of 25 students. Should we expect to find a mean of exactly 500 and an SD of 100 for this sample? It would be extremely unlikely to obtain the exact population value. Let us say that instead we calculated a mean of 505. If a completely new sample were drawn and another mean computed, we might obtain a value such as 497. The tendency for the statistics to fluctuate from one sample to another is known as **sampling error**. The challenge for a researcher is to determine whether sample values are good estimates of population parameters.

A researcher works with only *one* sample on which statistics are computed and inferences made. However, to understand inferential statistics, we must perform a small mental exercise. With the population of 10,000 nursing students, consider drawing a sample of 25 individuals, calculating a mean, replacing the 25 students, and drawing a new sample. Consider each mean computed in this fashion as a separate piece of data. If we draw 5000 such samples, we will have 5000 means or data points, which could then be used to construct a frequency polygon, such as the one shown in Figure 19-1. This kind of frequency distribution has a special name: it is called a sampling distribution of the mean. A **sampling distribution** is a theoretical rather than actual distribution because one does not in practice draw consecutive samples from a population and plot their means. The concept of a theoretical distribution of sample values is basic to inferential statistics.

Characteristics of Sampling Distributions

When an infinite number of samples are drawn from an infinite population, the sampling distribution of the mean has certain known characteristics. Our example of a population of 10,000 students, and 5000 samples with 25 students each, deals with finite quantities, but the numbers are large enough to approximate these characteristics.

Statisticians have been able to demonstrate that sampling distributions of means are nor-

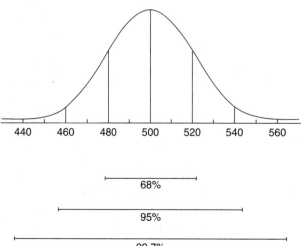

Figure 19-1. Sampling distribution

mally distributed. Furthermore, the mean of a sampling distribution consisting of an infinite number of sample means is always equal to the population mean. In the example shown in Figure 19-1, the mean of the sampling distribution is 500, the same value as the mean of the population.

In Chapter 18, we discussed the standard deviation in terms of percentages of cases falling within a certain distance from the mean. When data values are normally distributed, 68% of the cases fall between +1 SD and −1 SD from the mean. Because a sampling distribution of means is normally distributed, we can assert that 68 out of 100 randomly drawn sample means will lie within the range of values between +1 SD and −1 SD of the mean on the sampling distribution. Thus, if we knew or could estimate the value of the SD of the sampling distribution, we could then interpret the accuracy of any single sample mean.

Standard Error of the Mean

The standard deviation of a theoretical distribution of sample means is called the **standard error of the mean** (SEM). The word *error* signifies that the various means in the sampling distribution contain some error in their estimates of the population mean. The term *standard* indicates the magnitude of a standard, or average, error. The smaller the standard error—that is, the less variable the sample means—the more accurate are those means as estimates of the population value.

But how can we compute the standard deviation of a sampling distribution without actually constructing such a distribution? Fortunately, there is a formula for estimating the SEM from the data from a single sample. It has been shown that the value of the standard error (often symbolized as $s_{\bar{x}}$) has a systematic relationship to the standard deviation of the population and to the size of the samples drawn from it. The population standard deviation is estimated by the sample standard deviation to yield the following equation:

$$s_{\bar{x}} = \frac{SD}{\sqrt{N}}$$

Where SD = the standard deviation
         of the sample
    N = sample size
    $s_{\bar{x}}$ = standard error of the mean

If we use this formula to calculate the SEM in our current example for a sample SD of 100, we obtain

$$s_{\bar{x}} = \frac{100}{\sqrt{25}} = 20.0$$

The standard deviation of the sampling distribution is 20, as shown in Figure 19-1. This SEM statistic is an estimate of how much sampling error there is from one sample mean to another.

Given that a sampling distribution of means follows a normal curve, we can use these calculations to estimate the probability of drawing a sample with a certain mean. With a sample size of 25, the chances are about 95 out of 100 that any sample mean would fall between the values of 460 and 540. Only five times out of 100 would we draw a sample whose mean exceeded 540 or was less than 460. In other words, only five times out of 100 would we be likely to draw a sample whose mean deviates from the population mean by more than 40 points. Thus, by estimating the SEM, we can estimate the likely accuracy of our sample mean.

Because the value of the standard error of the mean is partly a function of sample size, we need only increase the sample size to increase the accuracy of our estimate of the population mean. Suppose that instead of using a sample of 25 nursing students to estimate the average SAT score, we used a sample of 100 students. With this many students, the SEM would be

$$s_{\bar{x}} = \frac{100}{\sqrt{100}} = 10.0$$

In such a situation, the probability of obtaining a sample mean greater than 520 or less than 480 would be about 5 in 100. The chances of drawing a sample with a mean very different from that of the population is reduced as the sample size increases because large numbers promote the likelihood that extreme cases will cancel each other out.

ESTIMATION OF PARAMETERS

Statistical inference consists of two major types of techniques: estimation of parameters and hypothesis testing. Of the two, hypothesis testing is more commonly encountered in research reports, but estimation plays an important role as well.

Estimation procedures are used to estimate a single population parameter, such as the mean value of some attribute. Suppose a new drug has been developed for people suffering from high blood pressure, and a researcher administers the drug to a sample of patients. The researcher could use estimation procedures to estimate the average blood pressure of a population of people with high blood pressure after administration of the drug. Estimation is the method used when no a priori prediction can be made about the attributes of a population, as might be the case for the effects of a new drug.

Estimation can take one of two forms: point estimation or interval estimation. **Point estimation** involves the calculation of a single statistic to estimate the population parameter. To continue with the SAT example, if we calculated the mean SAT score for a sample of 25 students and found that it was 510, then this number would represent the point estimate of the population mean.

The problem with point estimates is that they convey no information about accuracy. **Interval estimation** of a parameter is more useful because it indicates a range of values within which the parameter has a specified probability of lying. When researchers use interval estimation, they construct a **confidence interval** (sometimes abbreviated **CI**), and the upper and lower limits of the range of values are called **confidence limits**.

The construction of a confidence interval around a sample mean establishes a range of values for a population parameter and also establishes a certain probability of being correct. In other words, we make the estimation with a certain degree of confidence. Although the degree of confidence one wishes to attain is somewhat arbitrary, researchers conventionally use either a 95% or a 99% confidence interval.

The calculation of the confidence limits involves the use of the SEM and the principles associated with the normal distribution. As shown in Figure 19-1, 95% of the scores in a normal distribution lie within about 2 SDs (more precisely, 1.96 SDs) from the mean.

Returning to our example, let us say once again that the point estimation of the mean SAT score is 510, with an SD of 100. The SEM for a sample of 25 would be 20. We can now build a 95% confidence interval by using the following formula:

$$\text{Conf. } (\overline{X} \pm 1.96\ s_{\overline{x}}) = 95\%$$

That is, the confidence is 95% that the population mean lies between the values equal to 1.96 times the standard error, above and below the sample mean. In the example at hand, we would obtain the following:

Conf. $(510 \pm (1.96 \times 20.0)) = 95\%$
Conf. $(510 \pm (39.2)) \qquad = 95\%$
Conf. $(470.8 \leq \mu \leq 549.2) = 95\%$

The final statement may be read as follows: the confidence is 95% that the population mean (symbolized by the Greek letter mu [μ] by convention) is greater than or equal to 470.8 but less than or equal to 549.2. Another way to interpret the confidence interval concept is in terms of a probabilistic statement. One could say that in 100 samples with an N of 25, 95 out of 100 such confidence intervals would contain the parameter (the population mean).

The confidence interval reflects the degree of risk the researcher is willing to take of being wrong. With a 95% confidence interval, the researcher accepts the probability that she or he will be wrong five times out of 100. A 99% confidence interval sets the risk at only 1% by allowing a wider range of possible values. The formula is as follows:

$$\text{Conf. } (\overline{X} \pm 2.58 \ s_{\overline{x}}) = 99\%$$

The 2.58 reflects the fact that 99% of all cases in a normal distribution lie within ± 2.58 SD units from the mean. In the example, the 99% confidence interval would be:

$$\text{Conf. } (510 \pm (2.58 \times 20.0)) = 99\%$$
$$\text{Conf. } (510 \pm (51.6)) \qquad = 99\%$$
$$\text{Conf. } (458.4 \le \mu \le 561.6) \quad = 99\%$$

In 99 out of 100 samples with 25 subjects, the confidence interval so constructed would contain the population mean. One accepts a reduced risk of being wrong at the price of reduced specificity. In the case of the 95% interval, the range between the confidence limits was only about 80 points; here, the range of possible values is more than 100 points. The risk of error that one is willing to accept depends on the nature of the problem. In research that could affect the well-being of humans, it is not unusual to use stringent 99.9% confidence intervals, but for most research projects, a 95% confidence interval is sufficient.

HYPOTHESIS TESTING

Statistical hypothesis testing is essentially a process of decision making. Suppose a nurse researcher hypothesized that cancer patients' participation in a stress management program would result in lower anxiety. The sample consists of 25 patients in a control group who do not participate in the stress management program and 25 subjects in the experimental group who do. All 50 subjects are administered a self-report scale of anxiety. The researcher finds that the mean anxiety level for the experimental group is 15.8 and that for the control group is 17.5. Should the researcher conclude that the hypothesis has been supported? True, the group differences are in the predicted direction, but the results might simply be the result of sampling fluctuations. Statistical hypothesis testing allows researchers to make objective decisions concerning the results of their studies. Scientists need such a mechanism for helping them to decide which outcomes are likely to reflect only chance differences between sample groups and which are likely to reflect true population differences.

The Null Hypothesis

The procedures used in testing hypotheses are based on rules of negative inference. This logic often seems somewhat awkward and peculiar to beginning researchers, so we try to convey the concepts with a concrete illustration. In the stress management program example, a nurse researcher tested the effectiveness of a special program designed to reduce stress and anxiety in cancer patients. The researcher found that those participating in the program had lower mean anxiety scores than those not participating in the program. There are two possible explanations for this outcome: (1) the experimental treatment was successful in reducing patients' anxiety or (2) the differences resulted from chance factors (such as differences in the anxiety levels of the two groups even before any special treatment). The first explanation corresponds to the researcher's scientific hypothesis, but the second explanation corresponds to the null hypothesis. The **null hypothesis** is a statement that there is no actual relationship between variables and that any such observed relationship is only a function of chance, or sampling fluctuations. The need for a null hypothesis lies in the fact that statistical hypothesis testing is basically a process of rejection. It is impossible to demonstrate directly and conclusively that the first explanation—the scientific hypothesis—is correct. However, it is possible to show that the null hypothesis has a high probability of being incorrect, and such evidence lends support to the scientific hypothesis. The rejection of the null hypothesis, then, is what the researcher seeks to accomplish through **statistical tests**.

The null hypothesis is sometimes stated as a formal proposition, using the following symbols:

$$H_0: \mu_A = \mu_B$$

The null hypothesis (H_0) asserts that the population mean for method A (μ_A) is the same as the population mean for method B (μ_B) with regard to, in this case, anxiety scores. The **alternative**, or research, **hypothesis** may also be stated in similar terms:

$$H_A: \mu_A \neq \mu_B$$

Although null hypotheses are accepted or rejected on the basis of data from a sample, the hypothesis is made about population values. The real interest in testing hypotheses, as in all statistical inference, is to use samples to draw conclusions about relationships within the population.

Type I and Type II Errors

The researcher's decision about whether to accept or reject the null hypothesis is based on a consideration of how probable it is that observed differences are the result of chance alone.

Because information concerning the entire population is unavailable, it is not possible to assert flatly that the null hypothesis is or is not true. The researcher must be content with the knowledge that the hypothesis is either probably true or probably false. We make statistical inferences based on incomplete information, so there is always a risk of error.

A researcher can make two types of errors: the rejection of a true null hypothesis or the acceptance of a false null hypothesis. The possible outcomes of a researcher's decision are summarized in Figure 19-2. An investigator makes a **Type I error** by rejecting the null hypothesis when it is, in fact, true. For instance, if we concluded that the experimental treatment was more effective than the control treatment in alleviating patients' anxiety, when in actuality the observed sample differences in anxiety scores resulted only from sampling fluctuations, then we would have made a Type I error. In the reverse situation, if we concluded that the differences in group anxiety levels were the result of chance, when in fact the experimental treatment *did* have an effect on anxiety, we would be committing a **Type II error** by accepting a false null hypothesis.

Level of Significance

The researcher does not know when an error in statistical decision making has been commit-

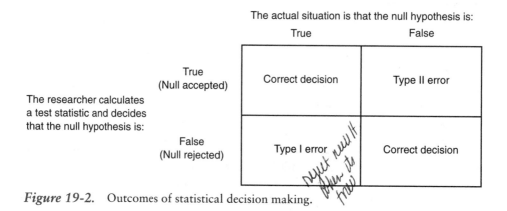

Figure 19-2. Outcomes of statistical decision making.

ted. The truth or falseness of a null hypothesis could only be definitively ascertained by collecting information from the entire population, in which case there would be no need for statistical inference. However, the researcher can directly establish the risk of a Type I error. **Level of significance** is the phrase used to signify the probability of committing a Type I error, and the probability is set by the investigator.

The two most frequently used levels of significance (often referred to as α, or alpha) are .05 and .01. If we say we are using a .05 significance level, this means that we are accepting the risk that out of 100 samples drawn from a population, a true null hypothesis would be rejected five times and accepted 95 times. With a .01 significance level, the risk of a Type I error is *lower*: in only 1 sample out of 100 would we erroneously reject the null hypothesis. By convention, the minimum acceptable level for α generally is .05. A stricter level may be desirable for statistical tests when the decision has important consequences.

Naturally, researchers would like to reduce the risk of committing both types of error. Unfortunately, lowering the risk of committing a Type I error increases the risk of a Type II error. The stricter the criterion we use for rejecting a null hypothesis, the greater the probability that we will accept a false null hypothesis. There is a kind of tradeoff that the researcher must consider in establishing criteria for statistical decision making. Procedures for addressing Type II errors are discussed later in this chapter.

Critical Regions

By designating a significance level, a researcher is establishing a decision rule. The decision is to reject the null hypothesis if the statistic being tested falls at or beyond a **critical region** on the applicable theoretical distribution, and to accept the null hypothesis otherwise. The critical region, which is defined by the significance level, indicates whether a result is improbable for a null hypothesis.

A simple example should help to clarify the statistical decision-making process. Suppose we were interested in determining the importance of religion among patients with AIDS. To address this issue, we ask a sample of 100 AIDS patients to rate the importance of religion to them on a scale that ranges from 0 (completely unimportant) to 10 (completely important). The goal is to determine whether the mean rating for the population of AIDS patients is different from 5.0, the score on the rating scale that represents neutrality. The null hypothesis is H_0: $\mu = 5.0$, and the alternate hypothesis is H_A: $\mu \neq 5.0$.

Now suppose that the data from the sample of 100 AIDS patients result in a mean rating of 5.50 with an SD of 2.0. This mean is consistent with the alternative hypothesis indicating that religion is not neutral to the average AIDS patient, but can we automatically reject the null hypothesis? Because of sampling error, we need to test for the possibility that the mean of 5.5 occurred simply because of a chance fluctuation and not because the population generally views religion as somewhat important to them.

In hypothesis testing, one assumes that the null hypothesis is true and then gathers evidence to disprove it. Thus, in this example, we need to construct a sampling distribution that assumes that the population mean is 5.0. Now we need to estimate the standard deviation of the sampling distribution (i.e., the SEM) by dividing the actual SD by the square root of the sample size. In this example, the SEM is 0.2 ($s_{\bar{x}} = 2.0 \div \sqrt{100}$).

The resulting sampling distribution is shown in Figure 19-3. Based on our knowledge of normal distribution characteristics, we can determine probable and improbable values of sample means drawn from the AIDS patient population. If, as is assumed, the population mean is actually 5.0, then 95% of all sample means would fall roughly between 4.6 and 5.4—that is, about 2 SDs above and below the mean. Thus, the obtained sample mean of 5.5 is improbable, if we use as our criterion of

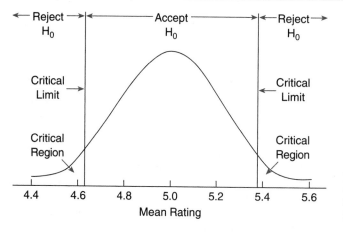

Figure 19-3. Critical regions in the sampling distribution for AIDS patients example.

improbability a significance level of .05. We would reject, therefore, the null hypothesis that the population mean equals 5.0. We would not be justified in saying that we have *proved* the alternative hypothesis because there is a 5% possibility of having made a Type I error. But we can *accept* the alternative hypothesis that AIDS patients are not, on average, neutral in the importance they attach to religion.

Statistical Tests

In practice, researchers do not construct a sampling distribution and calculate the critical regions on the distribution. Rather, the data collected for the study are used to compute a **test statistic**, using an appropriate formula. For every test statistic, there is a related theoretical distribution. The researcher can compare the value of the computed test statistic to values in a table that specify the **critical limits** for the applicable distribution.

When researchers calculate a test statistic that is beyond a tabled value, the results can be described as being **statistically significant**. This terminology has a precise meaning. The word *significant* should not be given the familiar interpretation of *important* or *meaningful* or *clinically relevant*. In statistics, significant means that the obtained results are unlikely to have been the result of chance, at some speci-

fied level of probability. A **nonsignificant result** means that any difference between an obtained statistic and a hypothesized parameter could have been the result of a chance fluctuation in the sample.

The remainder of this section provides an overview of different types of statistical tests.

ONE-TAILED AND TWO-TAILED TESTS

In most hypothesis-testing situations, researchers apply what are known as **two-tailed tests**. This means that both ends, or tails, of the sampling distribution are used to determine the range of improbable values. In Figure 19-3, for example, the critical region that contains 5% of the area of the sampling distribution really involves 2.5% at one end of the distribution and 2.5% at the other. If the level of significance were .01, then the critical regions would involve .5% of the distribution at both tails.

When the researcher has a strong basis for using a directional hypothesis (see Chapter 3), it may be justifiable to use what is referred to as a **one-tailed test**. For example, if a nurse researcher instituted an outreach program to improve the prenatal practices of low-income rural women, then it might be hypothesized that women in the experimental program would not just be *different* from control women not exposed to the intervention (in terms of outcomes such as pregnancy complications, infant birth-weight, and so on); one would expect the experimental subjects to have an *advantage*. It might make little sense to use the tail of the distribution that would signify *worse* outcomes among the experimental than the control mothers. In a one-tailed test, the critical region of improbable values is entirely in one tail of the distribution—the tail corresponding to the direction of the hypothesis, as illustrated in Figure 19-4. When a one-tailed test is used, the critical area of .05 covers a bigger region of the specified tail, and for this reason, one-tailed tests are less conservative. This means that it is easier to reject the null hypothesis with a one-tailed test than with a two-tailed test.

The use of one-tailed tests has been the subject of considerable controversy. Most researchers follow the convention of using a two-tailed test, even if they have stated a directional hypothesis. In reading research reports, one can assume that a two-tailed test has been used, unless the investigator specifically mentions a one-tailed test. However, when there is a strong logical or theoretical reason for using a directional hypothesis and for assuming that findings opposite to the direction hypothesized are virtually impossible, a one-tailed test may be warranted.

In the remainder of this chapter, the examples use two-tailed tests. If a computer is used to perform statistical analyses, then two-tailed hypothesis testing is almost always assumed.

PARAMETRIC AND NONPARAMETRIC TESTS

A distinction is often made between two classes of statistical tests. The bulk of the tests that we consider in this chapter—and also most tests used by researchers—are called parametric tests. **Parametric tests** are characterized by three attributes: (1) they involve the estimation of at least one parameter; (2) they require measurements on at least an interval scale; and (3) they involve several underlying assumptions about the variables under consideration, such as the assumption that the variables are normally distributed in the population.

Nonparametric tests, by contrast, are not based on the estimation of parameters. They are usually applied when the data have been measured on a nominal or ordinal scale. Nonparametric methods also involve less restrictive assumptions concerning the shape of the distribution of the critical variables than do parametric tests. For this reason, nonparametric tests are sometimes called **distribution-free statistics.**

Statisticians disagree about the utility and virtues of nonparametric tests. Purists insist that if the strict requirements of parametric tests are not met, then parametric procedures

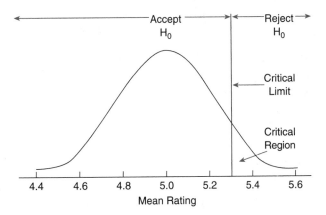

Figure 19-4. Critical region for a one-tailed test: AIDS patients example.

are inappropriate. Many statistical research studies have shown, however, that the violation of the assumptions for parametric tests usually fails to affect statistical decision making or the number of errors made. The more moderate position in this debate, and the one that we think is reasonable, is that nonparametric tests are most useful when the data under consideration cannot in any manner be construed as interval-level measures or when the distribution of data is markedly nonnormal. Parametric tests are usually more powerful and offer more flexibility than nonparametric tests and are, for these reasons, generally preferred.

BETWEEN-SUBJECTS TESTS AND WITHIN-SUBJECTS TESTS

Another distinction in statistical tests concerns the nature of the comparisons being made. Hypothesis testing involves making some type of comparison. When the comparison involves different people (e.g., men versus women), the research design is a between-subjects design, and the statistical test must be a **between-subjects test** (sometimes referred to as a **test for independent groups**).

There are research designs, however, that involve using a single group of subjects. For example, if a researcher used a repeated measures design, the same subjects would be exposed to two or more different experimental treatments. In this situation, the comparisons across treatments are not independent because the same subjects are used in all conditions. The appropriate statistical tests for such designs are **within-subjects tests** (sometimes referred to as **tests for dependent groups**).

Most research situations call for between-subjects tests, but both types are described in this chapter.

Overview of Hypothesis-Testing Procedures

In the pages that follow, various types of statistical procedures for testing research hypotheses

are examined. The discussion emphasizes the applications of statistical tests rather than actual computations. One computational example is worked out to illustrate that numbers are not just pulled out of a hat. However, computers have virtually eliminated the need for manual calculations, and so computational examples have been minimized. Those of you who will be performing statistical analyses are urged to pursue other references for a fuller appreciation of statistical methods. In this basic text on research methods, our primary concern is to alert researchers to the potential use (or misuse) of statistical tests for different purposes.

Although each of the statistical tests described in the remaining sections of this chapter has a particular application and can be used only with particular kinds of data, the overall process of testing hypotheses is basically the same. The seven steps are essentially as follows:

1. *Determine the test statistic to be used.* The researcher must select an appropriate statistical test, based on a number of factors (e.g., whether a parametric test is justified, whether the design is between- or within-subjects, and so on). Table 19-10, presented later in this chapter, offers assistance in selecting the appropriate test.

2. *Establish the level of significance.* The researcher must establish the criterion for the decision rule (whether to accept or reject the null hypothesis) *before* the analyses are undertaken. An α level of .05 will usually be acceptable. If a more stringent test is required, then α may be set at .01 or .001.

3. *Select a one-tailed or two-tailed test.* In most cases, a two-tailed test should be used, but if the researcher has a firm basis for hypothesizing not only a difference or a relationship but also the *nature* of that difference or relationship, then a one-tailed test may be warranted.

4. *Compute a test statistic.* Using the values from the collected data, calculate a test

statistic using the appropriate computational formulas. Or, alternatively, have the computer calculate the statistic using a program designed for this purpose.

5. *Calculate the degrees of freedom* (symbolized as *df*). **Degrees of freedom** is a concept used throughout hypothesis testing to refer to the number of observations free to vary about a parameter. The concept is too complex for full elaboration here, but fortunately the computation is extremely easy. (The formulas for the *df* vary from one test statistic to another).

6. *Obtain a tabled value for the statistical test.* Theoretical distributions have been developed for all test statistics. These theoretical distributions enable the researcher to discover whether obtained values of the test statistic are beyond the range of what is probable if the null hypothesis is true. That is, at some probability level specified by the researcher, the obtained value of the test statistic reflects a true relationship between variables (or a reliable estimate of a hypothesized population parameter) and not just a relationship or value that occurred in the sample by chance. The researcher examines a table appropriate for the test statistic and then obtains the critical value by entering the table at a point corresponding to the relevant degrees of freedom and level of significance.

7. *Compare the test statistic to the tabled value.* In the final step, the researcher compares the value found in the table with the computed value of the statistic. If the absolute value of the test statistic is *larger* than the tabled value, then the results are statistically significant. If the computed value is *smaller,* then the results are nonsignificant.

When a computer program is used to analyze the data, the researcher really only needs to follow the first two steps and then make the necessary commands to the computer. The computer will calculate the test statistic, the degrees of freedom, and the *actual* probability that the relationship being tested results from chance. For example, the computer may print that the probability (*p*) of an experimental group doing better on a measure of postoperative recovery than the control group on the basis of chance alone is .025. This means that fewer than 3 times out of 100 (or only 25 times out of 1000) would a difference between the two groups as large as the one obtained reflect haphazard sampling differences rather than differences resulting from an experimental intervention. This computed probability level can then be compared with the investigator's desired level of significance. If the significance level desired were .05, then the results would be said to be significant, because .025 is more stringent than .05. If .01 were the significance level, then the results would be nonsignificant (sometimes abbreviated *NS*). Any computed probability level greater than .05 (e.g., .20) indicates a nonsignificant relationship—that is, one that could have occurred on the basis of chance alone in more than 5 out of 100 samples.

In the sections that follow, a number of specific statistical tests and their applications are described. Examples of hypothesis tests using computerized computations are provided at the end of the chapter.

TESTING DIFFERENCES BETWEEN TWO GROUP MEANS

A common research situation is the comparison of two groups of subjects with respect to mean values on a dependent variable. For instance, we might wish to compare an experimental and control group of patients on a physiologic measure such as heart rate or blood pressure. Or, perhaps we would be interested in contrasting the average number of school days missed owing to illness among children who had been born preterm versus full-term. This section describes methods for testing the statistical significance of differences between two group means.

The basic parametric procedure for testing differences in group means is the *t*-test (sometimes referred to as **Student's *t***). The *t*-test can be used both in situations in which there are two independent groups (such as an experimental and control group, or male versus female subjects) and in situations in which the sample is paired or dependent (as when a single group yields pretreatment and posttreatment scores). Procedures for handling independent groups are described below to illustrate the computation of the *t*-statistic.

t-Tests for Independent Groups

Suppose that a researcher wanted to test the effect of early discharge of maternity patients on their perceived maternal competence. The researcher administers a scale of perceived maternal competence 1 week after delivery to 10 primiparas who were discharged early (i.e., within 24 hours of delivery) and to 10 primiparas who remained in the hospital for longer periods. The researcher finds that the mean scale scores for these two groups are 19 and 25, respectively. The question is, are these differences real (i.e., are they likely to be replicated in other samples of early-discharge and later-discharge mothers?), or are the group differences the result of chance fluctuations? The hypotheses being tested are

$$H_0: \mu_A = \mu_B \qquad H_A: \mu_A \neq \mu_B$$

To test these hypotheses, a *t*-statistic is computed. With independent samples such as in the current example, the formula is

$$t = \frac{\overline{X}_A - \overline{X}_B}{\sqrt{\dfrac{\Sigma_{x_A^2} + \Sigma_{x_B^2}}{n_A + n_B - 2}\left(\dfrac{1}{n_A} + \dfrac{1}{n_B}\right)}}$$

This formula looks rather complex and intimidating, but it boils down to simple components that can be calculated with elementary

arithmetic. Let us work through one example with data shown in Table 19-1.

The first column of numbers presents the scores of the regular-discharge group (group A), whose mean score of 25.0 is shown at the bottom of column 1. In column 4, similar scores are shown for the early-discharge group, whose mean is 19.0. The 20 scores shown in this table vary from one person to another. Some of the variability simply reflects individual differences in perceived maternal competence. Some may also be due to measurement error (i.e., the unreliability of the scale), whereas some may be the result of the subjects' moods on that particular day, and so forth. The research question is: "Can a significant portion of the 6-point mean group difference be attributed to the independent variable—time of discharge from the hospital?" The calculation of the *t*-statistic allows the researcher to answer this question in an objective fashion.

After calculating mean group scores, deviation scores are obtained for each subject, as shown in columns 2 and 5: 25.0 is subtracted from each score in group A, and 19.0 is subtracted from each score in group B. Then, each deviation score is squared (columns 3 and 6), and the squared deviation scores are added. We now have all the components for the formula presented above, as follows:

$$\overline{X}_A = 25.0 \text{ mean of group A}$$
$$\overline{X}_B = 19.0 \text{ mean of group B}$$
$$\Sigma_{x_A^2} = 242 \text{ sum of group A squared deviation scores}$$
$$\Sigma_{x_B^2} = 154 \text{ sum of group B squared deviation scores}$$
$$n_A = 10 \text{ number of subjects in group A}$$
$$n_B = 10 \text{ number of subjects in group B}$$

When these numbers are used in the *t*-equation, the value of the *t*-statistic is computed to be 2.86, as shown in Table 19-1.

To ascertain whether this *t*-value is statistically significant, we need to consult a table that specifies the probability points associated with different *t*-values for the theoretical *t*-distributions. To make use of such a

TABLE 19-1 Computation of the *t*-Statistic for Independent Samples

GROUP A (REGULAR-DISCHARGE GROUP)			GROUP B (EARLY-DISCHARGE GROUP)			
(1)	(2)	(3)	(4)	(5)	(6)	
X_A	x_A	x^2_A	X_B	x_B	x^2_B	
30	5	25	23	4	16	$t = \dfrac{25 - 19}{\sqrt{\dfrac{242 + 154}{(10 + 10 - 20)}\left(\dfrac{1}{10} + \dfrac{1}{10}\right)}} =$
27	2	4	17	-2	4	
25	0	0	22	3	9	
20	-5	25	18	-1	1	
24	-1	1	20	1	1	$t = \dfrac{6}{\sqrt{(22)(.2)}} =$
32	7	49	26	7	49	
17	-8	64	16	-3	9	
18	-7	49	13	-6	36	$t = \dfrac{6}{\sqrt{4.4}} =$
28	3	9	21	2	4	
29	4	16	14	-5	25	
$\Sigma X_A = 250$ $\overline{X}_A = 25.0$		$\Sigma x^2_A = 242$	$\Sigma X_B = 190$ $\overline{X}_B = 19.0$		$\Sigma x^2_B = 154$	$t = \dfrac{6}{2.1} = 2.86$

table, the researcher must have two pieces of information: (1) the α level sought, that is, the degree of risk of making a Type I error that one is willing to accept; and (2) the number of degrees of freedom available. For a *t*-test with independent samples, the formula for degrees of freedom is

$$df = n_A + n_B - 2$$

That is, the *df* is equal to the number of subjects in the two groups, minus 2. Thus, in the present example, the *df* is equal to 18 [(10 + 10) − 2].

A table of *t*-values is presented in Table B-1, Appendix B. The left-hand column lists various degrees of freedom, and the top row specifies different α values. If we use as our decision-making criterion a two-tailed probability (*p*) level of .05, we find that with 18 *df*, the tabled value of *t* is 2.10. This value is the upper limit to what is probable, if the null hypothesis were true; values in excess of 2.10 would be considered improbable. Thus, our

calculated *t* of 2.86* is improbable, that is, statistically significant. We are now in a position to say that the primiparas discharged early had significantly lower perceptions of maternal competence than those who were not discharged early. The probability that the mean difference of 6 points was the result of chance factors and not early discharge is less than 5 in 100 (*p* < .05). The null hypothesis is rejected, therefore, and the alternative hypothesis is accepted.

Paired *t*-Tests

In some studies, the researcher obtains two measures from the same subjects, or measures from paired sets of subjects (such as two siblings). Whenever two sets of scores on the dependent variable are not independent, then the

---

*The tabled *t*-value should be compared with the absolute value of the calculated *t*. Thus, if the calculated *t*-value had been −2.86, then the results would still be significant.

researcher must use a **paired *t*-test**—a *t*-test for dependent groups.

Suppose that we were interested in studying the effect of a special diet on the cholesterol level of adult men older than age 60 years. A sample of 50 men is randomly selected to participate in the study. The cholesterol levels are measured before the start of the investigation and measured again after 2 months on the special diet. The central concern here is the average difference in cholesterol values before and after the treatment. The hypotheses being submitted to a statistical test are

$$H_0: \mu_X = \mu_Y \qquad H_A: \mu_X \neq \mu_Y$$

where X = pretreatment cholesterol levels
Y = posttreatment cholesterol levels

As in the previous example, a *t*-statistic would be computed from the pretest and posttest measures (using, however, a different formula).* The obtained *t* would be compared with the *t*-values in Table B-1, Appendix B. For this particular type of *t*-test, the degrees of freedom equals the number of paired observations minus one ($df = N - 1$).

Other Two-Group Tests

In certain two-group situations, the *t*-statistic may be inappropriate. If the dependent variable is on an ordinal scale, or if the distribution is markedly nonnormal, then a nonpara-

---

*The paired *t*-statistic is computed according to the following formula:

$$t = \frac{D_{X-Y}}{\sqrt{\dfrac{\Sigma d^2}{N(N-1)}}}$$

where D_{x-y} = the difference between two paired scores
$\bar{D}_{x-y}$ = the mean difference between the paired scores
d = the deviation scores for the difference measure
Σd^2 = the sum of the squared deviation scores
n = number of pairs

metric test may be preferred. We mention a few such tests here without actually working out examples.

The **median test** involves the comparison of two independent groups on the basis of deviations from the median rather than the mean. In the median test, the scores for both samples are combined and the overall median calculated. Then, the number of cases above and below this median is counted separately for each sample, resulting in a 2 × 2 contingency table; (above/below median) × (group A/group B). From such a contingency table, a chi-square statistic (described in a subsequent section) can be computed to test the null hypothesis that the medians are the same for the two populations.

The **Mann-Whitney *U* test** is another nonparametric procedure for testing the difference between two independent samples when the dependent variable is measured on an ordinal scale. The test is based on the assignment of ranks to the two groups of measures. The sum of the ranks for the two groups can be compared by calculating the *U* statistic. The Mann-Whitney *U* test tends to throw away less information than a median test and, therefore, is more powerful.

When ordinal-level data are paired rather than independent, either the sign test or the Wilcoxon signed-rank test can be used. The **sign test** is an extremely simple procedure, involving the assignment of a "+" or "−" to the differences between a pair of scores, depending on whether X is larger than Y, or vice versa. The **Wilcoxon signed-rank test** involves taking the difference between paired scores and ranking the absolute difference.

Compared with *t*-tests, all these nonparametric tests are computationally easy. Because they are generally less powerful, however, the ease of computation should not be used as the basis for choosing which statistic is most appropriate, especially if a computer is being used to analyze the data.

TESTING DIFFERENCES BETWEEN THREE OR MORE GROUP MEANS

The procedure known as **analysis of variance** (**ANOVA**) is another commonly used statistical test. Like the *t*-test, ANOVA is a parametric procedure used to test the significance of differences between means. However, ANOVA is not restricted to two-group situations: The means of three or more groups can be compared with ANOVA.

The statistic computed in an ANOVA is the **F-ratio** statistic. ANOVA decomposes the total variability of a set of data into two components: (1) the variability resulting from the independent variable and (2) all other variability, such as individual differences, measurement unreliability, and so on. Variation *between* treatment groups is contrasted with variation *within* groups to yield an *F*-ratio. If the differences between groups receiving different treatments is large relative to fluctuations within groups, then it is possible to establish the probability that the treatment is related to, or has resulted in, the group differences.

One-Way Analysis of Variance

Suppose that we were interested in comparing the effectiveness of different interventions to help individuals stop smoking. One group of smokers will undergo behavior modification therapy, which is based on reinforcement theory (group A). A second group will be treated by hypnosis (group B). A third group will serve as a control and will receive no special treatment (group C). The dependent variable in this experiment will be cigarette consumption during the week following the intervention. Thirty smokers who wish to stop smoking are randomly assigned to one of the three conditions. The ANOVA will permit a test of the following hypotheses:

$$H_0: \mu_A = \mu_B = \mu_C \qquad H_A: \mu_A \neq \mu_B \neq \mu_C$$

The null hypothesis asserts that the population means for posttreatment cigarette smoking will be the same for all three groups, and the alternative (research) hypothesis predicts inequality of means. Table 19-2 presents some hypothetical data for such a study.

For each of the three groups, the raw score for each subject and the mean group score are shown. The mean numbers of posttreatment cigarettes consumed are 20, 25, and 33 for groups A, B, and C, respectively. These means are different, but are they significantly different—or are the differences attributable to random fluctuations?

The underlying concepts and terms for a one-way ANOVA are briefly explained without working out the computations for this example. Again, the reader is urged to consult a statistics text for formulas and more detailed explanations. In calculating an *F*-statistic, the total variability in the data is broken down into two sources. The portion of the variance resulting from group membership (i.e., from

TABLE 19-2	Fictitious Data for a One-Way ANOVA	
GROUP A	**GROUP B**	**GROUP C**
28	22	33
0	31	44
17	26	29
20	30	40
35	34	33
19	37	25
24	0	22
0	19	43
41	24	29
16	27	32
$\Sigma X_A = 200$	$\Sigma X_B = 250$	$\Sigma X_C = 330$
$\overline{X}_A = 20.0$	$\overline{X}_B = 25.0$	$\overline{X}_C = 33.0$

exposure to different treatments) is determined by calculating a component known as the **sum of squares between groups**, or SS_B. This SS_B represents the sum of squared deviations of the individual group means from the overall mean for all subjects (often referred to as the **grand mean**). The SS_B term reflects the variability in individual scores attributable to group membership.

The second component is the **sum of squares within groups**, or SS_W. This is an index of the sum of the squared deviations of each individual score from its own group mean. The SS_W term indicates variability attributable to individual differences, measurement error, and so on.

Recall from Chapter 18 that the formula for calculating a variance is $Var = \Sigma x^2 \div N - 1$. The two sums of squares described above are analogous to the numerator of this equation. The sums of squares represent sums of squared deviations from means. Therefore, to compute the variance within and the variance between groups, we must divide by a quantity analogous to $(N - 1)$. This quantity is the degrees of freedom associated with each sum of squares. For between groups, $df = G - 1$, which is the number of groups minus one. For within groups, $df = (n_A - 1) + (n_B - 1) + \ldots (n_G - 1)$. That is, degrees of freedom within is found by adding together the number of subjects less 1 for each group.

In an ANOVA context, the variance is conventionally referred to as the **mean square** (MS). The formulas for the mean square between groups and the mean square within groups are

$$MS_B = \frac{SS_B}{df_B} \qquad MS_W = \frac{SS_W}{df_W}$$

The *F*-ratio is the ratio of these mean squares, or

$$F = \frac{MS_B}{MS_W}$$

All these computations for the data in Table 19-2 are presented in the ANOVA summary table shown in Table 19-3. As this table shows, the calculated *F*-statistic for our fictitious example is 3.84.

The last step is to compare the obtained *F*-statistic with the value from a theoretical *F*-distribution. Table B-2, Appendix B, contains the upper limits of probable values for distributions with varying degrees of freedom. The first part of the table lists these values for a significance level of .05, and the second and third parts list those for .01 and .001 significance levels. Let us say that, for the current example, we have chosen the .05 probability level. To enter the table, we find the column headed by our between-groups *df* (2), and go down this column until we reach the row corresponding to the within-groups *df* (27). The tabled value of *F* with 2 and 27 *df* is 3.35. Because our obtained *F*-value of 3.84 exceeds

SOURCE OF VARIANCE	SS	df	MEAN SQUARE	F	p
Between groups	860.0	2	430.00	3.84	<.05
Within groups	3,022.0	27	111.93		
TOTAL	3,882.0	29			

TABLE 19-3   ANOVA Summary Table

3.35, we reject the null hypothesis that the population means are equal. The differences in the number of cigarettes smoked after treatment are beyond chance expectations. In fewer than 5 samples out of 100 would differences of this magnitude be obtained by chance alone. The data support the hypothesis that the interventions affected cigarette-smoking behaviors.

The ANOVA procedure does not allow us to say that each group differed significantly from all other groups. We cannot tell from these results if treatment A was significantly more effective than treatment B. Some researchers incorrectly use *t*-tests to compare the different pairs of means (A versus B, A versus C, B versus C) when this type of information is required. Methods known as **multiple comparison procedures** should be used in such situations. The function of these procedures is to isolate the differences between group means that are responsible for the rejection of the ANOVA null hypothesis. Multiple comparison methods are described in most intermediate statistical textbooks, such as that by Polit (1996).

Multifactor Analysis of Variance

The type of problem described previously is known as a **one-way ANOVA** because it deals with the effect of one independent variable (the different interventions) on a dependent variable. Chapter 3 pointed out that hypotheses are sometimes complex and make predictions about the effect of two or more independent variables on a dependent variable. The analysis of data from such studies is often performed by means of a **multifactor ANOVA**. In this section, we describe some of the principles underlying a two-way ANOVA. The actual computations, however, are not worked out here.

Suppose that we were interested in determining whether the two smoking cessation treatments were equally effective in helping men and women stop smoking, with no control group in the study. We could design an experiment using a randomized block design, with four groups: Women and men would be randomly assigned, separately, to the two treatment conditions. After the experimental period, each subject would be required to report the number of cigarettes smoked. Some fictitious data for this problem are shown in Table 19-4.

With two independent variables, there are several hypotheses to be tested. First, we are testing whether, for both genders, behavior modification is more effective than hypnosis as a means of reducing smoking, or vice versa. Second, we are testing whether smoking behavior after an intervention is different for men and women, irrespective of the type of treatment. Third, we are examining the differential effect of the two treatments on men and women. This last hypothesis is the **interaction hypothesis**. Interaction is concerned with whether the effect of one independent variable is consistent for every level of a second independent variable. In other words, do the two interventions have the same effect on both genders?

The data in Table 19-4 reveal that, overall, subjects in treatment 1 smoked less than those in treatment 2 (19.0 versus 25.0); that women smoked less than men (21.0 versus 23.0); and that men smoked less when exposed to treatment 1, but women smoked less when exposed to treatment 2. By performing a two-way ANOVA on these data, it would be possible to ascertain the statistical significance of these differences.

Multifactor ANOVA is an extremely important analytic technique. Human behaviors, conditions, and feelings are complex, and the ability to examine the combined effects of two or more independent variables permits this complexity to be incorporated into research designs. Multifactor ANOVA is not restricted to two-way schemes. Theoretically, any number of independent variables is possible, although in practice, studies with more than three or four factors are rare because of the

TABLE 19-4   Fictitious Data for a Two-Way (2 × 2) ANOVA

FACTOR B—GENDER	FACTOR A—TREATMENT			
	Behavior Modification (1)		Hypnosis (2)	
Female (1)	24 28 22 19 27 25 18 21 0 36	Group 1 $\overline{X} = 22.0$	27 0 45 19 22 23 18 20 12 14	Group 2 $\overline{X} = 20.0$	Females $\overline{X}_{B1} = 21.0$
Male (2)	10 21 17 0 33 16 18 13 15 17	Group 3 $\overline{X} = 16.0$	36 31 28 32 25 22 19 30 35 42	Group 4 $\overline{X} = 30.0$	Males $\overline{X}_{B2} = 23.0$
	Treatment 1 $\overline{X}_{A1} = 19$		Treatment 2 $\overline{X}_{A2} = 25$	$\overline{X}_T = 22$

large number of subjects required and the complexity of the design.

Repeated-Measures Analysis of Variance

Repeated-measures ANOVA (sometimes referred to as **within-subjects ANOVA**) is used in several circumstances. First, it is used when there are three or more measures of the same dependent variable for each subject. As discussed in Chapter 8, a repeated-measures experimental design is sometimes used to expose subjects to two or more treatment conditions, with subjects essentially acting as their own controls. When there are only two such conditions—that is, when subjects are exposed to

both treatment A and treatment B, with order of exposure determined at random—then a paired *t*-test can be used. However, when there are three or more treatment conditions, a repeated-measures ANOVA is required.

Second, repeated-measures ANOVA is used when multiple measures of the same dependent variable are collected longitudinally at several points in time. For instance, in some studies, physiologic measures such as blood pressure or heart rate might be collected before, during, and after a certain medical procedure.

In many applications of repeated-measures ANOVA, there are two or more groups, with two or more measures of the dependent variable collected for each subject. For example, suppose we collected heart rate data before (T1), during (T2), and after (T3) surgery for subjects randomly assigned to an experimental and a control group. Structurally, the ANOVA for analyzing these data would look similar to a multifactor ANOVA, although the calculations would differ. An *F*-statistic would be computed to test for differences in the treatment factor (experimental subjects versus controls), known as the **between-subjects effect**. This statistic would indicate whether, across all time periods, the mean heart rate differed for experimental subjects and controls. Another *F*-statistic would be computed to test for differences across time (T1, T2, T3), known as the **within-subjects effect**. This statistic would indicate whether, across both treatment groups, the mean heart rates differed before, during, and after surgery. Finally, an interaction effect would be tested to determine whether there was a differential treatment effect at different points in time. Given the many situations in which nurse researchers collect data from subjects at multiple time points, repeated-measures ANOVA represents an important analytic tool.

Nonparametric "Analysis of Variance"

Nonparametric tests do not, strictly speaking, analyze variance. There are, however, nonparametric procedures analogous to the parametric ANOVA for use with ordinal-level data or when a markedly nonnormal distribution renders parametric tests inadvisable. When the number of groups is greater than two and a one-way test for independent samples is desired, one may use a statistic developed by statisticians Kruskal and Wallis. The **Kruskal-Wallis test** is a generalized version of the Mann-Whitney *U* test, based on the assignment of ranks to the scores from the various groups. When the researcher is working with paired groups, or when several measures are obtained from a single sample, then the **Friedman test** for "analysis of variance" by ranks may be applied. These tests are described in Polit (1996).

TESTING DIFFERENCES IN PROPORTIONS

The tests we have examined thus far all involve dependent variables measured on an interval or ratio scale, when mean differences between groups are being compared. In this section, we examine procedures for testing group differences when the dependent variable is measured on a nominal scale.

The Chi-Square Test

The **chi-square test** is used when we have categories of data and hypotheses concerning the proportions of cases that fall into the various categories. In Chapter 18, we discussed the construction of contingency tables to describe the frequencies of cases falling in different classes. The chi-square (χ^2) statistic is computed from contingency tables to test the significance of different proportions.

Consider the following example. A researcher is interested in studying the effect of planned nursing instruction on patients' compliance with a self-medication regimen. An experimental group of 100 patients is instructed by nurses who are implementing the new instructional approach. A control group of 100 patients is cared for by nurses who continue their usual mode of instruction. The hypothesis being tested is that a higher proportion of subjects in the experimental group will report self-medication compliance than will subjects in the control group.

The chi-square statistic is computed by comparing two sets of frequencies: observed frequencies (i.e., those observed in the data) and expected frequencies. **Observed frequencies** for the example are shown in Table 19-5. As this table shows, 60 out of 100 experimental subjects (60%), but only 40 out of 100 controls (40%), reported self-medication compliance. The chi-square test will enable us to decide whether a difference in proportions of

TABLE 19-5 Observed Frequencies for Chi-Square Example			
PATIENT COMPLIANCE	**EXPERIMENTAL GROUP**	**CONTROL GROUP**	**TOTAL**
Compliant	60	40	100
Noncompliant	40	60	100
TOTAL	100	100	200

this magnitude is likely to reflect a real experimental effect or only chance fluctuations. **Expected frequencies** are calculated on the basis of the observed total frequencies for the rows and columns of a contingency table: They represent the values in the cells of the contingency table that would be obtained if there were *no* relationship between the two variables. In this example, if there were no relationship between treatment group and compliance, the expected frequency would be 50 subjects per cell.

The chi-square statistic is computed* by summarizing differences between observed and expected frequencies for each cell. In our example, there are four cells, and thus χ^2 will be the sum of four numbers. More specifically, $\chi^2 = 8.00$ in the current case. As usual, we need to compare this test statistic with the value from a theoretical chi-square distribution. A table of chi-square values for various degrees of freedom and significance levels is provided in Table B-3, Appendix B. For the chi-square statistic, the degrees of freedom are equal to $(R - 1) \times$

---

*The formula for the χ^2 statistic is

$$\chi^2 = \Sigma \frac{(f_O - f_E)^2}{f_E}$$ where f_O = observed frequency for a cell
f_E = expected frequency for a cell
Σ = sum of the $(f_O - f_E)^2/f_E$ ratios for all cells

$$f_E = \frac{f_R f_C}{N}$$ where f_R = observed frequency for the given row
f_C = observed frequency for the given column
N = total number of subjects

$(C - 1)$, or the number of rows minus 1 times the number of columns minus 1. In the current case, $df = 1 \times 1$, or 1. With 1 df, the value that must be exceeded to establish significance at the .05 level is 3.84. The obtained value of 8.00 is substantially larger than would be expected by chance. Thus, we can conclude that a significantly larger proportion of patients in the experimental group than in the control group complied with self-medication instructions.

Other Tests of Proportions

In certain situations, it may be inappropriate to calculate a chi-square statistic. When the total sample size is small (total N of 30 or less) or when there are cells with a value of 0, **Fisher's exact test** is usually used to test the significance of differences in proportions. Also, when the proportions being compared are derived from two dependent or paired groups (e.g., when a pretest–posttest design is used to compare changes in proportions on a nominal-level dichotomous variable), then the appropriate test is the **McNemar test**.

✍ TESTING RELATIONSHIPS BETWEEN TWO VARIABLES

All the procedures we have discussed thus far involve the comparison of two or more *groups*; that is, they involve situations in which the independent variable is a nominal-level variable with a fairly small number of values. In this section, we consider statistical tests for situations in which the independent variable is measured on a higher level of measurement.

Pearson's *r*

In Chapter 18, the computation and interpretation of the Pearson product–moment correlation coefficient were explained. Pearson's *r*, which is calculated when two variables are measured on at least the interval scale, is both a descriptive and inferential statistic. As a descriptive statistic, the correlation coefficient summarizes the magnitude and direction of a relationship between two variables. As an inferential statistic, *r* is used to test hypotheses concerning population correlations, which are ordinarily symbolized by the Greek letter rho, or ρ. The most commonly tested null hypothesis is that there is no relationship between two variables. Stated formally,

$$H_0: \rho = 0 \qquad H_A: \rho \neq 0$$

For instance, suppose we were studying the relationship between patients' self-reported level of stress (higher stress scores imply more stress) and the pH level of their saliva. With a sample of 50 subjects, we find that $r = -.29$. This value implies that there was a modest tendency for people who received higher stress scores to have lower pH levels than those with lower stress scores. But we need to question whether this finding can be generalized to the population. Does the coefficient of $-.29$ reflect a random fluctuation, reflecting only the particular group of subjects sampled, or is the relationship significant? The table of significant values (see Table B-4) in Appendix B allows us to make the determination. Degrees of freedom for correlation coefficients are equal to the number of subjects minus 2, or $(N - 2)$. With $df = 48$, the critical value for *r* (for a two-tailed test with $\alpha = .05$) lies between .2732 and .2875, or about .2803. Because the absolute value of the calculated *r* is .29, the

null hypothesis can be rejected. Therefore, we may conclude that there is a significant relationship between a person's self-reported level of stress and the acidity of his or her saliva.

It should be noted that Pearson's *r* can be used in both within-group and between-group situations. The previous example regarding the relationship between stress scores and the pH of people's saliva was a between-group situation: the question essentially is whether people with high stress scores tend to have significantly lower pH levels than people with low stress scores. An example of a within-group situation would be to correlate patients' stress scores before and after surgery, or to correlate patients' oral and rectal temperature measurements.

Other Tests of Bivariate Relationships

Pearson's *r* is a parametric statistic. When the assumptions for a parametric test are violated, or when the data are inherently ordinal level, then the appropriate coefficient of correlation is either **Spearman's rho** or **Kendall's tau**. The values of these statistics range from -1.00 to $+1.00$, and their interpretation is similar to that of Pearson's *r*.

Measures of the magnitude of relationships can also be computed with nominal-level data. For example, the **phi coefficient** (ϕ) is an index describing the relationship between two dichotomous variables. **Cramér's V** is an index of relationship applied to contingency tables larger than 2×2. Both of these statistics are based on the chi-square statistic and yield values that range between .00 and 1.00, with higher values indicating a stronger association between variables.

POWER ANALYSIS

Many published (and even more unpublished) nursing studies result in nonsignificant findings. Although standard statistical texts pay considerable attention to the problem of Type I errors (wrongly rejecting a *true* null hypothesis), little attention has been paid to Type II errors (wrongly accepting a *false* null hypothesis). **Power analysis** represents a method for reducing the risk of Type II errors and for estimating their occurrence.

As indicated earlier in this chapter, the probability of committing a Type I error is established by the investigator as the level of significance, or alpha (α). The probability of a Type II error is beta (β). The complement of (1 − β) is the *probability of obtaining a significant result* and is referred to as the **power** of a statistical test. It has been shown that many nursing studies have insufficient power (Polit & Sherman, 1990) and are therefore at high risk of committing a Type II error.

In performing a power analysis, there are four components, at least three of which must be known or estimated by the researcher; power analysis solves for the fourth component. The four major factors are as follows:

1. *The significance criterion,* α. Other things being equal, the more stringent this criterion, the lower is the power.
2. *The sample size, N.* As sample size increases, power increases.
3. *The population effect size, gamma* (γ). Gamma is a measure of how wrong the null hypothesis is, that is, how strong the effect of the independent variable is on the dependent variable in the population.
4. *Power, or* 1 − β. This is the probability of rejecting the null hypothesis.

Researchers typically use power analysis for two purposes: (1) to solve for the sample size needed in a study to increase the likelihood of demonstrating significant results and (2) to determine the power of a statistical test, after it has been applied. In this section, which is only a brief summary of power analysis, we focus on the first of these purposes.

To solve for an estimate of the needed sample size, the researcher must specify α, γ, and 1 − β. Usually, the researcher establishes α, the risk of a Type I error, as .05; in some cases, a lower (stricter) criterion, such

as .01, may be required. Just as .05 has been adopted as the standard for the α criterion, a conventional standard for 1 − β is .80. With power equal to .80, there is a 20% risk of committing a Type II error. Although this risk may seem high, a stricter criterion would require sample sizes much larger than most nurse researchers could manage. Most nursing studies being conducted have a power well below .80, making it difficult to avoid a Type II error.

With α and 1 − β specified, the only other piece of information needed to solve for N is γ, the population effect size. The **effect size** is an estimate of the magnitude of the relationship between the research variables. When relationships are strong, large samples are not needed to detect the effect at statistically significant levels. When the relationships are modest, then large sample sizes are needed to avoid Type II errors.

The value of γ is arrived at differently depending on the nature of the data and the statistical test to be performed. However, the principles for arriving at the estimate of γ are the same for all tests. The researcher needs to use available evidence to estimate the magnitude of the effect size. Sometimes, this evidence comes from the researcher's own pilot study, a procedure that is highly recommended when the main study is likely to be costly. More often, the researcher uses evidence from other published studies on the same or a similar problem. That is, an effect size is calculated (through procedures that follow) based on other researchers' data.* When there are *no* data that could reasonably be construed as relevant, the researcher may be forced to use

---

*Usually, a researcher will be able to find more than one piece of research from which the effect size can be estimated. In such cases, the estimate should be based on the study that yields the most stable and reliable results or whose design most closely approximates that of the new study. In some cases in which equally good (or equally bad) prior research is available, it may be desirable to combine information from multiple studies (through averaging or weighted averaging) to develop an effect size estimate.

conventions based on whether the effect size is expected to be small, medium, or large. In using these conventions, it is wise to be conservative because most nursing studies have modest effect sizes.

The procedures for estimating effects and the relevant power tables vary from one statistical test to another. We provide formulas for four situations that are especially common in nursing research: (1) testing the difference between two group means (i.e., situations requiring a *t*-test); (2) testing the difference between three or more group means (i.e., situations requiring an ANOVA); (3) testing the significance of a bivariate linear relationship (i.e., situations requiring Pearson's *r*); and (4) testing the significance of differences in proportions between two groups (i.e., situations requiring a chi-square test). Cohen (1977) and Jaccard and Becker (1990) discuss power analysis in the context of many other situations.*

Sample Size Estimates for Test of Difference Between Two Means

Suppose we were interested in testing the hypothesis that cranberry juice reduces the urinary pH of diet-controlled patients. In our study, we plan to assign some subjects randomly to a control condition (no cranberry juice) and others to an experimental condition in which they would be given 200 milliliters of cranberry juice with each meal for 5 days. How large a sample is needed for this study, given an α of .05 and power equal to .80?

To answer this question, we must first estimate γ. In a two-group situation in which the difference of means is of interest, the formula for the effect size is

$$\gamma = \frac{\mu^1 - \mu^2}{\sigma}$$

That is, γ is the difference between the two population means, divided by the population standard deviation. But how can the researcher know this information in advance? If we knew, for example, the mean urinary pH of all subjects who had or had not ingested cranberry juice, there would be little point in doing the study. Nevertheless, as explained above, the researcher must *estimate* the population means and standard deviation, based on whatever information is available. In our present example, suppose we found an earlier ex post facto study that compared the urinary pH of subjects who had or had not ingested cranberry juice in the previous 24 hours. The earlier and current studies are different. In the ex post facto study, the diets are uncontrolled; there may be selection biases in who drinks or does not drink cranberry juice, the length of ingestion is only one day, and so on. However, this study is a reasonable starting point. Suppose the results of the earlier study were as follows:

$\overline{X}_1$ (no cranberry juice) = 5.70
$\overline{X}_2$ (cranberry juice) = 5.50
σ (pooled SD) = .50

Thus, the value of γ would be .40:

$$\gamma = \frac{5.70 - 5.50}{.50} = .40$$

Table 19-6 presents approximate sample size requirements for various effect sizes and powers, and two values of α (for two-tailed tests), in a two-group mean-difference situation. In part A of the table for α = .05, we find that the estimated N needed for an effect size of .40 and a power of .80 is 98 subjects per group. That is, assuming that the earlier study provided a roughly accurate estimate of the population effect size, the total number of subjects required in the new study would be about 200, with half assigned to the control group (no cranberry juice) and the other half assigned to the experimental

*Computer software for performing power analyses is available for personal computers (Borenstein & Cohen, 1988).

TABLE 19-6   Approximate Sample Sizes* Necessary To Achieve Selected Levels of Power as a Function of Estimated Effect Size for Test of Difference of Two Means

POWER	ESTIMATED EFFECT†									
	.10	.15	.20	.25	.30	.40	.50	.60	.70	.80
PART A: α = .05										
.60	977	434	244	156	109	61	39	27	20	15
.70	1230	547	308	197	137	77	49	34	25	19
.80	1568	697	392	251	174	98	63	44	32	25
.90	2100	933	525	336	233	131	84	58	43	33
.95	2592	1152	648	415	288	162	104	72	53	41
.99	3680	1636	920	589	409	230	147	102	75	58
PART B: α = .01										
.60	1602	712	400	256	178	100	64	44	33	25
.70	1922	854	481	308	214	120	77	53	39	30
.80	2339	1040	585	374	260	146	94	65	48	37
.90	2957	1324	745	477	331	186	119	83	61	47
.95	3562	1583	890	570	396	223	142	99	73	56
.99	4802	2137	1201	769	534	300	192	133	98	

*Sample size requirements for *each* group; total sample size would be twice the number shown.

†Estimated effect (γ) is the estimated population mean group difference divided by the estimated population standard deviation, or:

$$\gamma = \frac{\mu_1 - \mu_2}{\sigma}$$

group. A sample size smaller than 200 would have a greater than 20% chance of resulting in a Type II error.

If there is *no* prior relevant research (which is rarely the case), then the researcher can, as a last resort, estimate on the basis of readings or experience whether the expected effect is small, medium, or large. By a convention developed by Cohen (1977), the value of γ in a two-group test of mean differences is estimated at .20 for small effects, .50 for medium effects, and .80 for large effects. With an α value of .05 and power of .80, the *total* sample size (number of subjects in both

groups) for studies with expected small, medium, and large effects would be 784, 126, and 50, respectively. Most nursing studies cannot expect effect sizes in excess of .50, and those in the range of .20 to .40 are especially common. In Polit and Sherman's (1990) analysis of effect sizes for all studies appearing in *Nursing Research* and *Research in Nursing & Health* in 1989, the average effect size for *t*-test situations was .35. Cohen noted that in new areas of research inquiry, effect sizes are likely to be small. A medium effect should be estimated only when the effect is so substantial that it can be detected by the naked eye (i.e., without formal research procedures).

Sample Size Estimates for Test of Difference Between Three or More Means

Suppose we wanted to study the effectiveness of three different modes of stimulation—auditory, visual, and tactile—on preterm infants' sensorimotor development. The dependent variable will be a standardized scale of infant development, such as the Denver Scale. With an α of .05 and power of .80, how many infants should be randomly assigned to the three groups?

There are alternative approaches to doing a power analysis in an ANOVA context, but the simplest approach is to calculate or estimate eta-squared, based on information from either other relevant studies or a pilot study. **Eta-squared** (η^2) is the index indicating the proportion of variance explained in ANOVA and is equal to the sum of squares between (SS_B) divided by the total sum of squares (SS_T). Eta-squared can be used directly as an estimate of the effect size.

In the modes of stimulation example, suppose we were able to find an earlier study that tested the same or a similar hypothesis, and that study yielded an η^2 of .05. Table 19-7 presents approximate sample size requirements

TABLE 19-7 Approximate Sample Sizes* Necessary To Achieve Selected Levels of Power for $\alpha = .05$ as a Function of Estimated Population Values of Eta-Squared

| POWER | \multicolumn{10}{c}{POPULATION ETA-SQUARED} |
	.01	.03	.05	.07	.10	.15	.20	.25	.30	.35
GROUPS = 3										
.70	255	84	50	35	24	16	11	9	7	6
.80	319	105	62	44	30	19	14	11	9	7
.90	417	137	81	57	39	25	18	14	11	9
.95	511	168	99	69	47	30	22	16	13	11
GROUPS = 4										
.70	219	72	43	30	21	13	10	8	6	5
.80	272	90	53	37	26	17	12	9	7	6
.90	351	115	68	48	33	21	15	12	9	8
.95	426	140	83	58	40	25	18	14	11	9
GROUPS = 5										
.70	193	64	38	27	18	12	9	7	6	4
.80	238	78	46	33	23	15	10	8	7	5
.90	306	101	59	42	29	18	13	10	8	7
.95	369	121	72	50	34	22	16	12	10	8

*The values are the number of subjects *per group.*

for various ANOVA situations. Note that, for the sake of economy and practicality, this table presents much more limited information in terms of power (the power ranges between .70 and .95) and α (only .05) than was true for the two-group situation because of the increased complexity: here, the sample size requirements vary as a function of the number of groups in the study. The table presents sample size estimates only for the most common group sizes: 3, 4, and 5. Jaccard and Becker (1990) provide expanded tables for different αs, powers, and group sizes.

Assuming that we desire a power of .80 and an α level of .05 in the hypothetical example, the number of subjects needed in each of the three stimulation groups would be 62 infants. If the experiment were undertaken with only 50 infants per group, there would be a 30% chance (power = .70) of finding nonsignificant results, even if the null hypothesis were false.

If no estimates of eta-squared could be developed on the basis of prior research, then the researcher would have to predict whether effects are likely to be small, medium, or large. For ANOVA-type situations, Cohen's conventional values of small, medium, and large effects would be values of η^2 equal to .01, .06, and .14, respectively. This would correspond to sample size requirements of about 319, 53, or 22 subjects *per group* (in a three-group study), assuming an α of .05 and power of .80.*

Sample Size Estimates for Bivariate Correlation Tests

Suppose we wanted to study the relationship between social support and primiparas' acceptance of the motherhood role. We plan to administer two scales to women who have had a normal vaginal delivery of a full-term infant. One scale measures the amount of so-

cial support available to the mother in her family and community; the other scale measures the woman's positive and negative reactions to her new role. The hypothesis is that women who have more social support available to them are more accepting of the role transition to motherhood. How many women should be included in the study, given an α of .05 and power of .80?

As in the previous cases, we need an estimate of γ. In this situation, we have two measures on an interval scale, and the relationship between them would be tested using Pearson's *r*. The estimated value of γ here is actually ρ, that is, the expected population correlation coefficient.

Suppose we found an earlier study that correlated a simple measure of social support (the number of people subjects felt they could count on in times of stress) with an observational measure of maternal warmth. Neither of these measures perfectly captures the variables in the new study, but they are conceptually close, and if no better information were available, they would provide a useful approximation. Suppose the completed study found *r* = .18, which we will use as our estimate of ρ and hence of γ. Table 19-8 shows sample size requirements for various powers and effect sizes in situations in which Pearson's *r* is used. With an α of .05 and power of .80, the sample size needed in the study would lie between 197 (for an effect size of .20) and 349 (for an effect size of .15). Extrapolating for an effect size of .18, we would need a sample of about 250 subjects to achieve a power of .80 with an α of .05. With a sample this size, we would wrongly reject the null hypothesis only 5 times out of 100 and wrongly retain the null hypothesis 20 times out of 100. To increase the power to .95 (wrongly retaining the null hypothesis only 5 times out of 100), we would need a sample of about 400 women.

When prior estimates of effect size are unavailable, the conventional values of small, medium, and large effect sizes in a bivariate correlation situation are .10, .30, and .50, re-

---

*When ANCOVA is used in lieu of *t*-tests or ANOVA, the sample size requirements are smaller—sometimes appreciably so—because of reduced error variance.

TABLE 19-8	Approximate Sample Sizes Necessary To Achieve Selected Levels of Power as a Function of Estimated Population Value of ρ

	POPULATION CORRELATION COEFFICIENT									
POWER	.10	.15	.20	.25	.30	.40	.50	.60	.70	.80
PART A: $\alpha = .05$										
.60	489	218	123	79	55	32	21	15	11	9
.70	616	274	155	99	69	39	26	18	14	11
.80	785	349	197	126	88	50	32	23	17	13
.90	1050	468	263	169	118	67	43	30	22	17
.95	1297	577	325	208	145	82	53	37	27	21
.99	1841	819	461	296	205	116	75	52	39	30
PART B: $\alpha = .01$										
.60	802	357	201	129	90	51	33	23	17	14
.70	962	428	241	155	108	61	39	28	21	16
.80	1171	521	293	188	131	74	48	33	25	19
.90	1491	663	373	239	167	94	61	42	31	24
.95	1782	792	446	286	199	112	72	50	37	28
.99	2402	1068	601	385	267	151	97	67	50	39

spectively. In Polit and Sherman's (1990) study, the average correlation found in nursing studies was in the vicinity of .20.

Sample Size Estimates for Testing Differences in Proportions

Estimating sample size requirements when differences in proportions between groups are being studied is more complex than in the previously described situations. For this reason, we present only a partial discussion of this topic here and recommend that other references, such as Cohen (1977) or Jaccard and Becker (1990), be consulted. We restrict our coverage to 2 × 2 contingency tables.

Suppose we were interested in comparing the rates of breastfeeding in two groups of women: (1) those receiving a special intervention—home visits by nurses during the third trimester, in which the advantages of breastfeeding would be described, and (2) those in a control group not receiving any home visits. How many subjects should be randomly assigned to the two groups?

The effect size for this type of situation is not arrived at in a straightforward fashion. This is because the effect size is influenced not only by expected differences in proportions (e.g., 60% in one group versus 40% in another, a 20 percentage point difference) but also by the absolute values of the proportions. In other words, the effect size for 60% versus 40% is *not* the same as that for 30% versus 10%. In general, the effect size is *larger* (and consequently, the sample size needs are *smaller*) at the extremes than near the midpoint: A 20 percentage point difference is easier to detect when the two percentages are 10% and 30% (or 70% and 90%) than when they are near the middle, such as 40% and 60%.

The computation of the effect size index involves a complex transformation (the arcsine transformation) that we do not fully elaborate on here. Rather than present sample size estimates based on effect size, Table 19-9 presents the approximate sample size requirements for detecting differences in various proportions, assuming an α of .05 and a power of .80. To use this table, we would need to have estimates of the proportions for both groups. Then we would find the proportion for one group in the first column and the proportion for the second group in the top row. The approximate sample size requirement *for each group* would be found at the intersection of the two appropriate proportions. Thus, in our example, if we had reason to expect (on the basis of a pilot study, say), that 20% of the control group mothers and 40% of the experimental group mothers would breastfeed their infants, then the sample size needed in the study (to keep the risk of a Type II error down to 20%) would be 80 subjects per group.

Because we have not presented information on the computationally complex effect size for the situation involving a 2 × 2 contingency table, we cannot conveniently identify Cohen's convention for small, medium, and large effects. We can, however, give *examples* of differences in proportions (i.e., the proportions in group 1 versus group 2) that conform to the conventions:

Small: .05 versus .10, .20 versus .29, .40 versus .50, .60 versus .70, .80 versus .87
Medium: .05 versus .21, .20 versus .43, .40 versus .65, .60 versus .82, .80 versus .96
Large: .05 versus .34, .20 versus .58, .40 versus .78, .60 versus .92, .80 versus .96

Thus, if the researcher expected a medium effect in which the proportion for group 1 could be expected to be in the vicinity of .40, then the number of subjects in each of the two groups would need to be about 70 to 75. As in other situations, researchers are encouraged to avoid the use of the conventions, if possible, in favor of more precise es-

TABLE 19-9 **Approximate Sample Sizes* Necessary To Achieve a Power of .80 for α = .05 for Estimated Population Difference Between Two Proportions**

GROUP II PROPORTIONS	GROUP I PROPORTIONS														
	.10	.15	.20	.25	.30	.35	.40	.45	.50	.55	.60	.70	.80	.90	1.00
.05	421	133	69	44	31	24	19	15	13	11	9	7	5	4	2
.10		689	196	97	59	41	30	23	18	15	12	9	6	5	3
.15			901	247	118	71	48	34	26	21	16	11	8	5	3
.20				1090	292	137	80	53	38	28	22	14	10	6	3
.25					1252	327	151	87	57	40	30	18	12	8	4
.30						1371	356	161	93	60	42	23	14	9	4
.35							1480	374	169	96	61	31	18	10	5
.40								1510	385	172	97	42	22	12	5
.45									1570	393	173	60	28	15	6
.50										1570	389	93	38	18	6
.55											1539	162	53	23	7
.60												356	80	30	8
.70													292	59	12
.80														195	18
.90															38

*The values are the number of subjects *per group.*

```
t-test for:  WEIGHT    INFANT BIRTH WEIGHT

                Number              Standard    Standard
                of Cases    Mean    Deviation     Error

     Group 1      15      107.5333   13.378       3.454
     Group 2      15      101.8667    7.239       1.869


            Pooled Variance Estimate

              t     Degrees of  2-Tail
            Value    Freedom     Prob.

             1.44      28         .160
```

Figure 19-5. SPSS Computer Printout: *t*-Test.

timates based on prior empirical evidence; when the use of the conventions is unavoidable, conservative estimates should be used to minimize the risk of finding nonsignificant results.

THE COMPUTER AND INFERENTIAL STATISTICS

As in Chapter 18, we have stressed the logic and uses of various statistics rather than their computational formulas and mathematic derivations.* Because the computer is increasingly called on to perform the computations for hypothesis testing, and because it is important to be able to make sense of the printed information produced by the computer, we include in this chapter examples of computer-produced information for two statistical tests.

We return to the example described in Chapter 18. A researcher has designed an experiment to test the effects of a special prenatal program designed for a group of young, low-income women. The raw data for the 30 subjects in this example were presented in Table 18–8 in Chapter 18. Given these data, let us test some hypotheses.

Hypothesis One: *t*-Test

Let us suppose that our first research hypothesis is as follows:

> The babies of the experimental subjects will have higher birthweights than the babies of the control subjects.

In this example, there are two independent groups of subjects, and differences in the mean birthweights are being compared. Therefore, the *t*-test for independent samples is used to test our hypothesis. The null and alternative hypotheses can be stated as follows:

H_0: μ experimental = μ control
H_A: μ experimental ≠ μ control

Figure 19-5 presents the computer printout for the *t*-test. The top of the figure presents some basic descriptive statistics for the birthweight variable, separately for the two groups. Thus, the mean birthweight of the babies in group 1 (the experimental group) was 107.53 ounces, compared with 101.87 ounces for the babies in group 2 (the control group). These data, then, are consistent with our research hypothesis—the average weight of the experimental subjects is higher than the average weight of the controls. But do the differences reflect the impact of the experimental intervention, or do they merely represent random fluctuations? To answer this, we examine the results of the *t*-test, shown under the heading "Pooled Variance Estimate." The computer

---

*Note that this introduction to inferential statistics has necessarily been superficial. We urge novice researchers to undertake further exploration of statistical principles.

```
Correlations:   WEIGHT      AGE

   WEIGHT        1.0000        .5938
               (   30)       (   30)
               P= .          P= .000

   AGE            .5938      1.0000
               (   30)       (   30)
               P= .000       P= .


(Coefficient / (Cases) / 1-tailed Significance)

" . " is printed if a coefficient cannot be computed
```

Figure 19-6. SPSS Computer Printout: Pearson Correlation Coefficients.

program calculated the value of t as 1.44. With 28 degrees of freedom $[(15 + 15) - 2]$, this value is not significant. The two-tailed probability (p value) for this t statistic is .16. This means that in 16 samples out of 100, one could expect to find a difference in weights at least this large as a result of chance alone. Therefore, since $p > .05$ (a nonsignificant result), we cannot conclude that the special intervention was effective in improving the birthweights of the experimental group.*

Hypothesis Two: Pearson Correlation

A second research hypothesis might involve the relationship between maternal age and the infant's birthweight, stated as follows:

Older mothers will have babies of higher birthweight than younger mothers.

In this case, both birthweight and age are measured on the ratio scale, and the appropriate test statistic is the Pearson product–moment correlation. The hypotheses subjected to the statistical test are

H_0: ρ birthweight—age $= 0$
H_A: ρ birthweight—age $\neq 0$

The printout for the test of the hypothesis is presented in Figure 19-6. The correlation matrix

*The average difference in birthweights is fairly sizable and in the hypothesized direction. The researcher may wish to pursue this study by increasing the sample size or by controlling some other variables, such as the mother's age, through analysis of covariance (see Chapter 20).

in Figure 19-6 shows, in row one, the correlation of weight with weight and of weight with age; and in row two, the correlation of age with weight and of age with age. The correlation of interest to us for testing the hypothesis is weight with age (or age with weight—the result is the same). At the intersection of these two variables, we find three numbers. The first is the actual correlation coefficient, and the second shows the number of cases. In our example, $r = .5938$ and $N = 30$. The correlation indicates a moderately strong positive relationship: The older the mother, the higher the baby's weight tended to be, as hypothesized. Again, the data are consistent with the research hypothesis, but does this reflect a true relationship or merely chance fluctuations in the data? The third number at the intersection of age and weight shows the probability that the correlation occurred by chance: P (for probability level) $= .000$. The printout only shows significance levels to the nearest thousandth. In this case, the actual p value might be .0004 or .000001; we do not know the real value. We *do* know, however, that $p < .001$. In other words, a relationship this strong would be found by chance alone in fewer than 1 out of 1000 samples of 30 young mothers. Therefore, the research hypothesis is accepted.

TIPS FOR USING INFERENTIAL STATISTICS

Most quantitative nursing studies use one of the statistical tests described in this chapter. It is essential for both consumers and producers of research to understand the logic underlying statistical tests and to be familiar with the interpretation of results from such tests. In this section, we offer further guidance relating to the use of inferential statistics.

- The selection and use of a statistical test depend on several factors, such as the measurement level of the variables, the sample size, the number of groups being compared, and the shape of the distribution of the dependent variable. To aid researchers in selecting a test statistic or evaluating statistical procedures used by researchers in the literature, a chart summarizing the major features of several commonly used tests is presented in Table 19-10.

- Among the more important factors to consider in selecting a statistical test is the level of measurement of the independent and dependent variables. Although we have advised that variables should generally be measured on as high a measurement scale as possible, there may be situations when it is appropriate to convert data to a lower level of measurement. For example, Parker, McFarlane, Soeken, Torres, and Campbell (1993) studied the incidence of physical and mental abuse among pregnant women, comparing pregnant women who were teenagers to women who were older. In this study, age—a continuous, ratio-level variable—was collapsed into a dichotomous variable (teenager versus adult). When there is reason to believe that a relationship between variables is not linear, it is often better to transform one of the variables. By **linear**, we mean that changes in one variable are not incrementally affected by changes in the other variable at every point along the measurement scale. In this case, for example, although the researchers hypothesized that very young women might be at especially high risk of abuse, they did not hypothesize differences at older ages (e.g., that 25-year-old women

would be at higher risk than 30-year-old women). If age and abuse were linearly related, abuse would diminish at successive ages, but this is clearly an unlikely situation. By collapsing ages into two groups, the researchers were better able to test their hypotheses.

- Statistical tests are designed to help researchers distinguish "real" relationships from random fluctuations that inevitably occur when data are collected from a sample. Statistical tests use the concept of a standard error to evaluate whether a result is likely to reflect random fluctuations, and all standard errors are directly affected by the size of the sample. Seen in this light, it should be clear that researchers run a risk of a large standard error when they use small samples. Or, put another way, a small sample size increases the likelihood that a Type II error will be committed. That is, when small samples are used, the researcher takes a sizable risk that the test will result in a rejection of the research hypothesis—even when the hypothesis is, in fact, correct. Thus, small samples should generally be avoided in quantitative studies that use inferential statistics.

- When a statistical test indicates that the null hypothesis should be retained (i.e., when the results are nonsignificant), this is sometimes referred to as a **negative result**. Negative results are often disappointing to researchers and may in some cases lead to the rejection of a manuscript by a journal editor. Research reports with negative results are not rejected because editors are prejudiced against certain types of outcomes; they are rejected because negative results are generally inconclusive and therefore difficult to interpret. A nonsignificant result simply indicates that the result *could* have occurred as a result of chance but offers no firm evidence that the research hypothesis is *not* correct.

TABLE 19-10   Guide to Widely Used Bivariate Statistical Tests

TEST NAME	TEST STATISTIC	BETWEEN OR WITHIN	PURPOSE	MEASUREMENT LEVEL IV	MEASUREMENT LEVEL DV*
Parametric Tests					
t-Test for independent groups	t	Between	To test the difference between two independent group means	Nominal	Interval, ratio
Paired *t*-test	t	Within	To test the difference between two related group means	Nominal	Interval, ratio
Analysis of variance (ANOVA)	F	Between	To test the difference among the means of 3+ independent groups, or of 2+ independent variables	Nominal	Interval, ratio
Repeated-measures ANOVA	F	Within	To test the difference among the means of 3 + related groups or sets of scores	Nominal	Interval, ratio
Pearson's product–moment correlation	r	Between, within	To test the existence of a relationship between two variables	Interval, ratio	Interval, ratio
Nonparametric Tests					
Mann-Whitney *U*-test	U	Between	To test the difference in ranks of scores of two independent groups	Nominal	Ordinal
Median test	χ^2	Between	To test the difference between the medians of two independent groups	Nominal	Ordinal
Kruskal-Wallis test	H	Between	To test the difference in ranks of scores of 3+ independent groups	Nominal	Ordinal

(continued)

TABLE 19-10 Guide to Widely Used Bivariate Statistical Tests (Continued)

TEST NAME	TEST STATISTIC	BETWEEN OR WITHIN	PURPOSE	MEASUREMENT LEVEL IV*	DV*
Nonparametric Tests					
Wicoxon signed-rank test	Z	Within	To test the difference in ranks of scores of two related groups	Nominal	Ordinal
Friedman test	χ^2	Within	To test the difference in ranks of scores of 3+ related groups	Nominal	Ordinal
Chi-square test	χ^2	Between	To test the difference in proportions in 2+ independent groups	Nominal	Nominal
McNemar's test	χ^2	Within	To test the difference in proportions for paired samples (2×2)	Nominal	Nominal
Fisher's exact test	—	Between	To test the difference in proportions in a 2×2 contingency table when $N < 30$	Nominal	Nominal
Spearman's rho	ρ	Between, within	To test that a correlation is different from zero (that a relationship exists)	Ordinal	Ordinal
Kendall's tau	τ	Between, within	To test that a correlation is different from zero (that a relationship exists)	Ordinal	Ordinal
Phi coefficient	ϕ	Between	To examine the magnitude of a relationship between two dichotomous variables	Nominal	Nominal
Cramér's V	V	Between	To examine the magnitude of a relationship between variables in a contingency table (not restricted to 2×2)	Nominal	Nominal

*IV, independent variable; DV, dependent variable.

- It is strongly recommended that power analysis be performed to estimate needed sample sizes during the design phase of the study. Once the study has been completed, however, power analysis is a useful tool for interpreting findings, especially when the statistical tests yield nonsignificant results that are often ambiguous.

RESEARCH EXAMPLES

The inferential statistics discussed in this chapter have been used in thousands of nursing studies. Some examples illustrating the use of these statistics are presented in Table 19-11. Two research examples are described in greater detail next.

TABLE 19-11 Examples of Statistical Tests Used by Nurse Researchers

STATISTICAL TEST	RESEARCH QUESTION OR HYPOTHESIS	VALUE OF STATISTIC	P
t-Test for independent groups	What is the effect of individualized developmental care by nurses compared with traditional care on preterm infants' time receiving mechanical ventilation? (Brown & Heermann, 1997)	$t = -2.26$	<.05
Paired t-test	Are there differences in the level of distress of fathers compared with mothers who have suffered the sudden death of a child? (Moriarty, Carroll, & Cotroneo, 1996)	$t = 4.57$	$p <.001$
ANOVA	What is the difference in functional status among women with breast cancer in three groups with different levels of depression? (Pasacreta, 1997)	$F = 8.7$	<.001
Mann-Whitney U test	What is the difference between healthy women and women with fibromyalgia with respect to disturbed sleep, fatigue, and memory deficits? (Söderberg, Lundman, & Norberg, 1997)	$U = 23.0$ $U = 70.5$ $U = 205.5$	<.001 <.001 <.001
Chi-square test	Rocking infants or giving them a pacifier will reduce bouts of persistent crying after the heelstick procedure (Campos, 1994)	$\chi^2 = 11.87$	<.01
Pearson's r	What is the relationship between Parkinson's disease patients' physical functioning and their spouse-caregivers' perception of their own health change? (Berry & Murphy, 1995)	$r = .42$	.02
Spearman's rho	What is the correlation between scores on three breastfeeding assessment tools? (Riordan & Koehn, 1997)	$\rho = .69$, .78, .68	<.001

Research Example With *t*-Tests and Correlations

Lattavo, Britt, and Dobal (1995) conducted a study designed to compare pulmonary artery (PA), oral, axillary, and two tympanic temperatures. A primary goal of the research was to investigate whether tympanic and core PA temperatures are interchangeable—that is, whether tympanic temperature is a reliable substitute for pulmonary artery temperature. The research sample consisted of 32 patients from a medical-surgical unit of an urban community hospital. The various temperature measurements were taken in the same order for all patients.

The researchers began by computing correlation coefficients between core PA temperature and all other temperature measures. The correlations ranged from a low of .68 (for axillary temperature) to a high of .84 (for tympanic temperature as measured by the IVAC Core-Check tympanic thermometer). All correlations were significant at $p <$ .01. However, the researchers reasoned that if the measures are equally reliable in measuring the same phenomenon (body temperature), the *r*s should be .90 or better. Because none of the measures met this criterion, the authors questioned using alternative temperature measurements as a substitute for core PA temperature.

As a further corroboration, the researchers performed a series of paired *t*-tests. If the PA and tympanic measures were truly comparable, there would be no significant differences between measures made on the same patients. However, most of the *t*-tests *were* statistically significant, indicating true (not spurious) differences between the measures. For example, the mean difference between core PA temperature and IVAC Core-Check tympanic temperature was 0.58°F ($t = 3.58$, $df = 31$, $p < .01$). The researchers reached the following conclusion: "Based on these data, the tympanic temperature measurements are not ideal substitutes for the PA temperature measurements" (p. 369).

Research Example With Repeated-Measures ANOVA

Fogel and Martin (1992) studied the mental health of incarcerated women who either were or were not mothers. Data were collected from a sample of 46 women (35 had children) at two points in time: within 1 week of the subjects' imprisonment, and then 6 months later. Two scales were administered to assess mental health: the Center for Epidemiological Studies Depression (CES-D) Scale and the Spielberger State Anxiety Inventory (STAI).

The data were analyzed using two repeated-measures ANOVAs—one for each dependent variable. In these analyses, motherhood status served as one factor, and time of administration of the scales (1 week versus 6 months after imprisonment) was the second factor. For the STAI scores, the analyses revealed a significant main effect for time ($F = 11.35$; $df = 1$, 44; $p = .002$). For the sample as a whole, anxiety levels decreased significantly over the 6 months of imprisonment. A significant interaction effect ($F = 5.06$; $df = 1$, 44; $p = .029$) indicated that, although anxiety declined over time for both groups, the mean STAI scores for the nonmothers declined more than that for the mothers. The main effect comparing mothers and nonmothers on the STAI scale was nonsignificant.

With respect to depression scores, there were no statistically significant main effects for time or motherhood, and no interaction effects. Levels of depression were found to be high for both groups at both testing points.

SUMMARY

Inferential statistics enable a researcher to make inferences about the characteristics of a population based on data obtained in a sample. The reason that we cannot make such inferences directly from the data is that sample statistics inevitably contain a certain degree of error as estimates of population parameters.

Inferential statistics offer the researcher a framework for deciding whether the sampling error is too high to provide reliable population estimates.

The **sampling distribution** of the mean is a theoretical distribution of the means of an infinite number of samples drawn from the same population. Because the sampling distribution of means follows a normal curve, it is possible to indicate the probability that a specified sample value will be obtained. The **standard error of the mean** is the standard deviation of the theoretical sampling distribution of the mean. This index indicates the degree of average error in a sample mean as an estimate of the population mean. The smaller the SEM, the more accurate are the estimates of the population value. Sampling distributions are the basis for inferential statistics.

Statistical inference consists of two major types of approaches: estimating parameters and testing hypotheses. When a researcher wants to discover the value of an unknown population characteristic, he or she may estimate the value by means of either point or interval estimation. **Point estimation** provides a single numeric value. **Interval estimation** provides the upper and lower limits of a range of values—the **confidence limits**—between which the population value is expected to fall, at some specified probability level. The researcher is able to establish the degree of confidence that the population value will lie within this **confidence interval**.

Statistical hypothesis testing enables researchers to make objective decisions concerning the results of their studies. The **null hypothesis** is a statement that no relationship exists between the variables and that any observed relationships are the result of chance or sampling fluctuations. Rejection of the null hypothesis lends support to the research hypothesis, and failure to reject the null hypothesis indicates that any observed differences may be due to chance fluctuations.

When a researcher fails to reject a null hypothesis that *should* be rejected, the error is re-ferred to as a **Type II error**. If a null hypothesis is rejected when it *should not* be rejected, then the error is called a **Type I error**. Researchers are able to control the risk of committing a Type I error by establishing a **level of significance**, which indicates the probability of making a Type I error. The two most commonly used levels of significance (designated as the α level) are .05 and .01. A significance level of .01 means that in only 1 out of 100 samples will the null hypothesis be rejected when, in fact, it should be retained.

In testing their hypotheses, researchers compute a **test statistic** and then determine whether the statistic falls at or beyond the **critical region** on the relevant theoretical distribution. If the value of the test statistic indicates that the null hypothesis is "improbable," the result is said to be statistically significant. The phrase **statistically significant** means that the obtained results are not likely to be the result of chance fluctuations at the specified level of probability (p level). Although most hypothesis testing involves **two-tailed tests**, in which both ends of the sampling distribution are used to define the region of improbable values, a **one-tailed test** may be appropriate if the researcher has a strong rationale for a directional hypothesis.

Statistical tests are classified as parametric and nonparametric. **Nonparametric tests** require less stringent assumptions than parametric tests and usually are used when the level of data is either nominal or ordinal or when the distribution is not normal. **Parametric tests** involve the estimation of at least one parameter, the use of data measured on an interval or ratio level, and assumptions concerning the distribution of variables. Parametric tests are usually more powerful than nonparametric tests and generally are preferred. Tests can also be classified as either a **between-subjects test** (sometimes called a **test for independent groups**) involving separate groups of subjects, or a **within-subjects test** (or a **test for dependent groups**) involving comparisons for either the same group of subjects over time or conditions or a related group of subjects.

Two frequently used parametric procedures are the *t*-test and **analysis of variance**, both of which can be used to test the significance of the difference between groups means. The *t*-test can only be applied to two-group situations, whereas the ANOVA procedure can handle three or more groups as well as more than one independent variable. Nonparametric analogues of these parametric tests include the **median test**, the **Mann-Whitney** *U* test, the **sign test** and the **Wilcoxon signed-rank test** (two-group situations), and the **Kruskal-Wallis** and **Friedman tests** (three-group or more situations). The nonparametric test that is used most frequently is the **chi-square test,** which is used in connection with hypotheses relating to differences in proportions. Statistical tests to measure the magnitude of bivariate relationships and to test whether the relationship is significantly different from zero include Pearson's *r* for interval-level data, **Spearman's rho** and **Kendall's tau** for ordinal-level data, and the **phi coefficient** and **Cramér's** *V* for nominal-level data.

Power analysis refers to techniques for estimating either the likelihood of committing a Type II error or sample size requirements. Power analysis involves four components: (1) a desired significance level (α), (2) power (1 − β), (3) sample size (N), and (4) an estimated **effect size** (γ). To calculate needed sample size, all three other components must be specified by the researcher.

▶ STUDY ACTIVITIES

Chapter 19 of the *Study Guide to Accompany Nursing Research: Principles and Methods, 6th ed.*, offers various exercises and study suggestions for reinforcing the concepts presented in this chapter. Additionally, the following study questions can be addressed:

1. A researcher has administered a Job Satisfaction Scale to a sample of 50 primary nurses and 50 team nurses. The mean score on this scale for each group was found to be 35.2 for the primary nurses and 33.6 for the team nurses. A *t*-statistic is computed and is found to be 1.89. Interpret this result, using the table for *t*-values in Appendix B.

2. Compute the chi-square statistic for the following contingency table:

GROUP	NUMBER OF COMPLICATIONS FOLLOWING SURGERY		
	None	One	More Than One
Experimental	38	72	54
Control	29	50	11

How many degrees of freedom are there? At the .05 level of significance, what may be concluded?

3. Given that:
   a. There are three groups of nursing school students, with 50 in each group
   b. Level of significance = .05
   c. Value of test statistic = 4.43
   d. Mean scores on test to measure motivation to attend graduate school: 25.8, 29.3, and 23.4 for groups A, B, and C, respectively

   Specify:
   a. What test statistic was used
   b. How many degrees of freedom there are
   c. Whether the test statistic is statistically significant
   d. What the test statistic means

4. What inferential statistic would you choose for the following sets of variables? Explain your answers. (Refer to Table 19-10.)
   a. Variable 1 represents the weights of 100 patients; variable 2 is the patients' resting heart rate.
   b. Variable 1 is the patients' marital status; variable 2 is the patient's level of preoperative stress.
   c. Variable 1 is whether an amputee has a leg removed above or below the knee;

variable 2 is whether or not the amputee has shown signs of aggressive behavior during rehabilitation.

5. Estimate the required total sample sizes for the following situations:
   a. Comparison of two group means: α = .01; power = .90; γ = .35.
   b. Comparison of three group means: α = .05; power = .80; η^2 = .07.
   c. Correlation of two variables: α = .01; power = .85; ρ = .27.
   d. Comparison of two proportions: α = .05; power = .80, P_1 = .35; P_2 = .50.

SUGGESTED READINGS

Methodologic References

Borenstein, M., & Cohen, J. (1988). *Statistical power analysis: A computer program.* Hillsdale, NJ: Erlbaum Associates.

Brogan, D. R. (1981). Choosing an appropriate statistical test of significance for a nursing research hypothesis or question. *Western Journal of Nursing Research, 3,* 337–363.

Cohen, J. (1988). *Statistical power analysis for the behavioral sciences* (2nd ed.). Mahwah, N. J.: L. Erlbaum.

Holm, K., & Christman, N. J. (1985). Post hoc tests following analysis of variance. *Research in Nursing & Health, 8,* 207–210.

Jaccard, J., & Becker, M. A. (1990). *Statistics for the behavioral sciences.* (2nd ed.). Belmont, CA: Wadsworth.

Jacobsen, B. S., Tulman, L., & Lowery, B. J. (1991). Three sides of the same coin: The analysis of paired data from dyads. *Nursing Research, 40,* 359–363.

Kanji, G. K. (1993). *100 statistical tests.* London: Sage.

McCall, R. B. (1997). *Fundamental statistics for behavioral sciences* (7th ed.). Pacific Grove, CA: Brooks-Cole.

Munro, B. H., & Page, E. B. (1997). *Statistical methods for health-care research* (3rd ed.). Philadelphia: Lippincott-Raven.

Polit, D. F. (1996). *Data analysis and statistics for nursing research.* Stamford, CT: Appleton & Lange.

Polit, D. F., & Sherman, R. (1990). Statistical power in nursing research. *Nursing Research, 39,* 365–369.

Sidani, S., & Lynn, M. R. (1993). Examining amount and pattern of change: Comparing repeated measures ANOVA and individual regression analysis. *Nursing Research, 42,* 283–286.

Triola, M. (1998). *Elementary statistics* (7th ed.). Menlo Park, CA: Addison-Wesley.

Welkowitz, J., Ewen, R. B., & Cohen, J. (1990). *Introductory statistics for the behavioral sciences* (4th ed.). New York: Academic Press.

Substantive References

Berry, R. A., & Murphy, J. F. (1995). Well-being of caregivers of spouses with Parkinson's disease. *Clinical Nursing Research, 4,* 373–386.

Brown, L. D., & Heermann, J. A. (1997). The effect of developmental care on preterm infant outcome. *Applied Nursing Research, 10,* 190–197.

Campos, R. G. (1994). Rocking and pacifiers: Two comforting interventions for heelstick pain. *Research in Nursing & Health, 17,* 321–331.

Fogel, C. I., & Martin, S. L. (1992). The mental health of incarcerated women. *Western Journal of Nursing Research, 14,* 30–47.

Lattavo, K., Britt, J., & Dobal, M. (1995). Agreement between measures of pulmonary artery and tympanic temperatures. *Research in Nursing & Health, 18,* 365–370.

Moriarty, H. J., Carroll, R., & Cotroneo, M. (1996). Differences in bereavement reactions within couples following the death of a child. *Research in Nursing & Health, 19,* 461–469.

Parker, B., McFarlane, J., Soeken, K., Torres, S., & Campbell, D. (1993). Physical and emotional abuse in pregnancy: A comparison of adult and teenage women. *Nursing Research, 42,* 173–178.

Pasacreta, J. V. (1997). Depressive phenomena, physical symptom distress, and functional status among women with breast cancer. *Nursing Research, 46,* 214–221.

Riordan, J. M., & Koehn, M. (1997). Reliability and validity testing of three breastfeeding assessment tools. *Journal of Obstetric, Gynecologic, and Neonatal Nursing, 26,* 181–187.

Söderberg, S., Lundman, B., & Norberg, A. (1997). Living with fibromyalgia. *Research in Nursing & Health, 20,* 495–503.

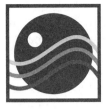

CHAPTER **20**

Multivariate Statistical Procedures

The phenomena of interest to nurse researchers are generally complex. Patients' preoperative anxieties, nurses' effectiveness in caring for people, the fears of cancer patients, or the abrupt elevation of patients' body temperature are phenomena that have multiple facets and multiple determinants. Scientists, in attempting to explain, predict, and control the phenomena that interest them, have recognized that a two-variable study is often inadequate for such purposes. The classic approach to data analysis and research design, which consists of studying the effect of a single independent variable on a single dependent variable, increasingly is being replaced by more sophisticated **multivariate*** procedures. Whether one structures a study to be multivariate or not, the fact remains that most nursing phenomena are essentially and unalterably multivariate in nature. The modern researcher who is unfamiliar with multivariate techniques is at a serious disadvantage both as a designer of research studies and as a consumer of research reports.

---

*We use the term *multivariate* in this chapter to refer generally to analyses dealing with at least three variables. Some statisticians reserve the term for problems involving more than one dependent variable.

Unlike the statistical methods reviewed in Chapters 18 and 19, multivariate statistics are computationally formidable. However, the widespread availability of computers has made complex manual calculations obsolete. Therefore, we make minimal reference to computational formulas. The purpose of this chapter is to provide a general understanding of how, when, and why multivariate statistics are used rather than to explain their mathematic basis. References are available at the end of this chapter for those desiring more comprehensive coverage.

MULTIPLE REGRESSION AND CORRELATION

Multiple regression analysis is a method used for understanding the effects of two or more independent variables on a dependent variable. The terms **multiple correlation** and **multiple regression** will be used almost interchangeably in reference to this technique, consistent with the strong bond between correlation and regression. To comprehend the nature of this bond, we first explain simple regression—that is, bivariate regression—before turning to multiple regression.

Simple Linear Regression

Regression analysis is usually performed with the intention of making predictions about phenomena. In the health care field, as in many other fields, the ability to make accurate predictions has important implications for the quality of services rendered. For example, whenever a costly or scarce resource (e.g., home visitation by nurses) is to be allocated, it is important to be able to predict who will benefit most from that resource.

In simple regression, one independent variable (X) is used to predict a dependent variable (Y). For instance, we could use simple regression to predict weight from height, blood pressure from age, nursing school achievement from Scholastic Assessment Test (SAT) scores, or stress from noise levels. An important feature of regression is that the higher the correlation between the two variables, the more accurate the prediction. If the correlation between diastolic and systolic blood pressure were perfect (i.e., if $r = 1.00$), then we would only need to measure one variable to be able to know the value of the other. Because most variables of interest to researchers are not perfectly correlated, most predictions made through regression analysis are imperfect.

A simple regression equation is a formula for making predictions about the numeric values of one variable, based on the scores or values of another variable. The basic linear regression equation is

$$Y' = a + bX$$

where Y' = predicted value of variable Y
a = intercept constant
b = regression coefficient (slope of the line)
X = actual value of variable X

Regression analysis solves for a and b, so for any value of X, a prediction about Y can be made. Those readers with recollection of high school algebra may remember that the above equation is the algebraic equation for a straight line. **Linear regression** is essentially a method for determining a straight line to fit the data in such a way that deviations from the line are minimized.

An illustration may help to clarify some of these points. Data for five subjects on two variables (X and Y) are shown in columns 1 and 2 of Table 20-1. Application of Pearson's r formula to these data reveals that the variables are strongly related, $r = .90$. What we wish to do is develop a way of predicting Y values for a *new* group of subjects from whom we will only have information on the variable X. To do this, we must use the five pairs of values to solve for a and b in the regression equation.

The formulas for these two components are as follows:

$$b = \frac{\Sigma xy}{\Sigma x^2} \qquad a = \overline{Y} - b\overline{X}$$

where b = regression coefficient
a = intercept constant
$\overline{Y}$ = mean of variable Y
$\overline{X}$ = mean of variable X
x = deviation scores from $\overline{X}$
y = deviation scores from $\overline{Y}$

The calculations required for the various elements of these equations are worked out for the current example in columns 3 through 7 of Table 20-1. As shown at the bottom of the table, the solution to the regression equation is $Y' = 1.5 + .9X$. What does one do with this information? Suppose for the moment that the X values in column 1 were the only data available for the five subjects, and that we wanted to predict the values for variable Y. For the first subject with an $X = 1$, we would predict that $Y' = 1.5 + (.9)(1)$, or 2.4. Column 8 shows similar computations for each X value. These numbers show that Y' does not exactly equal the actual values obtained for Y. Most of the errors of prediction (e) are small, as shown in column 9. The errors of prediction result from the fact that the correlation between X and Y is not perfect. Only when $r = 1.00$ or -1.00 does $Y' = Y$. The regression equation

TABLE 20-1	Computations for Simple Linear Regression

(1) X	(2) Y	(3) x	(4) x²	(5) y	(6) y²	(7) xy	(8) Y'	(9) e	(10) e²
1	2	−4	16	−4	16	16	2.4	−.4	.16
3	6	−2	4	0	0	0	4.2	1.8	3.24
5	4	0	0	−2	4	0	6.0	−2.0	4.00
7	8	2	4	2	4	4	7.8	.2	.04
9	10	4	16	4	16	16	9.6	.4	.16
$\Sigma X = 25$	$\Sigma Y = 30$		40		40	36		0.0	7.60
$\overline{X} = 5.0$	$\overline{Y} = 6.0$								$\Sigma e^2 = 7.60$

$$r = .90$$

$$b = \frac{\Sigma xy}{\Sigma x^2} = \frac{36}{40} = .90$$

$$a = \overline{Y} - b\overline{X} = 6.0 - (.9)(5.0) = 1.5$$
$$Y' = a + bX$$
$$Y' = 1.5 + .9X$$

solves for a and b in such a way as to minimize such errors. Or, more precisely, the solution minimizes the sums of squares of the prediction errors, which is why standard regression analysis is said to use a **least-squares principle** (standard regression is sometimes referred to as **ordinary least squares**, or **OLS**, regression). In column 10 of Table 20-1, the error terms—usually referred to as the **residuals**—have been squared and summed to yield a value of 7.60. Any values of a and b other than those obtained above would have yielded a larger sum of the squared residuals.

The solution to this regression analysis example is displayed graphically in Figure 20-1. The actual X and Y values from the table are plotted on the graph with circles. The line running through these points is the representation of the regression solution. The intercept (a) is the point at which the line crosses the Y axis, which in this case is 1.5. The slope (b) is the angle of the line, relative to the X and Y axes. With $b = .90$, the line slopes in such a fashion that for every 4 units on the X axis, we must go up 3.6 units ($.9 \times 4$) on the Y axis. The line,

then, embodies the whole regression equation. To find a predicted value for Y, we could go to the point on the X axis for an obtained X score, find the point on the regression line vertically above the score, and read the predicted Y value horizontally from the Y axis. For example, with an X value of 5, we would predict a Y' of 6, as shown by the star designating that point on the figure.

The connection between correlation and regression can be made more evident by pointing out an important aspect of a correlation coefficient. The correlation coefficient, it may be recalled, is an index of the degree to which variables are related. Relationships, from a statistical point of view, are concerned with how variations in one variable are associated with variations in another. The r statistic enables us to specify how much variability can be explained or accounted for by two correlated variables. The square of r (r^2) tells us the proportion of the variance in Y that can be accounted for by X. In the previous example, $r = .90$, so $r^2 = .81$. This means that 81% of the variability in the Y values can be understood

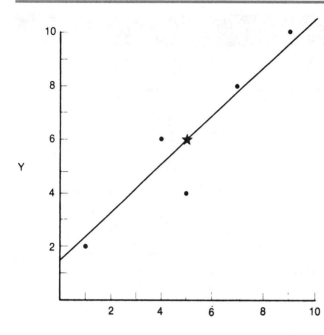

Figure 20-1. Example of simple linear regression.

in terms of the variability in the *X* values. The remaining 19% constitutes variability resulting from other sources.

Returning to the regression problem, it was found that the sum of the squared residuals (error terms) was 7.6. Column 6 of Table 20-1 also informs us that the sum of the squared deviations of the *Y* values from the mean of *Y* (Σy^2) was 40. To demonstrate that the residuals constitute 19% of the unexplained variability in *Y*, we can compute the following ratio:

$$\frac{7.6}{40} = .19 = 1 - r^2$$

Although the computations are not shown, the sum of the squared deviations of the *Y'* values from the mean of *Y'* ($\Sigma y'^2$) is equal to 32.4. As a proportion of the variability in the *actual Y* values, this would equal

$$\frac{32.4}{40} = .81 = r^2$$

These calculations reinforce a point made earlier: The stronger the correlation, the better is the prediction; the stronger the correla-

tion, the greater is the percentage of variance explained.

Multiple Linear Regression

Because the correlation between two variables is rarely perfect, it is often desirable to try to improve one's ability to predict a *Y* value by including more than one *X* as predictor variables. Suppose that we were interested in predicting graduate nursing students' grade-point averages (GPA). Because there are a limited number of students who can be accepted into graduate programs, there is naturally a concern for selecting those individuals who will have the greatest chance of success. Suppose that, from previous experience, it had been found that those students who performed well on the verbal portion of the Graduate Record Examination (GRE) tended to obtain higher grades in graduate school than those with lower GRE scores. The correlation between the GRE verbal scores (GRE-V) and graduate GPAs has been calculated as .50. With only 25% (.50^2) of the variance of graduate GPA accounted for, there will be many errors of prediction: many admitted students will not perform as well as desired, and many rejected applicants would have made successful students. It may be possible, by using additional information about students, to make more accurate predictions. Multiple regression can assist us by developing an equation that provides the best prediction possible, given the correlations among several variables. The basic multiple regression equation is

$$Y' = a + b_1X_1 + b_2X_2 + \ldots b_kX_k$$

where Y' = predicted value for variable Y
a = intercept constant
k = number of predictor (independent) variables
b_1 to b_k = regression coefficients for the k variables
X_1 to X_k = scores or values on the k independent variables

When the number of predictor variables exceeds two, the computations required to solve this equation are prohibitively laborious and complex. Therefore, we will restrict our discussion to hypothetical rather than worked-out examples.

In the example in which we wished to predict graduate nursing students' GPAs, suppose we decided that information on undergraduate GPA (GPA-U) and scores on the quantitative portion of the GRE (GRE-Q) would improve our ability to predict graduate GPA. The resulting equation might be

$$Y' = .4 + .05(\text{GPA-U}) + .003(\text{GRE-Q}) + .002(\text{GRE-V})$$

For instance, suppose an applicant had a GRE-V score of 600, a GRE-Q score of 550, and a GPA-U of 3.2. The predicted graduate GPA would be

$$Y' = .4 + (.05)(3.2) + .003(550) + .002(600) = 3.41$$

We can assess the degree to which the addition of two independent variables improved our ability to predict graduate school performance through the use of the multiple correlation coefficient. In bivariate correlation, the index expressing the magnitude of a relationship is Pearson's r. When two or more independent variables are used, the index of correlation is the **multiple correlation coefficient**, symbolized as **R**. Unlike r, R does not have negative values. R varies only from .00 to 1.00, showing the *strength* of the relationship between several independent variables and a dependent variable but not *direction*. It would make no sense to indicate direction, because X_1 could be positively related to Y, and X_2 could be negatively related to Y. The R statistic, when squared, indicates the proportion of variance in Y accounted for by the combined simultaneous influence of the independent variables. Sometimes, R^2 is referred to as the **coefficient of determination**.

The calculation of R^2 provides a direct means of evaluating the accuracy of the prediction equation. Let us say that with the three predictor variables used in the current example, the value of $R = .71$. This means that 50% ($.71^2$) of the variability in graduate students' grades can be explained in terms of their verbal and quantitative GRE scores and their undergraduate grades. The addition of two predictors doubled the variance accounted for by the single independent variable, from .25 to .50.

The multiple correlation coefficient cannot be less than the highest bivariate correlation between the dependent variable and one of the independent variables. Table 20-2 presents a correlation matrix that shows the Pearson correlation coefficients for all the variables in this example, taken as pairs. The independent variable that is correlated most strongly with graduate performance is GPA-U, $r = .60$. The value of R could not have been less than .60.

Another important point is that R tends to be larger when the independent variables have relatively low correlations among themselves. In the current case, the lowest correlation coefficient is between GRE-Q and GPA-U ($r = .40$), and the highest is between GRE-Q and

TABLE 20-2 Correlation Matrix

	GPA-GRAD	GPA-U	GRE-Q	GRE-V
GPA-GRAD	1.00			
GPA-U	.60	1.00		
GRE-Q	.55	.40	1.00	
GRE-V	.50	.50	.70	1.00

GPA-GRAD, graduate GPA; GPA-U, undergraduate GPA; GRE-Q, GRE quantitative score; GRE-V, GRE verbal score.

GRE-V ($r = .70$). All correlations here are fairly substantial, a fact that helps to explain why R is not much higher than the r between the dependent variable and undergraduate grades alone (.71 compared with .60). This somewhat puzzling phenomenon can be explained in terms of redundancy of information among predictors. When the correlations among the independent variables are high, they tend to add little predictive power to each other because they are redundant. When the correlations among the predictor variables are low, each variable has the ability to contribute something unique to the prediction of the dependent variable.

In Figure 20-2, a Venn diagram illustrates this concept. Each circle represents the total variability inherent in a variable. The circle on

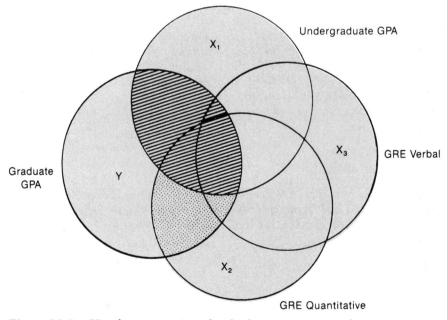

Figure 20-2. Visual representation of multiple regression example.

the left (Y) is the dependent variable, graduate GPA, whose values we are trying to predict. The overlap between this circle and the other circles represents the amount of variability that the variables have in common. If the overlap were complete—that is, if the entire graduate GPA circle were covered by the other circles—then R would equal 1.00. As it is, only 50% of the circle is covered, because $R^2 = .50$. The hatched area on this figure designates the independent contribution of undergraduate GPA toward explaining graduate performance. This contribution amounts to 36% of Y's variance ($.60^2$). The remaining two independent variables do not contribute as much as one would anticipate by considering their bivariate correlation with graduate GPA (r for GRE-V = .50; r for GRE-Q = .55). In fact, their combined additional contribution is only 14% ($.50 - .36 = .14$), designated by the dotted area on the figure. The contribution is small because the two GRE scores have redundant information once the undergraduate grades are taken into account.

A related point about multiple correlation is that, as more independent variables are added to the regression equation, the increment to R tends to decrease. It is rare to find many predictor variables that correlate well with a criterion measure and correlate only slightly with one another. Redundancy is difficult to avoid as more and more variables are added to the prediction equation. The inclusion of independent variables beyond the first four or five typically does little to improve the proportion of variance accounted for or the accuracy of prediction.

The dependent variable in multiple regression analysis, as in analysis of variance (ANOVA), should as a rule be measured on an interval or ratio scale. The independent variables, on the other hand, can either be continuous interval-level or ratio-level variables *or* dichotomous variables. A text such as that by Polit (1996) should be consulted for information on how to handle and interpret dichotomous **dummy variables.**

TESTS OF SIGNIFICANCE

In multiple correlation, as in bivariate correlation, researchers wishing to generalize their results must ask, Is the calculated R the result of chance fluctuations, or is does it reflect true (i.e., statistically significant) relationships? To test the null hypothesis that the population multiple correlation coefficient is equal to zero, we can compute a statistic that can be compared with tabled values for the F distribution.

We stated in Chapter 19 that the general form for calculating an F-ratio is as follows:

$$F = \frac{SS_{between}/df_{between}}{SS_{within}/df_{within}}$$

In the case of multiple regression, the form is similar:

$$F = \frac{SS_{due\ to\ regression}/df_{regression}}{SS_{of\ residuals}/df_{residuals}}$$

In both cases, the basic principle is the same: The variance resulting from the independent variables is contrasted with variance attributable to other factors or error. To calculate the F-statistic for regression, we can use the following alternative formula:

$$F = \frac{R^2/k}{(1 - R^2)/(N - k - 1)}$$

where k = number of predictor variables
N = total sample size

In the example relating to the prediction of graduate GPAs, suppose that a multiple correlation coefficient of .71 (an R^2 of .50) had been calculated for a sample of 100 graduate students. The value of the F-statistic would be

$$F = \frac{.50/3}{.50/96} = 32.05$$

The tabled value of F with 3 and 96 degrees of freedom for a significance level of .01 is about 4.0. Thus, the probability that the R of .71 resulted from chance fluctuations is considerably less than .01.

Another question that researchers often seek to answer is: Does adding X_k to the regression equation significantly add to the prediction of Y over that which is possible with X_{k-1}? In other words, how effective is, say, a third predictor in increasing our ability to predict Y after two predictors have already been used? An F-statistic can also be computed for answering this question.

Let us number each independent variable in the example at hand, in order according to its correlation with Y: $X_1 = $ GPA-U; $X_2 = $ GRE-Q; and $X_3 = $ GRE-V. We can then symbolize various correlation coefficients as follows:

$R_{y.1} = $ the correlation of Y with GPA-U
$R_{y.12} = $ the correlation of Y with GPA-U *and* GRE-Q
$R_{y.123} = $ the correlation of Y with all three predictors

The values of these Rs are as follows:

$R_{y.1} = .60$	$R^2_{y.1} = .36$
$R_{y.12} = .71$	$R^2_{y.12} = .50$
$R_{y.123} = .71$	$R^2_{y.123} = .50$

These figures show at a glance that the GRE-V scores made no independent contribution to the multiple correlation coefficient. The value of $R_{y.12}$ is identical to the value of $R_{y.123}$. Figure 20-2 illustrates this point: if the circle for GRE-V were completely removed, then the area of the Y circle covered by X_1 and X_2 would remain the same.

We cannot tell at a glance, however, whether adding X_2 to X_1 *significantly* increases the prediction of Y. What we want to know, in effect, is whether X_2 would be likely to improve predictions in a new sample, or if its added predictive power in this particular sample resulted from chance. The general formula for the F-statistic for testing the significance of variables added to the regression equation is

$$F = \frac{(R^2_{y.12...k_1} - R^2_{y.12...k_2})/(k_1 - k_2)}{(1 - R^2_{y.12...k_1})/(N - k_1 - 1)}$$

where $R^2_{y.12...k_1} = $ squared multiple correlation coefficient for Y correlated with k_1 predictor variables
$\qquad k_1 = $ the number of predictors for the larger of the two sets of predictors
$R^2_{y.12...k_2} = $ squared R for Y correlated with k_2 predictor variables
$\qquad k_2 = $ the number of predictors for the smaller of the two sets of predictors

In the current example, the calculated F-statistic for testing whether the addition of GRE-Q scores results in significant improvement of prediction over GPA-U alone would be

$$F = \frac{(.50 - .36)/1}{.50/97} = 27.16$$

Consulting Table B-2 in Appendix B, we find that with $df = 1$ and 97 and a significance level of .01, the critical value is about 6.90. Therefore, the addition of GRE-Q to the regression equation significantly improved the accuracy of predictions of GPA-GRAD, beyond the .01 level of significance.

STEPWISE MULTIPLE REGRESSION

If the researcher had 10 independent variables available for use in a regression equation, then the process of testing all possible combinations to determine which set of variables was significant and yielded the highest R^2 would be exceedingly time-consuming. **Stepwise multiple regression** is a method by which all potential predictors can be considered and through which the combination of variables providing the most predictive power can be chosen.

In stepwise multiple regression, predictors are stepped into the regression equation sequentially, in the order that produces the greatest increments to R^2. The first step involves the selection of the single best predictor of the dependent variable, which is the independent variable with the highest bivariate correlation coefficient with Y. The second variable to enter the regression equation is the one that produces the largest increase to R^2 when used simultaneously with the variable selected in the first step. The procedure continues until no additional predictor can significantly increase the value of R^2.

The basic principles of stepwise multiple regression are illustrated in Figure 20-3. The first variable to enter the regression, X_1, is correlated .60 with Y ($r^2 = .36$). No other predictor variable is correlated more strongly with the dependent variable. The variable X_1 accounts for the portion of the variability of Y represented by the hatched area in step 1 of the figure. This hatched area is, in effect, removed from further consideration as far as subsequent predictors are concerned. This portion of Y's variability is explained or accounted for. Therefore, the variable chosen in step 2 is not necessarily the X variable with the second largest correlation with Y. The selected variable is the predictor that explains the largest portion of what *remains* of Y's variability after X_1 has

been taken into account. Variable X_2, in turn, removes a second part of Y so that the independent variable selected in step 3 is the variable that accounts for the most variability in Y after *both* X_1 and X_2 are removed.

RELATIVE CONTRIBUTION OF PREDICTORS

Scientists are concerned not only about the prediction of phenomena but also about their explanation. Predictions can be made in the absence of understanding. For instance, in our graduate school example, we could predict performance moderately well without really understanding how the variables were functioning or what underlying factors were responsible for students' success. For practical applications, it may be sufficient to make accurate predictions, but scientists typically desire to understand phenomena and to make contributions to knowledge.

In multiple regression problems, one aspect of understanding the phenomenon under investigation is the determination of the relative importance of the independent variables. Unfortunately, the problem of determining the relative contributions of various independent variables

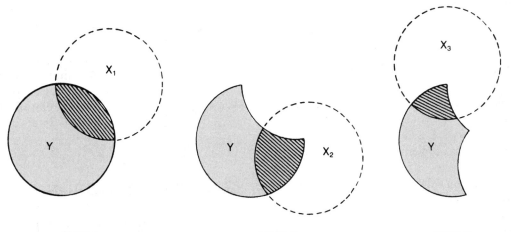

STEP 1 **STEP 2** **STEP 3**

Figure 20-3. Visual representation of stepwise multiple regression analysis.

in predicting a dependent variable is one of the thorniest issues in regression analysis. When the independent variables are correlated, as they usually are, there is no ideal way to disentangle the effects of the variables in the equation.

It may appear that a solution can be found by comparing the contributions of the independent variables to R^2. In our graduate school example, GPA-U accounted for 36% of Y's variance, and GRE-Q explained an additional 14% of the variance. Should we conclude that undergraduate grades are about two and one half times as important as GRE-Q scores in explaining graduate school grades? This conclusion would be inaccurate because the order of entry of variables in a regression equation affects their apparent contribution. If these two predictor variables were entered in reverse order, with GRE-Q first, then the R^2 would remain unchanged at .50; but GRE-Q's share would then be .30 ($.55^2$), and GPA-U's contribution would be .20 ($.50 - .30$). This circumstance results from the fact that whatever variance the independent variables have in common is attributed to the first variable entered in the regression analysis.

Another approach to assessing the relative importance of the predictors is to compare the regression coefficients. Earlier, the regression equation was given as

$$Y' = a + b_1X_1 + b_2X_2 + ... b_kX_k$$

where b_1 to b_k = regression coefficients

These b values are not directly comparable because they are in the units of raw scores, which differ from one X to another. X_1 might be in milliliters, X_2 in degrees Fahrenheit, and so forth. The use of **standard scores** (or z scores) eliminates this problem by transforming all variables to scores with a mean of 0.0 and a standard deviation (SD) of 1.00. The formula that accomplishes this standardization* is

$$z_X = \frac{X - \overline{X}}{SD_X}$$

In standard score form, the regression equation is

$$z_{Y'} = \beta_1 z_{X_1} + \beta_2 z_{X_2} + ... \beta_k z_{X_k}$$

where $z_{Y'}$ = predicted value of the standard score for Y

β_1 to β_k = standardized regression weights for k independent variables

z_{X_1} to z_{X_k} = standard scores for the k predictors

With all the βs (referred to as **beta [β] weights**) in the same measurement units, is it possible that their relative size could shed light on how much weight or importance to attach to the predictor variables? Many researchers have interpreted beta weights in this fashion, but there are problems in doing so. These regression coefficients will be the same no matter what the order of entry of the variables. The difficulty, however, is that regression weights are highly unstable. The values of β tend to fluctuate considerably from sample to sample. Moreover, when a variable is added to or subtracted from the regression equation, the beta weights change. Because there is nothing absolute about the values of the regression coefficients, it is difficult to attach much theoretical importance to them.

Another method of disentangling relationships is through causal modeling, which represents an important tool in the testing of theoretical expectations about relationships. Causal modeling is described later in this chapter.

ANALYSIS OF COVARIANCE

A significant portion of this chapter has been devoted to multiple regression analysis both because it is the most widely used multivariate

---

*For a complete discussion of standard scores, an elementary statistical text should be consulted.

technique and because an understanding of it should facilitate comprehension of other related multivariate statistics. **Analysis of covariance (ANCOVA)** is a good example of a related procedure: it combines features of ANOVA and regression.

Uses of Analysis of Covariance

A central feature of ANCOVA is that it permits statistical control of extraneous variables, as indicated in Chapter 9. ANCOVA is especially appropriate in certain types of research situations. For example, when random assignment to treatment groups is not feasible, a quasi-experimental design is often adopted. The initial equivalency of the comparison groups in such studies is always questionable; therefore, the researcher has to consider whether the obtained results were influenced by preexisting differences between the experimental and comparison groups. When experimental control, such as the ability to randomize, is lacking, ANCOVA offers the possibility of post hoc statistical control. Even in true experiments, ANCOVA can play a role in permitting a more precise estimate of group differences. This is because even when randomization procedures are used, there are typically slight differences between groups. ANCOVA can adjust for initial differences so that the final analysis will reflect more precisely the effect of an experimental intervention.

In both these situations, the researcher is concerned with the possibility that the comparison groups differ in some respect at the beginning of the study. That is, the groups may differ with regard to an attribute or attributes that affect the dependent variable and thereby obscure the relationship between the independent and dependent variables.

Strictly speaking, ANCOVA should not be used with intact groups because one of the underlying assumptions of ANCOVA is randomization. However, this assumption is frequently violated because no other alternative analysis works as effectively. Random assignment should always be done when possible, but in many situations in which randomization is not feasible, ANCOVA could make an important contribution to the internal validity of a study.

Analysis of Covariance Procedures

To use ANCOVA, a researcher must anticipate the extraneous variables to be controlled and must measure them at the outset of the study. For instance, suppose a researcher wanted to test the effectiveness of biofeedback therapy on patients' anxiety. An experimental group in one hospital is exposed to the treatment, and a comparison group of patients in another hospital is not. If the researcher wanted to test the initial equivalence of the two groups, then the anxiety levels of all subjects could be measured both before and after the intervention. The initial anxiety score could be statistically controlled through ANCOVA. In such a situation, the posttest anxiety score is the dependent variable, experimental/comparison group status is the independent variable, and the pretest anxiety score is referred to as the **covariate**. Covariates can either be continuous variables (e.g., anxiety test scores) or dichotomous variables (male/female). However, in ANCOVA, the independent variables are always categorical, that is, nominal-level variables.

ANCOVA tests the significance of differences between group means after first adjusting the scores on the dependent variable to eliminate the effects of the covariate. The adjustment of scores uses regression procedures. In essence, the first step in ANCOVA is the same as the first step in a stepwise multiple regression analysis. The variability in the dependent measure that can be explained by the covariate is removed from further consideration. ANOVA is performed on what remains of Y's variability to see whether, once the covariate is controlled, significant differences between the groups remain. Figure 20-4 illustrates this two-step process. Pursuing the example just cited, Y would be patients' posttest anxiety

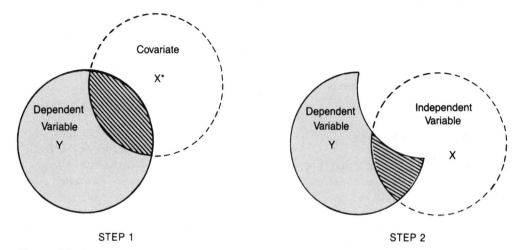

STEP 1   STEP 2

Figure 20-4.   Visual representation of analysis of covariance.

scores, the covariate X^* would be the pretest anxiety scores, and the independent variable X would designate whether the patients were exposed to the biofeedback therapy.

Another example may help to further explore aspects of the ANCOVA procedure. Suppose that we wanted to test the effectiveness of three different types of diets on overweight individuals. Although the sample of 30 subjects is randomly assigned to one of the three treatment groups, an ANCOVA, using pretreatment weights as the covariate, permits a more sensitive analysis of weight change than a simple ANOVA. Some hypothetical data for such a study are displayed in Table 20-3.

Two aspects of the weight scores in this table are immediately discernible. First, despite random assignment to the treatment groups, the initial group means are different. Subjects assigned to diet B differ from those assigned to diet C by an average of 10 pounds (175 versus 185 pounds). This difference is not significant* but rather reflects chance sampling fluctuations. Second, the posttreatment means are similarly different by a maximum of only 10

pounds. However, the mean number of pounds *lost* ranged from 10 pounds for diets A and B to 25 pounds for diet C.

An ordinary ANOVA for group differences in posttreatment means results in a nonsignificant *F*-value. The ANOVA summary table is presented in part A of Table 20-4. Based on the ANOVA results, we would conclude that all three diets had equal effects on weight loss.

Part B of Table 20-4 presents the summary table for the ANCOVA. The first step of the analysis breaks the total variability of the posttreatment weights into two components: (1) variability that can be accounted for by the covariate, the pretreatment weights; and (2) residual variability. As the table shows, the covariate accounted for a significant amount of the variance, which is not surprising in light of the strong relationship between the pretreatment and posttreatment weights ($r = .91$). This merely indicates that people who started out especially heavy (or light) tended to stay that way, relative to others in the sample. In the second phase of the analysis, the residual variance is broken down to reflect the between-group and within-group contributions. With 2 and 26 degrees of freedom, the *F* of 17.54 is significant beyond the .01 level. The

---

*Calculations demonstrating nonsignificance are not shown. The calculated $F = .45$. With 2 and 27 df, $p > .05$.

conclusion is that, after controlling for the initial weight of the subjects, there is a significant difference in weight loss resulting from exposure to different diets.

This fictitious example was deliberately contrived so that a result of "no difference" could be altered by the addition of a covariate to yield a significant difference. Most actual results are less dramatic than this example might suggest. Nonetheless, it is true that if the researcher can select meaningful covariates, then a more sensitive statistical test will always be made than if an ordinary ANOVA were performed. The increase in sensitivity results from the fact that the covariate reduces the error term (the within-group variability) against which treatment effects are compared. In part A of Table 20-4, it can be seen that the within-group term is extremely large, thereby masking the contribution made by the experimental treatments.

Theoretically, it is possible to use any number of covariates. It is probably unwise, however, to use more than five or six in practice. For one thing, the inclusion of more than five or six covariates is probably unnecessary be-cause of the typically high degree of redundancy beyond the first few variables. Moreover, it may be to the researcher's disadvantage to add covariates that do not explain a statistically significant portion of the variability of a dependent variable. Each covariate uses up a degree of freedom, leaving the balance for the within-group term. Fewer degrees of freedom means that a higher computed F is required for significance. For instance, with 2 and 26 df, an F of 5.53 is required for significance at the .01 level, but with 2 and 23 df (i.e., adding three covariates), an F of 5.66 is needed.

Adjusted Means

As shown in part B of Table 20-4, an ANCOVA table provides information relating to significance testing. The table indicates that at least one of the three groups had a posttreatment weight that is significantly different from the overall grand mean, after adjusting for pretreatment weights. Sometimes, it is extremely useful to examine **adjusted means**, that is, mean values on the dependent variable by group, after adjusting for (i.e., removing the effect of)

TABLE 20-3 Fictitious Data for ANCOVA Example					
DIET A (X_A)		**DIET B (X_B)**		**DIET C (X_C)**	
X_A^*	Y_A	X_B^*	Y_B	X_C^*	Y_C
195	185	205	200	175	160
180	170	150	140	210	165
160	150	145	135	150	130
215	200	210	190	185	170
155	145	185	185	205	180
205	195	160	150	190	165
175	165	190	175	160	135
180	170	165	150	165	140
140	135	180	165	180	160
195	185	160	160	230	195
1800	1700	1750	1650	1850	1600
$\overline{X}_A^* = 180.0$	$\overline{Y}_A = 170.0$	$\overline{X}_B^* = 175.0$	$\overline{Y}_B = 165.0$	$\overline{X}_C^* = 185.0$	$\overline{Y}_C = 160.0$

X, independent variable (diet); X*, covariate (pretreatment weight); Y, dependent variable (posttreatment weight).

TABLE 20-4 Comparison of ANOVA and ANCOVA Results

SOURCE OF VARIATION	SUM OF SQUARES	DF	MEAN SQUARE	F	P
A. SUMMARY TABLE FOR ANOVA					
Between groups	500.0	2	250.0	0.55	> .05
Within groups	12,300.0	27	455.6		
TOTAL	12,800.0	29			
B. SUMMARY TABLE FOR ANCOVA					
Step 1 { Covariate	10,563.1	1	10,563.1	132.23	< .01
Residual	2236.9	28	79.9		
TOTAL	12,800.0	29			
Step 2 { Between groups	1284.8	2	642.4	17.54	< .01
Within groups	952.1	26	36.6		
TOTAL	2236.9	28			

covariates. Means can be adjusted through a process that is sometimes referred to as **multiple classification analysis** (MCA). Adjusted means allow researchers to observe **net effects** (i.e., group differences on the dependent variable that are *net* of the effect of the covariate.)

MCA is a versatile supplement to ANCOVA (and multiple regression) that produces information about the mean value of a dependent variable after adjustment for covariates, for every level of one or more independent variables. MCA is versatile because it allows for dichotomous or continuous covariates, correlated independent variables or covariates, and nonlinear relationships between dependent and predictor variables. A subsequent section of this chapter, which discusses computer examples of multivariate statistics, provides more information about adjusted means.

FACTOR ANALYSIS

Factor analysis is a somewhat controversial multivariate procedure because it involves a

higher degree of subjectivity than one ordinarily finds in a statistical technique. It is, nevertheless, a highly powerful and widely applied procedure and, therefore, merits attention.

Factor analysis* is similar to the other multivariate procedures thus far described in that factor analysis also involves the formation of linear combinations of variables. However, the major purpose of factor analysis is to reduce a large set of variables into a smaller, more manageable set of measures, and not to test hypotheses. Factor analysis disentangles complex interrelationships among variables and identifies which variables "go together" as unified concepts. The underlying dimensions thus identified are called factors.

As an example, consider a researcher who has prepared 100 Likert-type items aimed at measuring women's attitudes toward meno-

---

*This section deals with a type of factor analysis that has come to be known as **exploratory factor analysis**. Another type—**confirmatory factor analysis**—uses more complex modeling and estimation procedures and more sophisticated computer programs, as briefly described in a subsequent section.

pause. Suppose that the research goal was to compare the attitudes of premenopausal and postmenopausal women. If the researcher does not combine some of the items to form a scale, it would be necessary to perform 100 separate statistical tests (such as chi-square tests or Mann Whitney *U*-tests) comparing the two groups of women on the 100 items. The formation of a scale is preferable, but it involves adding together the scores from several individual items. The problem is, which items are to be combined? Would it be meaningful to combine all 100 items? Probably not, because the 100 items are not all tapping exactly the same thing. There are various aspects or themes to a woman's attitude toward menopause. One aspect may relate to the aging process, and another aspect is concerned with a loss of the ability to reproduce. Other questions may touch on the general issue of sexuality, and yet others may concern avoidance of monthly pain or bother. There are, in short, multiple dimensions to the issue of attitudes toward menopause, and each dimension should be captured by a separate scale; a woman's attitude toward one dimension may be independent of her attitude toward another. The identification of these dimensions can be made a priori by the researcher, but the difficulty is that different researchers may read different concepts into the items. Factor analysis offers an empirical method of elucidating the underlying dimensionality of a large number of measures.

A factor, mathematically, is a linear combination of the variables in a data matrix. A data matrix contains the scores of N people on k different measures. For instance, a factor might be defined by the following equation:

$$F = b_1 X_1 + b_2 X_2 + b_3 X_3 + \ldots b_k X_k$$

where F = a factor score
X_1 to X_k = values on the k original variables
b_1 to b_k = weights

The development of such an equation for a factor permits the reduction of the X_k scores to one or more factor scores.

Factor Extraction

Most factor analyses consist of two separate phases. The first step is to condense the variables in the data matrix into a smaller number of factors. This first phase is sometimes referred to as the **factor extraction phase**. The factors usually are derived from the intercorrelations among the variables in the correlation matrix. The general goal is to extract clusters of highly interrelated variables within the matrix. There are various methods of performing the first step, each of which uses different criteria for assigning weights to the variables. Probably the most widely used method of factor extraction is called **principal components** (or principal factor or principal axes), but other methods that a researcher may come across are the image, alpha, centroid, maximum likelihood, and canonical techniques.

The result of the first step of the factor analysis is a **factor matrix** (sometimes called the **unrotated factor matrix**), which contains coefficients or weights for each variable in the original data matrix on each extracted factor. Because unrotated factor matrixes are difficult to interpret, we will postpone a detailed discussion of factor matrixes until the second factor analysis phase is described. In the principal components method, weights for the first factor are defined such that the average squared weight is a maximum, thereby permitting a maximal amount of variance to be extracted by the first factor. The second factor, or linear combination, is formed in such a way that the highest possible amount of variance is again extracted from what *remains* after the first factor has been taken into account. The factors thus delineated represent independent sources of variation in the data matrix.

In extracting factors in this fashion, some criterion must be applied to delimit the number of factors or underlying dimensions. Factoring should continue until there is no further meaningful variance left. There are several criteria available from which the researcher can choose to specify when factoring should cease. It is partly the availability of so many different criteria or justifications for halting factor extraction that makes factor analysis a semisubjective process. Several of the most commonly used criteria can be described by illustrating information that is usually output from factor analysis programs. Table 20-5 presents hypothetical values for eigenvalues, percentages of variance accounted for, and cumulative percentages of variance accounted for, for 10 factors. **Eigenvalues** are values equal to the sum of the squared weights for each factor. Many researchers establish as their cutoff point for factor extraction eigenvalues greater than 1.00. In the example in the table, this would mean that the first five factors or dimensions would meet this criterion. Another cutoff rule that is sometimes adopted is a minimum of 5% of explained variance, in which case six factors would qualify for inclusion in our current example. Yet another criterion is based on a principle of discontinuity. According to this procedure, a sharp drop in the percentage of explained variance indicates the appropriate termination point. In Table 20-5, one might argue that there is considerable discontinuity between the third and fourth factors. The general consensus appears to be that

it is probably better to extract too many factors than too few.

Factor Rotation

The factor matrix produced in the first phase of factor analysis is usually difficult to interpret. For this reason, a second phase, known as **factor rotation**, is almost invariably performed on those factors that have met one or more of the criteria for inclusion. The concept of rotation is complex and can be best explained graphically. Figure 20-5 shows two coordinate systems, marked by axes A1 and A2 and B1 and B2. The primary axes (A1 and A2) represent factors I and II, respectively, as they are defined before rotation. The points 1 through 6 represent six variables in this two-dimensional space. The weights associated with each variable can be determined in reference to the appropriate axis. For instance, before rotation, variable 1 is assigned a weight of .80 on factor I and .85 on factor II, and variable 6 has a weight of −.45 on factor I and .90 on factor II. The unrotated axes are designed to account for a maximum of variance but rarely provide a structure that has conceptual meaning. However, by rotating the axes in such a way that clusters of variables are distinctly associated with a factor, inter-

TABLE 20-5	Summary of Factor Extraction Results		
FACTOR	**EIGENVALUE**	**PERCENTAGE OF VARIANCE EXPLAINED**	**CUMULATIVE PERCENTAGE OF VARIANCE EXPLAINED**
1	12.32	29.2	29.2
2	8.57	23.3	52.5
3	6.91	15.6	68.1
4	2.02	8.4	76.5
5	1.09	6.2	82.7
6	.98	5.8	88.5
7	.80	4.5	93.0
8	.62	3.1	96.1
9	.47	2.2	98.3
10	.25	1.7	100.0

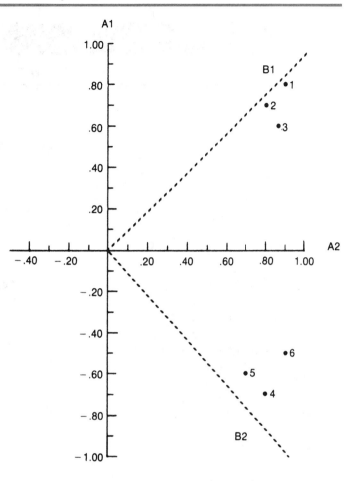

Figure 20-5. Illustration of factor rotation

pretability is enhanced. In the figure, B1 and B2 represent the rotated factors. The rotation has been performed in such a way that variables 1, 2, and 3 would be assigned large weights on factor I and small weights on factor II, and the reverse would be true for variables 4, 5, and 6.

The researcher must choose from two general classes of rotation procedures. Figure 20-5 illustrates **orthogonal rotation,** in which the factors are kept at right angles to one another. Orthogonal rotations maintain the independence of factors. That is, orthogonal factors are uncorrelated with one another. **Oblique rotations,** on the other hand, permit the rotated axes to depart from a 90-degree angle. In our figure, an oblique rotation would have put

axis B1 between variables 2 and 3 and axis B2 between variables 5 and 6. This placement of the axes strengthens the clustering of variables around an associated factor. The result is that oblique rotation produces correlated factors. Some researchers insist that orthogonal rotation leads to greater theoretical clarity; others claim that it is unrealistic. Those advocating oblique rotation point out that if the concepts *are* correlated, then the analysis should be permitted to reflect this fact. In practice, studies have revealed that similar conclusions are often reached by both rotational procedures.

The **rotated factor matrix** is what the researcher normally works with in interpreting the factor analysis. An example of such a matrix is displayed in Table 20-6 for discussion

TABLE 20-6	Rotated Factor Matrix		
VARIABLE	**FACTOR I**	**FACTOR II**	**FACTOR III**
1	.75	.15	.23
2	−.02	.61	.18
3	−.59	−.11	.03
4	.05	.08	.48
5	.21	.79	.02
6	−.07	−.52	−.29
7	.08	.19	.80
8	.68	.12	−.01
9	−.04	.08	−.61
10	−.43	−.13	.06

purposes. To make this discussion less abstract, let us say that the 10 variables listed in the table are the first 10 of the 100 items measuring attitudes toward menopause. The entries under each factor are the weights on that factor, which are called **factor loadings**. For orthogonally rotated factors, factor loadings can be readily interpreted. Like correlation coefficients, they range from −1.00 to +1.00. In fact, they can be interpreted in much the same way as a correlation coefficient. Factor loadings express the correlations between individual variables and factors (underlying dimensions). In this example, variable 1 is fairly highly correlated with factor 1, .75. Therefore, it is possible to find which variables "belong" to a factor. For factor I, variables 1, 3, 8, and 10 have fairly sizable loadings. Normally, a cutoff value of about .40 or .30 is used for such determinations. The researcher is now in a position to interpret the underlying dimensionality of the data. By inspecting items 1, 3, 8, and 10, it is usually possible to find some common theme that makes the variables go together. Perhaps these four questions have to do with the link between menopause and infertility, and perhaps items 2, 5, and 6 (i.e., the items with high loadings on factor II) are related to sexuality. The naming of factors is essentially a process of identifying theoretical constructs.

Factor Scores

In some cases in which the main purpose of factor analysis is to delineate the conceptual makeup of a set of measures, the analysis may end at this point. Frequently, however, the researcher wants to use the information obtained to develop **factor scores** for use in subsequent analyses. For instance, the factor analysis of the 100 menopause items might demonstrate that there are five principal dimensions or concepts being tapped. By reducing 100 variables to 5 new variables, the analysis of differences between premenopausal and postmenopausal women using some procedure such as *t*-tests or ANCOVA will be greatly simplified.

Several methods can be used to form factor scores. One procedure is to weight the variables according to their factor loading on each factor. For example, a factor score for the first factor in Table 20-6 could be computed for each subject by the following formula:

$$F_1 = .75X_1 - .02X_2 - .59X_3 + .05X_4 + .21X_5 - .07X_6 + .08X_7 + .68X_8 - .04X_9 - .43X_{10} \cdots b_{100}X_{100}$$

where the X values* = subject's scores on the 100 items

---

*Standardized (*z*) scores are often used in lieu of raw scores in computing factor scores when the means and standard deviations of the variables differ substantially.

Some factor analysis computer programs can directly compute this type of factor score.

A second method of obtaining factor scores is to select certain variables to represent the factor and to combine them with unit weighting. This composite estimate method would produce a factor score on the first factor of our example in the following fashion:

$$F_1 = X_1 - X_3 + X_8 - X_{10} \pm \ldots$$

The variables here are those with high loadings on factor I (the "$\pm \ldots$" indicates the inclusion of any of the other 90 variables with high loadings). This procedure is both computationally and conceptually simpler than the first approach; both have been found to yield similar results.

To illustrate the composite estimate approach more concretely, consider the rotated factor matrix in Table 20-6 and assume that factor scores were to be computed on the basis of this 10-item analysis, omitting for the sake of simplicity the remaining 90 items on the menopause scale. Suppose that two respondents had the following scores on these 10 items:

Subject 1: 7, 1, 1, 5, 1, 6, 7, 6, 3, 2
Subject 2: 2, 5, 6, 3, 7, 3, 2, 3, 4, 4

Factor I has fairly high loadings on variables 1, 3, 8, and 10. Thus, the two subjects' factor scores on factor 1 would be

$$7 - 1 + 6 - 2 = 10$$
$$2 - 6 + 3 - 4 = -5$$

The minus signs reflect the negative loadings on variables 3 and 10.* The same procedure would be performed for all three factors, yielding the following factor scores:

Subject 1: 10, −3, 9
Subject 2: −5, 9, 1

Factor scores would similarly be computed for all respondents, and these scores could then be used in the subsequent analyses as measures of different dimensions of attitudes toward menopause.

OTHER LEAST-SQUARES MULTIVARIATE TECHNIQUES

In addition to ANCOVA, several other multivariate techniques are closely related to least-squares multiple regression analysis. In this section, the methods known as discriminant function analysis, canonical correlation, and multivariate analysis of variance are introduced. The introduction is brief, and computations are entirely omitted because these procedures are exceedingly complex. The intent of this review is to acquaint the reader with the types of research situations for which these methods are appropriate. Advanced statistical texts such as the ones listed in the references may be consulted for additional information.

Discriminant Analysis

In multiple regression, the dependent variable being predicted is normally a measure on either the interval or ratio scale of measurement. The regression equation makes predictions about scores that take on a large range of values, such as heart rate, weight, or scores on a depression scale. **Discriminant analysis**, in contrast, makes predictions about membership in categories or groups. The purpose of the analysis is to distinguish groups from one another on the basis of available independent variables. For instance, we may wish to develop a means of predicting membership in or affiliation with such groups as complying versus noncomplying cancer patients, graduating nursing students versus dropouts, or normal

---

*Researchers forming scale scores with Likert items often reverse the direction of the scoring on negatively loaded items before forming the factor score to eliminate negative scores. Direction of an item can be reversed by subtracting the raw score from the sum of 1 + the maximum item value. For example, in a 7-point scale, a score of 2 would be reversed to 6 [(1 + 7) − 2]. When such reversals have been done, all raw scores can be added in forming factor scores.

pregnancies versus those terminating in a miscarriage.

Discriminant analysis develops a regression equation—called a **discriminant function**—for a categorical dependent variable, with independent variables that are either categorical or continuous. The researcher begins with data from subjects whose group membership is known. The intent is to develop an equation that can be used to predict membership for new subjects for whom only measures of the independent variables are available. The discriminant function indicates to which group each subject will probably belong.

Discriminant analysis that is used to predict membership into only two groups (e.g., nursing school dropouts versus graduates) is relatively simple and can be interpreted in much the same fashion as a multiple regression. When there are more than two groups or categories, the calculations and interpretations are more complicated. With three or more groups (e.g., very-low-birthweight, low-birthweight, and normal-birthweight infants), the number of discriminant functions is either the number of groups minus 1 or the number of independent variables, whichever is smaller. The first discriminant function is the linear combination of predictors that maximizes the ratio of between-group variance to within-group variance. The second function derived is the linear combination that maximizes this ratio, after the effect of the first function is removed. Because the independent variables are assigned different weights on the various functions, it is possible to develop theoretical interpretations based on the knowledge of which predictors are important in discriminating among different groups.

Discriminant analysis has several features in common with multiple regression analysis, aside from the fact that prediction equations based on a linear combination of independent variables are developed. For one thing, it is possible to use a stepwise approach in entering predictors into the equation. Also, the analysis produces an index designating the proportion of variance in the dependent variable accounted for by the predictor variables. The index is known as **Wilks' lambda** (λ). Actually, λ indicates the proportion of variance *unaccounted for* by predictors, or $\lambda = 1 - R^2$. In sum, discriminant analysis has potential for being useful to researchers, particularly those with practical problems of classification or diagnosis.

Canonical Correlation

Canonical correlation is the most general multivariate technique, of which other procedures are special cases. **Canonical correlation** analyzes the relationship between two or more independent variables and two or more dependent variables. Conceptually, one can think of this technique as an extension of multiple regression to more than one dependent variable. Mathematically and interpretatively, the gap between multiple regression and canonical correlation is greater than this statement suggests.

Like other techniques described thus far in this chapter, canonical correlation uses the least-squares principle to partition and analyze variance. Basically, two linear composites are developed, one of which is associated with the dependent variables, the other of which is for the independent variables. The relationship between the two linear composites is expressed by the **canonical correlation coefficient, R_C**. As in the case of the coefficient of determination (R^2), R^2_C indicates the proportion of variance accounted for in the analysis. When there is more than one source or dimension of covariation in the two sets of variables, more than one canonical correlation can be found.

Examples of research utilizing canonical correlation are not common. Perhaps the method is not well known, and it requires a higher degree of mathematic sophistication than is needed for most statistical techniques. Still, when a study involves multiple dependent and independent variables, canonical correlation may be the most suitable way to analyze the data.

Multivariate Analysis of Variance

Multivariate analysis of variance, sometimes abbreviated **MANOVA**, is the extension of ANOVA procedures to more than one dependent variable. This procedure is used primarily to test the significance of differences between the means of two or more dependent variables, considered simultaneously. Like ordinary ANOVA, MANOVA was developed for use in experimental situations in which at least one independent variable was manipulated. For instance, if we wanted to examine the effect of two methods of exercise (A_1 and A_2) and two lengths of exercise treatment (B_1 and B_2) on both diastolic and systolic blood pressure (Y_1 and Y_2), then a MANOVA would be appropriate. Researchers often analyze such data by performing two separate univariate ANOVAs. Strictly speaking, this practice is incorrect. Separate ANOVAs imply that the dependent variables have been obtained independently of one another. In fact, the dependent measures have been obtained from the same subjects and are, therefore, correlated. MANOVA takes the intercorrelations of the dependent variables into account in computing the test statistics. However, ANOVA is a more widely understood procedure than MANOVA, and thus its results may be more easily communicated to a broad audience.

MANOVA can be readily extended in ways analogous to ANOVA. For example, it is possible to perform **multivariate analysis of covariance** (**MANCOVA**), which allows for the control of extraneous variables (covariates) when there are two or more dependent variables. MANOVA can also be used in situations when there are repeated measures of the dependent variables (sometimes abbreviated **RMANOVA**).

Links Among Least-Squares Multivariate Techniques

The analogy might be made that multiple regression is to canonical correlation what ANOVA is to MANOVA. This analogy, although correct, obscures a point that the astute reader has perhaps already suspected, and that is the close affinity between multiple regression and ANOVA.

In fact, ANOVA and multiple regression are virtually identical. Both techniques are concerned with analyzing the total variability in a dependent measure and contrasting the proportion of the variability attributable to one or more independent variables with that attributable to unexplained sources of variation, or error. Multiple regression and ANOVA use a different approach and use different symbols and terminology, but both analyses boil down to a final *F*-ratio. By tradition, experimental data are typically analyzed by ANOVA, and correlational data are analyzed by regression procedures. Nevertheless, any data for which ANOVA is appropriate could also be analyzed by multiple regression, although the reverse is not true. In many cases, multiple regression is preferable because it can be used with a broader range of data and because it provides more information, such as a prediction equation and an index of association, *R*. With respect to the index of association issue, however, a formula can easily be applied to ANOVA results to derive **eta-squared** (η^2), the statistic that summarizes, like R^2, the strength of association between variables. Eta-squared is simply the sum of squares between groups divided by the total sum of squares. The value of η^2 is computed routinely by most ANOVA computer programs.

CAUSAL MODELING

Causal modeling involves the development of a hypothesized causal explanation of a phenomenon and the testing of that explanation through statistical procedures. In a causal model, the researcher posits explanatory linkages among three or more variables and then tests whether the hypothesized pathways from the causes to the effect are consistent with the data. Causal modeling is a complex topic to which entire books have been devoted. Therefore, we briefly describe some of the key concepts of two approaches to causal modeling without discussing actual analytic procedures.

Path Analysis

Path analysis, which relies on multiple linear regression, is a method for studying patterns of causation among a set of variables in ex post facto studies. As discussed in Chapter 8, path analysis usually begins with a theory or causal model that dictates the type of data to be collected. It is not a method for discovering causes; rather, it is a method applied to a prespecified model formulated on the basis of prior knowledge and theory.

Path analytic reports often use a **path diagram** to display their results; we use such a diagram (Fig. 20-6) here to illustrate important concepts. This model postulates that the dependent variable, patients' length of hospitalization (V4), is the result of their capacity for self-care (V3); this, in turn, is affected by nursing actions (V1) and the severity of their illness (V2).

In path analysis, a distinction is often made between exogenous and endogenous variables. An **exogenous variable** is a variable whose determinants lie outside the model. In Figure 20-6, nursing actions (V1) and illness severity (V2) are exogenous; no attempt is made in the model to elucidate what causes different nursing actions or different degrees of illness. An **endogenous variable,** by contrast, is one whose variation is determined by other variables in the model. In our example, self-care capacity (V3) and length of hospitalization (V4) are endogenous.

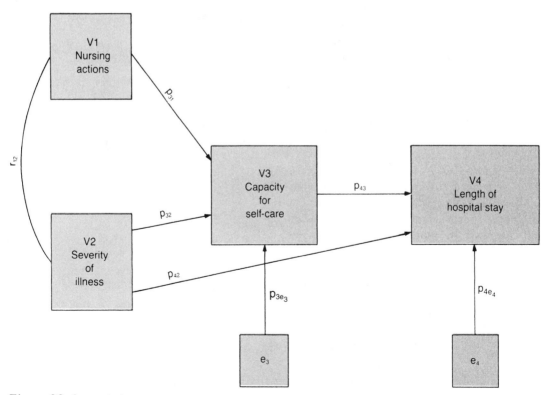

Figure 20-6. Path diagram.

In path analysis, causal linkages are illustrated by arrows, drawn from the presumed causes to the presumed effects. In our illustration, severity of illness is hypothesized to affect length of hospitalization both directly (path p_{42}) and indirectly through the **mediating variable** self-care capacity (paths p_{32} and p_{43}). Correlated exogenous variables are indicated by curved lines, as shown by the curved line between nursing actions and illness severity.

Ideally, the model would totally explain the outcome of interest, which in this case is length of hospitalization. In practice, this almost never happens because causal theories are rarely comprehensive when dealing with human phenomena. There are usually other determinants, which are generally referred to as **residual variables.** In Figure 20-6, there are two boxes labeled *e*, which denote a composite of all determinants of self-care capacity and hospital stay that are not in the model. The residuals summarize our lack of understanding of other determinants of endogenous variables. If we can identify and measure additional causative forces and incorporate them into the overarching theory, then they should be in the model.

Figure 20-6 represents what is referred to as a **recursive model.** This means that the causal flow is unidirectional and without feedback loops. In other words, it is assumed that variable 2 is a cause of variable 3, and that variable 3 is *not* a cause of variable 2.

In Figure 20-6, causal paths are indicated by symbols denoting that a given variable (e.g., V3) is caused by another (e.g., V2), yielding a path labeled p_{32}. In research reports, the path symbols would be replaced by actual numbers developed by applying regression procedures. The numbers shown are called **path coefficients,** which are standardized partial regression slopes. For example, path p_{32} is equal to $\beta_{32.1}$—the beta weight between variables 2 and 3, holding variable 1 constant. Because path coefficients are in standard form, they indicate the proportion of a standard deviation difference in the caused variable that is

directly attributable to a 1.00-SD difference in the specified causal variable. Thus, the path coefficients give us some indication of the relative importance of various determinants.

Path analysis involves estimation of the path coefficients through the use of **structural equations.** The structural equations for Figure 20-6 are as follows:

$$z_1 = e_1$$
$$z_2 = e_2$$
$$z_3 = p_{31}z_1 + p_{32z2} + e_3; \text{ and}$$
$$z_4 = p_{43}z_3 + p_{42}z_2 + e_4$$

These equations indicate that z_1 and z_2 (standard scores for variables 1 and 2) are determined by outside variables; that z_3 depends directly on z_1 and z_2 plus outside variables; and that z_4 depends directly on z_2, z_3, and outside variables. In our example, the structural equations could be solved to yield path coefficients by performing two multiple regressions: by regressing variable 3 on variables 1 and 2; and by regressing variable 4 on variables 2 and 3.

The model presented in Figure 20-6 may or may not be a reasonable construction of the hospitalization process. Path analysis involves a number of procedures for testing causal models and for determining effects. Polit (1996) provides an overview of path analytic techniques, and the advanced student should refer to books such as that by Blalock (1972).

Linear Structural Relations Analysis—LISREL

One of the drawbacks of using ordinary least-squares regression in doing path analysis is that the validity of the method is based on a set of restrictive assumptions, most of which are virtually impossible to meet. First, it is assumed that the variables are measured without error. As we discussed in Chapter 17, most measures used by nurse researchers contain some degree of error. Second, it is assumed that any of the residuals (error terms) in the different regression equations are uncorrelated. However, because error terms often represent untapped sources of individual differences—differences that are not entirely random—this assumption is seldom tenable. Third, traditional path analysis assumes that the causal flow is unidirectional or recursive. In reality, causes and effects are often reciprocal or iterative.

A more general and powerful approach that avoids these problems is known as **linear structural relations analysis**, which is usually abbreviated as **LISREL**.* Unlike path analysis, LISREL can accommodate measurement errors, correlated errors, correlated residuals, and **nonrecursive models** that allow for reciprocal causation. Another attractive feature of LISREL is that it can be used to analyze causal models involving latent variables. A **latent variable** is an unmeasured variable that corresponds to an abstract construct in which the researcher is interested. For example, factor analysis yields information about underlying, latent dimensionalities that are not directly measured by the variables in the analysis. In LISREL, latent variables are captured by two or more measured variables—sometimes referred to as the **manifest variables**—that serve as indicators of the underlying construct.

Path analysis uses least-squares estimation with its associated assumptions and restrictions. LISREL, by contrast, uses a different estimation procedure known as **maximum likelihood estimation**. Although a full elaboration is beyond the scope of this text, we note that maximum likelihood estimators are ones that estimate the parameters most likely to have generated the observed measurements (Hanushek & Jackson, 1977).

LISREL proceeds in two sequential phases. In the first phase, a measurement model is tested. This first phase corresponds to a confirmatory factor analysis (CFA). When there is evidence of an adequate fit of the data to the hypothesized measurement model, the causal

model can be tested by structural equation modeling. The causal model is also subjected to a goodness-of-fit test before the overall analysis is considered complete.

THE MEASUREMENT MODEL PHASE

The **measurement model** stipulates the hypothesized relationships among the latent and manifest variables. In path analysis, it is assumed—unrealistically—that underlying constructs on the one hand and the scales or instruments used to measure them on the other are identical. In LISREL, the constructs are treated as unobserved variables measured by two or more fallible indicators. Thus, a major advantage of LISREL is that it enables the researcher to separate latent variables from errors, and to then proceed to study causal relationships among the latent variables. However, the process depends on the judicious selection of indicators. An inadequate selection of measured variables to represent a latent variable will lead to questions about whether the theory's constructs are really embedded in the causal model.

During the measurement model phase, LISREL tests three things: (1) causal relationships between the measured variables and latent variables; (2) correlations between pairs of latent variables; and (3) correlations among the errors associated with the measured variables. The measurement model is essentially a factor analytic model that seeks to confirm a hypothesized factor structure. Thus, loadings on the factors (latent variables) provide a method for evaluating relationships between the observed and unobserved variables.

We can illustrate with a simplified example that involves the relationship between two latent variables: a person's cognitive ability and academic success. In our example, depicted in Figure 20-7, cognitive ability is captured by two indicators: scores on the verbal and quantitative portions of the GRE. According to the model, people's test scores are *caused by* their cognitive ability (and thus the arrows indicating a hypothesized causal path) and are also

---

*LISREL is actually the name of a specific computer program for analyzing covariance structures and for performing structural equations modeling, but the software has come to be almost synonymous with the approach.

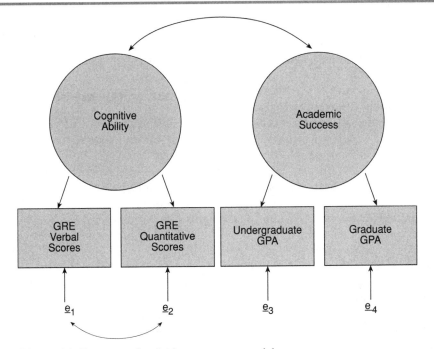

Figure 20-7.   Example of a measurement model.

affected by error (e_1 and e_2). Moreover, it is hypothesized that the error terms are correlated, as indicated by the curved line with double arrows connecting e_1 and e_2. Correlated measurement errors on the GRE might arise, for example, as a result of the person's test anxiety or level of fatigue—factors that would systematically depress test scores on both portions of the exam. The second latent variable is academic success, which is captured by undergraduate and graduate GPAs. The error terms associated with these two manifest variables are presumed not to be correlated. Within the measurement model, the two latent variables are hypothesized to be correlated.

After its specification, the hypothesized measurement model would be tested against the research data using LISREL. The analysis would provide information on loadings of the observed variables on the latent variables, the correlation between the two latent variables, and

the correlation between e_1 and e_2. The analysis would also indicate whether the overall model fit is good, based on a **goodness-of-fit statistic**. If the hypothesized model is not a good fit to the study data, the measurement model would need to be respecified and retested.

THE STRUCTURAL EQUATIONS MODEL PHASE

Once an adequate measurement model has been found, the second phase of the LISREL analysis can proceed. As in path analysis, the researcher must specify the theoretical causal model to be tested. As an example, we could use LISREL to test a causal model in which we hypothesized that the latent variable cognitive ability caused the latent variable academic success. The model to be tested would look similar to the one shown in Figure 20-7, except that there would be a straight line and an arrow (i.e., a path) from cognitive ability to academic success. There would also be another arrow leading to academic success representing the residual term.

In this part of the analysis, LISREL would yield information about the hypothesized causal parameters—that is, the path coefficients, which are presented as beta weights. The coefficients indicate the expected amount of change in the latent endogenous variable that is caused by a change in the latent causal variable. The LISREL program provides information on the significance of individual paths. The residual terms—the amount of unexplained variance for the latent endogenous variables—can also be calculated from the LISREL analysis. The overall fit of the causal model to the research data can be tested by means of several alternative statistics. Two such statistics that LISREL offers are the **goodness-of-fit index (GFI)** and the **adjusted goodness-of-fit index (AGFI)**. For both of these indexes, a value of .90 or greater indicates a good fit of the model to the data.

LISREL is an analytic approach that has gained considerable popularity among nurse researchers. However, it is a highly complex procedure, and its computer program (LISREL 7) is not easy to learn. Readers interested in further information on LISREL are urged to consult Jöreskog and Sörbom (1989) or Hayduk (1987).

OTHER MULTIVARIATE STATISTICAL PROCEDURES

The statistical procedures described in this chapter and in Chapters 18 and 19 cover most of the techniques for analyzing quantitative data used by nurse researchers today. However, the widespread use of computers and new developments in statistical analysis have combined to give researchers more options for analyzing their data than were available in the past. Although a full exposition of other sophisticated statistical procedures is beyond the scope of this book, we briefly describe a few of these advanced techniques and provide references for readers interested in more comprehensive discussions.

Life Table and Event History Analysis

Life table analysis is a procedure that is widely used by epidemiologists and medical researchers. It is used when the dependent variable represents the time interval between an initial event and a termination event. Life table analysis is often applied to situations in which mortality is the termination event—such as when the initial event is the onset of a disease or the initiation of treatment for the disease, and death is the end event. Because of this fact, life table analysis is also referred to as **survival analysis**. Life table analysis involves the calculation of a survival score, which compares the survival time for one subject with that for all other subjects. When the researcher is interested in group comparisons—for example, comparing the survival function of subjects in a special treatment versus a control group—a statistic can be computed to test the null hypothesis that the groups are samples from the same survival distribution.

Life table analysis can be applied to many situations that are unrelated to mortality. For example, a life table analysis could be used to analyze such time-related phenomena as length of time in labor, length of time elapsed between release from a psychiatric hospital and reinstitutionalization, and length of time between the termination of a first pregnancy and the onset of a second one. Further information about life table analysis may be found in Gross and Clark (1975) and Lee (1980).

More recently, extensions of life table analysis have been developed that allow researchers to examine the determinants of survival-type transitions in a multivariate framework. In these analyses, independent variables are used to model the risk (or hazard) of experiencing an event at a given point in time, given that one has not experienced the event before that time. The most common specification of the hazard is known as the **proportional hazards model**. These **event history** methodologies are likely to prove useful to nurse researchers in the future. A relatively straightforward explanation and illustration of this technique is presented in Teachman (1982), and further discussion may be found in Allison (1984) or Tuma and Hannan (1984).

Logistic Regression

Logistic regression (sometimes referred to as **logit analysis**) is a procedure that uses maximum likelihood estimation for analyzing relationships between multiple independent variables and a dependent variable that is categorical (i.e., a nominal-level measure). Logistic regression transforms the probability of an event occurring (e.g., that a woman will practice breast self-examination) into its odds. The **odds** of an event is defined as the ratio of two probabilities: the probability of an event occurring to the probability that it will not occur. As a result, probabilities that range between zero and one in actuality are transformed into continuous variables that range between zero and infinity. Because this range is still restricted, a further transformation is performed, namely calculating the logarithm of the odds. The range of this new variable (known as the **logit**) is now transformed from minus to plus infinity. Using the logit as a continuous dependent variable, maximum likelihood approaches are then used to estimate the coefficients of the independent variables. These techniques can also be used in the case of a categorical dependent variable that has more than two categories.

Logistic regression is based on the assumption that the underlying relationships among variables can be represented as an S-shaped probabilistic function—an assumption that is generally more tenable than the least-squares assumption of linearity and multivariate normality. Logistic regression thus is often more technically appropriate than discriminant analysis—although in practice, logistic regres-

sion and discriminant analysis often yield the same results. However, logistic regression may be better suited to many research questions because it is concerned with modeling the probability of an outcome rather than with the prediction of group membership. Also, logistic regression enables the researcher to generate odds ratios that can be meaningfully interpreted and graphically displayed. An **odds ratio** is the ratio of one odds to another odds and thus is an index of relative risk—that is, the risk of an event occurring given one condition, versus the risk of it occurring given a different condition. Although logit analysis was avoided by researchers for many years because of the unavailability of convenient computer programs, that is no longer the case.

THE COMPUTER AND MULTIVARIATE STATISTICS

Multivariate analyses are invariably done by computer because the computations are laborious. To illustrate computer analyses for two multivariate techniques, we return to the example described in Chapters 18 and 19, involving the implementation of a special prenatal intervention for low-income young women. All the data for the examples below were presented in Table 18–8.

Example of Multiple Regression

In Chapter 19, we tested the hypothesis that older mothers in the sample would have infants with higher birthweights than younger mothers, using Pearson's r. The computer calculated the value of r to be .5938, which was highly significant, thereby supporting the research hypothesis.

Suppose now that we want to test whether we can significantly improve our ability to predict infant birthweight by adding two other variables to the equation by means of multiple regression: whether or not the mother smoked

```
* * * *   M U L T I P L E   R E G R E S S I O N   * * * *

Correlation:

              WEIGHT      AGE       NPREGS      SMOKE

WEIGHT        1.000       .594       .324       -.244
AGE            .594      1.000       .522       -.301
NPREGS         .324       .522      1.000       -.054
SMOKE         -.244      -.301      -.054       1.000

Equation Number 1    Dependent Variable..   WEIGHT   INFANT BIRTH WEIGHT

Block Number  1.  Method: Stepwise     Criteria   PIN  .0500   POUT  .1000


Variable(s) Entered on Step Number
   1..   AGE        AGE OF MOTHER

Multiple R           .59383
R Square             .35264
Adjusted R Square    .32952
Standard Error      8.97022

Analysis of Variance
                    DF        Sum of Squares     Mean Square
Regression           1           1227.28336      1227.28336
Residual            28           2253.01664        80.46488

F =     15.25241       Signif F =  .0005


------------------ Variables in the Equation ------------------

Variable              B         SE B        Beta         T   Sig T

AGE            3.118890      .798603     .593833     3.905   .0005
(Constant)   48.040159    14.600097                  3.290   .0027

------------- Variables not in the Equation -------------

Variable      Beta In  Partial  Min Toler       T  Sig T

NPREGS         .019634  .020811   .727277     .108  .9147
SMOKE         -.072164 -.085540   .909592    -.446  .6591


End Block Number   1   PIN =     .050 Limits reached.
```

Figure 20-8. SPSS computer printout: multiple regression.

during the pregnancy (SMOKE), and the number of prior pregnancies (NPREGS). Figure 20-7 presents a part of the Statistical Package for the Social Sciences (SPSS) printout for a stepwise multiple regression in which WEIGHT is the dependent variable and in which AGE, SMOKE, and NPREGS are the predictor variables. We will explain some of the most noteworthy aspects of this printout.

Figure 20-8 shows (under Equation Number 1) that the first variable stepped into the regression equation is AGE and that the multiple $R = .59383$—the same value shown in Figure 19–6 in Chapter 19 for the bivariate correlation. The value of R^2 is .35264 ($.59383^2$), which represents the amount of variance in birthweight accounted for by the mother's age.* AGE was the first of the three available predictor variables stepped into the equation because it had the highest bivariate correlation with WEIGHT. (As shown in the correlation

---

*The adjusted R^2 of .32925 is the R^2 after it has been adjusted to reflect more closely the goodness of fit of the regression model in the population, through a formula that involves sample size and number of independent variables.

matrix at the top of Figure 20-7, the *r* between WEIGHT and NPREGS is .324, and the *r* between WEIGHT and SMOKE is −.244).

The next panel (under the Analysis of Variance) shows the calculation of the *F*-ratio in which the variability due to regression (i.e., to the relationship between WEIGHT and AGE) is contrasted with residual variability. The value of *F* (15.25241) with 1 and 28 *df* is significant at the .0005 level, consistent with the information from Figure 19–6.

The actual regression equation is presented in the next panel under Variables in the Equation. If we wanted to predict new values of WEIGHT from the same population as this sample based on maternal age at birth, the equation would be:

$$WEIGHT' = (3.118890 \times AGE) + 48.040159$$

That is, predicted values of WEIGHT would be equal to the regression coefficient (*b*) times values of AGE, plus the value of the intercept constant.

In regression, a statistical test can be performed for each regression coefficient by dividing *b* by the standard error for *b*; this is shown here under the columns T and Sig T. The value of T for the AGE coefficient is 3.905, which is significant at the .0005 level.

The final panel shows the predictor variables not yet in the equation (NPREGS and SMOKE). Among other pieces of information shown here, the T values for the regression coefficients for these two predictors are both nonsignificant (*p* = .9147 and .6591, respectively), once variation due to AGE is taken into account. Because of this fact, the stepwise regression procedure ends at this point, without adding either of the two additional predictors. Given the significance level of .05 (shown as PIN = .050, i.e., the *P* value for variables going *IN* the equation), the inclusion of either of the two predictor variables would not have significantly added to the prediction of WEIGHT, over and above that which was already achieved with AGE alone.

It is, of course, possible to *force* the two additional predictors into the regression equation by conducting a nonstepwise regression. When this is done (this is not shown in the table), the value of *R* increases from .59383 to .59836, a negligible and nonsignificant increase. Thus, we must conclude that we cannot improve our ability to predict infant birthweight in this sample, based on the two additional predictors available here.

Example of Analysis of Covariance

In Chapter 19, we tested the hypothesis that infants in the experimental group would have higher birthweights than infants in the control group, using a *t*-test. The computer calculated the value of *t* to be 1.44, which, with 28 *df*, was nonsignificant. The research hypothesis was therefore rejected.

Now that more sophisticated statistical procedures are available to us, we can test the same hypothesis using ANCOVA. Through ANCOVA, we can control for the effect of AGE, which, as we have just seen, is significantly correlated with WEIGHT. Figure 20-9 presents the printout for both ANCOVA and MCA for this analysis, with WEIGHT as the dependent variable, AGE as the covariate, and GROUP (experimental versus control) as the independent variable. At the top of the first panel, we see that the *F*-value for the covariate AGE is 19.457, significant at the .000 level (i.e., beyond the .001 level). After controlling for the effect of AGE, the *F*-value for the independent variable GROUP (the main effect) is 8.719, which is significant at the .006 level. In other words, once AGE is controlled, our research hypothesis about experimental versus control differences is supported rather than rejected. The total amount of variability explained with the two variables, when contrasted with residual variability, is also significant (*F* = 14.088, *p* < .000).

The next panel shows the results of the MCA. For the sample as a whole, the overall mean (grand mean) is 104.700. The original, unadjusted means for the experimental and

```
        * * *  A N A L Y S I S   O F   V A R I A N C E  * * *

            WEIGHT    INFANT BIRTH WEIGHT
        BY  GROUP
        WITH AGE      AGE OF MOTHER


                          Sum of                  Mean         Signif
    Source of Variation   Squares    DF          Square     F    of F

    Covariates           1227.283     1         1227.283  19.457  .000
      AGE                1227.283     1         1227.283  19.457  .000

    Main Effects          549.945     1          549.945   8.719  .006
      GROUP               549.945     1          549.945   8.719  .006

    Explained            1777.228     2          888.614 ·14.088  .000

    Residual             1703.072    27           63.077

    Total                3480.300    29          120.010


        30 Cases were processed.
         0 Cases (   .0 PCT) were missing.

    * * *  M U L T I P L E   C L A S S I F I C A T I O N   A N A L Y S I S  * * *

            WEIGHT    INFANT BIRTH WEIGHT
        By  GROUP
        With AGE      AGE OF MOTHER


    Grand Mean =      104.700                                Adjusted for
                                           Adjusted for     Independents
                                Unadjusted Independents     + Covariates
    Variable + Category     N   Dev'n Eta  Dev'n   Beta     Dev'n   Beta

    GROUP
      1 EXPERIMENTAL       15     2.83                        4.38
      2 CONTROL           15     -2.83                       -4.38
                                        .26                         .41

    Multiple R Squared                                              .511
    Multiple R                                                      .715
```

Figure 20-9. SPSS computer printout: analysis of covariance and multiple classification analysis.

control groups can be calculated by taking the unadjusted deviations from the grand mean. For example, the original mean for the experimental group was 107.53 (104.70 + 2.83), consistent with the information presented earlier in Figure 19–5 in Chapter 19. After adjusting for maternal age, however, the experimental mean is 109.08 (104.70 + 4.38), and the control mean is 100.32 (104.70 − 4.38), a much more sizable difference. The multiple R^2 for predicting birthweight, based on both AGE and GROUP, is .511—substantially more than the R^2 between AGE and WEIGHT alone (.352).

TIPS FOR USING MULTIVARIATE STATISTICS

With the widespread availability of computers and user-friendly programs for performing statistical analysis, multivariate statistics have become increasingly common in nursing studies.

In this section, we offer a few suggestions with regard to multivariate statistics.

- As with bivariate statistical tests, the selection of a multivariate procedure depends on several factors, including the nature of the research question and the measurement level of the variables. Table 20-7 summarizes some of the major features of several of the multivariate statistics discussed in this chapter and thus serves as an aid to the selection of an appropriate procedure.
- If you are using a computer to analyze data, you should definitely consider the use of a multivariate procedure in lieu of a bivariate one for testing your hypotheses because the commands to the computer are not appreciably more complicated. As we have seen, researchers can come to the wrong conclusions about their hypotheses (i.e., commit Type I errors) when extraneous variables are not controlled. Moreover, because the power of statistical tests is enhanced with multivariate procedures, sample size requirements are usually lower.
- With regard to the previous point, ANCOVA is a particularly good technique for researchers without extensive statistical training to use as a substitute for ANOVA and *t*-tests. ANCOVA is relatively easy to run on the computer, and the output is also relatively easy to interpret. Covariates are almost always available: at a minimum, you can use important background characteristics, such as age, gender, and so on. The covariates should be ones that the researcher suspects are correlated with the dependent variable, and demographic characteristics are usually related to a wide variety of other attributes and behaviors. A pretest measure is an excellent choice for a covariate, if one is available. In this context, a **pretest** is a measure of the dependent

variable, taken before the occurrence of the independent variable.

- One of the difficulties with using a multivariate procedure is that the findings may be less readily accessible to statistically unsophisticated readers, such as many practicing nurses or undergraduate nursing students. Thus, in some instances, you may opt to use a simpler analysis to enhance the utilizability of the findings. For example, three separate ANOVAs might be used in lieu of a single MANOVA. However, if the primary reason for *not* using the appropriate multivariate procedure is for communication purposes—rather than your own discomfort with complex procedures—you may want to consider some alternatives. For example, you could describe the bivariate analyses (e.g., ANOVA) in the report, but also perform the appropriate procedure (e.g., MANOVA) and note in the report that the results remained the same with the multivariate tests (if this is true). Another strategy is to make an extra effort to explain multivariate results in terms that are readily comprehensible. Complex analyses can often be boiled down to relatively straightforward statements about the research hypotheses.

RESEARCH EXAMPLES

Table 20-8 illustrates some of the applications of multivariate statistics within recent nursing studies. This section presents two studies in greater detail.

Example of a Study Using Factor Analysis and Logistic Regression

Kocher and Thomas (1994) used survey data from a random sample of 158 female junior nurse-officers in the Army to examine the fac-

TABLE 20-7   Guide to Selected Multivariate Analyses

TEST NAME	PURPOSE	MEASUREMENT LEVEL OF VARIABLES*			NUMBER OF VARIABLES†		
		IV	DV	Cov	IVs	DVs	Covs
Multiple regression/ correlation	To test the relationship between 2+ IVs and 1 DV; to predict a DV from 2+ IVs	N, I, R	I, R	—	2+	1	—
Analysis of covariance (ANCOVA)	To test the difference between the means of 2+ groups, while controlling for 1+ covariate	N	I, R	N, I, R	1+	1	1+
Multivariate analysis of variance (MANOVA)	To test the difference between the means of 2+ groups for 2+ DVs simultaneously	N	I, R	—	1+	2+	—
Multivariate analysis of covariance (MANCOVA)	To test the difference between the means of 2+ groups for 2+ DVs simultaneously, while controlling for 1+ covariate	N	I, R	N, I, R	1+	2+	1+
Discriminant analysis	To test the relationship between 2+ IVs and 1 DV; to predict group membership; to classify cases into groups	N, I, R	N	—	2+	1	—
Canonical correlation	To test the relationship between 2 sets of variables	N, I, R	N, I, R	—	2+	2+	—
Factor analysis	To determine the dimensionality and structure of a set of variables	—	—	—	—	—	—
Logistic regression	To test the relationship between 2+ IVs and 1 DV; to predict the probability of an event; to estimate relative risk	N, I, R	N	—	2+	1	—

*Variables: IV, independent variable; DV, dependent variable; Cov, covariate.

†Measurement levels: N, nominal; I, interval; R, ratio.

TABLE 20-8 Examples of Nursing Studies Using Multivariate Statistics	
RESEARCH QUESTION	**MULTIVARIATE PROCEDURE**
What is the relationship between postural control among older adults and their ankle strength, knee strength, age, alertness, and mood? (Topp, Estes, Dayhoff, & Suhrheinrich, 1997)	Stepwise multiple regression
What is the effect of a self-management program for asthmatic adults on asthmatic symptoms and airway obstruction, controlling for initial levels of symptoms and obstruction? (Berg, Dunbar-Jacob, & Sereika, 1997)	Analysis of covariance
What is the structure of symptom distress in women living with advanced lung cancer? (Sarna & Brecht, 1997)	Factor analysis
To what extent do characteristics of percutaneous central venous catheter use in neonates (e.g., length of time catheters were in place) predict sepsis? (Trotter, 1996)	Discriminant analysis
What is the effect of a self-efficacy information intervention for men newly diagnosed with prostate cancer on the men's anxiety and depression levels? (Davison & Degner, 1997)	Multivariate analysis of variance
What is the relationship between the adjustment responses of mothers and the adjustment responses of their children with cancer? (Moore & Mosher, 1997)	Canonical correlation analysis
What is the relationship between self-rated social support network conflict and self-report measures of occupational stressors, job satisfaction, and health outcomes among professional firefighters and paramedics? (Beaton, Murphy, Pike, & Corneil, 1997)	Path analysis
How successful is the Price-Mueller model in explaining job satisfaction and organization attachment among doctorally prepared nurses? (Gurney, Mueller, & Price, 1997)	LISREL
What are the predictors or mortality among intensive care unit patients? (Kollef, 1995)	Logistic regression
What is the effect of chlorhexidine on days to onset of chemotherapy-induced oral mucositis? (Dodd et al., 1996)	Survival analysis

tors that might explain the nurses' turnover behavior. The dependent variable in their analysis was nurse retention—whether the nurse remained on active duty 3 years after the survey was completed. The predictor variables available for the analysis included a range of demographic characteristics (e.g., race/ethnicity, age, marital status) as well as 10 items relating to the nurse's satisfaction with various aspects of her job.

For purposes of parsimony, the 10 job satisfaction items were factor analyzed. The analysis indicated that the 10 job satisfaction items could be reduced to four factors. The first factor, which the researchers labeled work/military life, consisted of three items that described various aspects of the nurses' work and working conditions. The second factor, labeled location/assignment stability, involved two items that relate to Army reassignments. The third factor, called advancement opportunities, involved three items (promotions, job training, job security). The fourth factor, called economic benefits, consisted of two items with an economic theme.

Scores on the four factors were then used in a logistic regression analysis designed to predict retention of the Army nurses. The results revealed that two of the satisfaction dimensions (satisfaction with work/military life and satisfaction with location/assignment stability) were significant predictors of retention of nurses in the Army, even when demographic characteristics and characteristics of the external job market were statistically controlled. Marital status and race were also significant predictors. For example, a married nurse who had children had about a one-third lower retention likelihood than a nurse who was not married with children.

Example of a Study Using Multiple Regression

Dibble, Bostrom-Ezrati, and Rizzuto (1991) conducted a study to describe the frequency of intravenous (IV) site symptoms among patients with an IV placement and to develop a predictive model to explain the number of such symptoms. The 514 research subjects were recruited from four hospitals in the San Francisco area. All patients were adults whose IV placement was distal to the antecubital fossa and whose placement was anticipated for more than 24 hours. The occurrence of IV site symptoms was assessed using a checklist with five symptoms: pain, redness, swelling, induration, and a venous cord. The dependent variable for the analyses was the total number of symptoms observed, which could range from 0 to 5. Additional data consisted of demographic characteristics as well as information about the insertion, maintenance, and removal of the IV.

The analyses revealed that 40% of the patients developed one or more site symptoms; the number of symptoms ranged from 0 to 4. Pain was the most common symptom, experienced by 65% of those with a symptom. Multiple regression was used to predict the total number of symptoms experienced, based on both clinical and demographic independent variables. The multiple regression analysis revealed that the most significant predictor was the duration of the IV placement: The longer the placement, the greater the number of symptoms ($p < .001$). Even with placement duration statistically controlled, however, other variables contributed significantly to the prediction of symptoms. For example, having no tape placed over the insertion site to anchor the device ($p < .05$) and receiving an IV solution with higher osmolarity ($p < .05$) tended to result in a significantly greater number of symptoms. Even with all these factors controlled, women had significantly more symptoms than men ($p < .01$). Other variables in the regression analyses (e.g., the gauge of the needle, the use of ointment at the IV site) were not significant predictors. Overall, the various independent variables taken together did only a modest job in explaining individual differences in the number of symptoms: the R^2 was only .18, meaning that 82% of the variability in the number of symptoms could not be explained in terms of the demographic and clinical factors used in the regression analysis. Thus, although several important predictive variables were identified in this study, the researchers concluded that further research is needed to explore other potential causes of IV site symptoms.

SUMMARY

The **multivariate statistical procedures** explored in this chapter are used to untangle complex relationships among three or more variables. One of the most versatile multivariate procedures is **multiple regression (multiple correlation)**, which is a statistical method for understanding the effects of two or more independent variables on a dependent variable. A simple regression equation is a formula for making predictions about the numeric values of one variable based on the values of a second variable. The researcher can often improve the precision of the predictions by including more than one predictor (independent) variable in the regression equation. The **multiple correlation coefficient** is symbolized by **R**. The multiple correlation coefficient, when squared (R^2), indicates the proportion of the variance of the dependent variable that is explained or accounted for by the combined influences of the independent variables. R^2 is sometimes referred to as the **coefficient of determination**. The versatility of multiple regression analysis is demonstrated by its various related analyses and special options. For example, in **stepwise multiple regression**, the researcher can identify from a pool of potential predictor variables those variables that in combination have the greatest predictive power.

Analysis of covariance (ANCOVA) is a procedure that permits the researcher to control extraneous or confounding influences on dependent variables. The effect of one or more variable (called the **covariate**) is statistically controlled or removed before testing for group differences by traditional ANOVA procedures. ANCOVA is often used in ex post facto or quasi-experimental designs to control for potential pretreatment differences but can also be used in experimental designs to provide more precise estimates of experimental effects. **Multiple classification analysis (MCA)** is a supplement to ANCOVA that yields information about a dependent variable after adjusting for covariates. The information is usually provided in the form of **adjusted means** of each group.

Factor analysis is used to reduce a large set of variables into a smaller set of underlying dimensions, called **factors**. Mathematically, each factor represents a linear combination of the variables contained in a data matrix. The first phase of factor analysis, called **factor extraction**, identifies clusters of variables with a high degree of communality and condenses the larger set of variables into a smaller number of factors. The second phase of factor analysis involves **factor rotation**, which enhances the interpretability of the factors by aligning variables more distinctly with a particular factor. The **factor loadings** shown in a rotated factor matrix can then be examined to identify and name the underlying dimensionality of the original set of variables and to compute **factor scores**.

Discriminant analysis is essentially a multiple regression analysis in which the dependent variable is categorical (i.e., nominal level of measurement). This procedure is useful for making predictions about membership in groups on the basis of two or more predictor variables. **Canonical correlation** is the most general of all the multivariate procedures: It analyzes the relationship between two or more independent *and* two or more dependent variables. **Multivariate analysis of variance (MANOVA)** is the extension of ANOVA principles to cases in which there is more than one dependent variable.

Causal modeling involves the development and testing of a hypothesized causal explanation of a phenomenon. **Path analysis** is a regression-based procedure for testing causal models. The researcher first prepares a **path diagram** that stipulates hypothesized causal linkages among variables. Using regression procedures applied to a series of **structural equations**, a series of

path coefficients are developed. These path coefficients represent weights associated with a causal path in standard deviation units. The simplest form of a causal model is one that is **recursive**, that is, one in which causation is presumed to be unidirectional.

Linear structural relations analysis (LISREL) is another approach to causal modeling that does not have as many assumptions and restrictions as path analysis. LISREL can accommodate measurement errors, **nonrecursive models** that allow for reciprocal causal paths, and correlated errors. LISREL can also analyze causal models involving **latent variables,** which are not directly measured but which are captured by two or more **manifest variables** (i.e., measured variables). LISREL proceeds in two sequential phases: the measurement model phase and the structural equations modeling phase. The **measurement model** stipulates the hypothesized relationship between latent variables and manifest variables. If the measurement model fits the data, the next phase involves the testing of the hypothesized causal model.

New statistical methodologies have gained in popularity among nurse researchers in the 1990s. These include such techniques as **life table analysis, event history analysis,** and **logistic regression.**

🐚 STUDY ACTIVITIES

Chapter 20 of the *Study Guide to Accompany Nursing Research: Principles and Methods, 6th ed.*, offers various exercises and study suggestions for reinforcing the concepts presented in this chapter. Additionally, the following study questions can be addressed:

1. Refer to Figure 20-1. What would the value of Y' be for the following X values: 8, 1, 3, 6?
2. A researcher has examined the relationship between preventive health care attitudes on the one hand and the person's educational level, age, and gender on the other. The multiple correlation coefficient is .62. Explain the meaning of this statistic. How much of the variation in attitudinal scores has been explained by the three predictors? How much is *unexplained?* What other variables might improve the power of the prediction?
3. Which multivariate statistical procedures would you recommend using in the following situations:
   a. A researcher wants to test the effectiveness of a nursing intervention for reducing stress levels among surgical patients, using an experimental group of patients from one hospital and a control group from another hospital.
   b. A researcher wants to predict which students are at risk of venereal disease by using background information such as sex, socioeconomic status, religion, grades in sex education course, and attitudes toward sex.
   c. A researcher wants to test the effects of three different diets on blood sugar levels and blood pH.

🐚 SUGGESTED READINGS

Methodologic References

Aaronson, L. S. (1989). A cautionary note on the use of stepwise regression. *Nursing Research, 38,* 309–311.

Aaronson, L. S., Frey, M., & Boyd, C. J. (1988). Structural equation models and nursing research: Part II. *Nursing Research, 37,* 315–318.

Allison, P. D. (1984). *Event history analysis: Regression for longitudinal event data.* Beverly Hills, CA: Sage.

Blalock, H. M., Jr. (1972). *Causal inferences in nonexperimental research.* New York: W. W. Norton.

Boyd, C. J., Frey, M. A., & Aaronson, L. S. (1988). Structural equation models and nursing research: Part I. *Nursing Research, 37,* 249–253.

Cleary, P. D., & Angel, R. (1984). The analysis of relationships involving dichotomous dependent variables. *Journal of Health and Social Behavior, 25,* 334–348.

Cohen, J., & Cohen, P. (1983). *Applied multiple regression: Correlation analysis for behavioral sciences* (2nd ed.). New York: Halsted Press.

Cox, D. R., & Oakes, D. (1984). *Analysis of survival data.* London: Chapman and Hall.

Goodwin, L. D. (1984). Increasing efficiency and precision of data analysis: Multivariate vs. univariate statistical techniques. *Nursing Research, 33,* 247–249.

Gross, A. J., & Clark, V. (1975). *Survival distributions: Reliability applications in the biomedical sciences.* New York: John Wiley.

Hanushek, E., & Jackson, J. (1977). *Statistical methods for social scientists.* New York: Academic Press.

Hayduk, L. A. (1987). *Structural equation modeling with LISREL: Essentials and advances.* Baltimore: Johns Hopkins University Press.

Jaccard, J., & Becker, M. A. (1990). *Statistics for the behavioral sciences.* (2nd ed.). Belmont, CA: Wadsworth.

Jöreskog, K. G., & Sörbom, D. (1989). *LISREL® 7: User's reference guide.* Mooresville, IN: Scientific Software.

Kerlinger, F. N. (1986). *Foundations of behavioral research* (3rd ed.). New York: Holt, Rinehart & Winston.

Knapp, T. R. (1994). Regression analysis: What to report. *Nursing Research, 43,* 187–189.

Knapp, T. R., & Campbell-Heider, N. (1989). Numbers of observations and variables in multivariate analyses. *Western Journal of Nursing Research, 11,* 634–641.

Lee, E. T. (1992). *Statistical methods for survival data analysis* (2nd ed.). New York: John Wiley.

Mason-Hawkes, J., & Holm, K. (1989). Causal modeling: A comparison of path analysis and LISREL. *Nursing Research, 38,* 312–314.

Maxwell, A. E. (1978). *Multivariate analysis in behavioral research: For medical and social science students* (2nd ed.). New York: Methuen.

Pedhazur, E. J. (1982). *Multiple regression in behavioral research* (2nd ed.). New York: Holt, Rinehart & Winston.

Polit, D. F. (1996). *Data analysis and statistics for nursing research.* Stamford, CT: Appleton & Lange.

Tatsuoka, M. (1970). *Discriminant analysis: The study of group differences.* Champaign, IL: Institute for Personality and Ability Testing.

Tatsuoka, M. (1987). *Multivariate analysis: Techniques for educational and psychological research.* (2nd ed.). New York: John Wiley and Sons.

Teachman, J. D. (1982). Methodological issues in the analysis of family formation and dissolution. *Journal of Marriage and the Family, 44,* 1037–1053.

Tuma, N. B., & Hannan, M. T. (1984). *Social dynamics: Models and methods.* New York: Academic Press.

Volicer, B. J. (1981). *Advanced statistical methods with nursing applications.* Bedford, MA: Merestat Press.

Weisberg, S. (1985). *Applied linear regression* (2nd ed.). New York: John Wiley and Sons.

Welkowitz, J., Ewen, R. B., & Cohen, J. (1982). *Introductory statistics for the behavioral sciences* (3rd ed.). New York: Academic Press.

Wu, Y. B., & Slakter, M. J. (1989). Analysis of covariance in nursing research. *Nursing Research, 38,* 306–308.

Substantive References

Beaton, R. D., Murphy, S. A., Pike, K. C., & Corneil, W. (1997). Social support and network conflict in firefighters and paramedics. *Western Journal of Nursing Research, 19,* 297–313.

Berg, J., Dunbar-Jacob, J., & Sereika, S. M. (1997). An evaluation of a self-management program for adults with asthma. *Clinical Nursing Research, 6,* 225–238.

Davison, J., & Degner, L. F. (1997). Empowerment of men newly diagnosed with prostate cancer. *Cancer Nursing, 20,* 187–196.

Dibble, S. L., Bostrom-Ezrati, J., & Rizzuto, C. (1991). Clinical predictors of intravenous site symptoms. *Research in Nursing & Health, 14,* 314–420.

Dodd, M. J., Larson, P. J., Dibble, S. L., Miaskowski, C., Greenspan, D., MacPhail, L., Hauck, W. W., Paul, S. M., Ignoffo, R., & Shiba, G. (1996). Randomized clinical trial of chlorhexidine versus placebo for prevention of oral mucositis in patients receiving chemotherapy. *Oncology Nursing Forum, 23,* 921–927.

Gurney, C. A., Mueller, C. W., & Price, J. L. (1997). Job satisfaction and organizational attachment of nurses holding doctoral degrees. *Nursing Research, 46*, 163–171.

Kocher, K. M., & Thomas, G. W. (1994). Retaining Army nurses: A longitudinal model. *Research in Nursing & Health, 17*, 59–65.

Kollef, M. H. (1995). The identification of ICU-specific outcome predictors. *Heart & Lung, 24*, 60–66.

Moore, J. B., & Mosher, R. B. (1997). Adjustment responses of children and their mothers to cancer. *Oncology Nursing Forum, 24*, 519–525.

Sarna, L., & Brecht, M. (1997). Dimensions of symptom distress in women with advanced lung cancer. *Heart & Lung, 26*, 23–30.

Topp, R., Estes, P. K., Dayhoff, N., & Suhrheinrich, J. (1997). Postural control and strength and mood among older adults. *Applied Nursing Research, 10*, 11–18.

Trotter, C. W. (1996). Percutaneous central venous catheters in neonates: A descriptive analysis and evaluation of predictors for sepsis. *Journal of Perinatal & Neonatal Nursing, 10*, 56–71.

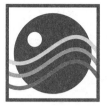

Designing and Implementing a Quantitative Analysis Strategy

The successful analysis of quantitative data requires considerable planning and attention to detail. This chapter provides an overview of the steps that normally have to be taken in designing and implementing a **data analysis plan**. The final phase of analyzing quantitative data involves the interpretation of the findings, and the interpretive process is discussed at some length.

PHASES IN THE ANALYSIS OF QUANTITATIVE DATA

The analysis of quantitative data normally proceeds through a number of different phases. The phases and the steps within the phases may vary from one project to another. For example, if the data set is an extremely simple one, then the researcher may be able to proceed fairly quickly from the collection to the analysis of the data. In most cases, however, a number of intermediary steps are necessary.

Figure 21-1 summarizes what the flow of tasks might look like when a researcher uses a computer, and when the final analyses involve the use of multivariate statistical procedures. Although we do not assume that most researchers

will use multivariate statistics, we do assume in this chapter that a computer will be used for the analysis. Computers are now ubiquitous, and applications are available to assist with every phase of a research project. Chapter 23 presents an overview of the use of computers in qualitative and quantitative studies.

Progress in the analysis of quantitative data may not always be as linear as Figure 21-1 suggests. For example, some backtracking may be required if data anomalies are discovered during the final analyses. However, the figure provides an adequate framework for discussing various steps in the analytic process. We begin with a brief discussion of some of the steps in the preanalysis phase.

PREANALYSIS PHASE

The first set of steps, shown in the Figure 21-1 as the Preanalysis Phase, involves a variety of clerical and administrative tasks. The tasks might include logging data in and maintaining appropriate administrative records, reviewing data forms for completeness and legibility, instituting steps to retrieve pieces of missing

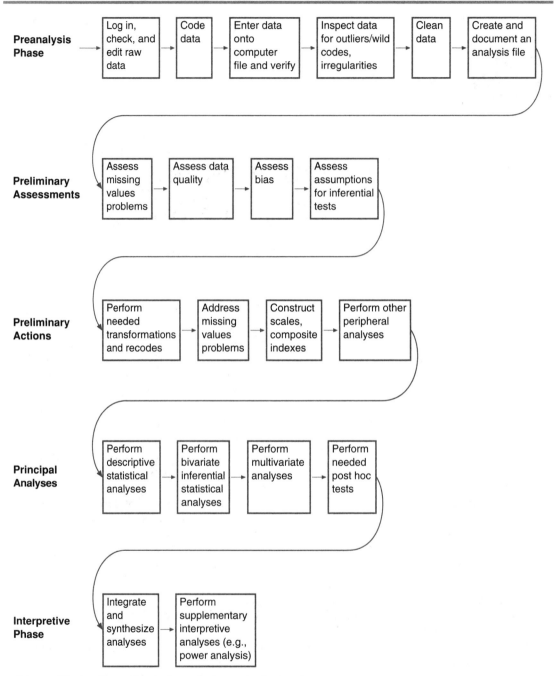

Figure 21-1. Flow of tasks in analyzing quantitative data.

information, and assigning identification (ID) numbers. Once these tasks have been performed, the researcher typically must code the data and enter them onto computer files to create a **data set** (the total collection of data for all sample members) for analysis.

Coding Quantitative Data

Data typically must be converted to a form amenable to computer analyses. Computers cannot process verbatim responses to open-ended questions, and it is also difficult for a computer to read and analyze information with verbal labels such as male or female, agree or disagree. **Coding** is the process by which basic research information is transformed into symbols compatible with computer analysis.

INHERENTLY QUANTITATIVE VARIABLES

Certain variables are inherently quantitative and therefore directly amenable to computer analysis. For example, variables such as age, weight, body temperature, and diastolic blood pressure do not normally require coding—the data are already in a quantitative form. Sometimes, the researcher may ask for information of this type in a way that *does* call for the development of a coding plan. If a researcher asks respondents to indicate whether they are younger than 30 years of age, between the ages of 30 and 49 years, or 50 years or older, then the responses would have to be coded before being entered into a computer file. When the responses to questions such as age, height, income level, and so forth are given in their full, natural form, the researcher should *not* reduce the information to coded categories for data entry purposes.

Information that is naturally quantitative thus may need no coding whatsoever, but the researcher nevertheless should inspect and edit the data. It is important that all the responses be of the same form and precision. For in-

stance, in entering a person's height, the researcher would need to decide whether to use feet and inches or to convert the information entirely to inches. Whichever method is adopted, it must be used consistently for all subjects. There must also be consistency in the method of handling information reported with different degrees of precision (e.g., coding a response such as 5 feet 2½ inches).

PRECATEGORIZED DATA

Much of the data from questionnaires, interviews, observation schedules, and psychological scales can be coded easily through precategorization (i.e., codes assigned even before data are collected). Closed-ended questions that provide for response alternatives can easily be preassigned a numeric code, as in the following example:

> From what type of program did you receive your basic nursing preparation?
> 1. Diploma school
> 2. Associate degree program
> 3. Baccalaureate degree program

Thus, if a nurse received his or her nursing preparation from a diploma school, the response to this question would be coded 1.

In many cases, the codes are arbitrary, as in the case of a variable such as gender. Whether a female is coded 1 or 2 will have no bearing on the subsequent analysis as long as females are consistently assigned one code and males another. Other variables will appear to have a more obvious coding scheme, as in the following example:

> How often do you experience insomnia?
> 1. Almost never
> 2. Once or twice a year
> 3. Three to 11 times a year
> 4. At least once a month but not weekly
> 5. Once a week or more

Sometimes, respondents may have the option of checking off more than one answer in reply to a single question, as in the following illustration:

> To which of the following journals do you subscribe?
> ( ) *Applied Nursing Research*
> ( ) *Clinical Nursing Research*
> ( ) *Nursing Research*
> ( ) *Qualitative Health Research*
> ( ) *Research in Nursing & Health*
> ( ) *Western Journal of Nursing Research*

With questions of this type, it is not appropriate to adopt a 1-2-3-4-5-6 code because respondents may check several, or none, of the responses. The most appropriate procedure for questions such as this is to treat each journal on the list as a separate question. In other words, the researcher would code the responses as though the item were six separate questions asking, "Do you subscribe to *Applied Nursing Research*? Do you subscribe to *Clinical Nursing Research*?" and so on. A check mark beside a journal would be treated as though the reply were yes. In effect, the question would be turned into six dichotomous variables, with one code (perhaps 1) signifying a "yes" response and another code (perhaps 2) signifying a "no" response.

CODING UNCATEGORIZED DATA

Qualitative data from open-ended questions, unstructured observations, and other narrative forms are not amenable to direct statistical analysis. When this type of information is to be statistically analyzed by the computer, it is necessary to categorize and code it. It is sometimes possible for the researcher to develop a coding scheme in advance of data collection. For instance, a question might ask, "What is your occupation?" If the researcher knew the sample characteristics, he or she could probably predict major categories (e.g., professional, managerial, clerical, and so on).

Usually, however, unstructured formats for data collection are adopted specifically because it is difficult to anticipate the kind of in-

formation that will be obtained. In such a situation, it is necessary to code responses after the data are collected. The researcher typically begins by reviewing a sizable portion of the data to get a feel for the nature of the content. The researcher can then proceed to develop a scheme to categorize the material. The categorization scheme should be designed to reflect both the researcher's theoretical and analytic goals as well as the substance of the information. The amount of detail in the categorization scheme can vary considerably, but the researcher should keep in mind that too much detail is better than too little detail. In developing a coding scheme for unstructured information, the only rule is that the coding categories should be both mutually exclusive and collectively exhaustive.

Precise instructions should always be developed for the coders and documented in a coding manual. Coders, like observers and interviewers, must be properly trained. Intercoder reliability checks are strongly recommended.

CODING MISSING VALUES

A code should be designated for every question or variable and for every sample member, even if in some cases no response or information is available. **Missing values** can be of various types. A person responding to an interview question may be undecided, refuse to answer, or say "Don't know." And, when a skip pattern is used, there is usually missing information for those questions that are irrelevant to a portion of the sample. In observational studies, an observer coding behavior may get distracted during a 10-second sampling frame, may be undecided about an appropriate categorization, or may observe behavior not listed on the observation schedule. In some studies, it may be important to distinguish between various types of missing data by specifying separate codes (e.g. distinguishing refusals and "don't knows"), and in other cases a single missing values code may suffice. This decision must be made with the conceptual aims of the research in mind. A person who replied "Don't know" to a question seeking to understand the public's familiarity with health maintenance organizations should probably be distinguished from a person who refused to answer the question.

Insofar as possible, it is desirable to code missing data in the same manner for all variables. If a nonresponse is coded as a 4 on variable 1, a 6 on variable 2, a 5 on variable 3, and so forth, there is a greater risk of error than if a uniform code is adopted. The choice of what number to use as the missing data code is fairly arbitrary, but the number must be one that has not been assigned to an actual piece of information. Many researchers follow the convention of coding missing data as 9 because this value is normally out of the range of codes for true information. Others use blanks, zeros, or negative values to indicate missing information.

Some software packages require a specific handling of missing information. Therefore, the researcher should decide what software will be used for data analysis before finalizing coding decisions.

Entering, Verifying, and Cleaning Data

Coded data must be entered onto a computer file for analysis and then verified and cleaned. This section provides an overview of these procedures. Technologic advances in data entry make it inevitable, however, that the information we provide here will need to be updated.

DATA ENTRY

For most types of computer analysis, the coded data are transferred onto a data file through a keyboard or a computer terminal. Various computer programs can be used for data entry, including spreadsheet or databases. The major software packages for statistical analysis (see Chapter 23) also have associated data entry programs. These sophisticated data entry programs can often be developed in conjunction with data collection instruments, so that the program actually generates both the forms and the format for data entry simultaneously. For example, a software package known as the Statistical Package for the Social Sciences (SPSS) has a data entry module (SPSS Data Entry) that can be used to design and customize self-report forms, automatically define variables to be used in statistical analyses, and establish data rules to check the accuracy of entered data and to deal with skip patterns.

When specialized data entry software is not used, the researcher must usually develop a data entry plan. It is often preferable to adopt what is known as a **fixed format**, which places the values for any specific variable in the same column of a data entry record for every case. The data that was used in the examples of computer analysis in the previous three chapters (and listed in Table 18-8 in Chapter 18) are shown in a fixed format data entry mode in Figure 21-2. In this example, the 30 lines of data correspond to the 30 study participants, with one line of data per person; the data for each person occupies 11 columns. (The variables entered for each case are as follows: identification number, experimental group status, infant birthweight, repeat pregnancy status, age of the mother, number of prior pregnancies, and smoking status.)

Most statistical programs also permit data to be entered in a **freefield format**, in which there is no necessary correspondence between the variables entered in any particular column from one case to the next, although the variables are always in the same order. In freefield format, the values for different variables are separated by a **delimiter**, such as a comma, one or more blank spaces, or a tab. For example, in freefield format, the first two lines of data that appear in Figure 21-2 might be entered as follows:

```
01 1 110 1 17 1 1
02  1  101 0 14 0 0
```

Although data entry is generally easier in freefield format, we recommend using a fixed format because checking for errors is simplified.

```
01110711711
02110101400
03111902130
04112812020
051 8901511
061 9901901
07111101910
08111711811
09110211700
10112002000
111 7601301
12111601801
13110011600
14111501800
15111302121
16211111900
17210802110
182 9501921
192 9901701
20210311900
212 9401501
22210111710
23211402120
242 9702010
252 9911801
26211301801
272 8901910
282 9802000
29210201700
30210501911
```

Figure 21-2. Data for 30 study participants.

Moreover, if a data value is inadvertently omitted during freefield entry, not only is it difficult to detect, but also the consequence is that the values for all subsequent variables would be incorrect.

With a fixed format, the researcher must specify in which columns all the data are to be entered. For many variables, the **field width** is a single column. If a variable has a code whose maximum value is one digit, then the variable can be assigned to one column. Examples include variables whose responses are agree/disagree and yes/no/maybe. Other variables, such as age, weight, and blood pressure measures, must occupy more than one column. Any time that the maximum value of a variable exceeds 9, the researcher must be sure to reserve two (or more, if the number is larger than 99) columns.

In a fixed format, the researcher must be careful in dealing with a variable whose values may be of different field widths for different subjects. For example, in recording data for infant birthweight, we would need only two digits for infants weighing less than 100 ounces but three digits for those weighing 100 ounces or more. Because the maximum value is three digits long, three columns on the record would be required for all subjects. To record the weight of an 89-ounce infant, for example (data record number 5 of Figure 21-2), it was necessary to enter 89 preceded by a blank space (or by a zero, as 089). This procedure is known as **right justification** of the data. Whenever a number smaller than the corresponding field is entered in fixed format, the number should be entered as far to the right as possible in the designated field. In the example shown in the figure, columns 4, 5, and 6 were reserved for the weight measurement, so 89 was entered in columns 5 and 6. If, instead, 89 were entered in columns 4 and 5, then the value would be read as 890.

In designing the layout for the data, the researcher should allocate space for recording an ID number. Each individual case (i.e., the information from a single questionnaire, test, observation, and so forth) should be assigned a unique ID number, and this number should be entered along with the actual data. This procedure permits the investigator to go back to the original source if there are any difficulties with the data file. The numbering is completely arbitrary and is used only as a label. Usually, a consecutive numbering scheme is used, running from number 1 to the number of actual cases. The ID number normally is entered in the first columns of the record—as we did in Figure 21-2. If there are fewer than 100 subjects, then the first two columns are used, starting with subjects 01, 02, and so on. As in the case of other variables, the field width for fixed format entry is determined by the maximum value of the ID number.

DATA VERIFICATION AND CLEANING

Once the data are coded and a scheme has been developed for the data file, the process of entering data onto the file can begin. Data entry is a tedious and exacting task that is usually subject to numerous errors. Therefore, it is necessary to verify or check the entries to correct the mistakes that are inevitably made. Several verification procedures exist. The first is to compare visually the numbers printed on a printout of the data file with the codes on the original source. A second possibility is to enter all the data twice and to compare the two sets of records. The comparison can be done either visually or with the assistance of the computer. Finally, there are special verifying programs that are designed to perform comparisons during direct data entry. The use of such verification is recommended as the best method for eliminating data entry inaccuracies.

Even after the records are verified, the data usually contain a few errors. These errors could be the result of data entry mistakes but could also arise from coding or reporting prob-

lems. Data are not ready for analysis until they have been cleaned. **Data cleaning** involves two types of checks. The first is a check for outliers and wild codes. **Outliers** are values that lie outside the normal range of values for other cases. Outliers can be found by inspecting frequency distributions, paying special attention to the lowest and highest values. In some cases, the outliers are true, legitimate values (e.g., an income of $2 million in a distribution where all other incomes are below $200,000). In other cases, however, outliers indicate an error in data entry that needs to be corrected, as when the frequency distribution reveals a **wild code**—that is, a code that is not possible. For example, the variable gender might have the following three defined code values: 1 for female, 2 for male, and 9 for not reported. If it were discovered that a code of 5 were entered for the gender variable, then it would be clear that an error had been made. The computer could be instructed to list the ID number of the culpable record, and the error could be corrected by checking the appropriate code on the original source. Another procedure is to use a program for data entry that automatically performs range checks.

Editing of this type, of course, will never reveal mistakes that look respectable or plausible. If the gender of a male is entered incorrectly as a 1, then the mistake may never be detected. Because errors can have a profound effect on the analysis and interpretation of data, it is naturally important to perform the coding, entering, verifying, and cleaning with great care.

The second data-cleaning procedure involves performing **consistency checks**, which focus on internal data consistency. In this task, the researcher looks for data entry or coding errors by testing whether data in one part of a record are compatible with data in another part. For example, one question in a questionnaire might ask respondents their current marital status, and another might ask how many times they had been married. If the data were internally consistent, then the respondents who answered "Single, never married" to the first question should have a zero (or a missing values code if there were a skip pattern) entered in the field for the second. As another example, if the respondent's gender were entered with the code for male and there was an entry of 2 for the variable "Number of pregnancies," then one of those two fields would contain an error. The researcher should identify as many opportunities for checking the consistency of entered data as possible.

Creating and Documenting the Analysis Files

Once the data set has been created and cleaned, the researcher must proceed to develop an appropriate analysis file, using one of the many available statistical software packages. Before analyses can begin, the computer must be told basic information about the data set, such as what variables are in it, where to find the values for those variables, and how to determine where one case ends and another one begins. As part of this process, the researcher must assign a name to each variable. The variable names are usually descriptive and informative (e.g., AGE and GENDER), but in some cases, they convey information about location in an instrument (e.g., Q1, Q2, and so on). As an example, in Figure 21-2, the variables were named as follows: ID, GROUP, WEIGHT, REPEAT, AGE, NPREGS, and SMOKE.

The decisions that a researcher makes concerning coding, field width, placement of data in columns, variable naming, and so on should be documented in full. Documentation is essential for the proper handling of any data set. The researcher's own memory should not be trusted to store all the required information. Several weeks after coding, the researcher may no longer remember if males were coded 1 and females 2, or vice versa. Moreover, colleagues may wish to borrow the data set to perform a secondary analysis. Whether one anticipates a secondary analysis or not, documentation

should be sufficiently thorough so that a person unfamiliar with the original research project could use the data.

A major portion of the documentation involves the preparation of a codebook. A **codebook** is essentially a listing of each variable, the column or columns in which the variable has been entered (for fixed format entry), and the codes associated with the various values of the variable. The codebook is often prepared before coding so that it can be used as a guide by coders. A codebook usually can be generated by statistical or data entry programs.

PRELIMINARY ASSESSMENTS AND ACTIONS

Researchers typically undertake a number of preliminary assessments of their data and several preanalytic activities before they proceed with the testing of their hypotheses. Several of these preparatory activities are discussed next.

Assessing and Handling Missing Values Problems

Researchers almost always find that their data set has missing values on some variables for some subjects. If the sample is large and the number of missing values is small, then the missing data should not cause problems. However, because many samples in nursing studies are small, missing data may be of considerable concern. The best overall strategy is to take steps to minimize data loss during the design and implementation of the data collection plan. Because it is usually inevitable to have some missing data—regardless of the vigilance of the researcher—various approaches have been used to deal with this situation after it has occurred.

In selecting one or more of these approaches, the researcher should first determine the distribution and patterning of the missing data. The appropriate solution will depend on such factors as the extensiveness of the missing data, the role that the variable with missing data plays in the analytic scheme (i.e., whether the missing values are in the dependent, independent, or descriptive variables), and the randomness of the missing data (i.e., whether missing values are related in any systematic way to important variables in the study). Obviously, the problem differs if only 2% of the values for a relatively minor variable are missing, as opposed to 20% of the values for the primary dependent variable. Also, if the missing values disproportionately come from people with certain characteristics, there is likely to be some bias.

The first step, then, is to determine the extent of the problem by examining frequency distributions on a variable-by-variable basis. (Most researchers routinely begin the data analysis process by running **marginals**—constructing frequency distributions—for all or most variables in their data set.) Another step is to examine the cumulative extent of missing values. If 10% of the cases have missing values for variable X and 10% of the cases have missing values for variable Y, there could be missing data for anywhere between 10% and 20% of the sample on these variables, depending on the degree of overlap. In statistical programs, it is possible to construct **flags** to count how many variables are missing for each sample member. Once a missing values flag has been created, a frequency distribution can be computed for this new variable; this would show how many cases had no missing values, one missing value, and so on.

Another assessment task is to evaluate the randomness of the missing values. A simple procedure is to divide the sample into two groups—those with missing data on a specified variable and those without missing data. These two groups can then be compared in terms of the other variables in the data set to determine if the two groups are comparable. Similarly, two groups can be created based on the missing values flag (e.g., those with no missing data versus those with *any* missing data) and compared on other variables.

Once the researcher has assessed the distribution and patterning of missing values, decisions must be made about how to address the problem. Some solutions are described next.

1. *Delete the missing cases.* One simple strategy is to delete a case (i.e., a subject) entirely if there is any missing information. However, particularly when samples are small, it is irksome to throw away an entire case—especially if information is missing for only one or two variables. If a person has extensive missing information, however, the deletion of this case is advisable. Also, if the missing information is for key dependent variables, it may be necessary to remove the entire case. This strategy is sometimes referred to as **listwise deletion** of missing values.

2. *Delete the variable.* Another option is to throw out information on a particular variable for all subjects. This option is especially suitable when a high percentage of cases have missing values on a specific variable. (This may occur if, for example, a question is objectionable and is left unanswered, or if there were problems in understanding directions and a question was inadvertently skipped by many.) When missing data on a variable are extensive, there may be systematic biases with regard to those subjects for whom data *are* available. Obviously, this approach is not attractive if the variable is a critical independent or dependent variable.

3. *Substitute the mean value.* When the missing values are reasonably random (and when the problem is not extensive), it is often useful to substitute real data values for the missing value codes. In essence, such a substitution represents a best guess as to what the value of the variable would have been, had the data

actually been collected. Because of this fact, researchers generally substitute a value that is typical for the sample, and typical values generally come from the center of the distribution. For example, if data for a subject's age were missing and if the average age of subjects in the sample were 45.2 years, the researcher might substitute the value 45 in place of the missing values code for subjects whose age is unknown.

This approach is especially useful when there are missing values for variables that comprise a multiple-item scale, such as a Likert scale. Suppose, for example, that we have a 20-item scale that measures anxiety, and that one person answered only 18 of the 20 items. It would be inappropriate to score the scale by adding together responses on the 18 items only, and it would be a waste of information on the 18 answered items to code the entire scale as missing. Thus, for the two missing items, the researcher could substitute the most typical responses (based on either the mean, median, or mode, depending on the distribution of scores), so that a scale score on the full 20 items could be computed. Needless to say, this approach only makes sense when a small proportion of scale items are missing. And, if the scale is a test of knowledge rather than a measure of a psychosocial characteristics, it usually is more appropriate to consider a missing value as a "don't know" and to mark the item as incorrect.

4. *Estimate the missing value.* When a researcher substitutes a mean value for a missing value, there is always the risk that the substitution is erroneous, perhaps dramatically so. For example, if the mean value of 45 is substituted for a missing value on a subject's age, but the range of ages in the sample is 25 to 70 years, then the substituted value could be wrong by 20 years or more. When only a couple of cases have missing data

for the variable age, an error of even this magnitude is unlikely to alter the findings. However, if missing values are more widespread, it is often worthwhile to substitute values that have a greater likelihood of being accurate.

Various procedures can be used to derive estimates of what the missing value should be. The simplest procedure is to use the mean for a subgroup that is most like the case that has the missing value, if there are subgroup differences with regard to the variable that has missing data. For example, suppose the mean age for women in the sample were 42.8 years and the mean age for men were 48.9 years. The researcher could then substitute 43 for women with missing age data and 49 for men with missing age data. This would likely result in improved accuracy, in comparison with the use of the overall mean of 45 for all subjects with missing age data.

Sometimes, multiple regression procedures are used to "predict" the correct value of the missing data. To continue with the example used previously, suppose that subjects' age was correlated with gender, heart rate, and length of hospital stay in this research sample. Based on the data from subjects without any missing values, these three variables could be used to develop a regression equation that could predict age for subjects whose age information is missing but whose values for the three other variables are not missing.

Some statistical software packages (such as SPSS) have a special procedure for estimating the value of missing data. These procedures can also be used to examine the relationship between the missing values and other variables in the data set.

5. *Delete cases selectively and pairwise.* Perhaps the most widely used (but not necessarily the best) approach is to delete

cases selectively, on a variable-by-variable basis. For example, in describing the characteristics of the sample, the researcher might use whatever information is available for each characteristic, resulting in a fluctuating number of cases across the range of descriptors. Thus, the mean age might be based on 95 cases, the gender distribution might be based on 102 cases, and so on. However, if the number of cases fluctuates widely across characteristics, the information is difficult to interpret because the sample of subjects is essentially a "moving target."

The same strategy is sometimes used to handle missing information for dependent variables. For example, an evaluation of an intervention to reduce patient anxiety might have blood pressure, self-reported anxiety, and an observational measure of stress-related behavior as the dependent variables. Suppose that 10 people out of a sample of 100 failed to complete the anxiety scale. The researcher might base the analyses of the anxiety data on the 90 subjects who completed the scale but use the full sample of 100 subjects in the analyses of the other dependent variables. The problem with this approach is that it can cause interpretive problems, especially if there are inconsistent findings across outcomes. For example, if there were experimental versus control group differences on all outcomes except the anxiety scale, one possible explanation is that the anxiety scale sample is simply not the same set of subjects as the full sample. Researchers generally strive for what is referred to as a **rectangular matrix** of data: data values for all subjects on all relevant and important variables. In the example just described, the researcher should, at a minimum, perform supplementary analyses using the rectangular matrix—that is, rerun all analyses using only the 90 subjects for whom complete

data are available. If the results are different from when the full sample was used, the researcher would at least be in a better position to interpret the findings.

In analyses involving a correlation matrix, researchers sometimes use what is referred to as **pairwise deletion** of cases with missing values. Figure 21-3 illustrates a correlation matrix with five variables in which pairwise deletion of missing values was used on a nonrectangular data matrix. As this figure shows, the correlations between pairs of variables are based on varying numbers of cases (shown in parentheses below the correlation coefficients), ranging from 18 subjects for the correlation between WEIGHT and STRESS to 25 subjects for the correlation between AGE and HEIGHT. Pairwise deletion is a tolerable procedure for descriptive purposes if the missing values are missing totally at random. But it is a risky procedure because data are often missing in some systematic fashion. It is especially imprudent to use this procedure for any multivariate analyses because the criterion correlations (i.e., the correlations between the dependent variable and the various predictors) are based on nonidentical subsets of subjects.

Each of these solutions has accompanying problems, so care should be taken in deciding how the missing data are to be handled. Procedures for dealing with missing values are discussed at greater length in Cohen and Cohen (1983) and Little and Rubin (1990).

Assessing Quantitative Data Quality

Steps are often undertaken to assess the quality of data in the early stage of the analyses. For example, when psychosocial scales or composite indexes are used, the researcher should generally assess the reliability of the measures, using either test–retest methods or,

```
Correlations:   AGE        WEIGHT      HEIGHT     HARTRATE    STRESS

    AGE         1.0000       .0453      -.0227       .2925      .4456
               (     0)     (    23)    (    25)    (    24)    (    20)
                P= .        P= .419     P= .457     P= .083     P= .024

    WEIGHT       .0453      1.0000       .8304       .3502      .0737
               (    23)     (     0)    (    23)    (    22)    (    18)
                P= .419     P= .        P= .000     P= .055     P= .386

    HEIGHT      -.0227       .8304      1.0000       .2197     -.0293
               (    25)     (    23)    (     0)    (    24)    (    20)
                P= .457     P= .000     P= .        P= .151     P= .451

    HARTRATE     .2925       .3502       .2197      1.0000      .5335
               (    24)     (    22)    (    24)    (     0)    (    19)
                P= .083     P= .055     P= .151     P= .        P= .009

    STRESS       .4456       .0737      -.0293       .5335     1.0000
               (    20)     (    18)    (    20)    (    19)    (     0)
                P= .024     P= .386     P= .451     P= .009     P= .


(Coefficient / (Cases) / 1-tailed Significance)

" . " is printed if a coefficient cannot be computed
```

Figure 21-3.   Correlation matrix with pairwise deletion of missing values.

more commonly, internal consistency methods (see Chapter 17).

The distribution of data values for key variables also should be examined to determine any anomalies, such as limited variability, extreme skewness, or the presence of ceiling or floor effects. For example, the use of a vocabulary test designed for 10-year-olds likely would yield a clustering of high scores in a sample of 11-year-olds, creating a **ceiling effect** that would tend to reduce correlations between test scores and other characteristics of the children. Conversely, there likely would be a clustering of low scores on the test with a sample of 9-year-olds, resulting in a **floor effect** with similar consequences. In such a situation, the data may need to be transformed to meet the requirements for certain statistical tests.

Assessing Bias

Researchers often undertake preliminary analyses designed to assess the direction and extent of any biases. A few examples illustrate the types of analysis that the researcher should consider.

- *Nonresponse bias.* Researchers are often interested in determining whether a biased subset of the population volunteered to participate in a study. If there is information available about the characteristics of all people who were asked to participate in a study (e.g., demographic information from hospital records), the researcher should compare the characteristics of those who did and did not agree to participate in the study to determine the nature and direction of any biases. This means, of course, that the data file for the study has to include a case for each respondent and each nonrespondent. Additionally, the data file should contain a variable that indicates the response status of each person (e.g., a variable could be coded 1 for participants and 2 for those who declined to participate).

- *Selection bias.* When a nonequivalent comparison group is used (in a quasi-experimental or ex post facto study), the researcher should always check for selection biases by comparing the background characteristics of the groups that are formed on the basis of the independent variable. It is particularly important to be aware of any possible group differences on extraneous variables that are strongly related to the dependent variable. These variables can (and should, if possible) then be controlled—for example, through analysis of covariance. Even when a true experimental design has been used, the researcher should check the success of the random assignment procedure. Random assignment does not guarantee equivalent groups across all characteristics, and the researcher should be aware of characteristics for which the different groups are not, in fact, comparable.

- *Attrition bias.* In longitudinal studies, it is always important to check for attrition biases, which involves a comparison of people who did and did not continue to participate in the study in later waves of data collection, based on characteristics of these two groups at the initial wave.

In performing any of these analyses, significant group differences are an indication of bias, and such bias must be taken into consideration in interpreting the results. Whenever possible, the biases should be controlled in testing the main hypotheses. Any detected biases should be discussed in the research report.

Testing Assumptions for Statistical Tests

Most statistical tests are based on a number of assumptions—conditions that are presumed to be true and, when violated, can lead to misleading or invalid results. For example, parametric tests assume that variables in the analysis are distributed normally. Frequency distributions, scatterplots, and other assessment procedures provide researchers with information about whether the underlying assumptions for statistical tests have been violated.

A frequency distribution can usually reveal whether the normality assumption is tenable. That is, the graphic or tabular presentation of the data values will indicate whether the distribution is severely skewed, multimodal, too peaked (**leptokurtic**), or too flat (**platykurtic**). Computer programs often have a special subcommand associated with the frequency distribution command that allows researchers to examine the extent to which the data approximate normality, by superimposing a normal distribution on the actual distribution of values. There are also various statistical indexes of skewness or peakedness that can be computed to determine whether the shape of the distribution deviates significantly from normality. However, it is not generally necessary to compute these indexes because most parametric tests are **robust** to violations of the normality assumption. By robust, we mean that the accuracy of our statistical decisions (the frequency of making Type I and Type II errors) is not greatly diminished when the underlying distribution of the variable is not normal. Thus, a visual inspection of a distribution is generally sufficient to determine if really gross violations of the normality assumption have occurred. (In general, the larger the sample, the less a researcher has to be concerned about normality.)

Performing Data Transformations

Raw data entered directly onto a computer file often need to be modified or transformed before the hypotheses can be tested using statistical analysis. **Data transformations** can be of various types and can easily be handled directly through instructions to the computer. All statistical software packages have the ability to create totally new variables through arithmetic manipulations of variables in the original data set. We present a few examples of such transformations in this section.

- *Performing item reversals.* Sometimes, response codes to certain items need to be completely reversed (i.e., high values becoming low, and vice versa), often for the purposes of combining items in the construction of a composite scale. For example, the widely used Center for Epidemiological Studies Depression (CES-D) scale consists of 20 items, 16 of which are statements indicating respondents' negative feelings in the prior week (e.g., item 9 states, "I thought my life had been a failure"), and four of which are statements worded positively (e.g., item 8 states, "I felt hopeful about the future"). To score the scale, the positively worded items must be reversed before all items can be added together, as discussed in Chapter 14. CES-D items have four response options, from 1 (rarely felt that way) to 4 (felt that way most days). To reverse an item (i.e., to convert a 4 to a 1, and so on), the raw value of the item is subtracted from the maximum possible value, plus 1. In SPSS, this could be accomplished through the "Compute" command, which could be used to set the value of a new variable to 5 minus the value of the original variable; for example, a new variable CESD8N could be computed as the value of $5 - CESD8$, where CESD8 was the original value of the eighth item on the CESD scale.

- *Constructing scales.* Transformations are also needed for the construction of composite scales or indexes, using responses to individual items. Commands in statistical software packages for creating such composite indexes are generally straightforward, using algebraic conventions. In SPSS, the "Compute" command could again be used to create a new variable, set equal to the sum of the values on the individual scale items; for example, a new variable STRESS could be set equal to $Q1 + Q2 + Q3 + Q4 + Q5$.

- *Performing counts.* Sometimes, composite indexes are created when the researcher is interested in a cumulative tally of the occurrence of some behavior or attribute. For example, suppose a researcher asked people to indicate which contraceptive methods they had used in the past 12 months, from a list of 10 different contraceptive options. Each question would be answered independently in a yes (coded 1) or no (coded 2) fashion. The researcher may want to create a variable indicating the total number of contraceptive methods used. In SPSS, the "Count" command would be used, creating a new variable equal to the sum of all the "1" codes to the 10 contraceptive items. Note that counting is the approach used to create missing values flags, described earlier in this chapter.

- *Recoding variables.* Other transformations involve recoding values that change the nature of the original data. For example, in some analyses, an infant's original birthweight (entered on the computer files in grams) might be used as a dependent variable. In other analyses, however, the researcher might be interested in comparing the subsequent morbidity of low-birthweight versus normal-birthweight infants. For example, in SPSS, the "Recode Into Same Variable" command could be used to recode the original variable (BWEIGHT) into a dichotomous variable with a code of 1 for a low-birthweight infant and a code of 2 for a normal-birthweight infant, based on whether the baby weighed less than 2500 grams.

- *Meeting statistical assumptions.* Transformations are also undertaken to render data appropriate for certain statistical tests. For example, if a distribution is markedly nonnormal, then a transformation can sometimes be done to make parametric procedures appropriate. A logarithmic transformation, for example, often tends to normalize the distribution. For example, in SPSS, the "Compute" command could be used to normalize the distribution of values on family income by computing a new variable (e.g., INCLOG) set equal to the natural log of the values on the original variable. Discussions of the use of transformations for changing the characteristics of a distribution can be found in Dixon and Massey (1983) and Ferketich and Verran (1994).

- *Creating dummy variables.* Multivariate statistical procedures often require data transformations for variables measured on the nominal scale. For example, for dichotomous variables, it is advisable to use a 0 versus 1 code (rather than, say, a 1 versus 2 code) to facilitate interpretation of the regression coefficients. Thus, if the original codes for gender were 1 for women and 2 for men, the variable should be recoded.

Clearly, we have not described all possible types of transformations, but these examples cover a range of realistic situations. Researchers can rarely analyze raw data that have been input directly onto a computer file, so the analysis plan must take into consideration the types of transformations that will be required to produce the most meaningful results.

Performing Additional Peripheral Analyses

Depending on the research project, additional peripheral analyses may need to be undertaken before proceeding to the substantive analyses. It is impossible to catalog all such peripheral analyses, but a few examples are provided to alert readers to the kinds of issues that need to be given some thought.

- *Manipulation checks.* In testing an experimental intervention, the primary research question is whether the treatment is effective in achieving the intended outcome. However, the researcher sometimes also wants to know whether the intended treatment was, in fact, received. Subjects may perceive a treatment, or respond to it, in unanticipated ways, and this can influence

the extent of the treatment's effectiveness. Therefore, researchers sometimes build in mechanisms to test whether the treatment was actually in place. For example, suppose we were testing the effect of noise levels on stress, exposing two groups of subjects to two different noise levels in a laboratory setting. As a **manipulation check**, we could ask subjects to rate how noisy they perceived the settings to be. If the subjects did not rate the noise levels in the two settings differently, it would probably affect our interpretation of the results—particularly if the stress in the two groups turned out not to be significantly different.

- *Data pooling.* Researchers sometimes obtain data from more than one source or from more than one type of subject. For example, to enhance the generalizability of their studies, researchers sometimes draw subjects from multiple sites, or they may recruit subjects with several different types of medical conditions. The risk in doing this is that the subjects may not really be drawn from the same population. Therefore, it is wise in such a situation to determine whether **pooling** of the data (combining data for all subjects) is warranted. This involves comparing the different subsets of subjects (i.e., the subjects from the different sites, and so on) in terms of key research variables. There are specific statistical tests that can be applied to evaluate whether pooling is justifiable (e.g., **Chow tests**); these tests are described in advanced textbooks on statistics.

- *Cohort effects.* Nurse researchers sometimes need to gather data over an extended period of time to achieve the sample sizes required to test the research hypotheses adequately. If sample members are recruited over a lengthy time period, it is possible that there will be **cohort effects**, that is, that relationships between research variables will vary over time. This might occur because the characteristics of the sample evolve over time or because of changes in the community, in families, in health care, and so on. If the research involves an experimental treatment, it may also be that the treatment itself is modified over time—for example, if early program experience is used to improve the treatment or if those administering the treatment simply get better at doing it. Thus, researchers with a long period of sample intake should consider testing for cohort effects because such effects can confound the results or even mask existing relationships. This activity usually involves splitting the sample into two or three groups based on the date of entry into the sample and comparing the cohorts on key research variables.

- *Sample representativeness.* Tests are sometimes performed to determine whether a research sample is representative of the population from which it has been drawn (e.g., the chi-square goodness-of-fit test; see Polit, 1996). For example, suppose a sample of teenage mothers were drawn for a research study from a hospital clinic, and the researcher wanted to know whether the sample was representative of teenage mothers statewide. If there are published statistics about the characteristics of the population (e.g., percentage on welfare), the goodness-of-fit test can be used to examine whether the sample is representative of that population.

PRINCIPAL ANALYSES

At this point, the researcher should have a data set that has been cleaned, has missing data problems resolved, and includes any needed transformed variables. The researcher should also at this point have some understanding of data quality and the extent of any biases. The researcher can now proceed with more substantive analyses of the data.

The Substantive Data Analysis Plan

In many research projects, the researcher collects data on dozens, and often hundreds, of variables. The researcher cannot realistically analyze every variable in relation to all others, and so a plan to guide data analysis must be developed. The researcher's hypotheses and research questions provide only broad and general direction.

One approach is to prepare a list of the analyses to be undertaken, specifying both the variables and the statistical test to be used. Another approach (which can be used in conjunction with a list of analyses) is to develop table shells. **Table shells** are layouts of how the researcher envisions presenting the research findings in a report, without any numbers in the table. Once a table shell has been prepared, the researcher can undertake whatever analyses are necessary to fill in the table entries.

Table 21-1 presents an example of an actual table shell created for an evaluation of an intervention for low-income women. This table guided a series of analyses of covariance that compared the experimental and control groups in terms of several indicators of emotional well-being, after controlling for various characteristics that were measured at random assignment. The completed table that eventually appeared in the research report was somewhat different than this table shell (e.g., another outcome variable was eventually added). Thus, a researcher does not need to be rigid in adhering to the table shells, but they provide an excellent mechanism for organizing the analysis of vast amounts of data.

Substantive Analyses

Once the researcher has developed an analytic plan, the next step involves performing the actual substantive analyses designed to answer the research questions. Typically, the task begins with descriptive analyses. For example, the researcher generally develops a descriptive

TABLE 21-1	Example of a Table Shell: Program Impacts on Indicators of Emotional Well-Being at the Time of the Follow-up Interview*			
OUTCOME	**EXPERIMENTAL GROUP**	**CONTROL GROUP**	**DIFFERENCE**	**P**
Mean score on the CES-D (depression) scale				
Percentage at risk of clinical depression (scores of 16 and above on the CES-D)				
Mean score, Master (self-efficacy) scale				
Mean score, Difficult Life Circumstances scale				
Percentage who cited no one as available as a social support				
Mean number of categories of social support cited as available				
Mean level of satisfaction with available social support				

*Note: Analyses to be performed using ANCOVA, controlling for 51 baseline characteristics.

profile of the sample and examines the distribution of values on all key variables. Also, the researcher often looks, in a descriptive fashion, at the correlations among the variables. These descriptive analyses may help to suggest further analyses (or further data transformations) that initially had not been envisioned. They also give the researcher an opportunity to become familiar with the data.

In the final stages of the substantive analyses, the researcher typically performs several statistical analyses to test the research hypotheses. In some cases, the researcher whose data analysis plan calls for multivariate analyses (e.g., MANOVA) will proceed directly to that procedure, but often the researcher will first perform various bivariate analyses (e.g., a series of ANOVAs). The primary statistical analyses are complete when all the research questions are addressed and, if relevant, when all the table shells have the applicable numbers in them.

The final phase of the data analysis task involves the interpretation of the findings and the conduct of any supplementary analyses that can aid in that endeavor. The interpretive phase is discussed in the next section.

INTERPRETATION OF RESULTS

The analysis of research data provides what are referred to as the **results** of the study. These results need to be evaluated and interpreted by the researcher with due consideration to the overall aims of the project, its theoretical underpinnings, the specific hypotheses being tested, the existing body of related research knowledge, and the limitations of the adopted research methods.

The interpretive task primarily involves a consideration of five aspects of the study findings: (1) their accuracy, (2) their meaning, (3) their importance, (4) the extent to which they can be generalized, and (5) their implications. In this section, we review issues relating to each of these five aspects.

Accuracy of the Results

One of the first tasks that the researcher faces in interpreting the results is assessing whether the findings are likely to be accurate. This assessment, in turn, requires a careful analysis of the study's methodologic and conceptual limitations. Whether one's hypotheses are supported or not, the validity and meaning of the results depend on a full understanding of the study's strengths and shortcomings.

Such an assessment relies heavily on the researcher's critical thinking skills as well as on an ability to be reasonably objective about one's own decisions. The researcher should carefully evaluate (e.g., using criteria such as those that we present in Chapter 25) all the major methodologic decisions made in planning and executing the study to determine whether alternative decisions might have yielded different results.

The assessment of accuracy, however, also depends on the ability of the researcher to assemble different types of evidence. One type of evidence is the body of prior research on the topic. The investigator should examine whether his or her results are consistent with those of other studies; if there are discrepancies, a careful analysis of the reasons for any differences should be undertaken.

Other types of evidence can often be developed through peripheral data analyses, some of which were discussed earlier in this chapter. For example, the researcher needs to assess carefully the quality of the data collected, the reliability of measures used, and the presence or absence of any biases.

Another highly recommended strategy in quantitative studies is the conduct of a power analysis. In Chapter 19, we described how power analysis is often used before a study is undertaken to estimate sample size requirements. The researcher can also determine the actual power of his or her own analyses to evaluate the likelihood of having committed a Type II error. It is especially useful to perform a power analysis when the results of the main hypothesis tests were not statistically significant.

For example, suppose we were testing the effectiveness of an intervention to reduce patients' perception of pain. The sample of 200 subjects (100 subjects each in an experimental and a control group) are compared in terms of pain scores, using a *t*-test. Suppose further that the mean pain score for the experimental group was 7.8 (SD = 1.3), whereas for the control group, the mean pain score was 8.2 (SD = 1.3), indicating lower reported pain among the experimental subjects. Although the results are in the hypothesized direction, the *t*-test was nonsignificant. We can provide a context for interpreting the accuracy of the nonsignificant results by performing a power analysis. First, we must estimate the effect size, using the formula presented in Chapter 19.

$$\gamma = \frac{8.2 - 7.8}{1.3} = .31$$

Table 19-6 in Chapter 19 shows us that, with an effect size of about .30, $\alpha = .05$, and a sample size of 100 per group (which is close to the N of 109 under the column headed .30 in the table), the power of the statistical test is about .60. This means that we had a 40% risk of committing a Type II error—that is, the incorrect retention of the null hypothesis. The power analysis also tells us that the next researcher testing the effectiveness of this intervention should use a sample of about 175 per group to reach power = .80, which is the conventional standard for acceptable risk with Type II errors.

A critical analysis of the research methods and conceptualization and an examination of various types of external and internal evidence will almost inevitably indicate some limitations. These limitations must be taken into account in interpreting the results.

Meaning of the Results

In qualitative studies, interpretation and analysis occur virtually simultaneously. In quantitative studies, however, the results are in the form of test statistic values and probability levels. It is the researcher's role to imbue these results with meaning. Sometimes, this involves supplementary analyses that were not originally planned. For example, if research findings are not what the researcher hypothesized, other types of information in the data set can often be examined to help the researcher understand what the findings mean.

In this section, we discuss the interpretation of various types of research outcomes within a hypothesis testing context. If the research was conceived on the basis of a theory or conceptual model, then it is important to relate the findings to that theoretical framework. That is, if a theoretical framework was truly the basis for the study, then it should also provide a basis for trying to understand the data.

INTERPRETING HYPOTHESIZED RESULTS

When the tests of statistical significance support the original research hypotheses, the task of interpreting the results is somewhat easier than when the hypotheses are challenged. In a sense, the interpretation has been partly accomplished beforehand in such a situation because the researcher has already had to bring together prior research findings, a theoretical framework, and logical reasoning in the development of the hypotheses. This groundwork can then form the context within which more specific interpretations are made.

Naturally, researchers are gratified when the results of many hours of effort offer support for their predictions. There is a decided preference on the part of individual researchers, advisers, and journal reviewers for studies whose hypotheses have been supported. This preference is understandable, but it is important not to let personal predilections interfere with the critical appraisal that is appropriate in all interpretive situations. A few cautionary suggestions should be kept in mind.

First, it is preferable to be somewhat conservative in drawing conclusions from the data. It is sometimes tempting to go far beyond the data in developing explanations for what the results mean, but this should be avoided. A simple example might help to explain what is meant by "going beyond" the data. Suppose a nurse researcher hypothesized that a relationship existed between a pregnant woman's level of anxiety about the labor and delivery experience and the number of children she has already borne. The data reveal that a negative relationship between anxiety levels and parity ($r = -.40$) does indeed exist. The researcher, therefore, concludes that increased experience with childbirth causes decreasing amounts of anxiety. Is this conclusion supported by the data? The conclusion appears to be logical, but in fact, there is nothing within the data that leads directly to this interpretation. An important, indeed critical, research precept is that *correlation does not prove causation*. The finding that two variables are related offers no evidence suggesting which of the two variables— if either—caused the other. In the example, perhaps causality runs in the opposite direction, that is, that a woman's anxiety level influences how many children she bears. Or perhaps a third variable not examined in the study, such as the woman's relationship with her husband, causes or influences both anxiety and number of children.

Alternative explanations for the findings should always be considered and, if possible, tested directly. If these competing interpretations can be ruled out on the basis of the data or previous research findings, so much the better. However, every angle should be examined to see if one's own explanation has been given adequate competition. Any evidence from the researcher's assessment of bias and data quality should be brought to bear at this point.

Empirical evidence supporting the research hypotheses never constitutes proof of their veracity. Hypothesis testing, as we have seen, is probabilistic. There always remains a possibility that the obtained relationships resulted from chance or from some artifact of the research methods. Therefore, one must be tentative about both the results and the interpretations given to those results. In summary, even when the findings are in line with expectations, the researcher should exercise restraint in drawing conclusions and should give due consideration to any limitations identified in the assessment of the accuracy of the results.

INTERPRETING NONSIGNIFICANT RESULTS

Failure to reject a null hypothesis is particularly problematic from an interpretative point of view. The statistical procedures currently prevalent are geared toward disconfirmation of the null hypothesis. The failure to reject a null hypothesis could occur for one or more reasons, and the researcher does not usually know which of these reasons pertains. The null hypothesis could actually be true. The nonsignificant result, in this case, would accurately reflect the absence of a relationship among the research variables. On the other hand, the null hypothesis could be false, in which case a Type II error would have been committed.

The retention of a false null hypothesis can be attributed to several things, such as internal validity problems, the selection of a deviant sample, the use of a weak statistical procedure, or the use of too small a sample. Unless the researcher has special justification for attributing the nonsignificant findings to one of these factors, interpreting such results is a tricky business. However, we suspect that in most cases, the failure to reject the null hypothesis is the consequence of insufficient power (usually reflecting too small a sample size). For this reason, the conduct of a power analysis can often come to the researcher's aid in interpretation when nonsignificant results are obtained, as indicated earlier.

In any event, there is never justification for interpreting a retained null hypothesis as proof of a *lack* of relationship among variables. *The safest interpretation is that nonsignificant findings represent a lack of evidence for either truth or falsity of the hypothesis.* Thus, one can see that if the researcher's actual research hypothesis states that no differences or no relationships will be observed, traditional hypothesis testing procedures will not permit the required inferences.

When no significant results are found, there is sometimes a tendency to be overcritical of one's research strategy and methods and undercritical of the theory or logical reasoning on which the hypotheses were based. This is understandable: It is easier to say, "My ideas were sound, I just didn't use the right approach to demonstrate this," than to admit that one has reasoned incorrectly. It is important to look for and identify flaws in the research methods, but it is equally important to search for theoretical shortcomings. The result of such endeavors should be recommendations for how the methods, the theory, or perhaps an experimental intervention could be improved.

INTERPRETING UNHYPOTHESIZED SIGNIFICANT RESULTS

Unhypothesized significant results can occur in two situations. The first involves findings about relationships that were not even considered in the design of the study. For example, in examining correlations among variables, the researcher might notice that two variables that were not central to the hypotheses or research question were nevertheless significantly correlated—and interesting. In determining how to interpret this finding, the researcher should try to evaluate whether the relationship is real or spurious. Sometimes, there are other indications within the data set that shed light on this issue, but in other cases, the researcher may need to consult the literature to determine if other investigators have observed similar relationships.

The second situation is more perplexing: obtaining results *opposite* to those hypothesized. For instance, a nurse researcher might hypothesize that individualized patient teaching of breathing techniques is more effective than group instruction, but the results might reflect that the group method was better. Or a positive relationship might be predicted between a nurse's age and level of job satisfaction, but a negative relationship might be found.

It is, of course, unethical to alter the hypothesis after the results are in. Although some researchers may view such situations as awkward or embarrassing, there is really little basis for such feelings. The purpose of research is not to corroborate the scientist's notions, but to arrive at truth and enhance understanding. There is no such thing as a study whose results "came out the wrong way," if the "wrong way" is the truth.

In the case of significant findings opposite to what was hypothesized, it is less likely, though not impossible, that the methods are flawed than that the reasoning or theory is incorrect. As always, the interpretation that the researcher gives to the findings should involve comparisons with other research, a consideration of alternate theories, and a critical scrutiny of the data collection and analysis procedures. The final result of such an examination should be a tentative explanation for the unexpected findings, together with suggestions for how such explanations could be tested in other research projects.

INTERPRETING MIXED RESULTS

The interpretive process is often confounded by mixed results. The investigator may find some hypotheses supported by the data and others that cannot be supported, or a hypothesis may be accepted when one measure of the dependent variable is used but rejected when using a different measure of the same construct. Of all the situations mentioned, mixed results are probably the most prevalent.

When only some results run counter to a theoretical position or conceptual scheme, the research methods are probably the first aspect of the study that deserves scrutiny. Differences in the validity and reliability of the various measures could account for such discrepancies, for example. On the other hand, mixed results could indicate how a theory needs to be

qualified or how certain constructs within the theory need to be reconceptualized. Mixed results often present opportunities for making conceptual advances because close scrutiny and attempts to make sense of disparate pieces of evidence may lead to breakthroughs that otherwise might have been impossible.

In summary, the interpretation of research findings is a demanding task, but it offers the possibility of unique intellectual rewards. The researcher must in essence play the role of a scientific detective, trying to make pieces of the puzzle fit together so that a coherent picture emerges.

Importance of the Results

In quantitative studies, results in support of the researcher's hypotheses are described as being significant. A careful analysis of the results of a study involves an evaluation of whether, in addition to being statistically significant, they are important.

The fact that statistical significance was attained in testing the hypothesis does not necessarily mean that the results were of value to the nursing community and their clients. Statistical significance indicates that the results were unlikely to be a function of chance. This means that the observed group differences or observed relationships were probably real but not necessarily important. With large samples, even modest relationships are statistically significant. For instance, with a sample of 500, a correlation coefficient of .10 is significant at the .05 level, but a relationship of this magnitude may have little practical value. Researchers, therefore, must pay attention to the numeric values obtained in an analysis in addition to the significance level when assessing the implications of the findings.

Conversely, the absence of statistically significant results does not mean that the results are unimportant—although because of the difficulty in interpreting nonsignificant results, the case is more complex. However, let us suppose that the study involved testing two alternative procedures for making a clinical assessment (e.g., body temperature). Suppose that a researcher retained the null hypothesis, that is, found no statistically significant differences between the two methods. If a power analysis revealed an extremely low probability of a Type II error (e.g., power = .99, a 1% risk of a Type II error), then the researcher might be justified in concluding that the two procedures yield equally accurate assessments. If one of these procedures was more efficient or less painful than the other, then the nonsignificant findings could indeed be clinically important.

Generalizability of the Results

Another aspect of the results that the researcher should assess carefully is their generalizability. Researchers are rarely interested in discovering relationships among variables for a specific group of people at a specific point in time. The aim of research is typically to reveal enduring relationships, the understanding of which can be used to improve human conditions. If a nursing intervention under investigation is found to be successful, others will want to adopt the procedure. Therefore, an important interpretive question is whether the intervention will "work" or whether the relationships will "hold" in other settings, with other people. Part of the interpretive process involves asking the question, "To what groups, environments, and conditions can the results of the study be applied?"

Implications of the Results

Once the researcher has formed conclusions about the accuracy, meaning, importance, and generalizability of the results, he or she is in a good position to draw inferences about the implications of the results and to make recommendations for how best to use and build on the study findings. The researcher should con-

sider the implications with respect to future research endeavors, theory development, and nursing practice.

The results of one study are often used as a springboard for additional research, and the investigator is typically in a good position to recommend "next steps." Armed with a comprehensive understanding of the study's limitations and strengths, the researcher can pave the way for studies that avoid the same pitfalls or that capitalize on known strengths. Moreover, the researcher is in a good position to assess how a new study could move a topic area forward. Is a replication needed, and, if so, with what groups? If observed relationships are significant, what do we need to know next for the information to be maximally useful?

If the study was based on a theoretical framework or conceptual model, then the researcher should also consider the implications of the study results for the theory. If the analysis of the study methods leads the researcher to conclude that the study had many flaws, then it may be difficult to make any inferences about the validity of the theory. However, if the study was reasonably rigorous methodologically, then the results should be used to either document support for the theory, suggest ways in which the theory ought to be modified, or discredit the theory as a useful approach for studying the topic under investigation.

Finally, the researcher should carefully consider the implications of the findings for nursing practice and nursing education. How can client outcomes or the nursing process be improved, based on the findings of the study? Specific suggestions for implementing the results of the study in a real nursing context are extremely valuable in the utilization process, as we discuss in Chapter 26. Of course, if the study is seriously flawed, it may be that the results are not usable within the nursing profession; nevertheless, they will probably be useful in designing an improved new study for the same research question.

TIPS FOR DEVELOPING AND IMPLEMENTING AN ANALYSIS PLAN

This chapter was designed to provide practical advice about the development and implementation of a data analysis plan. A few additional suggestions are offered next.

- Whenever you create transformed or recoded variables, it is important to check that the computer is performing the intended manipulation by examining a sample of values for the original and transformed variables. This can be done by instructing the computer to list the values of newly created variables and the original variables used to create them for a sample of cases in the data set.
- When transformed and recoded variables become an integral part of your data set, you should remember to document the transformations in the codebook carefully. This will facilitate secondary analysis by other researchers. It will also enable you to use your own data set at some later date.
- When you begin to undertake analyses designed to acquaint you with your data set, you should resist the temptation to go on a "fishing expedition," that is, to hunt for *any* interesting relationships between variables, even if they were not anticipated or even contemplated. The facility with which computers can generate statistical information certainly can free you from laborious (and error-prone) manual calculations. But it also permits you to run analyses in a rather indiscriminate fashion. The risk is that you will serendipitously find significant correlations between variables that are simply a function of chance. It is important to remember that if you adopt the conventional .05 probability level for a Type I error, there is a strong possibility that there will be some significant correlations that do not reflect true relationships in the population. To make this more concrete, in a correlation matrix with 10 variables (which will result in 45 nonredundant correlations), there are likely to be two or three spurious significant correlations ($.05 \times 45 = 2.25.$)

- In formulating your interpretation of the data, you should remember that others will be reviewing your interpretation with a critical and perhaps even a skeptical eye. Part of your job will be to convince others, in a fashion not dissimilar to convincing a jury in a judicial proceeding. Your hypotheses and interpretations are, essentially, on trial—and it must be remembered that the null hypothesis is considered "innocent" until proven "guilty." The evidence for your interpretation may come primarily from the statistical tests of the hypotheses, but you should look for opportunities to gather and present supplementary evidence in support of your conclusion. This includes evidence from other studies as well as internal evidence from your own study. You should scrutinize your data set and ask if there are any further analyses that could support your tentative explanation of the findings.

RESEARCH EXAMPLE

Researchers typically undertake many of the steps depicted in Figure 21-1 without reporting on them in their research reports. Thus, the research literature does not offer many examples that fully describe the design and implementation of an analysis plan. A few examples of the types of analyses described in this chapter are presented in Table 21-2.

Considerable analytic detail, however, was provided in a study published by Davis, Maguire, Haraphongse, and Schaumberger

TABLE 21-2 Examples of Non-Substantive Analyses Undertaken in Research Projects	
RESEARCH QUESTION	**TYPE OF ANALYSIS**
What are the effects of multiple sclerosis as perceived by afflicted people and their family members at different points in the trajectory of the illness? (Gulick, 1998)	Comparison of study participants who remained in the study for 10 years and those who dropped out, to test for attrition bias; replacement of missing values with means; analysis of data quality (reliability and validity)
What are the effects of a transmural home care intervention program for terminal cancer patients on the caregivers' quality of life, compared with standard care programs? (Smeenk et al., 1998)	Comparison of study dropouts to those who remained in the study; comparison of patients and caregivers in the two treatment groups to test for selection bias
What is the relationship between stress appraisal, coping, and characteristics of individuals responsible for older adults recently placed in nursing homes? (Kammer, 1994)	Comparison of subjects from two sites on key variables to determine if the data could be pooled
What is the validity and reliability of the Prenatal Psychosocial Profile? (Curry, Campbell, & Christian, 1994)	Listwise deletion to remove cases with missing data on key variables (for supplementary analyses performed on data merged from two studies)
To what extent do demographic variables and attachment predict quality of life in community-dwelling older men? (Rickelman, Gallman, & Parra, 1994)	Analysis of data quality (internal consistency reliability); recoding of variables for multiple regression
What is the effect of alternative types of information on coping with unplanned child hospitalization? (Melnyk, 1994)	Analysis of questions to determine whether subjects processed information they received—a manipulation check
What are the effects of ambulation at 3 versus 6 hours after cardiac anglogram on delayed bleeding, pain, and anxiety? (Barkman & Lunse, 1994)	Comparison of experimental and control group members on pretreatment variables to test the integrity of randomization

(1994), who examined whether the type of preparatory information provided to cardiac catheterization (CC) patients was equally effective in reducing anxiety for patients with different coping styles. The coping styles of the 145 patients who served as the subjects in this study were first assessed, and patients were then categorized as either "monitors" (i.e., people who coped through information-seeking strategies) or "blunters" (i.e., people who coped through an information-avoiding strategy). Using a randomized block design, the two coping-style groups were then randomly assigned to one of three preparatory information treatment conditions: (1) procedural information presented on videotape, (2) procedural–sensory information presented on videotape, and (3) procedural–sensory information presented in a booklet. Anxiety was measured at four points in time: preintervention, postintervention, pre-CC procedure, and post-CC procedure.

The central hypothesis regarding effects on patient anxiety was tested with a $2 \times 3 \times 4$ ANOVA (coping style $\times$ preparatory treatment $\times$ time period). In addition, the researchers undertook the following analyses:

- The six treatment groups (2 coping styles $\times$ 3 treatment groups) were compared in terms of basic demographic characteristics (age and education) and preintervention anxiety—an analysis aimed at assessing potential selection effects. One significant difference emerged: monitors reported more preintervention anxiety than blunters.
- The researchers then wondered whether gender might be implicated in the observed preintervention anxiety differences. A $2 \times 3 \times 2$ ANOVA (coping style $\times$ treatment group $\times$ gender) yielded a significant gender effect on preintervention anxiety scores (women were significantly more anxious than men). The researchers concluded that gender should be taken into account in their analyses but realized that they had too few women in the sample to analyze results for women separately.
- A subgroup analysis was, however, undertaken with the 107 men in the sample. This analysis revealed a significant coping style by treatment interaction in terms of preintervention anxiety. The male blunters randomly assigned to the three treatment groups were found to be comparable in terms of pretreatment anxiety, whereas the male monitors were not. This analysis, then, indicated that the random assignment did not result in the sought-after anxiety equivalency among the subgroup of male blunters. (A further analysis was performed to determine whether the nonequivalence among groups was the result of only one or two extreme scores on the preintervention anxiety measure, but this proved not to be the case).
- The investigators then examined whether it made sense to use preintervention anxiety as a covariate in subsequent analyses, which would allow them to control statistically the differences in preintervention anxiety among male blunters. However, they found that the correlations between preintervention anxiety and postintervention anxiety varied both across time and across groups, which precluded using preintervention anxiety as a covariate. Therefore, the researchers used ANOVA (rather than ANCOVA) for the main analyses. However, their knowledge of the pretreatment differences was taken into consideration in interpreting the results.
- The investigators calculated effect sizes as a means of assessing effects that were both statistically and clinically significant. They determined that any mean difference on the anxiety scale of 3 points or greater constituted an effect size of .30, which they established as their criterion for clinical significance.

As hypothesized, the researchers found that there was a significant three-way ANOVA interaction. Essentially, the results indicated that the procedural–sensory videotape treatment was especially beneficial for the monitors. The procedural modeling video was the optimal treatment for blunters. Over time, the monitors and blunters in each treatment group reported decreases in anxiety.

The researchers' results, then, include both expected and unexpected findings, which they addressed in the Discussion section of their report. The finding that coping styles moderated the effects of the preparation strategies was predicted on the basis of theory and prior research. The finding that women were significantly more anxious than their male counterparts in both coping-style groups led the researchers to recommend that gender be considered as a primary rather than an incidental variable in CC preparatory intervention research.

The nonequivalence among male monitors led the researchers to consider the following theoretical implications:

From a theoretic standpoint, it was determined that the observed nonequivalence in state anxiety among the male monitor groups might reflect an important and heretofore unexamined aspect of coping style: the relationship between subjects' monitoring and blunting repertoires and their procedural anxiety levels. (p. 136)

The researchers then pursued the implications of this suggestion with several supplementary analyses.

In summary, the researchers appear to have implemented a thorough and thoughtful analysis plan that took unexpected findings and design quality issues into account in interpreting the findings.

SUMMARY

Researchers who have collected quantitative data typically must progress through a series of steps in the analysis and interpretation of their data. The careful researcher lays out a **data analysis plan** in advance to guide that progress.

Quantitative data must be converted to a form amenable to computer analysis through the process of **coding**, which typically transforms all research data into numbers. Special codes need to be developed for coding **missing values.**

The researcher often plans in advance the layout of information into a computer file for each subject. In a **fixed format** arrangement, the values for any specific variable are entered in the same column of a data entry record for each case. In **freefield format**, variables are not necessarily entered in the same columns, but rather are separated by **delimiters** such as blank spaces. In fixed format mode, the **field width** for each variable is determined by the maximum numeric value for that variable, and the data are generally **right justified,** or entered as far to the right as possible in the designated field. Researchers typically document the decisions made concerning coding, variable naming, and field placement in a **codebook.**

Data entry is an error-prone process that requires **verification** and **cleaning.** The cleaning process involves a check for **outliers** (values that lie outside the normal range of values) and **wild codes** (codes that are not legitimate).

The focus of much of this chapter has been on the preliminary analysis steps that pave the way for substantive statistical analysis. An important early step is the implementation of procedures to address missing data problems. These steps include the deletion of cases with missing values (i.e., **listwise deletion**), deletion of variables with missing values, substitution of mean values, estimation of missing values, and selective and **pairwise deletion** of cases. Researchers strive to achieve a **rectangular matrix** of data (valid information on all variables for all cases), and several of these strategies can help the researcher to reach this goal.

Raw data entered directly onto a computer file often need to be modified for analysis. **Data transformations** can be of many types and are usually handled directly through commands to the computer. Examples of transformations include reversing of the coding of items, combining individual variables to form a composite scale, recoding the values of a variable, performing mathematic transformations for the purpose of meeting statistical assumptions, and creating dichotomous dummy variables for multivariate analyses.

Before the main analyses can proceed, the researcher usually has to undertake a number of additional steps to assess data quality and to maximize the value of the data. These steps include evaluating the reliability of measures, examining the distribution of values on key variables for any anomalies, and analyzing the magnitude and direction of any biases. Sometimes, peripheral analyses involve **manipulation checks,** tests to determine whether **pooling** of subjects is warranted, or tests for **cohort effects.**

Once the data are fully prepared for the substantive analysis, the researcher should develop a formal plan to reduce the temptation to go on a "fishing expedition." One of the mechanisms that researchers sometimes use in the planning process is the development of

table shells, that is, fully laid-out tables that do not yet have any numbers in them.

The interpretation of research findings basically represents the researcher's attempts to understand the research results. The interpretation typically involves five subtasks: (1) analyzing the accuracy of the results, (2) searching for the meaning underlying the results, (3) considering the importance of the findings, (4) analyzing the generalizability of the findings, and (5) assessing the implications of the study regarding future research, theory development, and nursing practice.

STUDY ACTIVITIES

Chapter 21 of the *Study Guide to Accompany Nursing Research: Principles and Methods, 6th ed.*, offers various exercises and study suggestions for reinforcing the concepts presented in this chapter. Additionally, the following study questions can be addressed:

1. Read the study by Coffman, Levitt, and Brown (1994) entitled "Effects of clarification of support expectations in prenatal couples" (*Nursing Research, 43,* 111–116). Indicate which steps in the process shown in Figure 21-1 are described in this report.
2. Suppose you were studying gender differences in physical health 6 months after loss of a spouse. Create a fictitious table shell for such a study.

SUGGESTED READINGS

Methodologic References

Cohen, J., & Cohen, P. (1983). *Applied multiple regression/correlation analysis for the behavioral sciences* (2nd ed.). New York: John Wiley and Sons.

Dixon, W. J., & Massey, F. J. (1983). *Introduction to statistical analysis* (4th ed.). New York: McGraw-Hill.

Ferketich, S., & Verran, J. (1994). An overview of data transformation. *Research in Nursing & Health, 17,* 393–396.

Harris, M. L. (1991). *Introduction to data processing* (3rd ed.). New York: John Wiley and Sons.

Jacobsen, B. S. (1981). Know thy data. *Nursing Research, 30,* 254–255.

Kim, J., & Curry, J. (1977). The treatment of missing data in multivariate analysis. In D. F. Alwin (Ed.), *Survey design and analysis.* Beverly Hills, CA: Sage.

Little, R. J. A., & Rubin, D. B. (1990). The analysis of social science data with missing values. In J. Fox & J. S. Long (Eds.), *Modern methods of data analysis.* Newbury Park, CA: Sage.

Polit, D. F. (1996). *Data analysis & statistics for nursing research.* Stamford, CT: Appleton & Lange.

Tabachnick, B. G., & Fidell, L. S. (1989). *Using multivariate statistics* (2nd ed.). New York: Harper & Row.

Substantive References

Barkman, A., & Lunse, C. P. (1994). The effect of early ambulation on patient comfort and delayed bleeding after cardiac angiogram. *Heart & Lung, 23,* 112–117.

Curry, M. A., Campbell, R. A., & Christian, M. (1994). Validity and reliability testing of the Prenatal Psychosocial Profile. *Research in Nursing & Health, 17,* 127–135.

Davis, T. M. A., Maguire, T. O., Haraphongse, M., & Schaumberger, M. R. (1994). Preparing adult patients for cardiac catheterization: Informational treatment and coping style interactions. *Heart & Lung, 23,* 130–139.

Ferketich S. L., & Mercer, R. T. (1994). Predictors of paternal role competence by risk status. *Nursing Research, 43,* 80–85.

Gulick, E. E. (1998). Symptoms and activities of daily living in multiple sclerosis: a 10-year study. *Nursing Research, 47,* 137–146.

Kammer, C. H. (1994). Stress and coping of family members responsible for nursing home placement. *Research in Nursing & Health, 17,* 89–98.

Melnyk, B. M. (1994). Coping with unplanned childhood hospitalization: Effects of informational interventions on mothers and children. *Nursing Research, 43,* 50–55.

Murata, J. (1994). Family stress, social support, violence, and sons' behavior. *Western Journal of Nursing Research, 16,* 154–168.

Rickelman, B. L., Gallman, L., & Parra, H. (1994). Attachment and quality of life in older, community-residing men. *Nursing Research, 43,* 68–72.

Smeenk, F. W., de Witte, L. P., van Haastregt, J. C., Schipper, R. M., Biezemans, H. P., & Crebolder, H. F. (1998). Transmural care of terminal cancer patients: Effects on the quality of life of direct caregivers. *Nursing Research, 47,* 129–136.

CHAPTER **22**

The Analysis of Qualitative Data

As we have seen, qualitative data take the form of loosely structured, narrative materials, such as verbatim dialogue between an interviewer and a respondent in a phenomenologic study, the field notes of a participant observer in an ethnographic study, or diaries used by historical researchers. These data are generally not amenable to the type of analyses we discussed in the chapters on statistical analysis. This chapter describes methods for analyzing such qualitative data.

INTRODUCTION TO QUALITATIVE ANALYSIS

Qualitative analysis is a very labor-intensive activity that requires insight, ingenuity, creativity, conceptual sensitivity, and sheer hard work. Qualitative analysis does not proceed in a linear fashion and is more complex and difficult than quantitative analysis because it is less standardized and formulaic. In this section, we discuss some general considerations relating to qualitative analysis.

Qualitative Analysis: General Considerations

The purpose of data analysis, regardless of the type of data one has and regardless of the tra-

dition that has driven its collection, is to impose some order on a large body of information so that the data can be synthesized, interpreted, and communicated. Although the overall aims of both qualitative and quantitative analysis are to organize, provide structure to, and elicit meaning from research data, an important difference is that, in qualitative studies, data collection and data analysis usually occur simultaneously, rather than after all the data are collected. The search for important themes and concepts begins from the moment data collection begins.

The data analysis task is almost always a formidable one, but it is particularly challenging for the qualitative researcher, for three major reasons. First, there are no systematic rules for analyzing and presenting qualitative data. It is at least partly because of this fact that qualitative methods have been described by some critics as "soft." The absence of systematic analytic procedures makes it difficult for the researcher engaged in qualitative analysis to present conclusions in such a way that their validity is patently clear. In addition, the absence of well-defined and universally accepted procedures makes replication difficult. Some of the procedures described in Chapter 17 (e.g., member checking and investigator triangulation) are extremely important tools for enhancing the trustworthiness not only of the data themselves but also of the analyses and interpretation of those data.

The second aspect of qualitative analysis that makes it challenging is the enormous amount of work that is required. The qualitative analyst must organize and make sense of pages and pages of narrative materials. In a qualitative study directed by one of the authors (Polit), the data consisted of transcribed, unstructured interviews with about 100 women who had recently divorced. The transcriptions ranged from 40 to 80 pages in length, resulting in more than 6000 pages that had to be read and re-read and then organized, integrated, and interpreted.

The final challenge comes in reducing the data for reporting purposes. The major results of quantitative research can often be summarized in a handful of tables. However, if one compresses qualitative data too much, the very point of maintaining the integrity of narrative materials during the analysis phase becomes lost. If one merely summarizes the conclusions reached without including numerous supporting excerpts directly from the narrative materials, then the richness of the original data disappears. As a consequence, it is sometimes difficult to do a thorough presentation of the results of qualitative research in a format that is compatible with space limitations in professional journals.

Analysis Styles

Crabtree and Miller (1992) observed that there are nearly as many qualitative analysis strategies as there are qualitative researchers. However, they have identified four major analysis styles or patterns that fall along a continuum. At one extreme is a style that is more objective, systematic, and standardized, and at the other extreme is a style that is more intuitive, subjective, and interpretive. The four prototypical styles they described are as follows:

- *Quasi-statistical style.* The researcher using a quasi-statistical style typically begins with some preconceived ideas about the analysis, and then uses those ideas to sort the data. This approach is sometimes referred to as **manifest content analysis**—the researcher reviews the content of the narrative data, searching for particular words or themes that have been specified in advance in a codebook. The result of the search is information that can be manipulated statistically—and hence the name quasi-statistics. For example, the analyst can count the frequency of occurrence of specific themes. This style is similar to the traditional, quantitative approach to performing content analysis.

- *Template analysis style.* In this style, the researcher develops a **template** or analysis guide to which the narrative data are applied. The units for the template are typically behaviors, events, and linguistic expressions (e.g., words or phrases). A template is more fluid and adaptable than a codebook in the quasi-statistical style. Although the researcher may begin with a rudimentary template before collecting any data, the template undergoes constant revision as more data are gathered. The analysis of the resulting data, once sorted according to the template, is interpretive and not statistical. This type of style is most likely to be adopted by researchers whose research tradition is ethnography, ethology, discourse analysis, and ethnoscience.

- *Editing analysis style.* The researcher using the editing style acts as an interpreter who reads through the data in search of meaningful segments and units. Once these segments are identified and reviewed, the interpreter develops a **categorization scheme** and corresponding codes that can be used to sort and organize the data. The researcher then searches for the patterns and structure that connect the thematic categories. The grounded theory approach typically incorporates this type of style. Researchers whose research tradition is phenomenology, hermeneutics, and ethnomethodology use procedures that fall within the editing analysis pattern.

- *Immersion/crystallization style.* This style involves the analyst's total immersion in and reflection of the text materials, resulting in an intuitive crystallization of the data. This highly interpretive and subjective style is exemplified in personal case reports of a semi-anecdotal nature and is less frequently encountered in the nursing research literature than the other three styles.

Qualitative nurse researchers are especially likely to use an analytic strategy that can best be characterized as an editing style. Most of the remainder of this chapter describes analytic activities that are consistent with that style.

The Qualitative Analysis Process

The analysis of qualitative data typically is an active and interactive process—especially at the interpretive end of the analysis style continuum. Qualitative nurse researchers typically scrutinize their data carefully and deliberatively. Insights and theories cannot spring forth from the data without the researcher becoming completely familiar with those data. Qualitative researchers often read their narrative data over and over again in a search for meaning and deeper understandings. Morse and Field (1995) note that qualitative analysis is a "process of fitting data together, of making the invisible obvious, of linking and attributing consequences to antecedents. It is a process of conjecture and verification, of correction and modification, of suggestion and defense"(p. 126).

Several intellectual processes play a role in qualitative analysis. Morse and Field (1995) have identified four such processes:

- *Comprehending.* Early in the analytic process, qualitative researchers strive to make sense of the data and to learn "what is going on." When comprehension is achieved, the researcher is able to prepare a thorough and rich description of the phenomenon under study, and new data do not add much to that description. In other words, comprehension is completed when saturation has been attained.

- *Synthesizing.* Synthesizing involves "sifting" the data and putting pieces together. At this stage, the researcher gets a sense of what is "typical" with regard to the phenomenon under study and what the range and variation are like. At the end of the synthesis process, the researcher can begin to make some generalized statements about the phenomenon and about the study participants.

- *Theorizing.* Another important process in qualitative analysis is theorizing, which involves a systematic sorting of the data. During the theorizing process, the researcher develops alternative explanations of the phenomenon under study and then holds these explanations up to determine their "fit" with the data. The theorizing process continues to evolve until the best and most parsimonious explanation is obtained.

- *Recontextualizing.* The process of **recontextualization** involves the further development of the theory such that its applicability to other settings or groups is explored. In qualitative inquiries whose ultimate goal is theory development, it is the theory that must be recontextualized and generalized.

Although the intellectual processes in qualitative analysis are not linear in the same sense that quantitative analysis is, it is nevertheless true that these four processes follow a rough progression over the course of the study. Comprehension occurs primarily while in the field. Synthesis begins in the field, but may continue well after the field work has been completed. Theorizing and recontextualizing are processes that are difficult to undertake before synthesis has been completed.

QUALITATIVE DATA MANAGEMENT AND ORGANIZATION

The intellectual processes of qualitative analysis are supported and facilitated by tasks that help to organize and manage the masses of narrative data. Data management tasks involve activities that prepare the data for subsequent analysis.

Developing a Categorization Scheme

The first step in analyzing qualitative data is to organize them; without some system of organization, there is only chaos. The main task in organizing qualitative data is developing a method to classify and index the materials. That is, the researcher must design a mechanism for gaining access to parts of the data, without having to repeatedly re-read the set of data in its entirety. This phase of data analysis is essentially a reductionistic activity—data must be converted to smaller, more manageable, and more manipulatable units that can easily be retrieved and reviewed.

The most widely used procedure is to develop a categorization scheme and to then code the data according to the categories. Different analysis styles proceed with this task somewhat differently, as previously noted. That is, a categorization system is sometimes prepared (at least in a preliminary version) before data collection. However, in most cases, the qualitative analyst develops categories based on a scrutiny of the actual data.

There are, unfortunately, no straightforward or easy guidelines for this task. The development of a high-quality categorization scheme for qualitative data involves a careful reading of the data, with an eye to identifying underlying concepts and clusters of concepts. Depending on the aims of the study, the nature of the categories may vary in level of detail or specificity as well as in level of abstraction.

Researchers whose aims are primarily descriptive tend to use categories that are fairly concrete. For example, the category scheme may focus on differentiating various types of actions or events, or different phases in a chronologic unfolding of an experience. The topical coding scheme used in Gagliardi's (1991) study of the family's experience of living with a child with Duchenne muscular dystrophy is presented in Box 22-1. (Gagliardi's study was described as a research example in Chapter 17). This is an example of a category system that is fairly concrete and descriptive. For example, it allows the coders to code specific relationships among family members, and events occurring in specific locations.

In developing a category scheme, related concepts are often grouped together to facilitate the coding process. As shown in Box 22-1, Gagliardi's system involved five major clusters of categories. For example, all of the excerpts illustrating how family members feel about living with a child with Duchenne muscular dystrophy are clustered under "Feeling Codes."

Studies that are designed to develop a theory (e.g., a grounded theory study) are more likely to develop abstract and conceptual categories. In designing conceptual categories, the researcher must break the data into segments, closely examine them, and compare them to other segments for similarities and dissimilarities to determine what types of phenomena are reflected in them and what the meaning of those phenomena are. (This is part of the process referred to as **constant comparison** by grounded theory researchers.) The researcher asks questions about discrete events, incidents, or thoughts that are indicated in an observation or statement, such as the following:

- What is this?
- What is going on?
- What does it stand for?

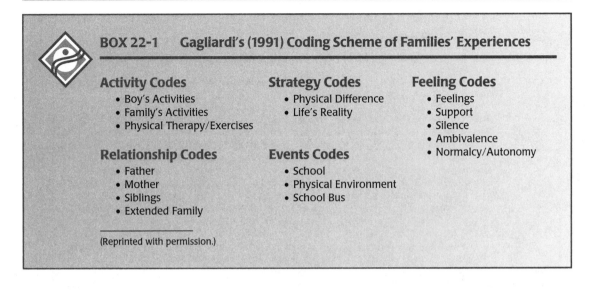

BOX 22-1   Gagliardi's (1991) Coding Scheme of Families' Experiences

Activity Codes
- Boy's Activities
- Family's Activities
- Physical Therapy/Exercises

Relationship Codes
- Father
- Mother
- Siblings
- Extended Family

Strategy Codes
- Physical Difference
- Life's Reality

Events Codes
- School
- Physical Environment
- School Bus

Feeling Codes
- Feelings
- Support
- Silence
- Ambivalence
- Normalcy/Autonomy

(Reprinted with permission.)

- What else is like this?
- What is this distinct from?

Important concepts that emerge from close examination of the data are then given names or labels that form the basis for a categorization scheme. These category names are necessarily abstractions, but the labels are generally sufficiently graphic that the nature of the material to which they refer is clear—and often provocative. Strauss and Corbin (1990), prominent grounded theory methodologists, advise qualitative researchers as follows: "The important thing is to name a category, so that you can remember it, think about it, and most of all begin to develop it analytically" (pp. 67–68).

Coding Qualitative Data

Once a categorization scheme has been developed, all of the data are then reviewed for content and coded for correspondence to or exemplification of the identified categories. In a grounded theory study, the entire initial process of breaking down, categorizing, and coding data is often referred to as **open coding**.

The actual codes corresponding to the category system are arbitrary. They can be an abbreviation of the category (e.g., B-ACT for

Boy's Activities in Gagliardi's category system), a code corresponding to an outline structure (e.g., Boy's Activities might be A.1 and Family's Activities might be A.2), or some other type of symbolic configuration. When a computer is used to index the data, the software being used often specifies requirements for labeling the codes.

This process of coding qualitative material is seldom an easy one, for several reasons. First, the researcher may have difficulty deciding which code is most appropriate or may not fully comprehend the underlying meaning of some aspect of the data. It may take a second or third reading of the material to grasp the nuances contained in some portions of the data.

Second, the researcher often discovers in going through the data that the initial category system was incomplete or otherwise inadequate. In many cases, this means going back and starting from scratch. For this reason, it is usually necessary to review a very large portion of the data before an adequate categorization scheme can be developed. It is not unusual for some topics to emerge that were not initially conceptualized. When this happens, it is risky to assume that the topic failed to appear in materials that have already been coded. That is, a concept might not be identified as salient until it has emerged three or four times

```
Subject 025
June 25, 1980
Page 32

Int:      How did you feel right after the separation?  Will you tell
          me a little more about that?

025:      Well, you know, when I look back...I mean I think anybody
          would have felt hopeless and helpless...because of, you
          know, emotionally...I think maybe it's a little easier if    2b
          you've got more security...more money.  I was really stuck.   9
          I caught myself thinking..."Oh, if it wasn't for the
          kids..."  I love them both dearly, but...I mean there have
          been times when I've said to myself--I think a lot of women   5c
          go through this too--I really had thought of giving them
          up.  In the beginning I used to think, too, they'd be so
          much better off with somebody that could, you know...When I
          was really struggling--I was on welfare----I used to think,
          "My God, how am I going to educate them?  What are they      1b
          going to have?  I can't make ends meet now."  It's kinda
          projecting the unknown...fear of the unknown.  I think you
          can get mixed up.
```

Figure 22-1.   Coded excerpt from an unstructured interview.

in the data. In such a case, it would be necessary to re-read all previously coded material to have a truly complete grasp of that category.

Another problem stems from the fact that narrative materials are generally not linear. For example, paragraphs from transcribed interviews may contain elements relating to three or four different categories, embedded in a complex fashion. An example of a multitopic segment of an interview from a study of divorced women by one of the authors, with codes in the margin, is shown in Figure 22-1.*

Methods of Organizing Qualitative Data

Traditionally, qualitative data have been organized manually through a variety of techniques. Although these manual methods have

a long and respected history, they are becoming increasingly outmoded as a result of the widespread availability of personal computers that can be used to perform the filing and indexing of qualitative material. Computer programs for managing qualitative data are described in Chapter 23. Here, we briefly describe some manual methods of data organization and management.

When the amount of data is small, or when a category system is fairly simple, researchers sometimes use color paper clips or color Post-It Notes to code the content of the narrative materials. For example, if we were analyzing responses to a single unstructured question about women's attitudes toward the menopause, we might use blue paper clips for comments relating to the topic of loss of reproductive capacity, red clips for comments relating to physical side effects such as hot flashes, yellow clips for comments relating to aging, and so on. Then the researcher could pull out all of the responses coded with a certain color clip to examine one aspect of menopausal attitudes at a time.

---

*Figure 22-1 does not show the categories that the alphanumeric codes in the margin represent. The code categories used in the figure are as follows: 2b—General psychologic state during the divorce; 9—Finances; 5c—Feelings about single parenting; and 1b—Divorce-induced problems.

Before the advent of computer programs for managing qualitative data, the most usual procedure was the development of **conceptual files.** In this approach, a physical file is developed for each of the various categories, and all of the materials relating to that topic are cut out and inserted into the file. To create conceptual files, the researcher must first go through all of the data and write the relevant codes in the margins, as in Figure 22-1. Then the researcher cuts up a copy of the material by category area, and places the cut-out excerpt into the file for that category. In this fashion, all of the content on a particular topic can be retrieved by going to the applicable file folder.

The creation of such conceptual files is clearly a cumbersome and labor-intensive task. This is particularly true when segments of the narrative materials have multiple codes, as is true in the excerpt shown in Figure 22-1. In such a situation, there would need to be four copies of the paragraph—one for each file corresponding to the four codes. The researcher must also be sensitive to the need to provide enough context that the cut-up material can be understood. For example, it might be necessary to include material preceding or following the directly relevant materials. Finally, the researcher must usually include pertinent administrative information on each item in the conceptual files. For example, if the data consisted of transcribed interviews, each informant would ordinarily be assigned an identification (ID) number. Each excerpt filed in the conceptual file would also need to include the appropriate ID number so that the researcher could, if necessary, obtain additional information from the master copy.

In lieu of conceptual files, some researchers use qualitative sort cards (also known as McBee cards) for indexing their data. These index cards have holes on all sides that can be used for easy retrieval of information on a given topic or concept. That is, the researcher places notches in the holes corresponding to coded topical categories or concepts. Then, when information relating to a particular topic or concept is needed, all of the cards notched for that category can easily be pulled from the deck of index cards. Some researchers directly paste their data on these cards, when the data set is of a manageable size, and then directly code each data segment using the notched holes to indicate a code. Others write an abstract of an entire case (e.g., one interview or one observational session) onto the card, and then indicate on the card the page numbers (e.g., pages of the observational notes or transcribed interview) where different codes may be found.

Clearly, such manual methods are labor intensive. Computer programs remove the drudgery of cutting and pasting pages and pages of narrative material and are fast becoming indispensable research tools. However, some people argue that beginning researchers should gain at least some experience with manually organizing qualitative data. Part of this argument stems from the sentiment that manual indexing provides a more hands-on type of experience that allows the researcher to get closer to the data. Other concerns have been expressed about the use of computers with qualitative data. For example, one potential pitfall is that the researcher might develop an overly elaborate coding system, resulting from the fact that retrieval of information is vastly simplified with a computer. The advent of sophisticated programs that aid in the analysis of data has also given rise to objections to having a process that is basically cognitive turned into an activity that is mechanical and technical. Despite these concerns, most qualitative researchers have switched to computerized management of their data, and this trend is unlikely to be reversed. Computerized data management frees up the researcher's time so that greater attention can be paid to more important conceptual issues.

ANALYTIC PROCEDURES

Data management tasks in qualitative research are typically reductionist in nature because they convert large masses of data into smaller, more manageable segments. By contrast, qualitative data analysis tasks are constructionist in nature: They involve putting together segments into a meaningful conceptual pattern. Although different approaches to qualitative data analysis have been advocated, there are some elements that are common to several of them. We provide some general guidelines, followed by a description of the analytic procedures used in two specific types of approach.

A General Analytic Overview

The analysis of qualitative materials generally begins with a search for **themes** or recurring regularities. In many cases, the thematic analysis begins in the field as the data are being collected. In other situations, the thematic analysis occurs after the data have been collected, during a reading (or re-reading) of the data set.

Themes often develop within categories of data (i.e., within categories of the coding scheme used for indexing materials) but sometimes cut across them. For example, in Gagliardi's (1991) study, six themes describing the families' experiences were identified, and these themes were further grouped under three headings corresponding to the stages in the process of adapting to the child's disability. The first theme, disillusionment, embraced content that had been coded under several topical codes (see Box 22-1), primarily the topics within the feeling category.

The search for themes involves not only the discovery of commonalities across subjects but also a search for natural variation in the data. Themes that emerge from unstructured observations and interviews are never universal. The researcher must attend not only to what themes arise but also to how they are patterned. Does the theme apply only to certain subgroups? In certain types of communities or organizations? In certain contexts? At certain periods? What are the conditions that precede the observed phenomenon, and what are the apparent consequences of it? In other words,

the qualitative analyst must be sensitive to *relationships* within the data.

The analyst's search for themes, regularities, and patterns in the data can sometimes be facilitated by charting devices that enable the researcher to summarize the evolution of behaviors, events, and processes. For example, for qualitative studies that focus on dynamic experiences—such as decision making—it is often useful to develop flow charts or timelines that highlight time sequences, major decision points and events, and factors affecting the decisions. An example of such a flow chart from a study of decision making among infertile couples is presented in Figure 22-2. The construction of such flow charts for all subjects would help to highlight any regularities in the subjects' evolving behaviors.

A further step frequently taken involves the validation of the understandings that the thematic exploration has provided. In this phase, the concern is whether the themes inferred are an accurate representation of the perspectives of the people interviewed or observed. Several procedures can be used in this validation step, some of which were discussed in Chapter 17. If there is more than one researcher working on the study, debriefing sessions in which the themes are reviewed and specific cases discussed can be highly productive. Multiple perspectives—what we referred to in Chapter 17 as investigator triangulation—cannot ensure the validity of the themes, but it can minimize any idiosyncratic biases. Using an iterative approach is almost always necessary. That is, the researcher derives themes from the narrative materials, goes back to the materials with the themes in mind to see if the materials really do fit, and then refines the themes as necessary. It is generally useful to undertake member checks—that is, to present the preliminary thematic analysis to some of the subjects or informants, who can be encouraged to offer suggestions that might support or contradict this analysis.

It is at this point that some researchers introduce quasi-statistics—a tabulation of the

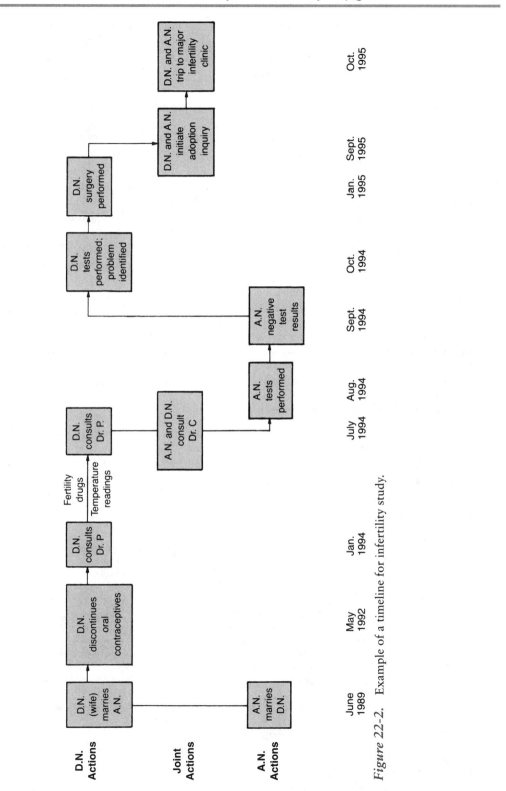

Figure 22-2.   Example of a timeline for infertility study.

frequency with which certain themes, relations, or insights are supported by the data. The frequencies cannot be interpreted in the same way as frequencies generated in survey studies, because of imprecision in the sampling of cases and enumeration of the themes. Nevertheless, as Becker (1970) pointed out,

> Quasi-statistics may allow the investigator to dispose of certain troublesome null hypotheses. A simple frequency count of the number of times a given phenomenon appears may make untenable the null hypothesis that the phenomenon is infrequent. A comparison of the number of such instances with the number of negative cases—instances in which some alternative phenomenon that would not be predicted by his theory appears—may make possible a stronger conclusion, especially if the theory was developed early enough in the observational period to allow a systematic search for negative cases. Similarly, an inspection of the range of situations covered by the investigator's data may allow him to negate the hypothesis that his conclusion is restricted to only a few situations, time periods, or types of people in the organization or community. (p. 81)

In the final stage of analysis, the researcher strives to weave the thematic pieces together into an integrated whole. The various themes need to be interrelated in a manner that provides an overall structure (such as a theory or integrated description) to the entire body of data. The integration task is an extremely difficult one because it demands creativity and intellectual rigor if it is to be successful. A strategy that sometimes helps in this task is to cross-tabulate dimensions that have emerged in the thematic analysis. For example, Barton (1991), in her study of parents' adaptations to their adolescent children's drug abuse problems, found that parental power and parental responsibility were two important dimensions that, when cross-tabulated, reflected important coping patterns among the parents in her sample. Her diagram displaying the cross-tabulated schema is presented in Figure 22-3.

Analytic Induction

The general procedures and steps previously described provide a general outline of how qualitative researchers make sense of their data and distill from them their understandings of processes and behaviors operating in naturalistic settings. However, there are some variations in the goals and underlying philosophies of qualitative researchers that also lead to variations in how the analytic task is handled. One of the strategies for analyzing qualitative data is referred to as **ana-**

	+ POWER −	
+	The parents feel guilty despite professionals' attempts to eliminate guilt Style is "committed"/ "correcting the flaw"	The parents are especially "fused" to the child Style is "stuck"/"secondary gains" or "protection from social responsibility"
−	The parents accept not feeling responsible and have power. Style is "successful"/ "mastery"	The parents accept not feeling responsible but let go of power. Style is "letting go"/"new meaning"

RESPONSIBILITY (label to the left of the grid)

Figure 22-3. Barton's (1991) schema describing parental adaptation to adolescent drug abuse (reprinted with permission).

lytic induction, an approach that was developed in the 1930s.

The analytic induction approach requires a careful scrutiny of all the researcher's data, usually according to the following six steps:

1. Define the phenomenon to be studied and explained.
2. Based on a review of the data, formulate a hypothetical explanation of the phenomenon; that is, develop an inductively derived hypothesis.
3. Conduct an intensive analysis of individual cases to see whether the hypothesis fits particular cases.
4. Search for negative cases that, if found, lead to a reformulation of the hypothesis *or* a redefinition of the phenomenon to exclude the particular case.
5. Continue the examination of cases, redefinition of the phenomenon, and reformulation of hypotheses until a universal pattern of relationships is established.
6. Create a higher level of abstraction or conceptualization through comparison with other settings or groups.

In practice, the use of analytic induction results in a procedure that alternates back and forth between tentative explanation and tentative definition, each refining the other so that a sense of closure can be achieved when an integral relation between the two is established. As an example from the nursing research literature, Mayo (1992) conducted an ethnographic study of the processes of managing physical activity among African American working women; she used analytic induction as the method of analyzing her qualitative data.

Grounded Theory Analysis

By far the most widely used analytic approach among nurse researchers is Glaser and Strauss's (1967) grounded theory method of generating theories from data. Because of its popularity, we describe here some of the specific analytic techniques of grounded theory.

As we have seen, the first step is the development of a categorization scheme and the substantive coding of data through the preliminary process referred to as open coding (or, sometimes, **level I coding**). Open coding allows the researcher to identify major categories and subcategories and to describe their major properties and dimensions.

Level II coding (often referred to as **axial coding**) is a reconstructive process that puts the data back together in new ways after open coding is completed by connecting a category and its subcategories. Constant comparison is used again in axial coding to refine theoretical categories. Strauss and Corbin (1990) noted that, in axial coding, the "focus is on specifying a category (*phenomenon*) in terms of the conditions that give rise to it; the *context* (its specific set of properties in which it is embedded; the action/interaction *strategies* by which it is handled, managed, carried out; and the consequences of those strategies" (p. 97). Axial coding is a complex process involving both inductive and deductive thinking and is designed to move the coding process to a higher level of abstraction.

Throughout the coding and analysis process, the grounded theory analyst documents his or her ideas, insights, and feelings about the data, themes, and the emerging conceptual scheme in the form of **memos**. Morse and Field (1995) note that the memos serve numerous functions in a grounded theory study. For example, memos help the researcher to identify underlying assumptions. They also preserve ideas that may initially not seem productive but may later prove valuable once further developed. An especially important function is that memos encourage a higher level of abstract thinking by getting the researcher to reflect on and describe themes and patterns in the data, relationships between categories, and emergent conceptualizations.

Once saturation has been achieved and both open coding and axial coding are completed, integration can begin. Here, the analyst reviews and sorts the memos to explore theoretical explanations and searches for the **core category**—the central phenomenon that is used to integrate all other categories. Level III coding (also referred to as **selective coding**) is the process of selecting the core category, systematically identifying and integrating relationships between the core category and other categories, and validating those relationships. The integrative process is similar to axial coding, except that it is done at a more highly abstract level of analysis.

Level III coding results in a description of a **basic social process (BSP)**, which is the central social process resulting from the data. Because of the activities in which the researcher has engaged, the emergent theory of what this process is and how it works is grounded in the data.

The grounded theory method is concerned with the generation of categories, properties, and hypotheses rather than with testing them

(as in the case of analytic induction). The product of the typical grounded theory study is a conceptual or theoretical model that endeavors to explain the phenomenon under study. As an example, Figure 22-4 presents the model developed by King and Jensen (1994) in their grounded theory study that conceptualized the process of women's "preserving the self" during cardiac surgery.

There are some obvious similarities between the grounded theory and analytic induction approaches, but there are also some important differences. Of particular importance is their overall aims. Analytic induction is concerned with the testing of inductively derived hypotheses; it is purported to be a method for coming to terms with the problem of causal inference while remaining faithful to qualitative, naturalistic data. The grounded theory method is concerned with the generation of categories, prop-

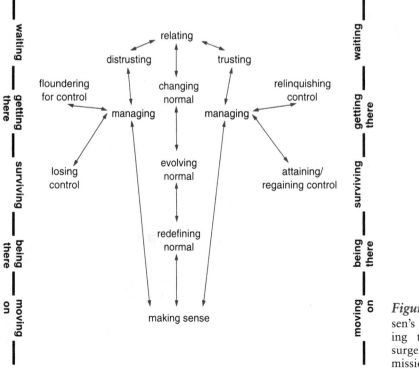

Figure 22-4. King and Jensen's (1994) model of preserving the self during cardiac surgery (reprinted with permission).

erties, and hypotheses rather than with testing them. The product of many grounded theory studies is a conceptual or theoretical model that endeavors to explain the phenomenon under study.

INTERPRETATION OF QUALITATIVE FINDINGS

In qualitative studies, interpretation and analysis of the data occur virtually simultaneously. That is, the researcher interprets the data as he or she categorizes it, develops a thematic analysis, and integrates the themes into a unified whole. Efforts to validate the qualitative analysis are necessarily efforts to validate the interpretation as well. Thus, in qualitative studies, the meaning of the data flows from the analysis.

Nevertheless, the prudent qualitative researcher holds his or her interpretation up for closer scrutiny—self-scrutiny as well as review by peers and outside reviewers. It might be noted that even when the researcher has undertaken procedures such as member checks and peer debriefings, this in itself does not constitute proof that the results and interpretations are credible. For example, in member checks, many participants might be too polite to disagree with the researcher's interpretations, or they may become intrigued with a conceptualization that they themselves would never have developed on their own—a conceptualization that is not necessarily accurate. Thus, for qualitative researchers as well as quantitative researchers, it is important to consider possible alternative explanations for the findings and to take into account methodologic or other limitations that could have affected the study results.

In drawing conclusions, the qualitative researcher should also consider the transferability of the findings. That is, whereas qualitative researchers rarely seek to make generalizations, they often strive to develop an understanding of how the study results can be usefully applied. The central question is, In what

other types of settings and contexts could one expect the phenomena under study to be manifested in a similar fashion?

The implications of the findings of qualitative studies, as with quantitative ones, are often multidimensional. First, there are implications for further research: Should the study be replicated in another study? Can the study be expanded (or circumscribed) in meaningful and productive ways? Do the results suggest that an important construct has been identified that merits the development of a more formal instrument? Does the emerging theory suggest hypotheses that could be tested through more controlled, quantitative research? Second, do the findings have implications for nursing practice? For example, could the health care needs of a subculture (e.g., the homeless) be identified and addressed more effectively as a result of the study? Finally, do the findings shed light on the fundamental processes that are incorporated into nursing theory?

ILLUSTRATION OF QUALITATIVE ANALYSIS ACTIVITIES

Qualitative researchers seldom discuss in any detail the ways in which they analyze their data. However, the steps undertaken by a research team that studied how the role of clinical nurse researchers was being defined, enacted, and evaluated was described by Knafl and Webster (1988). This study involved in-depth telephone interviews with 34 clinical nurse researchers (CNRs) and their corresponding chief nurse executives (CNEs). The data consisted of about 1000 pages of interview transcripts.

The researchers undertook six major tasks during the data management phase and five major tasks during the data analysis phase:

Phase I: Data Management

1. Independent reading of a sample of interview transcripts by team members; collaborative development of six major

descriptive coding categories; development of a codebook to ensure consistent application of final coding categories

2. Independent coding of all interviews in margins of transcripts by two coders; collaborative review of codes and resolution of differences in coding
3. Cut-and-paste transfer of all data onto color-coded 5- × 8-inch index cards, with colors corresponding to the six major categories
4. Identification of subcategories reflecting narrower topical areas within the major categories
5. Coding of the index cards according to the subcategories identified
6. Construction of descriptive summary grids for each subcategory across all subjects, with each cell of the grid containing a brief summary of pertinent content

Phase II: Data Analysis

1. Description of the content of each subcategory and identification of major themes; preparation of a written analysis summary
2. Description of the content of each major category, constructed from the subcategory summary
3. Description of the CNR group, synthesizing and integrating relevant material
4. Description of the CNE group, synthesizing and integrating relevant material
5. Description of CNR–CNE pairs, contrasting of within-pair themes

TIPS FOR ANALYZING QUALITATIVE DATA

Qualitative analysis is a challenging—but often a very rewarding—enterprise. In this section, we offer a few additional tips to beginning students regarding the conduct of a qualitative analysis.

- In developing a category system for coding qualitative data, a substantial sample of the data should be carefully read before the scheme is finalized. To the extent possible, the researcher should try to read materials that vary along important dimensions, in an effort to capture the full range of content. The dimensions might include informant characteristics (e.g., transcripts of men versus women, articulate versus less articulate informants) or aspects of the data collection experience (e.g., shorter versus longer interviews, observations in different types of settings). If the researcher can identify in advance what the important dimensions might be, methods should be used to facilitate identification of good exemplars (e.g., by appending written comments on the relevant dimensions at the end of an interview).

- Even when a category system is "finalized," the researcher should be prepared to amend or even totally revise it. Even simple changes may mean re-reading all previously coded material. Making changes midway is often painful and frustrating, but without a highly effective category system, the researcher will be unable to identify and integrate important themes adequately.

- In most studies, it is wise to develop a codebook, that is, written documentation describing the exact definition of the various categories used to code the data. Good qualitative codebooks usually include two or three actual excerpts that typify materials coded in each category.

- Even if you have little experience using a computer, the available programs for qualitative data management are relatively easy to learn and should not be a cause of anxiety. In selecting a program (see Chapter 23), try to discuss the merits of various programs with other researchers who have experience using them.

• Many researchers engage in qualitative studies on their own rather than with a co-investigator. However, collaborative efforts are becoming more common, as journal editors and peers have come to demand that greater attention be paid to validating qualitative data and the meanings associated with them. Having one or more team member ensures that the data will not be analyzed and interpreted in a totally subjective fashion.

RESEARCH EXAMPLES

The number of qualitative studies that have been published in nursing journals during the past decade has risen dramatically. Two research examples are described below.

Research Example of a Grounded Theory Analysis

Bright (1992) studied the birth of a first child as an intergenerational experience with the aim of discovering the basic social process associated with this event and generating a theory on normative family process. She collected in-depth interview and observational data over a 15-month period from three families: three first-born infants and their parents and six sets of grandparents. Data collection began during the last trimester of pregnancy and continued until the child's first birthday. The families differed in terms of whether the pregnancy was planned and wanted.

Within each family, the interviews were initially conducted in a group setting, which allowed the researcher to observe family interactional patterns and to learn about family beliefs and customs as well as expectations about the anticipated birth event. Subsequent interviews were conducted with individual family members, with dyads, and with small groups as deemed needed on the basis of the developing hypotheses. Interviews and ob-

servations occurred in parental and grand-parental homes, on the hospital maternity ward, and at other locations, such as baptismal ceremonies. Telephone interviews were used to clarify data and to check on the validity of the emerging hypotheses.

The analysis of data was done as an ongoing process, integrated with data collection and coding. Interviews were audiotaped, transcribed, and then coded line by line. One three-generation family interaction was videotaped to provide recorded nonverbal as well as verbal data for coding. Coded data were grouped into related categories and then compared with one another and with new data to refine and discard emerging hypotheses continually. Memoranda were prepared concurrently to record the researcher's theoretical analysis of the data. Several methods were used to validate the themes emerging from the analysis, including review by members of the families.

The analysis resulted in the identification of an evolutionary family process that reflected reorganized interpersonal patterns. "Making place," the central social process that emerged from Bright's analysis, was defined as the family process through which a newborn individual receives recognition as a member of that family. The family made place both physically and socially for the new and expanded relationships created by the child's birth.

Research Example of an Analysis for an Ethnographic Study

Russell (1996) conducted an ethnographic study that focused on the care-seeking process used by elders residing in a continuing-care retirement community. During 8 months of field work in the retirement community, Russell collected data on the elders' process of eliciting care and engaging caregivers in care interactions. Data were collected through in-depth semistructured interviews with 12 elders, participant observation in the facility's adult care center where 34 elders were observed, and a focus group interview with four elders. Each of the data collection methods yielded different perspectives about the participants' care seeking. The interviews and focus group sessions were taped and fully transcribed, and the researcher took field notes after observational sessions. Data collection and data analysis were done concurrently. The data were entered into computer files for organization and management.

The first step involved comparing and contrasting data elements from different sources to generate a categorization scheme. The result was the development of a codebook with more than 150 codes and definitions. The codes were then organized and reorganized into larger units that enabled the researcher to identify patterns, features, sequences, and relationships in elders' care seeking. Field notes and memos were maintained to document new ideas about the analysis, including both theoretical and methodologic insights.

The basic unit of analysis was a specific care encounter. More than 275 such units were demarcated in the textual database. Each case was characterized in terms of certain structural elements, such as actors, contexts, and behaviors. These cases were used to develop and test an emerging conceptualization of the care-seeking process.

According to Russell's analysis, the care-seeking process comprises two phases, which she labeled "Care Eliciting" and "Care Engaging." Figure 22-5 shows Russell's diagram of the care-seeking process. The Initiating Stage, which began when elders decided that assistance was needed, was shaped by the elders' preferences (i.e., their desires and expectations relating to care) and their beliefs in terms of the appropriateness of a potential caregiver. Stage 2, the Alerting Stage, involved both verbal and nonverbal strategies designed to alert others of their desire for assistance. Stage 3, the Negotiating Stage, began when a caregiver become engaged in an elder's care. The negotiations between the elder and caregiver varied in terms of content, history of the relationship, and "doing"—the extent to which elders did for themselves or worked with caregivers to accomplish their care. Finally, stage 4 was the Evaluation Stage, the periodic appraisal that the elders undertook to make further decisions regarding the care taking. This stage was characterized by the elders' perceptions about the care settings, caregivers, and the care itself. Russell concluded that the findings supported viewing elders' care seeking as an interactional and developmental process.

SUMMARY

Qualitative analysis is a more challenging and labor-intensive activity than quantitative analysis—and one that is guided by fewer standardized rules. Although there are no universally adopted strategies for analyzing qualitative data, four prototypical styles have been identified that fall on a continuum from objective and systematic to interpretive and subjective: (1) a **quasi-statistical style** that begins

CARE-ELICITING PHASE	CARE-ENGAGING PHASE
1. Initiating Stage	3. Negotiating Stage
Preferences	Content
Beliefs	History
	Doing
2. Alerting Stage	4. Evaluating Stage
Verbal	Care Settings
Nonverbal	Caregivers
	Care

Figure 22-5. Russell's (1996) diagram of sequences in the care-seeking process.

with a preestablished codebook of themes or words and that lends itself to basic descriptive statistical analysis; (2) a **template analysis style** that involves the development of an analysis guide (**template**) used to sort the data; (3) an **editing analysis style** that involves an interpretation of the data on which a **categorization scheme** is based; and (4) an **immersion/ crystallization style** that involves the analyst's total immersion in and reflection of text materials. Most nurse researcher use a strategy that is best characterized as an editing analysis style—a style that typically requires four types of intellectual processes: comprehending, synthesizing, theorizing, and **recontextualizing** (exploration of the developed theory in terms of its applicability to other settings or groups).

The first major step in analyzing qualitative data is to organize the materials according to some plan, so that portions of the data can be readily retrieved. Typically, qualitative researchers develop a categorization scheme based on a reading of a portion of the data and then code the content of the data based on this system. Traditionally, researchers have developed **conceptual files** for organizing their data. In using this system, researchers first code their data in the margins of the printed narrative materials (e.g., observational notes or transcripts of interviews); cut out the coded excerpts; and finally place each excerpt into a file corresponding to each of the topics covered in the coding scheme. Then the researcher can retrieve all of the information on a topic by going to a single file. However, the widespread availability of personal computers and appropriate software has lessened the burden of indexing, organizing, and retrieving qualitative materials. There are now a wide variety of programs that not only perform basic indexing functions but also offer various enhancements that can facilitate analysis of the data.

The actual analysis of data begins with a search for **themes**. The search for themes involves not only the discovery of commonalities across subjects, but also of natural variation in the data. The next step generally involves a validation of the thematic analysis. Some researchers use **quasi-statistics**, which involves a tabulation of the frequency with which certain themes or relations are supported by the data. In a final step, the analyst tries to weave the thematic strands together into an integrated picture of the phenomenon under investigation.

Although this overview summarizes some of the major steps, there are a number of different philosophies underlying qualitative analysis. **Analytic induction** refers to an approach in which the researcher alternates back and forth between tentative definition of emerging hypotheses and tentative explanation, with each iteration making refinements. However, the most widely used approach by nurse researchers is grounded theory. Grounded theory begins with **open coding** (**level I coding**)—the development of a categorization scheme (using constant comparison) and subsequent initial coding of the data. **Level II coding** (also referred to as **axial coding**) is a reconstructive process that puts data back together in new ways by connecting categories and subcategories. The analyst begins the process of integration by reviewing and sorting the **memos** that have been used to document conceptual ideas throughout the data collection and data analysis process. During **level III coding** (or **selective coding**) the grounded theory analyst searches for the **core category**—the central phenomenon used to integrate all others. This phase results in an emerging theory of a **basic social process** (**BSP**) that is grounded in the data.

STUDY ACTIVITIES

Chapter 22 of the *Study Guide to Accompany Nursing Research: Principles and Methods, 6th ed.*, offers various exercises and study suggestions for reinforcing the concepts presented in this chapter. Additionally, the following study questions can be addressed:

1. Suggest a research problem amenable to qualitative research. Explain why you think the problem is better suited to a qualitative than to a quantitative approach.
2. Read a qualitative nursing study (several are suggested under Substantive References). Do you think that if a different investigator had gone into the field to study the same problem, the conclusions would have been the same? How generalizable are the researcher's findings? What did the researcher learn that he or she would probably not have learned with a more structured and quantified approach?
3. As a class assignment, have each student ask two people to describe their conception of preventive health care and what it means in their daily lives. Pool all the narrative descriptions, and develop a coding scheme to organize the reasons. What are the major themes that emerge?

✎ SUGGESTED READINGS

Methodologic References

Becker, H. S. (1970). *Sociological work*. Chicago: Aldine.

Carey, M. A., & Smith, M. W. (1994). Capturing the group effect in focus groups: A special concern in analysis. *Qualitative Health Research, 4,* 123–127.

Chenitz, W. C., & Swanson, J. M. (1986). *From practice to grounded theory: Qualitative research in nursing*. Menlo Park, CA: Addison-Wesley.

Crabtree, B. F., & Miller, W. L. (Eds.). (1992). *Doing qualitative research*. Newbury Park, CA: Sage.

Gephart, R. P., Jr. (1988). *Ethnostatistics: Qualitative foundations for quantitative research*. Newbury Park, CA: Sage.

Glaser, B. G., & Strauss, A. L. (1967). *The discovery of grounded theory: Strategies for qualitative research*. Chicago: Aldine.

Knafl, K. A., & Webster, D. C. (1988). Managing and analyzing qualitative data: A description of tasks, techniques, and materials. *Western Journal of Nursing Research, 10,* 195–218.

Lofland, J., & Lofland, L. H. (1984). *Analyzing social settings: A guide to qualitative observation and analysis* (2nd ed.). Belmont, CA: Wadsworth.

Miles, M. B., & Huberman, A. M. (1994). *Qualitative data analysis: An expanded sourcebook* (2nd ed.). Thousand Oaks, CA: Sage.

Morgan, D. L. (1993). Qualitative content analysis: A guide to paths not taken. *Qualitative Health Research, 3,* 112–121.

Morse, J. M., & Field, P. A. (1995). *Qualitative research methods for health professionals* (2nd ed.). Thousand Oaks, CA: Sage.

Strauss, A., & Corbin, J. (1990). *Basics of qualitative research*. Newbury Park, CA: Sage.

Substantive References

Barton, J. A. (1991). Parental adaptation to adolescent drug abuse: An ethnographic study of role formulation in response to courtesy stigma. *Public Health Nursing, 8,* 39–45.

Bright, M. A. (1992). Making place: The first birth in an intergenerational family context. *Qualitative Health Research, 2,* 75–78.

Gagliardi, B. A. (1991). The family's experience of living with a child with Duchenne muscular dystrophy. *Applied Nursing Research, 4,* 159–164.

King, K. M., & Jensen, L. (1994). Preserving the self: Women having cardiac surgery. *Heart & Lung, 23,* 99–105.

Mayo, K. (1992). Physical activity practices among American black working women. *Qualitative Health Research, 2,* 318–333.

Russell, C. K. (1996). Elder care recipients' care-seeking process. *Western Journal of Nursing Research, 18,* 43–62.

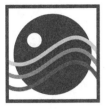

CHAPTER **23**

Computers and Nursing Research

Computers have evolved and expanded at a tremendous rate since their development in the 1940s. Few aspects of American society have remained untouched by the impact of computers, and with the advent of personal computers, they have become ubiquitous.

The use of computers in research, as one might suspect, is substantial. Computers have, in fact, revolutionized research by making possible certain operations that could not have been attempted with human labor alone. Computers are now used by researchers throughout the research process—to conduct bibliographic searches, to learn about funding opportunities for research projects, to collect and store data of all types, to maintain administrative research records, to analyze data, to write research reports and other documents, and to produce professional-looking charts and tables. Although there are numerous applications of computer technology in research, the discussion in this chapter focuses primarily on the use of computers to analyze research data.

One of the most striking features of modern computer technology is that computer users do not need to understand in detail how a computer works to benefit from its labor-saving computations. Computers have become accessible to broader and broader classes of users. It is hoped that an acquaintance with some of the basic characteristics of computers will be sufficient to demonstrate that computer analysis is within the reach of all readers of this book.

INTRODUCTION TO COMPUTERS

Most students have used computers for one purpose or another, and many of you own a computer and are familiar with their operation. Therefore, this section presents only a brief overview regarding several important computer features.

Powers and Limitations of Computers

Computers are machines of tremendous power. The most noteworthy characteristic of computers is unquestionably their remarkable speed. The speed of computers removes the drudgery and delays of doing computations manually and can increase researcher productivity. Not only are computers fast, but they also are accurate. Highly complex calculations can be performed without error. By contrast, humans are fallible. The person who spends an hour calculating a statistic such as a correlation coefficient would probably have to spend at least as much time checking for computational errors. A computer could perform the same calculation, error free, in less than 1 second. An additional advantage of computers is that they are *dependably* accurate. They can work hour after hour without making a mistake.

The memory capacity of most computers is impressive. The memory of a computer can store immense files of symbols to which it can gain access in a fraction of a second. Some memory devices can store millions of digits. What is even more impressive is that the information stored in memory is not permanent but can be erased and replaced with new information. In other words, the memory can be used over and over again to solve new problems.

Finally, although computers do break down, they behave for the most part as our faithful servants. They do exactly what they are told to do, day in and day out, no matter how boring or repetitive the task might be.

On the other hand, computers are not on the verge of making human intelligence obsolete. One of the most conspicuous limitations of computers is their utter and complete stupidity. Computers are sometimes referred to as giant brains, but computers have no innate intelligence. They do only those operations that they are told to do by humans. The computer's inability to think sometimes can result in frustrating experiences for its users. Unlike humans, a computer is unable to make even the simplest of inferences. A related limitation is the detail with which instructions must be described. When a human is confronted with the task $2 + 2 = X$, the solution is—at the conscious level at least—straightforward and simple. A computer normally requires several instructions to process such a computation. Every logical and arithmetic operation must be explained to the computer in detail. Fortunately, the average researcher does not have to worry about such matters. The de-

tailed instructions are developed by experts who have taken pains to simplify the use of computers.

Types of Computers

Broadly speaking, computers are either special-purpose or general-purpose machines. A **special-purpose computer** is dedicated to a single function: controlling the machines in which they are embedded. Many pieces of hospital equipment contain special-purpose computers. A **general-purpose computer** can be used for a wide variety of applications. **Applications** are the things that computers can be used to do.

There are two major types of general purpose computers that nurse researchers are likely to use: microcomputers and mainframes. Many universities, hospitals, and other large institutions own what is referred to as a **mainframe computer**, which is a large multiuser system that usually can be accessed from multiple locations. Mainframes typically have huge memory capacities and operate at very high rates of speed.

Microcomputers, or **personal computers** (**PCs**), are becoming increasingly popular both in institutions and in private homes and offices. PCs are slower and have less memory than mainframes, yet PCs are inexpensive, generally easy to use, and useful for many research applications, such as word processing and the analysis of most data sets. Personal computers vary in size from hand-held and lap-top models with rather restricted uses to relatively powerful desktop models with sophisticated applications.

Computer Components

The components of a computer system can be classified as either hardware or software. **Hardware** refers to the physical equipment that stores, processes, and controls information. **Software** refers to the instructions and procedures required to operate the computer.

COMPUTER HARDWARE

Essentially, the computer hardware consists of five types of components: input devices, output devices, memory, a control unit, and an arithmetic/logic unit. Information is fed into the computer through some type of **input device**—the device that allows you to "talk to" the computer. The information read in through an input device for data analysis comprises data, on the one hand, and instructions concerning how the data are to be processed, on the other. A keyboard or terminal typically serves as the primary input device. After the computer has performed the analyses, the resulting information comes out through an **output device**—the device that allows the computer to "talk back" to you. A common output device is a printer. In a mainframe environment, input/output devices (sometimes abbreviated **I/O devices**) are generally the only parts of the machine with which a researcher comes in direct physical contact.

The information that is read into the computer is stored in a device called **memory**. One way to conceptualize memory is as a series of pigeon holes or post office boxes. Each mailbox can store either an instruction or a numeric value. The memory unit of a computer is designed to store large amounts of information and to allow rapid access to any specific portion of that information. Memory capacity is measured in kilobytes (K), megabytes (MB) or gigabytes (GB). A **byte** is equivalent to a single character, such as a number, letter, or specialized symbol, such as a "+" sign. One kilobyte equals 1000 bytes, 1 megabyte equals 1 million bytes, and 1 gigabyte equals 1 billion bytes.

From the memory, the instructions are sent to the **control unit**. This component coordinates the functions of the other components. The control unit interprets the instructions, determines the sequence of operations of the computer, and controls the movements of information from one component to another. The **arithmetic/logic unit** is the component in which arithmetic operations are accomplished. The control unit and arithmetic/logic unit are together referred to as the **central processing unit** (CPU), which is where all the decisions are made and calculations performed.

COMPUTER SOFTWARE

The software components of a computer include the instructions for performing operations (referred to as a **program**) and the documentation for those instructions. The ability of a computer to solve problems depends on computer programs, which specify clearly and precisely what operations the machine is to perform and how to perform them.

People must be able to communicate with computers to give them programmed commands. Computers, unfortunately, do not directly understand natural languages such as English. Direct machine language that a computer *can* comprehend is extremely complex and accessible to only programming experts. Happily, various **programming languages** have been developed that are reasonably easy to learn and that are structured in a manner comfortable to human communicators. Most researchers can easily use computers without ever having to learn a programming language. This is because there are standard programs available for widely used applications. The applications software most commonly used by nurse researchers include the following:

- **Word processing**—software used for composing, revising, storing, and printing written documents, such as research reports, questionnaires, or research proposals
- **Desktop publishing**—software for printing documents, charts, and graphs at near-typeset quality
- **Spreadsheets**—programs that perform a variety of mathematic calculations and organize numeric information

- **Database management**—programs used for storing, retrieving, and manipulating large collections of data or information
- **Communications**—programs that allow computers to talk to one another over telephone lines
- **Data analysis**—software for organizing and analyzing data

Various data analysis software packages are discussed later in this chapter.

PERSONAL COMPUTERS

Most nurse researchers today enter and analyze their research data (and perform other functions as well) on PCs rather than on mainframes. Therefore, we devote this section to a discussion of the main features of PCs.

The Two Personal Computer Camps

Most personal computers currently used by researchers fall into two camps: (1) IBM PCs and compatible computers; and (2) Apple Macintosh computers (Macs). The IBM line of PCs have been widely imitated by other manufacturers. The terms **IBM clone** and **IBM compatible** indicate a computer not made by IBM, but one that uses similar design and components and that can use the same programs as IBM PCs. Clones of Macintosh computers are, by contrast, rare.

The main difference between IBM PCs and Macs concerns their **user interface**—the software that passes information to and from the person using the computer. Macs use a **graphical user interface** (GUI, pronounced "gooey"), which is a user-friendly interface centered around pictures (**icons**), graphic symbols, and **menus** (lists of options). The Mac's interface also uses **windows**—a method for dividing the display screen into rectangles for viewing two or more applications or parts of a single application at the same time.

Traditional IBM interfaces tended to be more text oriented. However, special windows programs for IBMs are now widespread, in effect making IBMs and their clones look and function more like Macs. Because most sophisticated analytic software for PCs have been designed for use on IBM-type computers, some of the discussion in this section is more relevant to IBM PCs than to Macs.

Personal Computer Systems

The basic hardware components of most PC systems consist of the following: a keyboard for inputting information, a display device, the systems unit, the disk drives and disks, and a printer for outputting information.

A **keyboard** is a device that converts keystrokes into codes that are intelligible to the computer. A PC keyboard looks like a typewriter but has a number of additional keys, including **function keys** (labeled F1 to F12) that perform special functions idiosyncratic to the application. Most keyboards also include a numeric keypad arranged like a calculator, for entering large amounts of numeric information. Most PCs also have a supplementary input device—a **mouse**—that allows you to point to words or objects on the computer screen.

The **display** (sometimes called a **monitor** or **computer screen**) is one of the output devices of a PC. The display gives you immediate feedback while you operate the computer (e.g., by displaying your keystrokes as you enter them) and is sometimes used for viewing the computer's output, such as the results of a statistical analysis.

The PC's **systems unit** houses both the memory and CPU. Most PCs today come with 32 to 64 megabytes of memory. In a PC, the CPU is a **microprocessor chip**. Microprocessors vary considerably in processing speed, measured in **megahertz** (MHz). One MHz represents 1 million cycles per second, so that in a 20-MHz microprocessor, there are 20 million cycles per second.

Disks are flat spinning objects, analogous to records, with magnetizable surfaces and concentric tracks. Disks are used to store information and can be used as either an input or output device. There are two types of magnetic disks—floppy disks and hard disks. **Hard disks** are large-capacity storage devices that are housed within the systems unit case, invisible to the computer user. **Floppy disks** have lower storage capacity and need to be inserted into the appropriate disk drive before use. Floppies are often used as **external storage** (i.e., for storing information outside the computer itself). Most PCs have a hard disk drive and one or two disk drives for floppies. The floppy drives are sometimes referred to as the **A drive** (and the **B drive** if there are two floppy drives), and the hard disk drive is the **C drive**. Both hard disks and floppy disks can be erased and used over and over again. Many PCs can also use **CD-ROMs** as input devices, which may be designated as the **D drive**.

For many applications, the primary output device is a **printer**, which produces paper-copy output from a computer program. Printers come in a variety of types, from relatively inexpensive **dot-matrix** printers that form characters with a pattern of dots, to **ink-jet** and **laser-jet** printers that create professional-looking output.

Operating System

An **operating system** is the software that controls the overall operation of the computer system. The operating system allows various parts of the computer system to talk to one another, and it also supports applications programs by managing the flow of information and keeping track of everything in memory. Applications software is designed for use with specific operating systems.

There are two basic types of operating systems: single-tasking and multitasking. A **single-tasking** operating system runs one application program or task at a time. **Multitasking** operating systems allow more than one application program or task to be active simultaneously. Several different operating systems are currently in use, but by far the most common are those produced by the Microsoft Corporation. In the 1980s, the most prevalent operating system was Microsoft's **MS-DOS** (*Microsoft Disk-Operating System*), a single-tasking system. During the 1990s, Microsoft released several new multitasking operating systems that use a graphical user interface, such as Windows 3.1, Windows 95, Windows 98, and Windows NT.*

Another widely used multitasking operating system is called **UNIX**, currently owned and marketed by Novell, Inc. UNIX is popular with computer programmers. Most computers that are networked on the Internet use the UNIX operating system.

Macintosh computers use completely different operating systems. The operating system used by today's Macintosh computers is System 8.

NETWORKS AND THE INTERNET

Communication among computers is becoming an increasingly important feature of contemporary computer use. This section discusses computer networking and the Internet.

Networks

A **network** is a group of two or more computers and related equipment that are linked together by communication devices and communication software. In a network, the main computer that manages the network is known

---

*Strictly speaking, the Windows software systems are not operating systems; there is still a DOS operating system running "underneath" Windows software, but it is usually invisible to users.

as the **server** (or **file server**). The server runs the network's operating system, which runs on top of the regular PC's operating system, and houses the files and programs that are shared.

There are several reasons for networking computers. First, networks allow computers to share data, files, and programs; thus, networks enhance communication. Relatedly, people connected by means of a computer network can exchange messages through the process of **electronic mail** (**e-mail**). Finally, networking allows multiple computers to share expensive peripheral equipment, such as laser-jet printers.

There are two types of networks: local-area and wide-area networks. A **local-area network** (**LAN**) is a network in which the computers are connected with wire cables. LANs are usually installed in relatively close proximity in a single building. Many universities and hospitals are replacing their mainframe computers with clusters of powerful PCs that are networked on an LAN.

In **wide-area networks** (**WAN**s), some of the links in the networking chain are connected by modems. A **modem** (short for *mo*dulate and *dem*odulate) is a hardware device that enables two computers to exchange information over standard telephone lines. Modems are sometimes external devices, separate from the computer, but in other cases, they may be built into the computer's system unit case. Through a modem and appropriate communications software, intercity and intercountry communication between computers is possible. WANs are used to tap **on-line information services**, such as America OnLine, CompuServe, Prodigy, and GEnie.

The Internet

The **Internet** is the electronic highway (the "information superhighway") that interconnects tens of thousands of networks around the world over telephone lines. The main difference between the Internet and a simple network is its scope. By connecting to the Internet

through a local service provider or university (or through one of the on-line information services), a user can send e-mail messages, chat online, search databases, receive (**download**) or send (**upload**) files, and share information with others throughout the world. The backbone of the Internet is a series of high-speed communication links between major supercomputer sites, such as the one maintained by the U.S. National Science Foundation. However, unlike every network that is part of the Internet, the Internet is not something under anyone's control. No person or organization is responsible for the Internet.

The **World Wide Web** is the "hottest" part of the Internet and has become the centerpiece of Internet activity. The World Wide Web facility on the Internet links resources (e.g., documents, graphic images, and video clips) around the world, providing an information exchange of unfathomable proportions. The Internet uses an addressing scheme called a **URL** (Uniform Resource Locator). Basic URLs are used as an initial address to access the **home page** (starting page of a document) of a World Wide Web **website**, which is a server on the Internet that contain documents.

The first part (prefix) of any URL is a keyword that indicates the Internet protocol that must be used. On the Internet, there are a dozen or so protocols, but for the World Wide Web, the Internet protocol is:

http://

All of the Internet addresses specified in this book have this http prefix. The second part of a full URL is the name of the computer where a file or document of interest is located. For example, the full URL (website address) for the American Nurses Association's "Nursing World" home page is: http://www.nursingworld.org.* The third part of a URL can specify a particular document or resource (des-

---

*In several places in this text, we have omitted the "http://" prefix because that prefix is always needed to gain access to sites on the World Wide Web.

tination); for example, http://nursingworld.org/aan/index.htm is the index page within the Nursing Times website for the American Academy of Nursing. Websites of interest to researchers have proliferated and are continuing to grow. Access to websites is facilitated by such **web browsers** as NetScape Navigator, Mosaic, and Microsoft's Internet Explorer, as well as through **search engines** such as Yahoo, which permit you to search for topics and names of interest.

Although the Internet is currently being used by researchers primarily to access various types of information supportive of the research process, the Internet also has potential as a resource for data collection (Murray, 1995; Fawcett and Buhle, 1995). Examples of studies that have used the Internet as a means of data collection have begun to appear in the literature (e.g., Igoe, 1997).

AVAILABLE PROGRAMS FOR STATISTICAL ANALYSIS

Computers have clearly created numerous opportunities for researchers, and nowhere is this more apparent than in relation to data analysis. Many statistical procedures are now routinely performed that would simply never have been attempted using manual computations. Ready-made programs for the statistical analysis of research data are widely available. The computer centers at universities are particularly likely to have a variety of software packages available to their users. Most computer centers have a professional staff that is accessible for consultation concerning the computer's library of programs. Sophisticated programs for performing statistical analysis are available for both mainframes and PCs.

Major Statistical Software Packages

The most widely used statistical software packages for use on mainframe and PCs include the Statistical Package for the Social Sciences (SPSS) and the Statistical Analysis System (SAS). Both of these packages contain programs to handle a broad variety of statistical analyses. Because these packages are updated, refined, and expanded frequently, readers are advised to check with personnel at their computer facility for any modifications to the description and listings provided in this chapter.

SPSS

SPSS was developed by researchers at the University of Chicago and National Opinion Research Center to assist researchers in the analysis of social science data. SPSS represents a highly flexible program with a syntax that is not technically oriented. For people with limited statistical and computer backgrounds, SPSS is relatively easy to learn. SPSS has a mainframe version, but the desktop version is adequate for performing analyses of all but the largest data sets. The current version of SPSS for PCs is SPSS 8.0 for Windows, which offers such features as pop-up definitions of statistical terms, online statistical advice for choosing statistical procedures or helping to interpret results, sophisticated graphing capabilities, and strong data and file management capabilities. As noted in Chapter 21, SPSS also has a data entry program that can be used to create data files for subsequent analysis.

SPSS can perform all of the basic descriptive and inferential statistical analyses, such as *t*-tests, analysis of variance (ANOVA), correlation analysis, and a wide range of nonparametric procedures. SPSS can also perform most widely used multivariate analyses, including multiple regression, analysis of covariance (ANCOVA), discriminant function analysis, factor analysis, multivariate analysis of variance (MANOVA), canonical correlation, logistic regression, life table analysis, proportional hazards modeling, and structural equations modeling. Further information about SPSS is available through SPSS Inc. in Chicago or through their website (www.spss.com).

SAS

SAS is a computer package that was developed at North Carolina State University. SAS is an integrated set of data management tools that includes a complete programming language as well as modules for multiple functions, including spreadsheets, project management, scheduling, and mathematic, engineering, and statistical applications. SAS's analytic programs (SAS/STAT) are generally considered to be somewhat more sophisticated, from a statistical point of view, than those of SPSS.

Like SPSS, the base SAS system is fairly easy to learn, even for those without a strong statistical or computer background. SAS is also available in both a mainframe and a PC version. At the time of preparing this book, the most recent release of the SAS System was version 6.12 for Windows. The SAS statistical package includes all basic descriptive and inferential statistics, plus additional programs for cluster analysis, Guttman scalogram analysis, multiple regression, factor analysis, discriminant function analysis, canonical correlation, logit/probit analysis, and psychometric analysis.

Further information about the SAS system is available through the SAS Institute in Cary, North Carolina or through the Internet. The URL for SAS is www.sas.com.

Using a Packaged Program

Researchers using packaged programs do not need to know a programming language, but they still must be able to communicate to the computer some basic information about what their variables are and how the data are to be analyzed. This is accomplished by means of certain commands that are unique to each software package. We can illustrate some aspects of the process using concepts from the menu-driven Windows version of SPSS.

The first step is to get your data file into SPSS through the Open command on the File menu. SPSS can read most spreadsheet files, dBASE files, and ASCII text files. (**ASCII files** are created through database and word processing programs, but are stripped of any proprietary codes, leaving only "plain vanilla" numbers and text.) Alternatively, the data can be entered directly into SPSS's Data Editor. As part of the process of getting the data into SPSS, you will in most cases need to define variable names and data formats. For example, if your data were in a text file in fixed format (see Chapter 21) and you had data for a person's gender in column 4, you would need to indicate this information through the "Define Fixed Variables" dialog box. (A **dialog box** is a small window that provides the options currently available to the user.) All variables would need to be assigned names (e.g., GENDER) that have a maximum of eight characters. Through the same dialog box, you would also indicate the value of the missing values codes for the variables in the file (e.g., 9 for the variable GENDER). Additional variable information can be specified through a different dialog box, such as adding labels for different values of a variable (e.g., 1 = "Male" and 2 = "Female") and adding labels to more fully describe variables (e.g. Q101 = "Number of prior hospitalizations").

Once all the data have been defined, any needed data transformations can be performed through various data transformation dialog boxes accessed through the Transform menu. Then, through the Statistics menu, a statistical procedure can be specified. For any specified statistical procedure, the variables in the data file would be displayed, and the relevant variables can be selected through standard mouse-clicking procedures. Finally, the procedure would be run, and the results would be displayed in SPSS's Output Navigator. In the Output Navigator window, you could browse the output results and could readily access whichever part of the output you wanted to see. Output files can be edited, saved, transferred to another application, and printed.

We hope that this brief discussion has made it clear that a researcher need not be a statistical expert or computer whiz to make use of a computer for quantitative analysis. The new graphical and menu-driven environments of SPSS and SAS are designed to be easy to learn by people with limited computer skills.

COMPUTERS AND THE ANALYSIS OF QUALITATIVE DATA

The traditional manual methods of organizing qualitative data, as described in Chapter 22, have a long and respected history. However, they are becoming increasingly outmoded as a result of the widespread availability of PCs that can be used to perform the filing and indexing of qualitative material.

The early attempts to computerize qualitative data involved numbering all paragraphs of the researcher's field notes or interviews, coding each paragraph for topical codes, and then entering the information into computer files. This is essentially an automated version of the manual indexing and retrieval systems described in the previous chapter. Sophisticated computer programs for managing qualitative data are now widely used. These programs permit the entire data file to be entered onto the computer, each portion of an interview or observational record coded and categorized, and then portions of the text corresponding to specified codes retrieved and printed (or shown on a screen) for analysis. The current generation of programs also has features that go beyond simple indexing and retrieval—they offer possibilities for actual analysis and integration of the data.

The most widely used computer programs for qualitative data have been designed for PCs, and most are for use with IBM-compatible computers rather than Macs. There are mainframe programs for managing large qualitative data sets (e.g., QUAL), but PCs now have sizable memories and operate at fast enough speeds that most qualitative data sets can be managed on a PC. The most widely used pro-

grams include the following: The Ethnograph, MARTIN, and QUALPRO (all for use with IBM-type PCs) and the HyperQual2 (for use with Macs). These programs have been debugged for computer problems and have user manuals that are relatively straightforward. The program NUD·IST (Nonnumerical Unstructured Data Indexing, Searching, and Theorizing) is an example of a program designed to support analysis and theory-building; it is available for both Macs and PCs using Windows. A new generation of programs, which Weitzman and Miles (1995) categorize as "conceptual network builders," are designed to help users formulate and represent conceptual schemes through a graphic network of links. Examples of this category of programs include MECA and SemNet.

It is beyond the scope of this text to describe the main features of all the available programs—and, in any event, the description would likely be quickly outdated because new releases of these programs become available almost yearly. However, we can describe some attractive features of programs for qualitative analysis so that such programs can be more readily appraised.

Typically, the researcher begins by entering the qualitative data onto a computer file using a word processing program (e.g., Word or WordPerfect). The data are then imported into the analysis program in ASCII format. A few qualitative data management programs (e.g., QUALPRO, HyperQual2) allow text to be entered directly rather than requiring an ASCII import file from a word processor.

Next, the researcher marks the boundaries (i.e., the beginning and end) of a segment of data, and then codes the data according to a previously developed category system. In some programs, this step can be done directly on the computer screen in a one-step process, but others require two steps. The first step involves the numbering of lines of text and the subsequent printing out of the text with the line numbers appearing in the margins. Then, after coding the paper copy, the researcher tells the computer which codes go with which lines of text. Most (but not all) programs permit overlapping coding and the nesting of segments with different codes within one another.

All the major qualitative analysis programs permit proofreading and editing. That is, codes can be altered, expanded, or deleted, and the boundaries of segments of text can be changed. All programs also provide screen displays or printouts of collated segments—however, some programs do this only on a file-by-file basis (e.g., one interview at a time), rather than allowing the researcher to retrieve all the segments with a given code across files.

Beyond these basic features, the available programs vary considerably in the enhancements they offer the researcher. The following is a nonexhaustive list of features that are available in some programs but not in others:

- Automatic coding according to words or phrases found in the data
- Compilation of a master list of all codes used
- Selective searches (i.e., restricted to cases with certain characteristics, such as searching for a code only in interviews with women)
- Searches for co-occurring codes (i.e., retrieval of data segments to which two or more specific codes are attached)
- Retrieval of information on the sequence of coded segments (i.e., on the order of appearance of certain codes)
- Frequency count of the occurrence of codes
- Calculation of code percentages, in relation to other codes
- Calculation of the average size of data segments
- Listing and frequency count of specific words in the data files
- Searches for relationships among coded categories

Several of these enhancements have lead to a blurring in the distinction between qualitative data management and data analysis.

TIPS FOR USING COMPUTERS

Unless your data set is very small and your analyses are very simple, we urge you to learn enough about computers to use a data analysis program. Here are a few suggestions regarding the use of a computer.

- You should *assume* that you have the capability of using the computer for data analysis. You do not need to know anything about electronic circuits. You do not need to learn any programming language. You will need to learn a few fairly simple procedures. For example, you can probably learn to produce simple statistical output, like frequency distributions, with a few hours of training. As you become more comfortable with the software, you can increase the repertoire of statistical procedures available to you.
- When learning a new software package, find out if there is a tutorial available. **Tutorials** are special programs that contain step-by-step instructions on how to use a software package and that make learning easier through real hands-on experience. Many applications software (e.g., SPSS) have tutorials.
- If someone is teaching you how to use a particular computer and software package through a demonstration, take very specific and detailed notes about every step in the process. Often, people who are adept at computers do a lot of things automatically, without giving much thought to the individual steps because the steps have become so routine to them. If the person instructing you has done something that you do not understand, ask him or her to slow down and back up. Also, be sure that your notes are precise.
- *Always* remember to make backup copies of the files you create, and store them in a secure place. It is a good protection against accidental erasures and also

against computer **viruses** that occasionally infect some machines.

- Do not be afraid to make mistakes—especially if you have all your files backed up! If you make a mistake, it can usually be corrected easily. For example, data files and analysis control files can readily be edited. If you make a mistake using the statistical software package, the computer will send you an **error message**, usually giving you some clues about what is wrong. If you cannot decipher an error message by yourself, ask someone who knows the software for help.

☜ SUMMARY

The advantages of computers to researchers include their speed, accuracy, and flexibility. On the other hand, computers require considerable attention to detail on the part of users because computers have no capacity to think.

Large, multiuser computer systems are often referred to as **mainframe computers**. Increasingly, people are using powerful **microcomputers**, also known as **personal computers** or **PCs**. The components of a computer system are broadly categorized as either hardware or software. **Hardware** refers to the physical equipment that stores, processes, and controls information. **Software** refers to the instructions and procedures required to operate the computer.

There are five components of computer hardware. The **input device** is the means by which the researcher feeds information into the computer. The **memory** is the device that stores the information. The **control unit** coordinates the functions of the other components. The **arithmetic/logic unit** performs the arithmetic or logic operations requested. Finally, the **output device** produces the resulting information. The control unit and the arithmetic/logic unit are collectively called the **central processing unit (CPU)**.

A **program**—the main part of a computer's software—is a set of instructions informing the computer what to do. **Programming languages** make it possible for humans to communicate with computers. Many packaged software programs exist for the researcher who is not greatly skilled in a programming language. Researchers are most likely to use software for several of the following **applications: word processing, desktop publishing, spreadsheets, database managers, communications software,** and **data analysis software**.

Researchers can now rely on PCs for most applications. PCs fall into two camps: IBMs (and their **clones**) and MacIntosh computers (**Macs**). These two types differ primarily with regard to their **user interface**—the software that passes information to and from the user of the computer. The availability of **windows** programs for IBM-type PCs has made these computers look more like a Mac, whose **graphical user interface (GUI)** has traditionally been considered more user friendly. The main input devices for PCs are the **keyboard** and the **mouse**, and the main output devices are the **display screen (monitor)** and **printers** that provide hard-copy printouts. Magnetic **disks** are used for both input and output as well as for **external storage**. Most PCs have both **hard disks**, embedded in the **systems unit** case, and **floppy disks**; many also use **CD-ROMs** as external storage. The **operating system** is the software that controls the overall operation of the computer system, and for IBM-type PCs, the most frequently used operating systems are **MS-DOS** and Microsoft's windows series (e.g., Windows 95)

PCs are often linked together in a **network**, either in the same building through cables (a **local-area network** or **LAN**) or through telephone lines by means of a **modem** (a **wide-area network** or **WAN**). Networking capabilities have given us the **Internet**, the information superhighway that interconnects thousands of networks around the world. Sites on the **World Wide Web**, the centerpiece of Internet activity, use an address (or **URL**) that begins with the prefix "http://"; these websites can be identified through the help of various **web browsers** and commercial **search engines**.

Researchers generally do not need to learn programming to analyze their data by computer because of the widespread availability of sophisticated statistical packages. The most widely used packages for quantitative data, for both mainframes and PCs, are **SPSS** and **SAS**.

There are also numerous programs that have lessened the burden of indexing, organizing, and retrieving qualitative data. The current generation of programs not only perform basic indexing functions but also offer enhancements that can facilitate the analysis of qualitative data and provide direction for theory building.

STUDY ACTIVITIES

Chapter 23 of the *Study Guide to Accompany Nursing Research, 6th ed.*, offers various exercises and study suggestions for reinforcing the concepts presented in this chapter. Additionally, the following study questions can be addressed:

1. If you have access to a PC, find out how much memory is available on your computer. Also, find out the speed of the microprocessor. Which operating system does it use?
2. If you have access to the Internet, find the URL for five nursing journals.

SUGGESTED READINGS

General References

Biow, L. (1993). *How to use your computer.* Emeryville, CA: Ziff-Davis Press.

Blissmer, R. H. (1993) *Introducing computers: Concepts, systems, and applications.* New York: John Wiley and Sons.

Cox, H., Harsanyi, B., & Dean, L. (1988). *Computers and nursing: Applications to practice, education and research.* Norwalk, CT: Appleton & Lange.

Fawcett, J., & Buhle, E. L. (1995). Using the Internet for data collection. *Computers in Nursing, 13,* 273–279.

Hutchinson, D. (1997). A nurse's guide to the Internet. *RN, 60,* 46–52.

Igoe, B. A. (1997). Symptoms attributed to ovarian cancer by women with the disease. *Nurse Practitioner, 22,* 122–128.

Jacobsen, B. S., Tulman, L., Lowery, B. J., & Garson, C. (1988). Experiencing the research process by using statistical software on microcomputers. *Nursing Research, 37,* 56–59.

Murray, P. J. (1995). Using the Internet for gathering data and conducting research. *Computers in Nursing, 13,* 206–208.

Norton, P., & Goodman, J. (1997) *Peter Norton's Inside the PC* (7th ed.) Indianapolis: Sams Publishing.

Prohaska, J. L., & Change, B. L. (1996). Using the Internet to enhance nursing knowledge and practice. *Western Journal of Nursing Research, 18,* 365–370.

Taft, L. B. (1993). Computer-assisted qualitative research. *Research in Nursing & Health, 16,* 379–383.

Tesch, R. (1991). Computer programs that assist in the analysis of qualitative data: An overview. *Qualitative Health Research, 1,* 309–325.

Walker, B. L. (1993). Computer analysis of qualitative data: A comparison of three packages. *Qualitative Health Research, 3,* 91–111.

Walker, G., Pullam, J., & Farmer, G. (1990). *Introduction to data analysis* (2nd ed.). Dubuque, IA: Kendall/Hunt Publishing.

Weitzman, E. A., & Miles, M. B. (1995). *Computer programs for qualitative data analysis.* Thousand Oaks, CA: Sage.

PART **VI**

Communication
in the Research Process

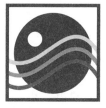

CHAPTER **24**

Writing a Research Report

No research project is ever complete until a research report has been prepared. The most brilliant piece of work is of little value to the nursing community unless that work is known. The task of preparing a research report may appear to be anticlimactic: after all, the researcher has satisfied his or her curiosity. Nevertheless, the reporting of results adds to knowledge on some issue and is a researcher's responsibility. It is also to the researcher's advantage to have research findings known by others because proper credit should be given to the work that has been completed. This chapter offers general guidelines for helping researchers to communicate their research results.

THE RESEARCH REPORT: CONTENT

Research reports are prepared for different audiences and for different purposes. A thesis or dissertation not only communicates the research strategy and results but also serves as documentation of the student's thoroughness and ability to perform scholarly empirical work. Theses and dissertations, therefore, are rather lengthy documents. Journal articles, on the other hand, are typically short because they must compete with other reports for limited journal space and

because they will be read by busy professionals. Oral reports and presentations at professional conferences are another mechanism for disseminating research results; they offer the possibility of immediate two-way communications and are therefore highly useful.

Despite differences among various types of research reports, their general form and content are similar. The major distinction lies in the amount of detail reported and the emphasis given to different parts. In this section, we expand on the information presented in Chapter 4 by reviewing in greater depth the type of material that is covered in four of the major sections of a research report: introduction, method, results, and discussion. The distinctions among the various kinds of reports are described later in the chapter.

The Introduction

The purpose of the introductory section of a research report is to acquaint readers with the research problem, the significance of the problem for nursing and for a field of knowledge, and the context within which the problem was developed. The introduction sets the stage for a description of the study through the inclusion of a brief literature review; description of the conceptual framework; presentation of the problem statement, hypotheses, and any underlying assumptions; and discussion of the rationale for studying the problem.

A precise and unambiguous problem statement is of immense value in communicating to the reader the major objectives of the study. If formal hypotheses have been developed, then they should also be identified in the introduction. It is often useful to number research questions or hypotheses so that they can be more readily referenced in reporting the results.

The researcher should explain enough of the background of the study to make clear the reasons that the problem was considered worth pursuing. The justification of a nursing research problem should ideally include both the practical and theoretical significance of the study. This ideal is not always feasible. Not all studies have a direct bearing on theoretical issues, nor should they all necessarily be expected to have such a bearing in a practicing profession such as nursing. With the current state of knowledge, no one should feel apologetic if a study can solve a practical problem but is not linked to a theory. Of course, studies that are framed within a theoretical context are most likely to make enduring contributions to knowledge about nursing and the nursing process. The introduction should make explicit such theoretical rationales when they exist. In most cases, the theoretical framework should be sufficiently explained that a reader who may be unfamiliar with the particular framework can nevertheless understand its main thrust and its link to the research problem.

The statement of the problem should also be accompanied by a summary of related research so that the research may be seen in an appropriate context. The review of the literature helps to clarify the theoretical and practical foundations of the research problem. Chapter 4 describes in greater detail the write-up of the literature review section.

Finally, the introduction should incorporate definitions of the concepts under investigation.

In quantitative studies, complete operational definitions are often reserved for the method section, but a reader should have a fairly good idea early in the report what the researcher had in mind with regard to such terms as "grief," "stress," "therapeutic touch," and so forth if they are the key concepts under study.

In many research reports, the introductory materials are not explicitly grouped under a heading labeled Introduction. In fact, research reports in journals typically begin without any header. Some introductory sections have headings or subheadings dedicated to specific aspects of the study's background, such as Literature Review, Conceptual Framework, or Hypotheses. In general, however, all the material before the method section is considered to be the introduction to the report.

In summary, the introduction should prepare readers for the description of what was done and what was discovered. The introduction should answer the questions, What did the researcher want to know? Why did he or she want to know it? and What is the likely theoretical and practical significance of such a study?

The Method Section

Consumers of a research report need to understand what the researcher did to address the problem identified in the introduction. The method section should have as its goal a description of what was done to collect and analyze the data in sufficient detail that another researcher could replicate the study if desired. In theses and final reports to funding agencies, this goal should almost always be satisfied. In journal articles, however, it is often necessary to condense the method section. For example, it is typically impossible to include a complete questionnaire, interview schedule, or observation schedule. Nevertheless, the degree of detail should be sufficiently adequate to permit a reader to evaluate the manner in which the research problem was solved.

The method section is often subdivided into several parts. The reader needs to know, first of all, who the people participating in the study were. The description of the study participants normally includes the specification of the population from which the sample was drawn and the setting for the research. The method of sample selection, the rationale for the sampling design, and the sample size should be clearly delineated so that the reader can understand the strengths and limitations of the sampling plan. It is also advisable to describe the basic characteristics of the participants, such as their age, gender, and other relevant attributes.

The design of the study also needs to be described. The design is often given more detailed coverage in an experimental project than in a nonexperimental one. In an experiment, the researcher should indicate what variables were manipulated, how subjects were assigned to groups, the nature of the experimental intervention, and the specific design adopted. In longitudinal studies, the report should indicate the amount of time elapsed between waves of data collection. Regardless of study design, the report should offer a rationale for its use. Also, in quantitative studies, it is important to identify what steps were taken to control the research situation in general and extraneous variables in particular.

A description of the method used to collect the data is a critical component of the method section. In rare cases, this description may be accomplished in three or four sentences, such as when a standard physiologic measure has been utilized. More often, a detailed explanation of the instruments or procedures and a rationale for their use are required to communicate to the reader the manner in which the data were gathered. When it is not feasible to include the actual research instrument within the report, its form and content should be outlined in as much detail as possible. If the measuring devices were constructed specifically for the research project, then the report should describe how they were developed, the methods used for pretesting, revisions made as a result

of pretesting, scoring procedures, and guidelines for interpretation. Any information relating to data quality and procedures used to evaluate data quality should also be mentioned. Such information is particularly important in a qualitative study because so much of the analysis depends on the researcher's interpretation of the data.

A procedures section provides information about what steps were followed in actually collecting the data. In an experiment, how much time elapsed between the intervention and the measurement of the dependent variable? In an interview study, where were the interviews conducted, who conducted them, and how long did the average interview last? In an observational study, what was the role of the observer in relationship to the subjects? When questionnaires are used, how were they delivered to respondents, were follow-up procedures used to increase the response rate, and what was the response rate? Any unforeseen events occurring during the collection of data that could affect the findings should be described and assessed. Those reading a report must be in a position to evaluate the quality of the data obtained, and a description of research procedures assists in this evaluation.

A delineation of the analytic procedures is sometimes incorporated into the method section and sometimes put with the results of the analyses. In qualitative studies, in which there is less standardization than is true in analyzing quantitative data, analytic procedures are often described in some detail. In quantitative studies, it is usually sufficient to identify the statistical procedures used. It is unnecessary to give computational formulas or even references for commonly used statistics. For unusual procedures or unusual applications of a common procedure, a technical reference justifying the approach should be noted.

Table 24-1 illustrates the content covered in the method section of quantitative research reports, using excerpts from several studies published in nursing research journals. Table 24-2

TABLE 24-1	Excerpts From Method Sections: Quantitative Nursing Research Reports
METHODOLOGIC ASPECT	**EXCERPT**
Research design	A prospective, repeated measures design was used. Data were collected in-hospital 5 to 6 days after surgery, and at 1, 6, and 12 months after hospital discharge. (King, Rowe, Kimble, & Zerwic, 1998, p. 16)
Sampling plan	A two-stage process was used to select the sample of nurses in this study. First, a random sample of hospitals in the state of Illinois was selected and, then, from each hospital a random sample of nurses was selected. Within the hospitals, nurses were sampled exclusively from the emergency rooms. (Keenan, Cooke, & Hillis, 1998, p. 62)
Measurements	At the follow-up visit, the following measures were obtained: (a) height and weight of child with a portable floor scale, (b) the HOME scale . . . , and (c) a 24-hour recall on the child's diet obtained from the parents. (Reifsnider, 1998, p. 21)
Data collection procedures	After obtaining informed consent, data collection took place during 2 home visits, one in the evening and one in the early morning. During the evening visit, questionnaire and interview data were collected and blood pressures were measured. Fasting blood samples, anthropometric measurements, and additional blood pressure readings were obtained during the morning visit. All the data were collected by nurse clinicians who followed a standardized protocol. (Meininger, Hayman, Coates, & Gallagher, 1998, p. 13)
Data quality	Cronbach's alpha coefficients were satisfactory for the whole (social support) scale (.87 for caregivers and .91 for supportive others). . . . A significant, positive relationship was found between the total score . . . and the actual size of the social network ($r = .50$), supporting the construct validity of the measure of received social support. (Robinson & Austin, 1998, p. 53)
Data analysis	Means and standard deviations were computed for the nine BSI dimensions and the GSI among the three groups. Repeated measures analysis of variance was used to test for differences among the three groups of care, changes over time, and time-by-group interaction for levels of psychological distress during bereavement. (McCorkle, Robinson, Nuamah, Lev, & Benoliel, 1998, p. 4)

presents analogous information for qualitative studies.

The Results Section

The results section summarizes the results of the analyses. In qualitative studies, the re-searcher presents a summary of the thematic analysis and the integration of the narrative materials, often including direct quotes to illustrate important points. Owing to space constraints in journals, quotes cannot be extensive, and great care must be exercised in selecting the best possible exemplars. Figures and dia-

TABLE 24-2	Excerpts from Method Sections: Qualitative Nursing Research Reports

METHODOLOGIC ASPECT	EXCERPT
Research design	This article reports a prospective, descriptive interpretive study that uses phenomenology, hermeneutics, and narrative ethics to explore values and beliefs that influence decision-making practices of 12 expectant couples who were eligible for prenatal genetic testing due to advanced maternal age. (Anderson, 1998, p. 171)
Sampling plan	Family members were purposively sampled with the assistance of two nurse managers and several staff nurses on the units. Participants were selected if they were described by nursing staff as "staying with" the patient. . . . Over a period of 5 months, 14 family members who were staying with hospitalized patients were approached for possible inclusion in the study and 8 agreed to participate. (Carr & Clarke, 1997, p. 728)
Data collection procedures	In open-ended interviews, participants were requested to tell their breast cancer stories. . . . After consent was obtained, interviews were conducted and audiotaped in a place of the interviewee's choice—her home, or the interviewer's home or office. We developed an interview guide to facilitate the emergence of the story, but it was most often not needed as each narrator told her story spontaneously with little prompting from the interviewer. (Langellier & Sullivan, 1998, p. 78)
Data quality	Strategies to ensure the trustworthiness of the data and findings were established using the framework described by Lincoln and Guba. . . . The four standards for assessing rigor in qualitative research are credibility, transferability, dependability, and confirmability. Table 2 briefly defines these criteria and describes the individual strategies used to establish trustworthiness in this study. (Herth, 1998, p. 211)
Data analysis	Qualitative analysis of the transcribed interviews followed [an] iterative process. . . . Initially, transcribed interviews were read and summary memos prepared. All interviews were reread and first-level codes were assigned. First-level codes were then clustered into categories, which were named using descriptive terminology. Interviews were recoded using the descriptive categories with new categories identified and added. Categories were then clustered into themes. (Bott, Cobb, Scheibmeir, & O'Connell, 1997, p. 259).

grams are often extremely useful in qualitative studies in summarizing an overall conceptualization of the phenomena under study.

In quantitative studies, if both descriptive and inferential statistics have been used, then the descriptive statistics ordinarily come first. If both quantitative and qualitative analysis has been performed, the qualitative analyses are often placed later because of their ability to explain the meaning of statistical analyses. On the other hand, in some cases, quantitative results may serve a useful summation or confirmatory function and may be more meaningful after a presentation of qualitative results.

The researcher must be careful to report all results as accurately and completely as possible, whether or not the hypotheses were supported. If there are too many analyses for inclusion in the report, then the criterion used to select analyses should be their relevance to the overall objectives of the study.

When the results of several statistical analyses are to be presented, it is frequently useful to summarize the findings in a **table**. Good tables, with precise headings and titles, are an important way to economize on space and to avoid dull, repetitive statements. Box 24-1 presents some suggestions regarding the con-struction of effective tables. **Figures** may also be used to summarize results. Figures that display the results in graphic form are used less as an economy than as a means of dramatizing important findings and relationships. Figures are especially helpful for displaying information on some phenomenon over time.

When the results of statistical tests are reported, three pieces of information are normally included: the value of the calculated statistic, the number of degrees of freedom, and the significance level. For instance, it might be stated, "A chi-square test revealed that patients who were exposed to the experimental

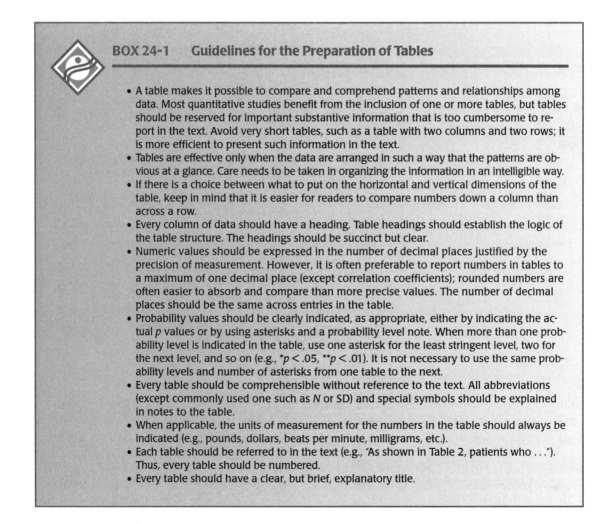

BOX 24-1   Guidelines for the Preparation of Tables

- A table makes it possible to compare and comprehend patterns and relationships among data. Most quantitative studies benefit from the inclusion of one or more tables, but tables should be reserved for important substantive information that is too cumbersome to re-port in the text. Avoid very short tables, such as a table with two columns and two rows; it is more efficient to present such information in the text.
- Tables are effective only when the data are arranged in such a way that the patterns are ob-vious at a glance. Care needs to be taken in organizing the information in an intelligible way.
- If there is a choice between what to put on the horizontal and vertical dimensions of the table, keep in mind that it is easier for readers to compare numbers down a column than across a row.
- Every column of data should have a heading. Table headings should establish the logic of the table structure. The headings should be succinct but clear.
- Numeric values should be expressed in the number of decimal places justified by the precision of measurement. However, it is often preferable to report numbers in tables to a maximum of one decimal place (except correlation coefficients); rounded numbers are often easier to absorb and compare than more precise values. The number of decimal places should be the same across entries in the table.
- Probability values should be clearly indicated, as appropriate, either by indicating the ac-tual *p* values or by using asterisks and a probability level note. When more than one prob-ability level is indicated in the table, use one asterisk for the least stringent level, two for the next level, and so on (e.g., *$p < .05$, **$p < .01$). It is not necessary to use the same prob-ability levels and number of asterisks from one table to the next.
- Every table should be comprehensible without reference to the text. All abbreviations (except commonly used one such as *N* or SD) and special symbols should be explained in notes to the table.
- When applicable, the units of measurement for the numbers in the table should always be indicated (e.g., pounds, dollars, beats per minute, milligrams, etc.).
- Each table should be referred to in the text (e.g., "As shown in Table 2, patients who . . ."). Thus, every table should be numbered.
- Every table should have a clear, but brief, explanatory title.

intervention were significantly less likely to develop decubitus ulcers than patients in a control group ($\chi^2 = 8.23$, $df = 1$, $p < .01$)."

Although we will discuss style in a later section, it is difficult to avoid the mention of style here. The write-up of statistical results is often a difficult task for beginning researchers because they are unsure both about what should be said and about the style in which to say it. A few suggestions may prove helpful. By now, it should be clear that research evidence does not constitute proof of anything, but the point bears repeating here. The research report should never claim that the data proved, verified, confirmed, or demonstrated that the hypotheses were correct or incorrect.

Hypotheses are supported or unsupported, accepted or rejected. It may seem a trivial point, but the presentation of results should be written in the past tense. For example, it is inappropriate to say, "Nurses who receive special training perform triage functions significantly better than those without training." In this sentence, "receive" and "perform" should be changed to "received" and "performed." The present tense implies that the results apply to all nurses, when in fact the statement pertains only to a particular sample whose behavior was observed in the past.

To further acquaint readers with the write-up of research results, Table 24-3 presents excerpts from the results sections of several quantitative

TABLE 24-3   Excerpts From Results Section: Quantitative Nursing Research Reports

TYPE OF ANALYSIS	EXCERPT
Descriptive statistics	Participants reported in the sleep diaries 0–12 awakenings during the night of the study ($M = 2.91$, $SD = 2.45$). Eighteen participants (54.5%) reported one or more daytime naps. (Redeker, Tamburri, & Howland, 1998, p. 32)
t-Tests	A paired *t* test revealed that Total Mood Disturbance Scores (TMDS) predischarge ($M = 65.37$) were significantly higher ($t = 3.76$, $df = 89$, $p < .01$) than 2 weeks postdischarge ($M = 54.59$) (Perkins & Jenkins, 1998, p. 41)
ANOVA	A 3 (ethnic) by 6 (visits) mixed repeated measures ANOVA was used to examine changes in the proportion of safety behaviors adopted over time. The change across time was significant ($F = 150.6$; $df = 5, 645$; $p < .001$), with no differences between ethnic groups ($F = 1.5$; $df = 2, 129$; $p = .23$) and no interaction of ethnicity and visit ($F = 0.3$; $df = 10$; $p = .98$). (McFarlane, Parker, Soeken, Silva, & Reel, 1998, p. 67)
Correlation	The correlation between the average caloric intake for the four highest-binge calorie days and the average caloric intake for the preceding days was $r = .67$ ($p < .001$). Using simple linear regression, 45% of the variance in the caloric intake of highest-calorie binge days was explained by the caloric intake for the preceding day. (Timmerman, 1998, p. 112)
Multiple regression	A full regression model predicting proportion agreement for the six behavioral variables was calculated to determine the degree to which the use of behavioral cues predicted the nurses' agreement with the pharmacological standard. Although this stepwise model accounted for 23% of the variance . . . the overall model was not significant. (Hudson-Barr, Duffey, Holditch-Davis, Funk, & Frauman, 1998, p. 9)

studies published in nursing journals. Excerpts from the results sections of qualitative and multimethod studies are presented in Table 24-4.

The Discussion Section

A bare report of the findings is never sufficient to convey their full implications. The meaning that a researcher gives to the results plays a rightful and important role in the report. The discussion section is typically devoted to a consideration of the study's limitations, the interpretation of the results, and recommendations that incorporate the study's implications.

In qualitative studies, the findings and the interpretation are typically presented together in the results section because the task of integrating qualitative materials is necessarily interpretive. In quantitative studies, however, the interpretation is reserved for the discussion.

In quantitative studies, the interpretation of the results involves the translation of statistical findings into practical and conceptual meaning. The interpretative process is a global one, encompassing the investigator's knowledge of the results, the methods, the sample characteristics, related research findings, clinical dimensions, and theoretical issues. The researcher should justify his or her interpre-

TABLE 24-4	Excerpts From Results Section: Qualitative and Mixed Method Nursing Research Reports
TYPE OF ANALYSIS	**EXCERPT**
Qualitative	African American and Mexican American women mentioned with equal frequency both personal and medical consequences of overweight. For Euro-Americans, the consequences of overweight were overwhelmingly personal as opposed to medical. They reported being unattractive, having difficulty buying clothes, and having poor self-image as the major consequences of overweight. (Allan, 1998, p. 57)
Mixed method	[In the survey], the lack of a doctor's recommendation was the single most frequently given reason for never having had a mammogram, but one in three responses concerned knowledge barriers. . . . The focus group findings echoed the survey findings, adding a few dimensions and providing more specific information on other dimensions. As in the survey, lack of provider recommendation was the single most frequently mentioned reason for not getting breast cancer screening. (Saint-Germain, Bassford, & Montano, 1993, p. 360)
Qualitative	We have discerned three approaches to taking care of oneself . . . These are (a) "do and think for yourself," (b) "what can I do? . . . others take care of me," or (c) I don't pay attention to myself. Doing and thinking for oneself involves taking charge of one's own health care and well-being. . . . Those who took this as a primary approach firmly believed one could do something about one's health and that one could control many aspects of the aging process. For example, a 76-year-old Korean woman talked extensively about how she increasingly took charge of her own health as she grew older saying, "Although I have gone through many changes, I adapt to new changes. For example, my eating habit changed. Now, I pay a lot of attention to avoid things that would hurt my health." (Berman & Iris, 1998, p. 228)

tations, explicitly stating why alternative explanations have been ruled out. If the findings conflict with those of earlier research investigations, then tentative explanations should be offered. A discussion of the generalizability of the study findings and an analysis of their importance should also be included.

Although the readers should be told enough about the methods of the study to identify its major weaknesses, report writers should point out the limitations themselves. The researcher is in the best position to detect and assess the impact of sampling deficiencies, design constraints, data quality problems, and so forth, and it is a professional responsibility to alert the reader to these difficulties. Moreover, if the writer shows that he or she is aware of the study's limitations, then the reader will know that these limitations were not ignored in the development of the interpretation.

The implications derived from a study are often speculative and, therefore, should be couched in tentative terms. For instance, the kind of language appropriate for a discussion of the interpretation is illustrated by the following sentence: "The results suggest that it may be possible to improve nurse–physician interaction by modifying the medical student's stereotype of the nurse as the physician's 'handmaiden.' " The interpretation is, in essence, a hypothesis and as such can presumably be tested in another research project. The discussion section, therefore, should include recommendations for studies that would help to test this hypothesis as well as suggestions for other research studies to answer questions raised by the findings.

Other Aspects of the Report

The materials covered in the four major sections are found in some form in virtually all research reports, although the organization might differ slightly. In addition to these major divisions, some other aspects of the report deserve mention.

Every research report should have a title. The phrases "Research Report" or "Report of a Nursing Research Investigation" are inadequate. The title should indicate to prospective readers the nature of the study. Insofar as possible, the dependent and independent variables (or central phenomenon under study) should be named in the title. It is also desirable to indicate the study population. However, the title should be brief (no more than about 15 words), so the writer must balance clarity with brevity. Some examples of titles include the following:

> The Effect of Advance Information on Pain Perception in Hospitalized Children

> Attitudes Toward Preventive Health Care in the Urban Working Class

> The Subjective Experience of Memory Loss Among Elderly Nursing Home Residents

If the title gets too unwieldy, its length can often be reduced by omitting unnecessary terms such as "A Study of . . ." or "An Investigation To Examine the Effects of . . ." and so forth. The title should communicate clearly and concisely the phenomena that were researched.

Research reports often include an abstract or a summary. Abstracts, it may be recalled, are brief descriptions of the problem, methods, and findings of the study, written so that a reader can assess whether the entire report should be read. Sometimes, a report concludes with a brief summary, and the summary, in such cases, usually substitutes for the abstract. Abstracts and summaries are typically only 100 to 200 words in length. Finally, each report concludes with a list of cited references so that the reader can locate other relevant materials.

THE STYLE OF A RESEARCH REPORT

Research reports are generally written in a distinctive style. Some stylistic guidelines were discussed previously in this chapter and in Chapter 4, but additional points are elaborated on in this section.

A research report is not an essay but rather a factual account of how and why a problem was studied and what results were obtained. The report should generally not include overtly subjective statements, emotionally laden statements, or exaggerations. When opinions are stated, they should be clearly identified as such, with proper attribution if the opinion was expressed by another writer.

In quantitative reports, personal pronouns such as "I," "my," and "we" are often avoided because the passive voice and impersonal pronouns suggest greater impartiality. Qualitative reports, by contrast, are often written in the first person and in an active voice. Some qualitative researchers (e.g., Webb, 1992) have argued that the the use of the neutral, anonymous third person in quantitative research is actually deceptive because it suggests greater objectivity than may be warranted. It is likely that the report-writing styles of researchers working within different paradigms will continue to diverge. However, even among quantitative researchers, there has been an increased tendency to strike a greater balance between active and passive voice and first-person and third-person narration. If a direct presentation can be made without suggesting bias, a more readable and lively product usually will result.

It is not easy to write simply and clearly, but these are important goals of scientific writing. The use of pretentious words or technical jargon does little to enhance the communicative value of the report, although colloquialisms should not be used. Avoiding jargon and highly technical terms is especially important in communicating research findings to practicing nurses. Also, complex sentence constructions are not necessarily the best way to convey ideas. The style should be concise and straightforward. If writers can add elegance to their reports without interfering with clarity and accuracy, so much the better, but the product is not expected to be a literary achievement. Needless to say, this does not imply that grammatical and spelling accuracy should be sacrificed. The research report should reflect scholarship, not pedantry.

With regard to references and specific technical aspects of the manuscript, various styles have been developed. The writer may be able to select a style, but often such considerations are imposed by journal editors and university regulations. Specialized manuals such as those of the University of Chicago Press (1993), the American Psychological Association (1994), and the American Medical Association (1989) are widely used. Most nursing research journals (e.g., *Nursing Research, Research in Nursing & Health, Western Journal of Nursing Research, Clinical Nursing Research*, and *Applied Nursing Research*) use the reference style recommended by the American Psychological Association, which is the reference style used in this book.

A common flaw in the reports of beginning researchers is inadequate organization. The overall structure is fairly standard and, therefore, should pose no difficulties, but the organization within sections and subsections needs careful attention. Sequences should be in an orderly progression with appropriate transition. Themes or ideas should not be introduced abruptly nor abandoned suddenly. Continuity and logical thematic development are critical to good communication.

TYPES OF RESEARCH REPORTS

Although the general form and structure of a research report are fairly consistent across different types of reports, certain requirements vary. This section describes the content, structure, and features of three major kinds of research reports: theses and dissertations, journal articles, and papers for professional meetings. Reports for class projects are excluded—not because they are unimportant but rather because they so closely resemble theses on a smaller scale. Final reports to agencies that have sponsored research are also not described. Most funding agencies issue guidelines for their reports, and these guidelines can be secured from project officers. In most cases, reports to funding agencies require nearly as much detail and documentation as dissertations.

Theses and Dissertations

Most doctoral degrees are granted on the successful completion of an empirical research project. Empirical theses are sometimes required of master's degree candidates as well. Theses and dissertations typically document completely the steps performed in carrying out the research investigation. Faculty members overseeing the project must be able to judge whether the student has understood the research problem both substantively and methodologically. The length of most doctoral dissertations is between 150 and 250 typed or printed double-spaced pages.

Most universities have a preferred format for their dissertations, but the following format is fairly typical:

    Preliminary Pages
        Title Page
        Acknowledgment Page
        Table of Contents
        List of Tables
        List of Figures
    Main Body
        Chapter I. Introduction
        Chapter II. Review of the Literature
        Chapter III. Methods
        Chapter IV. Results
        Chapter V. Discussion and Summary
    Supplementary Pages
        Bibliography
        Appendix

The preliminary pages for a dissertation are much the same as those for a scholarly book. The title page indicates the title of the study, the author's name, the degree requirement being fulfilled, the name of the university

awarding the degree, the date of submission of the report, and the signatures of the dissertation committee members. The acknowledgment page gives the writer the opportunity to express appreciation to those who contributed to the completion of the project. The table of contents outlines the major sections and subsections of the report, indicating on which page the reader will find those sections of interest. The lists of tables and figures identify by number, title, and page the tables and figures that appear in the text.

The main body of a dissertation incorporates those sections that were described earlier. The literature review often is so extensive for doctoral dissertations that a separate chapter may be devoted to it. When a short review is sufficient, the first two chapters may be combined. In some cases, a separate chapter may also be required to elaborate the study's conceptual framework.

The supplementary pages include a bibliography or list of references used to prepare the report and one or more appendixes. An appendix contains information and materials relevant to the study that are either too lengthy or too unimportant to be incorporated into the body of the report. Data collection instruments, listings of special computer programs, detailed scoring instructions, cover letters, permission letters, listings of the raw data, codebooks, category schemes, and peripheral statistical tables are examples of the kinds of materials included in the appendix. Some universities also require the inclusion of a brief *curriculum vitae*, or autobiography, of the author.

Journal Articles

Progress in nursing research depends on researchers' efforts to share their work with others. Dissertations and final reports to funders are rarely read by more than a handful of individuals. They are too lengthy and too inaccessible for widespread use. Publication in a professional journal ensures the broadest possible circulation of scientific findings. From a personal point of view, it is exciting and professionally advantageous to have one or more publications.

A journal article generally follows the same form as the main body of a thesis, but articles are much shorter. The purpose of an article is not to demonstrate research competence but rather to communicate the contribution that the study makes to knowledge. Because readers are particularly interested in the findings of a research project, a relatively large proportion of the journal report normally is devoted to the results and discussion sections. For the sake of economy of journal space, the typical research article is only about 10 to 25 typewritten double-spaced pages.

Several nursing journals accept research articles for publication. *Nursing Research,* which is published six times annually, is a major communication outlet for research in the field of nursing and has been published for almost five decades. Other nursing journals that focus primarily on empirical studies are *Advances in Nursing Science, Applied Nursing Research, Clinical Nursing Research, Qualitative Health Research, Research in Nursing & Health,* and the *Western Journal of Nursing Research.* Nursing journals that are not devoted exclusively or even primarily to research are now increasingly publishing research reports. Many journals that do not directly focus on nursing also publish articles by nurse authors, such as *The American Journal of Public Health, Journal of School Health, Journal of Adolescent Health,* and numerous others.

The prospective author should check through recent issues of journals under consideration for guidance concerning the journals' stylistic requirements and content coverage. Many publications make an explicit statement concerning the type of manuscripts they are seeking. Swanson, McCloskey, and Bodensteiner (1991) prepared a valuable report on publishing opportunities for nurses in journals. This article includes information on the circulation of the journal, number of copies of a manuscript required for submission, typical article word length, time needed to arrive at an editorial decision, and acceptance rate for 92 U.S. journals in nursing and related health fields.

When the manuscript is finally prepared for journal submission, the required number of copies should be sent to the editor with a brief cover letter indicating the mailing address of at least one author.* Generally, the receipt of the manuscript is acknowledged immediately, but the final decision concerning the paper's acceptance or rejection may require several months.

Many journals have a policy of independent, anonymous (sometimes referred to as **blind**) **peer reviews** by two or more knowledgeable people. By anonymous, we mean that the reviewers do not know the identity of the authors of the article, and the authors do not learn the identity of the reviewers. Journals that have such a policy are sometimes described as **refereed journals** and are generally more prestigious than nonrefereed journals.

Accepted manuscripts almost invariably are revised somewhat, either by the authors at the editor's request or by the editorial staff of the journal. If the manuscript is not accepted, authors are usually sent copies of the reviewers' comments or a summary of the reasons for its rejection. This information can be used to revise a manuscript before submitting it to another journal.

Presentations at Professional Conferences

Numerous professional organizations sponsor annual national meetings at which research activities are presented, either through the reading of a research report or through visual display in a poster session. The American Nurses' Association is an example of an organization

---

*By convention, the ordering of authors' names on a research report usually is alphabetic if authors have contributed equally, or in order of the importance of their contribution if otherwise. See Waltz, Nelson, & Chambers (1985) and Hanson (1988) for a discussion of author credits.

that holds meetings where nurses have an opportunity to share their knowledge with others interested in their research topic. Many local chapters of Sigma Theta Tau devote one or more of their annual activities to research reports. Examples of regional organizations that sponsor research conferences are the Western Society for Research in Nursing, the Southern Council on Collegiate Education for Nursing, the Eastern Nursing Research Society of MARNA/NEON, and the Midwest Nursing Research Society. Other nursing organizations, such as the Society for Research in Nursing Education, the American Association of Critical Care Nurses, the American Association of Neurosurgical Nurses, and the Congress of Nursing in Child Health, sponsor research conferences.

Presentation of research results at a conference has at least two advantages over journal publication. First, there is generally less time elapsed between the completion of a research project and its communication to others when a presentation is made at a meeting. Second, there is an opportunity for dialogue between the researcher and the audience at a professional conference. The listeners can request clarification on certain points and can suggest interesting modifications to the research paradigm. For this reason, a professional conference is a particularly good forum for presenting results to a clinical audience. At professional conferences, researchers also can take advantage of meeting and talking with others who are working on the same or similar problems in different parts of the country.

The mechanism for submitting a presentation to a conference is somewhat simpler than in the case of journal submission. The association sponsoring the conference ordinarily publishes a **Call for Papers** in its newsletter or journal about 6 to 9 months before the meeting date. The notice indicates requirements and deadlines for submitting a paper. The journal *Nursing Research* publishes a Call for Papers section as one of its regular departments, and most universities and major health care agencies also receive and post Call for Papers notices. Usually, an abstract of 500 to 1000 words is submitted rather than a full paper. If the submission is accepted, the researcher is committed to appear at the conference to make a presentation.

Research reports presented at professional meetings follow much the same format as a journal article. The report is typically condensed because the time allotted for presentation usually ranges from 10 to 20 minutes. Therefore, only the most important aspects of the study can be included in the paper. A handy rule of thumb is that a page of double-spaced text requires 2½ to 3 minutes to read aloud. Presentations are usually more effective, however, if they are informal summaries of research than if they are read verbatim from a written text.

Researchers sometimes elect to present their findings in a **poster session**. In such a session, several researchers simultaneously present visual displays summarizing the highlights of the study, and conference attendees circulate around the room perusing these displays. In this fashion, those interested in a particular topic can devote considerable time to discussing the study with the researcher and avoid those posters dealing with topics of less personal interest. Poster sessions are thus efficient and encourage one-on-one discussions. Several nurse researchers have prepared useful tips for poster sessions (e.g., Lippman & Ponton, 1989; McDaniel, Bach, & Poole, 1993; Ryan, 1989).

TIPS FOR WRITING RESEARCH REPORTS

If you are beginning to write a research report for the first time, the following suggestions may help you to get started:

- Do not begin to write until you have carefully examined a high-quality research report that you can use as a model. If you are writing a manuscript for submission to a journal, select as a model a journal article on a topic similar to your own. If you are preparing a dissertation, you are less likely to be able to find a model on a similar topic—but it is more important to find a dissertation that is considered to be of exceptional quality. Your adviser may be able to suggest a good example.

- If you are reporting quantitative findings, do not repeat all statistical information in both the text and in tables. Tables should be used to display information that would be monotonous to present in the text—and to display it in such a way that the numbers and patterns among the numbers are more comprehensible. The text can then be used to highlight the major thrust of the tables.

- It is usually best to limit the number of tables in a manuscript for journal submission to 4 or 5 because tables are complicated and expensive to typeset. Tables (and figures) should be numbered for easy reference. If you use tables, be sure that you reference each one in the text.

- It is often useful to study carefully tables presented in research journals to acquaint yourself with the format and content normally considered appropriate for reporting the kinds of analysis other researchers have undertaken. Because some people do not like to read tables, it is best to keep them as simple as possible. A cluttered table with hundreds of numbers in it is daunting to even a seasoned researcher—and even more so to a clinical nurse who is reading research to keep up with a field. It is usually unnecessary to report numbers beyond one decimal point (e.g., 10.2 rather than 10.18), and in some cases it might be better to round to the nearest whole number. Every table should have a concise but clearly explanatory title. Care should also be taken to use column headings that are clearly labeled and comprehensible.

- First drafts of research reports are almost never perfect. The assistance of a colleague or an adviser can be invaluable in improving the quality of a scientific paper. Objective criticism can often be achieved by simply putting the report aside for a few days and then re-reading it with a fresh outlook. As a final check, you might want to subject your own manuscript to an evaluation according to the guidelines presented in Chapter 25.

- If you are hoping to publish your report in a journal, do not be too disheartened by a rejection. A rejection by one journal should not discourage you from sending the manuscript to another journal. The competition for journal space is keen, and a rejection does not necessarily mean that a study is unworthy of publication. Although it is considered unethical to submit an article to two journals simultaneously, manuscripts may need to be reviewed by several journals before final acceptance.

SUMMARY

A research project is not complete until the results have been communicated in the form of a report. Despite some differences in the length, purposes, and audience of different types of research reports, the general form and content are similar. In general, the four major sections of a research report are the introduction, methods, results, and discussion.

The purpose of the introduction is to acquaint the reader with the research problem. This section includes the problem statement, the research hypothesis, a justification of the importance or value of the research, a summary of relevant related literature, the identification of a theoretical framework, and definitions of the concepts being studied. The methods section acquaints the reader with what the researcher did to solve the research problem. This section normally includes a description of the study participants, how they were selected, the instruments and procedures used to collect the data, and the techniques used to analyze the data. In the results section, the findings obtained from the analyses are summarized. Finally, the discussion section of a research report presents the researcher's interpretation of the results, a consideration of the study's limitations, and recommendations for future research and for utilization of the findings.

Research reports should be written as simply and clearly as possible. Emotionally laden statements and overtly subjective statements should be excluded from research reports. Various reference manuals exist to assist the researcher in selecting a consistent and acceptable style for noting references and handling other technical aspects of report writing. The style should be congruent with that of the university or journal to which the report is submitted.

The major types of research reports are theses and dissertations, reports to funding agencies, journal articles, and presentations at professional meetings. When space or time are at a premium—as in the case of journal articles and conference papers—detail should be kept to a minimum. In other types of reports, however, extensive documentation may be required.

STUDY ACTIVITIES

Chapter 24 of the *Study Guide to Accompany Nursing Research: Principles and Methods, 6th ed.*, offers various exercises and study suggestions for reinforcing the concepts presented in this chapter. Additionally, the following questions can be addressed:

1. Write an abstract for an article appearing in a 1992 or 1993 issue of the *Western Journal of Nursing Research*. Compare your abstract with that written by a classmate.

2. What are the similarities and differences of research reports that are written for journal publication and for presentation at a professional meeting?

3. Read a research report. Now write a two- to three-page summary of the report that communicates the major points of the report to a clinical audience with minimal research skills.

SUGGESTED READINGS

Methodologic/Stylistic References

Aaronson, L. S. (1994). Milking data or meeting commitments: How many papers from one study? *Nursing Research, 43,* 60–62.

American Medical Association. (1989). *American Medical Association manual of style* (8th ed.). Baltimore: Williams & Wilkins.

American Psychological Association. (1994). *Publication manual of the American Psychological Association* (4th ed.). Washington, DC: Author.

Burns, N. (1989). Standards for qualitative research. *Nursing Science Quarterly, 2,* 44–52.

Gay, J. T., & Edgil, A. E. (1989). When your manuscript is rejected. *Nursing and Health Care, 10,* 459–461.

Hanson, S. M. H. (1988). Collaborative research and authorship credit: Beginning guidelines. *Nursing Research, 37,* 49–52.

Hayes, P. (1992). "De-jargonizing" research communication. *Clinical Nursing Research, 1,* 219–220.

Huth, E. J. (1990). *How to write and publish papers in the medical sciences.* (2nd ed.). Philadelphia: Institute for Scientific Information.

Jackle, M. (1989). Presenting research to nurses in clinical practice. *Applied Nursing Research, 2,* 191–193.

Johnson, S. H. (1982). Selecting a journal. *Nursing and Health Care, 3,* 258–263.

Juhl, N., & Norman, V. L. (1989). Writing an effective abstract. *Applied Nursing Research, 2,* 189–191.

Knafl, K. A., & Howard, M. T. (1984). Interpreting and reporting qualitative research. *Research in Nursing & Health, 7,* 17–24.

Kolin, P. C., & Kolin, J. L. (1980). *Professional writing for nurses in education, practice, and research*. St. Louis: C. V. Mosby.

Lippman, D. T., & Ponton, K. S. (1989). Designing a research poster with impact. *Western Journal of Nursing Research, 11*, 477–485.

Markman, R. H., & Waddell, M. J. (1994). *Ten steps in writing the research paper* (5th ed.). Woodbury, NY: Barron's Educational Series.

McDaniel, R. W., Bach, C. A., & Poole, M. J. (1993). Poster update: Getting their attention. *Nursing Research, 42*, 302–304.

McKinney, V., & Burns, N. (1993). The effective presentation of graphs. *Nursing Research, 42*, 250–252.

Miracle, V. A., & King, K. C. (1994). Presenting research: Effective paper presentations and impressive poster presentations. *Applied Nursing Research, 7*, 147–151.

Ryan, N. M. (1989). Developing and presenting a research poster. *Applied Nursing Research, 2*, 52–55.

Strunk, W., Jr., & White, E. B. (1979). *The elements of style* (3rd ed.). New York: Macmillan.

Swanson, E., McCloskey, J., & Bodensteiner, A. (1991). Publishing opportunities for nurses: A comparison of 92 U.S. journals. *Image—The Journal of Nursing Scholarship, 23*, 33–38.

Tornquist, E. M. (1986). *From proposal to publication: An informal guide to writing about nursing research*. Menlo Park, CA: Addison-Wesley.

Tornquist, E. M., Funk, S. G., & Champagne, M. T. (1989). Writing research reports for clinical audiences. *Western Journal of Nursing Research, 11*, 576–582.

University of Chicago Press. (1993). *The Chicago manual of style* (14th ed.). Chicago: Author.

Waltz, C. F., Nelson, B., & Chambers, S. B. (1985). Assigning publication credits. *Nursing Outlook, 33*, 233–238.

Webb, C. (1992). The use of the first person in academic writing. *Journal of Advanced Nursing, 17*, 747–752.

Substantive References

Allan, J. D. (1998). Explanatory models of overweight among African American, Euro-American, and Mexican American women. *Western Journal of Nursing Research, 20*, 45–66.

Anderson, G. (1998). Creating moral space in prenatal genetic services. *Qualitative Health Research, 8*, 168–187.

Berman, R. L., & Iris, M. A. (1998). Approaches to self-care in late life. *Qualitative Health Research, 8*, 224–236.

Bott, M. J., Cobb, A. K., Scheibmeir, M. S., & O'Connell, K. A. (1997). Quitting: Smokers relate their experiences. *Qualitative Health Research, 7*, 255–269.

Carr, J. M., & Clarke, P. (1997). Development of the concept of family vigilance. *Western Journal of Nursing Research, 19*, 726–739.

Herth, K. (1998). Integrating hearing loss into one's life. *Qualitative Health Research, 8*, 207–223.

Hudson-Barr, D. C., Duffey, M. A., Holditch-Davis, D., Funk, S., & Frauman, A. (1998). Pediatric nurses' use of behaviors to make medication administration decisions in infants recovering from surgery. *Research in Nursing & Health, 21*, 3–13.

Keenan, G. M., Cooke, R., & Hillis, S. L. (1998). Norms and nurse management of conflicts. *Research in Nursing & Health, 21*, 59–72.

King, K. B., Rowe, M. A., Kimble, L. P., & Zerwic, J. J. (1998). Optimism, coping, and long-term recovery from coronary artery surgery in women. *Research in Nursing & Health, 21*, 15–26.

Langellier, K. M., & Sullivan, C. F. (1998). Breast talk in breast cancer narratives. *Qualitative Health Research, 8*, 76–94.

McCorkle, R., Robinson, L., Nuamah, I., Lev, E., & Benoliel, J. Q. (1998). The effects of home nursing care for patients during terminal illness on the bereaved's psychological distress. *Nursing Research, 47*, 2–10.

McFarlane, J., Parker, B., Soeken, K., Silva, C., & Reel, S. (1998). Safety behaviors of abused women after an intervention during pregnancy. *Journal of Obstetric, Gynecologic, and Neonatal Nursing, 27*, 64–69.

Meininger, J. C., Hayman, L. L., Coates, P. M., & Gallagher, P. R. (1998). Genetic and environmental influences on cardiovascular disease risk factors in adolescents. *Nursing Research, 47*, 11–18.

Perkins, S., & Jenkins, L. S. (1998). Self-efficacy expectation, behavior performance, and mood state in early recovery from percutaneous transluminal coronary angioplasty. *Heart & Lung, 27*, 37–46.

Redeker, N. S., Tamburri, L., & Howland, C. L. (1998). Prehospital correlates of sleep in patients hospitalized with cardiac disease. *Research in Nursing & Health, 21,* 27–37.

Reifsnider, E. (1998). Follow-up study of children with growth deficiency. *Western Journal of Nursing Research, 20,* 14–29.

Robinson, K., & Austin, J. K. (1998). Wife caregivers' and supportive others' perceptions of the caregivers' health and social support. *Research in Nursing & Health, 21,* 51–57.

Saint-Germain, M. A., Bassford, T. L., & Montano, G. (1993). Surveys and focus groups in health research with older Hispanic women. *Qualitative Health Research, 3,* 341–367.

Timmerman, G. M. (1998). Caloric intake patterns of nonpurge binge-eating women. *Western Journal of Nursing Research, 20,* 103–118.

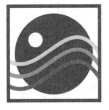

CHAPTER **25**

Evaluating Research Reports

Research in a practicing profession such as nursing contributes not only scholarly knowledge but also information concerning how that practice can be improved. Nursing research, then, has relevance for all nurses, not just the minority of nurses who actually engage in research projects. As professionals, nurses should possess skills to evaluate reports of research in their field. We hope that this text has provided a foundation for the development of such skills. In this chapter, more specific guidelines for the critical and intelligent review of research are presented.

THE RESEARCH CRITIQUE

If nursing practice is to be based on a solid foundation of knowledge, then the worth of studies appearing in the nursing literature must be critically appraised. Consumers sometimes have the mistaken belief that if a research report was accepted for publication, then it must be a good study. Unfortunately, this is not the case. Indeed, *most* research has limitations and weaknesses, and for this reason, no single study can provide unchallengeable answers to research inquiries. Nevertheless, disciplined empirical research continues to provide us with the best possible means of

answering certain questions. Knowledge is accumulated not by an individual researcher conducting a single, isolated study but rather through the conduct—and the evaluation—of several studies addressing the same or similar research questions. Thus, consumers who can thoughtfully critique research reports also have a role to play in the advancement of nursing knowledge.

Critiquing Research Decisions

Although no single study is infallible, there is a tremendous range in the quality of studies—from nearly worthless to exemplary. The quality of the research is closely tied to the kinds of decisions the researcher makes in conceptualizing, designing, and executing the study and in interpreting and communicating the study results. Each study tends to have its own peculiar flaws because each researcher, in addressing the same or a similar research question, makes somewhat different decisions about how the study should be done. It is not uncommon for researchers who have made different research decisions to arrive at different answers to the same research question. It is precisely for this reason that research consumers must be knowledgeable about the research process. As a consumer of research reports, you must be able to

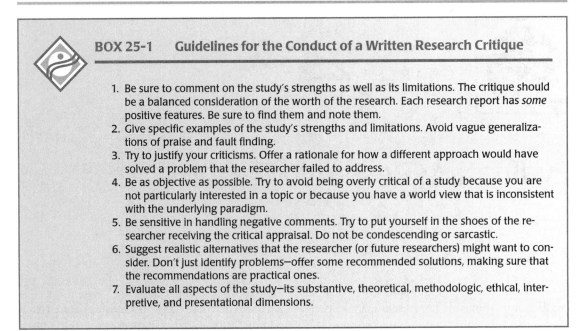

BOX 25-1   Guidelines for the Conduct of a Written Research Critique

1. Be sure to comment on the study's strengths as well as its limitations. The critique should be a balanced consideration of the worth of the research. Each research report has *some* positive features. Be sure to find them and note them.
2. Give specific examples of the study's strengths and limitations. Avoid vague generalizations of praise and fault finding.
3. Try to justify your criticisms. Offer a rationale for how a different approach would have solved a problem that the researcher failed to address.
4. Be as objective as possible. Try to avoid being overly critical of a study because you are not particularly interested in a topic or because you have a world view that is inconsistent with the underlying paradigm.
5. Be sensitive in handling negative comments. Try to put yourself in the shoes of the researcher receiving the critical appraisal. Do not be condescending or sarcastic.
6. Suggest realistic alternatives that the researcher (or future researchers) might want to consider. Don't just identify problems—offer some recommended solutions, making sure that the recommendations are practical ones.
7. Evaluate all aspects of the study—its substantive, theoretical, methodologic, ethical, interpretive, and presentational dimensions.

evaluate the decisions that investigators made so that you can determine how much faith should be put in their conclusions. The consumer must ask, What other approaches could have been used to study this research problem? and If another approach had been used, would the results have been more reliable, believable, or replicable? In other words, you must evaluate the impact of the researcher's decisions on the study's ability to reveal the truth.

Much of this book has been designed to acquaint students with a range of methodologic options for the conduct of research—options on how to develop a research design, collect and analyze data, select a study sample, operationalize variables, and so on. We hope that an acquaintance with these options has provided you with the tools to challenge a researcher's decisions and to suggest alternative methods.

Purpose of a Research Critique

Research reports are evaluated for a variety of purposes. Students are often asked to prepare a critique to demonstrate their mastery of

methodologic and analytic skills. Seasoned researchers are sometimes asked to write critiques of manuscripts to help journal editors make publication decisions or to accompany the report as published commentaries.* Journal clubs in clinical or other settings may meet periodically to critique and discuss research studies. For all these purposes, the goal is generally to develop a balanced evaluation of the study's contribution to knowledge.

A research critique is not just a review or summary of a study; rather, it is a careful, critical appraisal of the strengths and limitations of a piece of research. A written critique should serve as a guide to researchers and practitioners. The critique should also inform the research community of the ways in which the study results may have been compromised, and it should alert researchers to how better to go about addressing the research question. The critique should thus help to advance a

---

*The *Western Journal of Nursing Research,* for example, usually publishes a research report followed by one or two commentaries that include appraisals of the report.

particular area of knowledge. When the audience is clinical nurses, the critique should help those who are practicing nursing to decide how the findings from the study can best be incorporated into their practice, if at all.

The function of critical evaluations of nursing studies is not to hunt for and expose mistakes. A good critique objectively and critically identifies adequacies and inadequacies, virtues as well as faults. Sometimes, the need for such balance is obscured by the terms *critique* and *critical appraisal,* which connote unfavorable observations. The merits of a study are as important as its limitations in coming to conclusions about the worth of its findings. Therefore, the research critique should reflect a thoughtful, objective, and balanced consideration of the study's validity and significance. If the critique is not balanced, then it will be of little utility to the researcher who conducted the study because it might engender defensiveness, and a practitioner may erroneously get the impression that the study has no merit at all.

Box 25-1 summarizes general guidelines to consider in preparing a written research critique. In the section that follows, we present some specific guidelines for evaluating various aspects of a research report.

ELEMENTS OF A RESEARCH CRITIQUE

Each research report has several important dimensions that should be considered in a critical evaluation of the study's worth. In this section, we review the substantive and theoretical, methodologic, interpretive, ethical, and presentational and stylistic dimensions of a study.

Substantive and Theoretical Dimensions

The reader of a research report needs to determine whether the study was an important one in terms of the significance of the problem studied, the soundness of the conceptualizations, and the creativity and appropriateness of the theoretical framework. The research problem is one that should have obvious relevance to some aspect of the nursing profession. It is not enough that a problem be interesting if it offers no possibility of contributing to nursing knowledge or improving nursing practice. Thus, even before you learn *how* a study was conducted, you should evaluate whether the study should have been conducted in the first place.

The reader's own disciplinary orientation should not intrude in an objective evaluation of the study's significance. A clinical nurse might not be intrigued by a study focusing on the determinants of nursing turnover, but a nursing administrator trying to improve staffing decisions might find such a study highly useful. Similarly, a psychiatric nurse might find little value in a study of the sleep–wake patterns of low-birthweight infants, but nurses in neonatal intensive care units might not agree. It is important, then, not to adopt a myopic view of the study's importance and relevance to nursing.

Many problems that are relevant to nursing are still not necessarily worthwhile substantively. You must ask a question such as, Given what we know about this topic, is this research the right next step? Knowledge tends to be incremental. Researchers must consider how to advance knowledge on a topic in the most beneficial way. They should avoid unnecessary replications of a study once a body of research clearly points to an answer, but they should also not leap several steps ahead when there is an insecure foundation. Sometimes, replication is exactly what is needed to enhance the believability or generalizability of earlier findings.

Another issue that has both substantive and methodologic implications is the congruence between the study question and the methods used to address it. There must be a good fit between the research problem on the one hand and the overall study design, the method of collecting research data, and the approach to

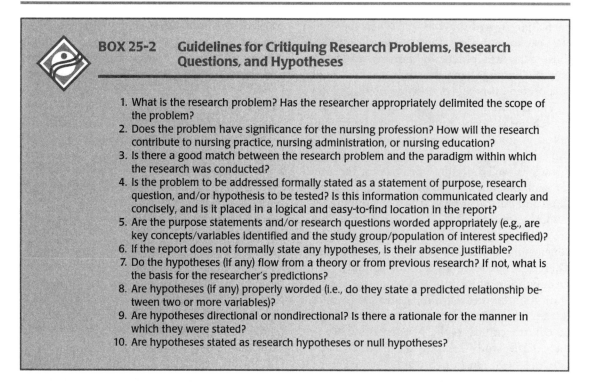

BOX 25-2   Guidelines for Critiquing Research Problems, Research Questions, and Hypotheses

1. What is the research problem? Has the researcher appropriately delimited the scope of the problem?
2. Does the problem have significance for the nursing profession? How will the research contribute to nursing practice, nursing administration, or nursing education?
3. Is there a good match between the research problem and the paradigm within which the research was conducted?
4. Is the problem to be addressed formally stated as a statement of purpose, research question, and/or hypothesis to be tested? Is this information communicated clearly and concisely, and is it placed in a logical and easy-to-find location in the report?
5. Are the purpose statements and/or research questions worded appropriately (e.g., are key concepts/variables identified and the study group/population of interest specified)?
6. If the report does not formally state any hypotheses, is their absence justifiable?
7. Do the hypotheses (if any) flow from a theory or from previous research? If not, what is the basis for the researcher's predictions?
8. Are hypotheses (if any) properly worded (i.e., do they state a predicted relationship between two or more variables)?
9. Are hypotheses directional or nondirectional? Is there a rationale for the manner in which they were stated?
10. Are hypotheses stated as research hypotheses or null hypotheses?

analyzing those data on the other. Questions that deal with poorly understood phenomena, with processes, with the dynamics of a situation, or with in-depth description, for example, are usually best addressed with flexible designs, unstructured methods of data collection, and qualitative analysis. Questions that involve the measurement of well-defined variables, cause-and-effect relationships, or the effectiveness of a specific intervention, however, are usually better suited to more structured, quantitative approaches using designs that offer control over the research situation.

A final issue to consider is whether the researcher has appropriately placed the research problem into some larger theoretical context. As we emphasized in Chapter 5, a researcher does little to enhance the value of the study if the connection between the research problem and a conceptual framework is artificial and contrived. However, a specific research problem that is genuinely framed as a part of some larger intellectual issue can generally go much further in advancing knowledge than a problem that ignores its theoretical underpinnings.

The substantive and theoretical dimensions of a study are normally communicated to readers in the introduction to a report. The manner in which the introductory materials are presented is vital to the proper understanding and appreciation of what the researcher has accomplished. Specific guidelines for critiquing the introduction of a research report are presented in Boxes 25-2 through 25-4.* Box 25-2 provides guidelines for critiquing the researcher's statement of the problem, re-

---

*The questions included in the boxes in this chapter are not exhaustive. Many additional questions will need to be raised in dealing with a particular piece of research. Moreover, the boxes include many questions that do not apply to every piece of research. The questions are intended to represent a useful point of departure in undertaking a critique.

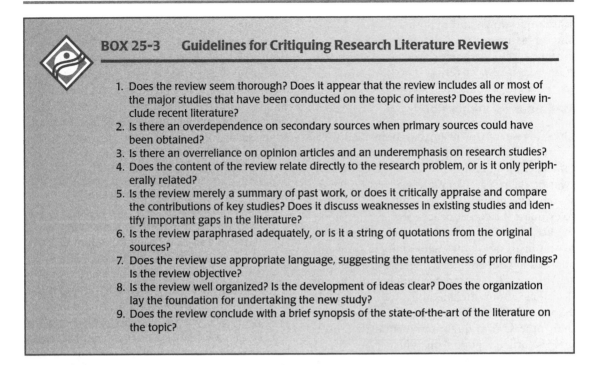

BOX 25-3   Guidelines for Critiquing Research Literature Reviews

1. Does the review seem thorough? Does it appear that the review includes all or most of the major studies that have been conducted on the topic of interest? Does the review include recent literature?
2. Is there an overdependence on secondary sources when primary sources could have been obtained?
3. Is there an overreliance on opinion articles and an underemphasis on research studies?
4. Does the content of the review relate directly to the research problem, or is it only peripherally related?
5. Is the review merely a summary of past work, or does it critically appraise and compare the contributions of key studies? Does it discuss weaknesses in existing studies and identify important gaps in the literature?
6. Is the review paraphrased adequately, or is it a string of quotations from the original sources?
7. Does the review use appropriate language, suggesting the tentativeness of prior findings? Is the review objective?
8. Is the review well organized? Is the development of ideas clear? Does the organization lay the foundation for undertaking the new study?
9. Does the review conclude with a brief synopsis of the state-of-the-art of the literature on the topic?

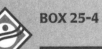

BOX 25-4   Guidelines for Critiquing Theoretical and Conceptual Frameworks

1. Does the research report describe a theoretical or conceptual framework for the study? If not, does the absence of a theoretical framework detract from the usefulness or significance of the research?
2. Does the report adequately describe the major features of the theory so that readers can understand the conceptual basis of the study?
3. Is the theory appropriate to the research problem? Would a different theoretical framework have been more appropriate?
4. Is the theoretical framework based on a conceptual model of nursing, or is it borrowed from another discipline? Is there adequate justification for the researcher's decision about the type of framework used?
5. Do the research problem and hypothesis flow naturally from the theoretical framework, or does the link between the problem and theory seem contrived?
6. Are the deductions from the theory or conceptual framework logical?
7. Are all the concepts adequately defined in a way that is consistent with the theory?
8. Does the researcher tie the findings of the study back to the framework at the end of the report? Do the findings support or undermine the framework?

search questions, and hypotheses. Boxes 25–3 and 25–4 suggest considerations relevant to a critique of the literature review and conceptual framework, respectively.

Methodologic Dimensions

Once a research problem has been identified, the researcher must make a number of important decisions regarding how to go about answering the research questions or testing the research hypotheses. It is your job as a critiquer to evaluate the consequences of those decisions. In fact, the heart of the research critique lies in the analysis of the methodologic decisions adopted in addressing the research question.

Although the researcher makes hundreds of decisions about the methods for conducting a study, there are some that are more critical than others. In a quantitative study, the four major decision points on which you should focus critical attention are as follows:

- *Decision 1*: What design will yield the most unambiguous and meaningful (internally valid) results about the relationship between the independent variable and dependent variable, or the most valid descriptions of the concepts under study?
- *Decision 2*: Who should participate in the study? What are the characteristics of the population to which the findings should be generalized? How large should the sample be, from where should participants be recruited, and what sampling approach should be used to select the sample?
- *Decision 3*: What method should be used to collect the data? How can the variables be operationalized and reliably and validly measured for each participant in the study?
- *Decision 4*: What statistical analyses will provide the most appropriate tests of the research hypotheses or answers to the research questions?

In a quantitative study, these methodologic decisions are typically made up-front, and the researcher then simply executes the prespeci-

fied plan. In a qualitative study, by contrast, the researcher makes ongoing methodologic decisions while in the process of collecting and analyzing data—once the very important decision about the research setting has been made. In a qualitative study, the major methodologic decisions that you should consider in your critique are as follows:

- *Decision 1*: Where should the study take place? What setting will yield the richest information about the phenomenon under study?
- *Decision 2*: What should the sources of data be, and how should the data be gathered? Should multiple sources of data (e.g., unstructured interviews and observations) be used to achieve method triangulation?
- *Decision 3*: Who should participate in the study? How can participants be selected so as to enhance the theoretical richness of the study? How many participants will be needed to achieve data saturation? How much time should be spent in the field to achieve "prolonged engagement"?
- *Decision 4*: What types of evidence can be obtained to support the credibility, transferability, dependability, and confirmability of the data, the analysis, and the interpretation?

Because of practical constraints, research studies almost always involve making some compromises between what is ideal and what is feasible. For example, the researcher might ideally like to work with a sample of 1000 subjects, but because of limited resources, he or she might have to be content with a sample of 200 subjects. The person doing a research critique cannot realistically demand that researchers attain these methodologic ideals but must be prepared to evaluate how much damage has been done by failure to achieve them.

After you evaluate the types of decisions that the researcher made, a further step is necessary: You must assess how well the research plan was actually executed. A well-conceived research plan may go awry because of time pressures, financial constraints, personnel changes, researcher inexperience, administrative problems, and so on. Therefore, the methodologic aspects of a study must be critiqued not only as they were conceived but also as they were put into operation.

Various guidelines are presented in the following displays to help you in performing a critical analysis of the research methods, which are generally described in the method section of a research report. Box 25-5 presents guidelines for critiquing the overall research design of quantitative studies, and Box 25-6 has guidelines for critiquing the design of qualitative and mixed-method studies. The sampling strategy can be evaluated using the questions included in Box 25-7 for quantitative studies or Box 25-8 for qualitative ones.

Six separate boxes are included here to assist with a critique of the researcher's data collection plan. Box 25-9 provides suggestions for critiquing the actual procedures used to collect the data. Explicit guidelines are provided for evaluating self-report approaches (Box 25-10), observational methods (Box 25-11), and biophysiologic measures (Box 25-12). Criteria are not provided for evaluating infrequently used data collection techniques, such as Q sorts and records. However, in addition to questions adapted from Boxes 25–10 through 25–12, other methods can be evaluated by considering one overarching question: Was the researcher's

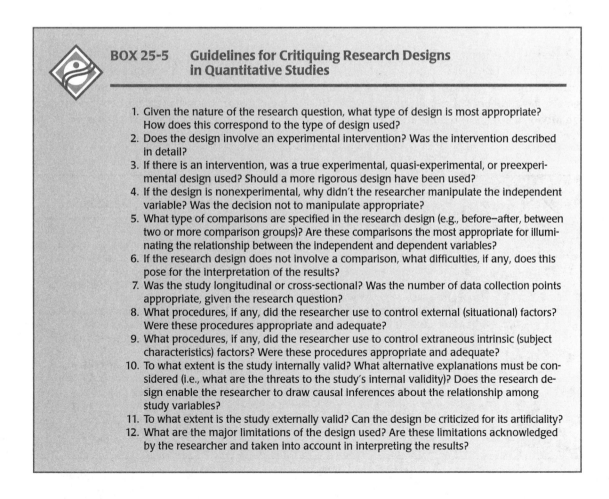

BOX 25-5   Guidelines for Critiquing Research Designs in Quantitative Studies

1. Given the nature of the research question, what type of design is most appropriate? How does this correspond to the type of design used?
2. Does the design involve an experimental intervention? Was the intervention described in detail?
3. If there is an intervention, was a true experimental, quasi-experimental, or preexperimental design used? Should a more rigorous design have been used?
4. If the design is nonexperimental, why didn't the researcher manipulate the independent variable? Was the decision not to manipulate appropriate?
5. What type of comparisons are specified in the research design (e.g., before–after, between two or more comparison groups)? Are these comparisons the most appropriate for illuminating the relationship between the independent and dependent variables?
6. If the research design does not involve a comparison, what difficulties, if any, does this pose for the interpretation of the results?
7. Was the study longitudinal or cross-sectional? Was the number of data collection points appropriate, given the research question?
8. What procedures, if any, did the researcher use to control external (situational) factors? Were these procedures appropriate and adequate?
9. What procedures, if any, did the researcher use to control extraneous intrinsic (subject characteristics) factors? Were these procedures appropriate and adequate?
10. To what extent is the study internally valid? What alternative explanations must be considered (i.e., what are the threats to the study's internal validity)? Does the research design enable the researcher to draw causal inferences about the relationship among study variables?
11. To what extent is the study externally valid? Can the design be criticized for its artificiality?
12. What are the major limitations of the design used? Are these limitations acknowledged by the researcher and taken into account in interpreting the results?

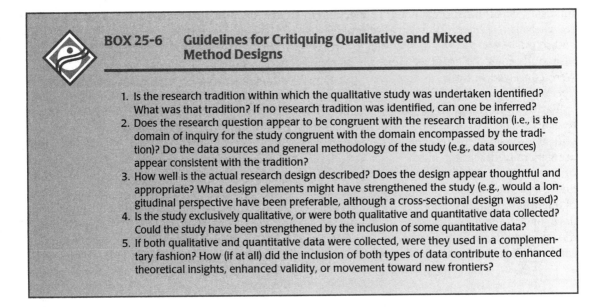

BOX 25-6   Guidelines for Critiquing Qualitative and Mixed Method Designs

1. Is the research tradition within which the qualitative study was undertaken identified? What was that tradition? If no research tradition was identified, can one be inferred?
2. Does the research question appear to be congruent with the research tradition (i.e., is the domain of inquiry for the study congruent with the domain encompassed by the tradition)? Do the data sources and general methodology of the study (e.g., data sources) appear consistent with the tradition?
3. How well is the actual research design described? Does the design appear thoughtful and appropriate? What design elements might have strengthened the study (e.g., would a longitudinal perspective have been preferable, although a cross-sectional design was used)?
4. Is the study exclusively qualitative, or were both qualitative and quantitative data collected? Could the study have been strengthened by the inclusion of some quantitative data?
5. If both qualitative and quantitative data were collected, were they used in a complementary fashion? How (if at all) did the inclusion of both types of data contribute to enhanced theoretical insights, enhanced validity, or movement toward new frontiers?

method of measurement and data collection the best possible approach to capturing the key research variables? Boxes 25–13 and 25–14 suggest some guidelines for evaluating the overall quality of the data in quantitative and qualitative studies, respectively.

The researcher's analytic plan is the final methodologic area that requires a critical analysis. The analytic strategy is sometimes presented in the methods section of a research report but is usually more fully explicated in the results section, where the actual findings are re-

BOX 25-7   Guidelines for Critiquing Quantitative Sampling Designs

1. Is the target or accessible population identified and described? Are the eligibility criteria clearly specified? Would a more limited population specification have controlled for important sources of extraneous variation not covered by the research design?
2. What type of sampling plan was used? Does the report make clear whether probability or nonprobability sampling was used?
3. How were subjects recruited into the sample? Does the method suggest potential biases?
4. How adequate is the sampling plan in terms of yielding a representative sample?
5. If the sampling plan is weak (e.g., a convenience sample), are potential biases identified? Is the sampling plan justified, given the research problem?
6. Did some factor other than the sampling plan itself (e.g., a low response rate) affect the representativeness of the sample? Did the researcher take steps to produce a high response rate?
7. Are the size and key characteristics of the sample described?
8. Is the sample sufficiently large? Was the sample size justified on the basis of a power analysis?
9. To whom can the study results reasonably be generalized?

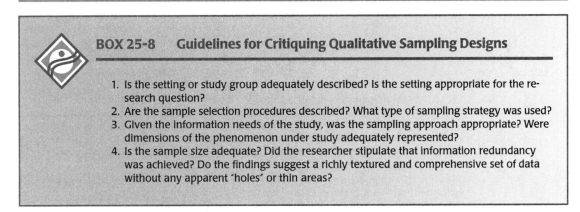

BOX 25-8   Guidelines for Critiquing Qualitative Sampling Designs

1. Is the setting or study group adequately described? Is the setting appropriate for the research question?
2. Are the sample selection procedures described? What type of sampling strategy was used?
3. Given the information needs of the study, was the sampling approach appropriate? Were dimensions of the phenomenon under study adequately represented?
4. Is the sample size adequate? Did the researcher stipulate that information redundancy was achieved? Do the findings suggest a richly textured and comprehensive set of data without any apparent "holes" or thin areas?

ported. Box 25-15 lists a number of guiding questions of relevance for evaluating quantitative analyses, and Box 25-16 identifies questions for qualitative analyses. When a study has used both qualitative and quantitative analyses, questions from both boxes are likely to be applicable.

Ethical Dimensions

In performing a research critique, you should consider whether there is any evidence that the rights of human subjects were violated during the course of the investigation. If there are any potential ethical problems, then you need to consider the impact of those problems on the scientific merit of the study on the one hand and on participants' well-being on the other. Guidelines for evaluating the ethical dimensions of a research report are presented in Box 25-17.

There are two main types of ethical transgressions in research studies. The first class consists of inadvertent actions or activities

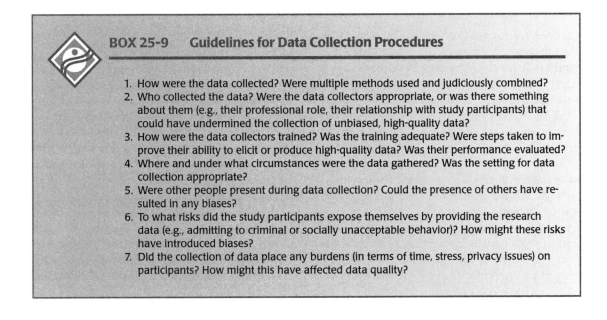

BOX 25-9   Guidelines for Data Collection Procedures

1. How were the data collected? Were multiple methods used and judiciously combined?
2. Who collected the data? Were the data collectors appropriate, or was there something about them (e.g., their professional role, their relationship with study participants) that could have undermined the collection of unbiased, high-quality data?
3. How were the data collectors trained? Was the training adequate? Were steps taken to improve their ability to elicit or produce high-quality data? Was their performance evaluated?
4. Where and under what circumstances were the data gathered? Was the setting for data collection appropriate?
5. Were other people present during data collection? Could the presence of others have resulted in any biases?
6. To what risks did the study participants expose themselves by providing the research data (e.g., admitting to criminal or socially unacceptable behavior)? How might these risks have introduced biases?
7. Did the collection of data place any burdens (in terms of time, stress, privacy issues) on participants? How might this have affected data quality?

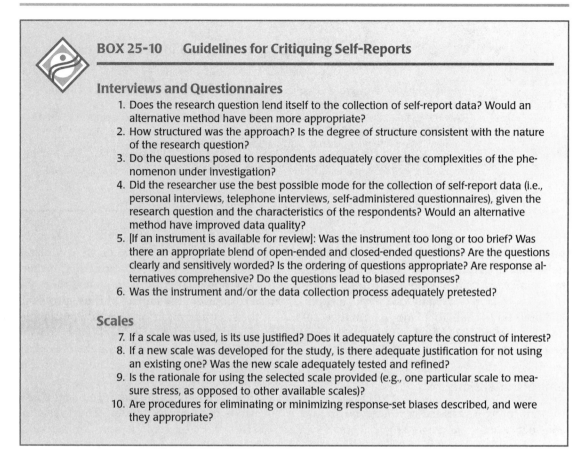

BOX 25-10   Guidelines for Critiquing Self-Reports

Interviews and Questionnaires

1. Does the research question lend itself to the collection of self-report data? Would an alternative method have been more appropriate?
2. How structured was the approach? Is the degree of structure consistent with the nature of the research question?
3. Do the questions posed to respondents adequately cover the complexities of the phenomenon under investigation?
4. Did the researcher use the best possible mode for the collection of self-report data (i.e., personal interviews, telephone interviews, self-administered questionnaires), given the research question and the characteristics of the respondents? Would an alternative method have improved data quality?
5. [If an instrument is available for review]: Was the instrument too long or too brief? Was there an appropriate blend of open-ended and closed-ended questions? Are the questions clearly and sensitively worded? Is the ordering of questions appropriate? Are response alternatives comprehensive? Do the questions lead to biased responses?
6. Was the instrument and/or the data collection process adequately pretested?

Scales

7. If a scale was used, is its use justified? Does it adequately capture the construct of interest?
8. If a new scale was developed for the study, is there adequate justification for not using an existing one? Was the new scale adequately tested and refined?
9. Is the rationale for using the selected scale provided (e.g., one particular scale to measure stress, as opposed to other available scales)?
10. Are procedures for eliminating or minimizing response-set biases described, and were they appropriate?

that the researcher did not interpret as creating an ethical dilemma. For example, in a study that examined married couples' experiences with sexually transmitted diseases, the researcher might inadvertently have scheduled the interview at a time when privacy for the members of the couple could not be ensured.

In other cases, the researcher may have been aware of having committed some violation of ethical principles, but made a conscious decision that the violation was relatively minor in relation to the knowledge that could be gained by doing the study in a certain way. For example, a researcher may decide not to obtain informed consent from the parents of minor children attending a family planning clinic because to require such consent would probably have dramatically reduce the number of minors willing to participate in the research and would lead to a biased sample of clinic users; it could also violate the minors' right to confidential treatment at the clinic. When the researcher knowingly elects not to follow the ethical principles outlined in Chapter 6, you must evaluate the decision itself *and* the researcher's rationale.

A reviewer who comments on the ethical aspects of a study based on a report of completed research is obviously too late to prevent an ethical transgression from occurring. Nevertheless, the critique can bring the ethical

BOX 25-11   Guidelines for Critiquing Observational Methods

1. Does the research question lend itself to an observational approach? Would an alternative method have been more appropriate?
2. Is the degree of structure of the observational method consistent with the nature of the research question?
3. To what degree were the observers concealed during data collection? What effect might their presence have had on the behaviors and events they were observing?
4. What was the unit of analysis in the study? How much inference was required on the part of the observers, and to what extent did this lead to a potential for bias?
5. Where did the observations actually take place? To what extent did the setting influence the "naturalness" of the behaviors being observed?
6. How were data actually recorded (e.g., on field notes or checklists)? Did the recording procedure appear appropriate?
7. What steps were taken to minimize observer biases? For example, how were observers trained? How detailed were the explanations of the behaviors to be recorded?
8. If a category scheme was developed, was it exhaustive? Was the scheme overly demanding of observers, leading to the potential for inaccurate data? If the scheme was not exhaustive, did the omission of large realms of subject behavior lead to an inadequate context for understanding the behaviors of interest? Do the categories included in the instrument adequately cover the relevant behaviors?
9. What was the plan by which events or behaviors were sampled for observation? Did this plan appear to yield a representative sample of relevant behaviors?

BOX 25-12   Guidelines for Critiquing Biophysiologic Measures

1. Does the research question lend itself to a biophysiologic approach? Would an alternative method have been more appropriate?
2. Was the proper instrumentation used to obtain the biophysiologic measurements? Would an alternative instrument or method have been more appropriate? Did the researcher present a rationale for the use of the particular method, and was that rationale convincing?
3. Were the procedures for data collection adequately described? Did the procedures appear to be appropriate?
4. Does the report suggest that care was taken to obtain accurate data? For example, did the researcher's activities permit accurate recording if an instrument system without recording equipment was used?
5. Does the researcher appear to have the skills necessary for proper interpretation of the biophysiologic measurements?

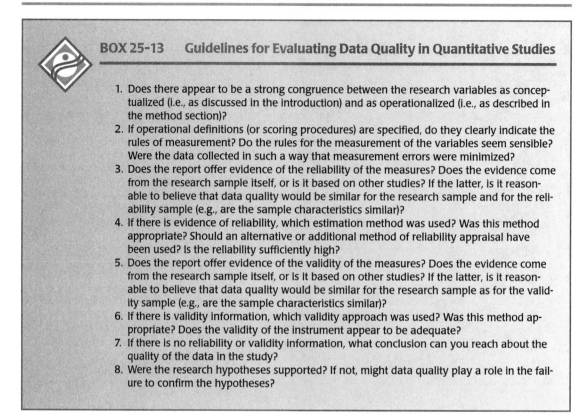

BOX 25-13   Guidelines for Evaluating Data Quality in Quantitative Studies

1. Does there appear to be a strong congruence between the research variables as conceptualized (i.e., as discussed in the introduction) and as operationalized (i.e., as described in the method section)?
2. If operational definitions (or scoring procedures) are specified, do they clearly indicate the rules of measurement? Do the rules for the measurement of the variables seem sensible? Were the data collected in such a way that measurement errors were minimized?
3. Does the report offer evidence of the reliability of the measures? Does the evidence come from the research sample itself, or is it based on other studies? If the latter, is it reasonable to believe that data quality would be similar for the research sample and for the reliability sample (e.g., are the sample characteristics similar)?
4. If there is evidence of reliability, which estimation method was used? Was this method appropriate? Should an alternative or additional method of reliability appraisal have been used? Is the reliability sufficiently high?
5. Does the report offer evidence of the validity of the measures? Does the evidence come from the research sample itself, or is it based on other studies? If the latter, is it reasonable to believe that data quality would be similar for the research sample as for the validity sample (e.g., are the sample characteristics similar)?
6. If there is validity information, which validity approach was used? Was this method appropriate? Does the validity of the instrument appear to be adequate?
7. If there is no reliability or validity information, what conclusion can you reach about the quality of the data in the study?
8. Were the research hypotheses supported? If not, might data quality play a role in the failure to confirm the hypotheses?

BOX 25-14   Guidelines for Evaluating Data Quality in Qualitative Studies

1. Does there appear to be a strong relationship between the phenomena of interest as conceptualized (i.e., as described in the introduction) and as described in the discussion of data collection approach?
2. Does the report discuss efforts made to enhance or evaluate the trustworthiness of the data? If not, is there other information that allows you to conclude that the data are of high quality?
3. Which techniques (if any) did the researcher use to enhance and appraise data quality? Was the investigator in the field an adequate amount of time? Was triangulation used, and, if so, of what type? Did the researcher search for disconfirming evidence? Were there peer debriefings and/or member checks? Do the researcher's qualifications enhance the credibility of the data?
4. Were the procedures used to enhance and document data quality adequate?
5. Given the procedures used to enhance data quality, what can you conclude about the credibility, transferability, dependability, and confirmability of the data? In light of this assessment, how much faith can be placed in the results of the study?

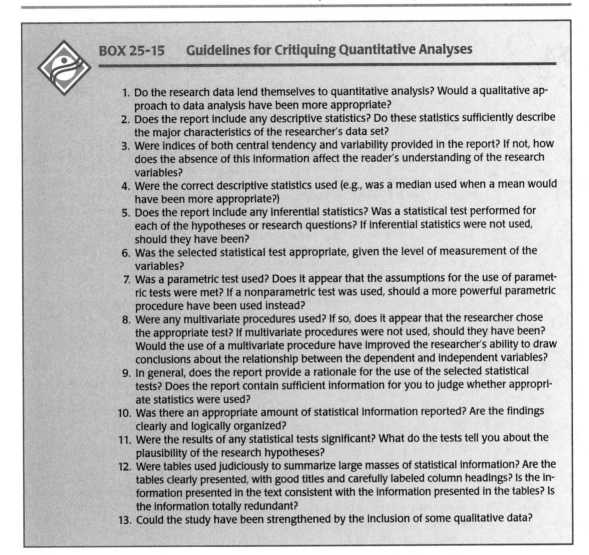

BOX 25-15   Guidelines for Critiquing Quantitative Analyses

1. Do the research data lend themselves to quantitative analysis? Would a qualitative approach to data analysis have been more appropriate?
2. Does the report include any descriptive statistics? Do these statistics sufficiently describe the major characteristics of the researcher's data set?
3. Were indices of both central tendency and variability provided in the report? If not, how does the absence of this information affect the reader's understanding of the research variables?
4. Were the correct descriptive statistics used (e.g., was a median used when a mean would have been more appropriate?)
5. Does the report include any inferential statistics? Was a statistical test performed for each of the hypotheses or research questions? If inferential statistics were not used, should they have been?
6. Was the selected statistical test appropriate, given the level of measurement of the variables?
7. Was a parametric test used? Does it appear that the assumptions for the use of parametric tests were met? If a nonparametric test was used, should a more powerful parametric procedure have been used instead?
8. Were any multivariate procedures used? If so, does it appear that the researcher chose the appropriate test? If multivariate procedures were not used, should they have been? Would the use of a multivariate procedure have improved the researcher's ability to draw conclusions about the relationship between the dependent and independent variables?
9. In general, does the report provide a rationale for the use of the selected statistical tests? Does the report contain sufficient information for you to judge whether appropriate statistics were used?
10. Was there an appropriate amount of statistical information reported? Are the findings clearly and logically organized?
11. Were the results of any statistical tests significant? What do the tests tell you about the plausibility of the research hypotheses?
12. Were tables used judiciously to summarize large masses of statistical information? Are the tables clearly presented, with good titles and carefully labeled column headings? Is the information presented in the text consistent with the information presented in the tables? Is the information totally redundant?
13. Could the study have been strengthened by the inclusion of some qualitative data?

problems to the attention of those who may be replicating the research.

Interpretive Dimensions

Research reports almost always conclude with a Discussion, Conclusions, or Implications section. It is in the final section that the researcher attempts to make sense of the analyses, to understand what the findings mean in relation to the research hypotheses, to consider whether the findings support or fail to support a theoretical framework, and to discuss what the findings imply for the nursing profession. Inevitably, the discussion section is more subjective than other sections of the report, but it must also be based on a careful consideration of the evidence.

As a reviewer, you should be somewhat wary if the discussion section fails to point

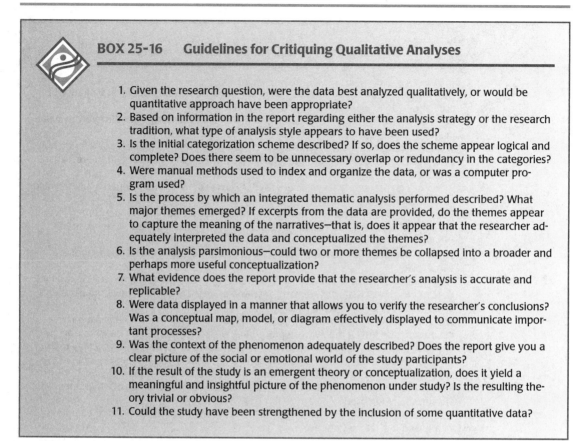

BOX 25-16   Guidelines for Critiquing Qualitative Analyses

1. Given the research question, were the data best analyzed qualitatively, or would be quantitative approach have been appropriate?
2. Based on information in the report regarding either the analysis strategy or the research tradition, what type of analysis style appears to have been used?
3. Is the initial categorization scheme described? If so, does the scheme appear logical and complete? Does there seem to be unnecessary overlap or redundancy in the categories?
4. Were manual methods used to index and organize the data, or was a computer program used?
5. Is the process by which an integrated thematic analysis performed described? What major themes emerged? If excerpts from the data are provided, do the themes appear to capture the meaning of the narratives—that is, does it appear that the researcher adequately interpreted the data and conceptualized the themes?
6. Is the analysis parsimonious—could two or more themes be collapsed into a broader and perhaps more useful conceptualization?
7. What evidence does the report provide that the researcher's analysis is accurate and replicable?
8. Were data displayed in a manner that allows you to verify the researcher's conclusions? Was a conceptual map, model, or diagram effectively displayed to communicate important processes?
9. Was the context of the phenomenon adequately described? Does the report give you a clear picture of the social or emotional world of the study participants?
10. If the result of the study is an emergent theory or conceptualization, does it yield a meaningful and insightful picture of the phenomenon under study? Is the resulting theory trivial or obvious?
11. Could the study have been strengthened by the inclusion of some quantitative data?

out the study's limitations. The researcher is in the best position to detect and assess the impact of sampling deficiencies, practical constraints, data quality problems, and so on, and it is a professional responsibility to alert readers to these difficulties. Moreover, when a researcher notes some of the methodologic shortcomings of the study, then readers have some assurance that these limitations were not ignored in the development of the interpretation of the results. As an example, Carty, Bradley, and Winslow (1996) conducted a study of women's perceptions of fatigue during pregnancy and postpartum. Women who were discharged within 3 days of delivery were compared with women who were discharged later with respect to fatigue levels. The researchers found few differences

between the two groups with regard to hours slept, perceptions of tiredness, and impact of tiredness on daily life. However, the researchers included a word of caution in their discussion section:

> The following limitations should be considered when interpreting the findings: The women in this study chose their discharge time, those who went home early had significant follow-up by nurses, and the questionnaire developed for this study does not have established reliability. (p. 77)

Of course, researchers are unlikely to note *all* relevant shortcomings of their own work. For instance, in the above example, the authors failed to point out that the absence of significant group differences could have resulted from the use of a relatively small sample. Thus, the inclusion of comments about study limitations in the discussion section, while important, does not relieve you of the responsibility of appraising methodologic decisions.

Your task as a reviewer is generally to contrast your own interpretation with that of the researcher and to challenge conclusions that do not appear to be warranted by the results. If your objective reading of the research methods and study findings leads to an interpretation that is notably different from that endorsed by the researcher, then the interpretive dimension of the study may well be faulty.

In addition to contrasting your interpretation with that of the researcher, your critique should also draw conclusions about the stated implications of the study. Some researchers make rather grandiose claims or offer unfounded recommendations on the basis of modest results. Some guidelines for evaluating the researcher's

interpretation and implications are offered in Box 25-18.

Presentational and Stylistic Dimensions

Although the worth of the study itself is reflected primarily in the dimensions we have reviewed thus far, the manner in which the information is communicated in the research report is also fair game in a comprehensive critical appraisal. Box 25-19 summarizes the major points that should be considered in evaluating the presentation of a research report.

An important consideration is whether the research report has provided sufficient information for a thoughtful critique of the other dimensions. For example, if the report does not describe how the sample was selected, then the reviewer cannot comment on the adequacy of the sampling plan, but he or she can criticize the researcher's failure to include information

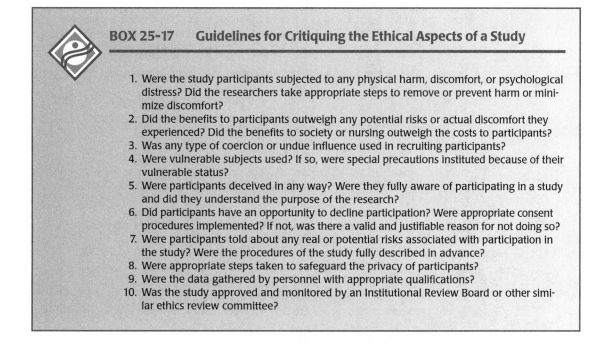

BOX 25-17   Guidelines for Critiquing the Ethical Aspects of a Study

1. Were the study participants subjected to any physical harm, discomfort, or psychological distress? Did the researchers take appropriate steps to remove or prevent harm or minimize discomfort?
2. Did the benefits to participants outweigh any potential risks or actual discomfort they experienced? Did the benefits to society or nursing outweigh the costs to participants?
3. Was any type of coercion or undue influence used in recruiting participants?
4. Were vulnerable subjects used? If so, were special precautions instituted because of their vulnerable status?
5. Were participants deceived in any way? Were they fully aware of participating in a study and did they understand the purpose of the research?
6. Did participants have an opportunity to decline participation? Were appropriate consent procedures implemented? If not, was there a valid and justifiable reason for not doing so?
7. Were participants told about any real or potential risks associated with participation in the study? Were the procedures of the study fully described in advance?
8. Were appropriate steps taken to safeguard the privacy of participants?
9. Were the data gathered by personnel with appropriate qualifications?
10. Was the study approved and monitored by an Institutional Review Board or other similar ethics review committee?

on sampling. When vital pieces of information are missing, the researcher leaves readers little choice but to assume the worst because this would lead to the most cautious interpretation of the results.

The writing in a research report, as in any published document, should be clear, grammatically correct, concise, and well-organized. Unnecessary jargon should be kept to a minimum, although colloquialisms should also be avoided. Inadequate organization is perhaps the most common presentation flaw in research reports. Continuity and logical thematic development are critical to good communication of scientific in-

formation, but these qualities are often difficult to attain.

Styles of writing do differ for qualitative and quantitative reports, and it is unreasonable to apply the standards considered appropriate for one paradigm to the other. Quantitative research reports are typically written in a more formal, impersonal fashion, using either the third person or passive voice to connote objectivity. Qualitative studies are likely to be written in a more literary style, using the first or second person and active voice to connote proximity and intimacy with the data and the phenomenon under study. Regardless of style,

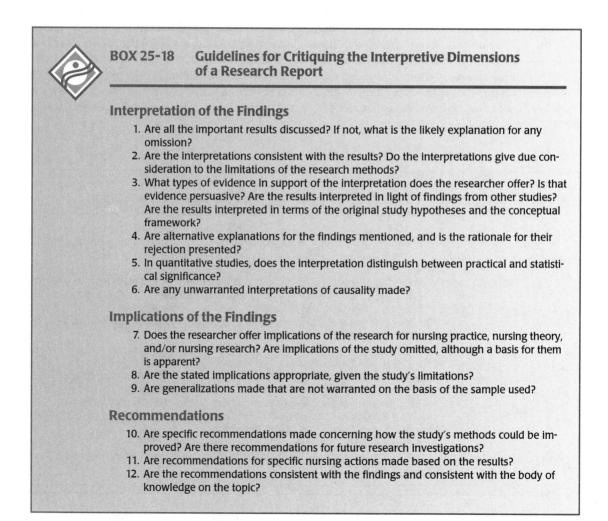

BOX 25-18   Guidelines for Critiquing the Interpretive Dimensions of a Research Report

Interpretation of the Findings

1. Are all the important results discussed? If not, what is the likely explanation for any omission?
2. Are the interpretations consistent with the results? Do the interpretations give due consideration to the limitations of the research methods?
3. What types of evidence in support of the interpretation does the researcher offer? Is that evidence persuasive? Are the results interpreted in light of findings from other studies? Are the results interpreted in terms of the original study hypotheses and the conceptual framework?
4. Are alternative explanations for the findings mentioned, and is the rationale for their rejection presented?
5. In quantitative studies, does the interpretation distinguish between practical and statistical significance?
6. Are any unwarranted interpretations of causality made?

Implications of the Findings

7. Does the researcher offer implications of the research for nursing practice, nursing theory, and/or nursing research? Are implications of the study omitted, although a basis for them is apparent?
8. Are the stated implications appropriate, given the study's limitations?
9. Are generalizations made that are not warranted on the basis of the sample used?

Recommendations

10. Are specific recommendations made concerning how the study's methods could be improved? Are there recommendations for future research investigations?
11. Are recommendations for specific nursing actions made based on the results?
12. Are the recommendations consistent with the findings and consistent with the body of knowledge on the topic?

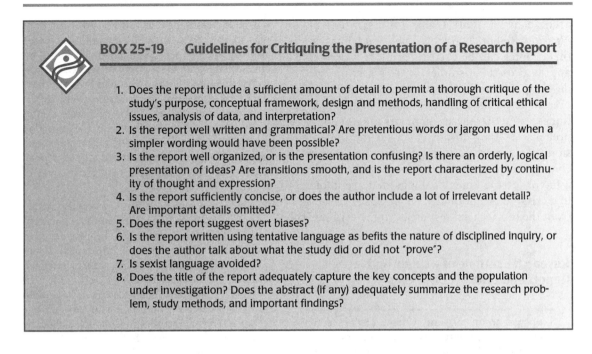

BOX 25-19   Guidelines for Critiquing the Presentation of a Research Report

1. Does the report include a sufficient amount of detail to permit a thorough critique of the study's purpose, conceptual framework, design and methods, handling of critical ethical issues, analysis of data, and interpretation?
2. Is the report well written and grammatical? Are pretentious words or jargon used when a simpler wording would have been possible?
3. Is the report well organized, or is the presentation confusing? Is there an orderly, logical presentation of ideas? Are transitions smooth, and is the report characterized by continuity of thought and expression?
4. Is the report sufficiently concise, or does the author include a lot of irrelevant detail? Are important details omitted?
5. Does the report suggest overt biases?
6. Is the report written using tentative language as befits the nature of disciplined inquiry, or does the author talk about what the study did or did not "prove"?
7. Is sexist language avoided?
8. Does the title of the report adequately capture the key concepts and the population under investigation? Does the abstract (if any) adequately summarize the research problem, study methods, and important findings?

however, as a reviewer, you should be alert to indications of overt biases, unwarranted exaggerations, emotionally laden comments, and melodramatic language.

In summary, the research report is meant to be an account of how and why a problem was studied and what results were obtained. The report should be accurate, clearly written, cogent, and concise. It should be written in a manner that piques the reader's interest and curiosity.

CONCLUSION

In concluding this chapter, several points about the research critique should be made. It should be apparent to those who have glanced through the questions in the boxes in this chapter that it will not always be possible to answer the questions satisfactorily on the basis of the research report. This is especially true for journal articles, in which the need for economy often translates into a severe abridgement of methodologic descriptions. Furthermore, there are many questions listed that may have little or no relevance for a particular study. The inclusion of a question in the list does not necessarily imply that all reports should have all the components mentioned. The questions are meant to suggest aspects of a study that often are deserving of consideration; they are not meant to lay traps for identifying omitted and perhaps unnecessary details.

It must be admitted that the answers to many questions will call on your judgment as much as, or even more than, your knowledge. An evaluation of whether the most appropriate data collection procedure was used for the research problem necessarily involves a degree of subjectiveness. Issues concerning the appropriateness of various strategies and techniques are topics about which even experts disagree. You should strive to be as objective as possible and to indicate your reasoning for the judgments made.

RESEARCH EXAMPLES

There are two complete research reports—one qualitative and the other quantitative—in the accompanying *Study Guide for Essentials of Nursing Research, 6th ed.* The guidelines in this chapter can be used to conduct a critical appraisal of these studies. In this section, we describe two studies by nurse researchers and present excerpts from published written critiques. Note that these comments are not comprehensive—they do not cover all the dimensions of a research critique as described in this chapter. However, the excerpts should provide a flavor for the kinds of things that are noted in a critique. Additionally, we present excerpts from the researchers' responses to the critique.

Research Example of a Quantitative Report and Critical Comments

Skoner, Thompson, and Caron (1994) conducted a retrospective case-control study to investigate risk factors for stress urinary incontinence (SUI) in women. A sample of 140 women (94 cases and 46 controls), who were recruited from three private physician practices, participated in the study. To be eligible, cases had to have symptoms of SUI, and controls had no evidence of SUI. Controls were selected from a list of potential patients without SUI, matched to cases by age within 5-year age intervals. The study was described to cases as an investigation of urinary incontinence in women, whereas it was described to controls as a study of women's health issues.

Telephone interviews were used to obtain data relating to various factors that the research literature suggested were associated with the risk of SUI. The questions covered family history of incontinence, reproductive events and menstrual history, gynecologic-related surgeries and infections, urinary tract infections and procedures, current health behaviors, and medications. No follow-up procedures were instituted for women who were nonrespondents to the telephone survey.

The data were analyzed using logistic regression with SUI status as the dependent variable. Age and other factors were statistically controlled. The results indicated that having a vagi-

nal birth versus having only cesarean sections was associated with a substantially increased risk for SUI. Other significant risk factors included having an episiotomy or tear during delivery, having a mother who had SUI, and having had multiple urinary tract infections.

Knapp and Nickel (1995) prepared a letter to the editor of *Nursing Research*, the journal in which Skoner and colleagues' report appeared, to comment on various aspects of the report. Their first concern related to the matching of the cases and controls:

> The group matching was apparently carried out before the cooperation of cases and controls had been obtained. The original plan called for 123 cases and 198 controls, but with the inevitable attrition and reclassification of some cases as controls, and some controls as cases, the final numbers of 94 and 46 were obtained. The initial matching on age was therefore lost to a considerable degree by the low response rates for both cases and controls and by the reclassifications. No information is provided regarding age distribution and the extent to which the matching was successful within each 5-year interval. (p. 58)

Skoner and Thompson (1995) offered a response to this criticism:

> Regarding age differences, we reported a mean of 51.5 for cases and a mean of 54.3 for controls. In order to control for the possible confounding effects of this modest difference, age was included in the multivariable logistic regression modeling. . . . Control for this and other potential confounding variables did not materially alter the estimates presented in Table 1. (p. 58)

Knapp and Nickel also commented on the operationalization of the dependent variable, namely status as a case with SUI or as a control without SUI. Specifically, they noted that information regarding diagnoses for the controls was not included in the report, and wondered why reclassification was based solely on SUI symptoms. The researchers responded that cystourethrograms were a means of expediting the identification of potential cases in only one of the three practices from which participants were recruited. However, for all subjects, the final classification was based on self-report. The researchers acknowledged the limitations of this approach: "Possible selection bias is of concern in any clinic-based case-control study, and we hope that population-based studies of stress urinary incontinence will be undertaken to avoid this potential methodological problem" (p. 58).

Knapp and Nickel also had concerns about the statistical analyses. For example, they noted that, "Given that 35 comparisons were made, some sort of procedure for protection from increased likelihood of Type I errors should have been employed" (p. 58). Skoner and Thompson (1995) responded as follows:

> Finally, regarding the issue of multiple comparisons, we do not feel that some sort of "protection" is warranted. We regard our confidence intervals as approximate indicators of the statistical uncertainty of estimating the odds ratios, and we have not adopted a strict adherence to the qualitative distinction between statistical significance versus non-significance. Of greater interest to us is the overall pattern of findings. . . . (p. 58)

Research Example of a Qualitative Report and Critical Comments

Vallerand and Ferrell (1995a) performed a secondary analysis of qualitative data to examine issues of control in patients with cancer pain. The original research that generated the data was an in-depth study of pain management at home among cancer patients. Ten patient–caregiver–nurse triads comprised the sample. Participants, who were cancer patients recruited from home health care agencies, had been experiencing cancer-related pain for at least 1 month. All patients had a primary caregiver who was older than 18 years of age. Nurses were the primary nurses for the patient and had at least 6 months' experience in home health care.

The data were collected through in-depth interviews, which were tape-recorded and transcribed. The interviews included questions about the patient's illness and pain experience, pain management at home, decision making, and ethical conflicts related to pain. All patient and caregiver interviews were conducted in the patients' homes; the nurses were interviewed at the home health care agencies. Each interview lasted 1 to 2 hours.

For the secondary analysis, Vallerand (who was not involved in the original study) read all the transcripts and coded the data with regard to control; she also coded the data according to a previously developed classification scheme that organized control into five distinct types: processual control, contingency control, cognitive control, behavioral control, and existential control. All data that related directly or indirectly to issues of control were coded, whereas other issues discussed in the interviews were unanalyzed for the purposes of this study. The second author (Ferrell, who was a lead researcher in the original study) independently recoded the data for control-related themes. Agreement between researchers was achieved before analysis.

Using the classification scheme to organize their analysis, the authors found that there were differences in the perception of control by the patient, the caregiver, and the nurse caring for the patient with cancer pain. For the patients, the main focuses were their attempt to maintain independence and control of their environment, the management of their pain, and the outcomes of their treatment. Both the primary family caregivers and the home care nurses were confronted with a struggle on a continuum ranging from helplessness to control. The authors concluded their report with some examples of interventions that could be used to increase patient control in the management of pain.

Fowler-Kerry (1995) prepared a commentary that was published in the same journal as this research report. Fowler-Kerry noted the importance of research relating to pain management in cancer patients. However, she expressed a few concerns regarding this research. A main concern was the adequacy of the data set for the conduct of this secondary analysis:

> The authors report that the concept of control emerged as a recurrent theme in the analysis

of the primary study transcripts. No in-depth questioning or probing of informants about control occurred in the primary study.... The authors provide an explanation of the methodology used in both the primary study and the secondary analysis. There is no discussion of any limitations inherent in the secondary analysis. (pp. 481–482)

In their response to the commentary (Vallerand & Ferrell, 1995b), the researchers noted that despite the absence of specific in-depth questioning relating to control, control emerged spontaneously as a central topic in the primary study. The absence of prompting, according to the researchers, underscored the importance of the concept:

> This approach allows for the respondents to select from their own personal experiences those elements that they want to discuss, and therefore the respondents are not biased by the questions of the researcher or early labeling of the concept. Although we have not specifically included the concept of control ... the participants in these studies consistently discussed the concept of control. (p. 482)

Fowler-Kerry commended the authors for including a detailed list of examples of interventions to increase control in pain management. However, she noted that the researchers did not identify which interventions emerged specifically as a result of the analysis: "Possibly the authors could comment about what novel results emerged from this study that would affect clinical practice or future research questions" (p. 482). The researchers acknowledged that this aspect of their report was not as well developed as might be desired but noted that there was indeed a link between the interventions and their ongoing research on pain management.

SUMMARY

Evaluating research reports involves critically appraising both the merits and the limitations of the published report. A systematic assessment of the various aspects of a research re-

port is essential in judging the utility and value of a study. This chapter offers suggestions for assessing the substantive, methodologic, interpretive, ethical, and stylistic aspects of a written research report.

STUDY ACTIVITIES

Chapter 25 of the *Study Guide to Accompany Nursing Research: Principles and Methods, 6th ed.*, offers various exercises and study suggestions for reinforcing the concepts presented in this chapter. Additionally, the following study questions can be addressed:

1. Read the article, "Weight-related distress in the early months after childbirth" by L. O. Walker (1998), *Western Journal of Nursing Research, 20, 30–44.* What limitations of the research methods did the authors identify? Do these limitations alter your acceptance of the findings?
2. Read an article from any issue of *Nursing Research* or any other nursing research journal and systematically assess the article according to the questions contained in this chapter. What are the merits and limitations of the report?
3. Read the article, "Some new dying trick: African American youths 'choosing' HIV/AIDS," by S. C. Tourigny (1998), *Qualitative Health Research, 8, 149–167.* Develop some practice implications based on this research.

SUGGESTED READINGS

Methodologic References

Aamodt, A. M. (1983). Problems in doing nursing research: Developing criteria for evaluating qualitative research. *Western Journal of Nursing Research, 5, 398–402.*

Becker, P. H. (1993). Common pitfalls in published grounded theory research. *Qualitative Health Research, 3, 254–260.*

Burns, N. (1989). Standards for qualitative research. *Nursing Science Quarterly, 2,* 44–52.

Field, W. E. (1983). Clinical nursing research: A proposal of standards. *Nursing Leadership, 6,* 117–120.

Gehlbach, S. H. (1992). *Interpreting the medical literature.* (3rd ed.). Lexington, MA: The Collamore Press.

Horsley, J., & Crane, J. (1982). *Using research to improve nursing practice: A guide.* New York: Grune & Stratton.

Morse, J. M. (1991). Evaluating qualitative research. *Qualitative Health Research, 1,* 283–286.

Ryan-Wenger, N. M. (1992). Guidelines for critique of a research report. *Heart & Lung, 21,* 394–401.

Topham, D. L., & DeSilva, P. (1988). Evaluating congruency between steps in the research process: A critique guide for use in clinical nursing practice. *Clinical Nurse Specialist, 2,* 97–102.

Substantive References

Carty, E. M., Bradley, C., & Winslow, W. (1996). Women's perceptions of fatigue during pregnancy and postpartum. *Clinical Nursing Research, 5,* 67–80.

Fowler-Kerry, S. (1995) Commentary on "Issues of control in patients with cancer pain." *Western Journal of Nursing Research, 17,* 481–482.

Knapp, T. R., & Nickel, J. T. (1995). Letter to the editor re "Factors associated with risk of stress urinary incontinence in women." *Nursing Research, 44,* 58.

Skoner, M. M., Thompson, W. D., & Caron, V. A. (1994). Factors associated with risk of stress urinary incontinence in women. *Nursing Research, 43,* 301–306.

Skoner, M. M., & Thompson, W. D. (1995). Response to letter to the editor re "Factors associated with risk of stress urinary incontinence in women." *Nursing Research, 44,* 58.

Vallerand, A. H., & Ferrell, B. R. (1995a). Issues of control in patients with cancer pain. *Western Journal of Nursing Research, 17,* 467–481.

Vallerand, A. H., & Ferrell, B. R. (1995b). Response to commentary by Fowler-Kerry on "Issues of control in patients with cancer pain." *Western Journal of Nursing Research, 17,* 482–483.

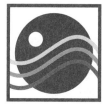

CHAPTER **26**

Utilization of Nursing Research

Most nurse researchers would like to see their research findings used to improve nursing practice. Moreover, most nurses working in clinical settings are aware of the benefits of having a **research-based** (or **evidence-based**) **practice.** That is, there is growing interest in developing a practice in which there is solid evidence from disciplined research that specific nursing actions and decisions are clinically appropriate and cost-effective and result in positive outcomes for clients.

During the past two decades, a number of changes in nursing education and in nursing research have been prompted by the desire to develop a better knowledge base for the practice of nursing. In education, most schools of nursing changed their curricula to include courses on nursing research; now, almost all baccalaureate and graduate nursing programs offer courses to instill some degree of research competence in their students. In the research arena, there has been a dramatic shift toward a focus on clinical nursing problems. There was an assumption—or at least a hope—that the production of clinically relevant studies would lead to improved nursing practice, if only there were an audience of practicing nurses who were competent in critically evaluating these studies. Changes in the nursing curriculum and in research focus, however, have not

in and of themselves resulted in sweeping changes in nurses' use of research findings. Research utilization, as the nursing community has increasingly begun to recognize, is a complex and nonlinear phenomenon and continues to be a serious professional challenge. In this chapter, we discuss various aspects of the utilization of nursing research.

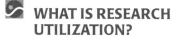

WHAT IS RESEARCH UTILIZATION?

Broadly speaking, **research utilization** refers to the use of some aspect of a scientific investigation in an application unrelated to the original research. Current conceptions of research utilization recognize a continuum in terms of the specificity of the use to which knowledge is put. At one end of the continuum are discrete, clearly identifiable attempts to base a specific action on the results of research findings. For example, a series of studies in the 1960s and 1970s demonstrated that the optimal placement time of a glass thermometer for accurate oral temperature determination is 9 minutes (e.g., Nichols & Verhonick, 1968). When nurses specifically altered their behavior from shorter placement times to the empirically based recommendation of 9 minutes, this constituted an instance of research utilization at this end of the continuum. Research utilization is sometimes defined in terms of such direct, specific actions. For example, Horsley, Crane, Haller, and Bingle (1983), who were involved in a major project on the utilization of research in nursing, defined research utilization as a "process directed toward transfer of specific research-based knowledge into practice through the systematic use of a series of activities" (pp. 100–101). This type of utilization has been referred to as **instrumental utilization** (Caplan & Rich, 1975).

There is growing recognition, however, that research can be utilized in a more diffuse manner—in a way that promotes cumulative awareness, understanding, or enlightenment. Caplan and Rich (1975) refer to this end of the utilization continuum as **conceptual utilization**. Thus, a practicing nurse may read a research report in which the investigators report that nonnutritive sucking among preterm infants in a neonatal intensive care unit had a beneficial effect on the number of days to the infant's first bottle feeding and on the number of days of hospitalization. The nurse may be reluctant to alter his or her own behavior or suggest an intervention based on the results of a single study. However, the nurse's reading of the research report may make the nurse more observant in his or her own work with preterm infants and may lead the nurse to collect informal data regarding the benefits of nonnutritive sucking in the nurse's own setting. Conceptual utilization, then, refers to situations in which users are influenced in their thinking about an issue based on their knowledge of one or more studies but do not put this knowledge to any specific, documentable use.

The middle ground of this continuum involves the partial impact of research findings on nursing activities. Here, nursing actions or decisions are based to some extent on research findings, but other factors, such as first-hand experience, tradition, and situational constraints, are also considered. This middle ground is frequently the result of a slow evolutionary process that does not reflect a conscious decision to use an innovative procedure but rather reflects what Weiss (1980) termed knowledge creep and decision accretion. **Knowledge creep** refers to an evolving "percolation" of research ideas and findings. **Decision accretion** refers to the manner in which momentum for a decision builds over time based on accumulated information gained through readings, informal discussions, meetings, and so on.

Research utilization at all points along this continuum appears to be an appropriate goal for nurses.

RESEARCH UTILIZATION IN NURSING

Numerous commentators have noted that progress in utilizing the results of nursing research studies in practice has proceeded slowly—too slowly for many who are anxious to establish a scientific base for nursing actions. In this section, we consider the possibilities for research utilization, and then review evidence on the extent to which utilization has occurred.

Incorporating Research Into Practice: The Potential

The nursing process is complex and requires nurses to engage in many decision-making activities. In the course of delivering patient care, nurses collect relevant information, make assessments and diagnoses, develop plans for appropriate nursing actions, initiate interventions, and evaluate the effects of these interventions. These activities correspond to the five phases of nursing outlined in the *Standards of Clinical Nursing Practice* established by the American Nurses' Association (1991). Within each of these phases, the findings from research can assist nurses in making more informed decisions and in taking actions that have a solid, research-based rationale. Thus, research conducted by nurses can potentially play a pivotal role in improving the quality of nursing care and the efficiency and costs with which it is delivered.

ASSESSMENT PHASE

Nurses collect information to assess patient needs from a variety of sources. The information may come from interviews with clients, family members, other nurses, and other types of health professionals as well as from records, charts, and nurses' observations. Each source contributes its unique part to the total assessment. Research can focus on how best to collect the information, what types of information need to be collected, how to integrate various pieces of assessment data, and how to improve the accuracy of gathering information. Research can also help nurses select alternative methods or forms for particular types of clients, settings, and situations. Through research, nurses can determine the extent to which the forms produce comparable information.

DIAGNOSIS PHASE

Based on an analysis of the information collected in the assessment phase of the nursing process, nurses are expected to develop nursing diagnoses. Research can play an important role in helping nurses make more accurate nursing diagnoses by validating the etiology of each diagnosis against the recorded assessment information. In addition, nursing research can help to determine the frequency of occurrence for each defining characteristic or cue associated with each diagnosis. The documentation can be helpful to the nursing profession, which has only recently begun the task of building up its taxonomy of diagnoses. Continued efforts in this area hold promise for the clustering of

nursing diagnostic groups and for the refinement of accepted nursing diagnoses.

PLANNING PHASE

The planning phase of the nursing process involves decisions concerning *what* nursing actions or interventions are needed; *when* the nursing actions are most appropriately instituted for each nursing diagnosis; *whom* the recipients of the nursing interventions should be; and under *which* conditions the interventions are to be implemented. Research findings can fruitfully be used by nurses in planning care by indicating the nursing interventions that are especially effective for particular cultural groups, settings, types of problems, and client characteristics. Research can also help nurses to evaluate the holism of the plan of care and to make more informed decisions about whether the established goals are realistic in a given situation.

INTERVENTION PHASE

Ideally, professionally accountable nurses would base as many of their nursing interventions as possible on research findings. Consider, for example, the many decisions made by nurses working the night shift in a nursing home. At what point do they decide that the nursing interventions are no longer producing the desired results for a resident in the process of dying? When is it time to notify the family or physician? What alterations in nursing interventions are available that facilitate, with as much ease as is possible, the transition from a state of life to a state of death? What approach might be used with families? What response might be expected from other residents of the home, and how might their stresses be appropriately alleviated? The systematic documentation of nursing interventions that have been found to have desirable outcomes may benefit other nurses facing the same kinds of situations.

EVALUATION PHASE

The last stage of the nursing process involves the evaluation of the degree to which the behavioral outcomes or goals developed at the planning stage have been met—and in the most cost-effective manner. Research can help document success or failure in achieving the various outcomes. When success occurs with relative frequency, it may offer other nurses the opportunity to implement the plan in other comparable situations with a fair degree of confidence. When the plan has been unsuccessful, nurses are redirected to examine the accuracy of the assessment, the nursing diagnoses, the plan, and the nursing interventions. Such information, collected systematically, may aid other nurses in avoiding the same dilemmas and should lead to improvements in nursing care.

Incorporating Research Into Practice: The Record

As we have just seen, there is ample potential for utilizing research throughout the various phases of the nursing process. Currently, however, there is considerable concern that nurses have thus far failed to realize this potential for using research findings as a basis for making decisions and for developing nursing interventions. This concern is based on some evidence suggesting that nurses are not always aware of research results and do not effectively incorporate these results into their practice.

One of the first pieces of evidence about the gap between research and practice was a study by Ketefian (1975), who reported on the oral temperature determination practices of 87 registered nurses. Ketefian's study was designed to learn what "happens to research findings relative to nursing practice after five or ten years of dissemination in the nursing literature" (p. 90). The results of a series of investigations in the late 1960s had clearly demonstrated that the optimal placement time for oral temperature determination using glass thermometers is 9 minutes. In Ketefian's study, only 1 out of 87 nurses reported the correct placement time, suggesting that these practicing nurses were unaware of or ignored the research findings about optimal placement time.

In another study investigating research utilization, Kirchhoff (1982) investigated the discontinuance of coronary precautions in a nationwide sample of 524 intensive care nurses. Several published studies had failed to demonstrate that the practices of restricting ice water and rectal temperature measurement were necessary, yet Kirchhoff's results indicated that these coronary precautions were still widely practiced. Only 24% of the nurses had discontinued ice water restrictions, and only 35% had discontinued rectal temperature restrictions.

Coyle and Sokop (1990) investigated practicing nurses' adoption of 14 nursing innovations that had been reported in the nursing research literature, replicating a study by Brett (1987). The utilization criteria suggested by Haller, Reynolds, and Horsley (1979) were used in selecting the 14 innovations: scientific merit of the study, significance and usefulness of the research findings to the practice setting, and the suitability of the finding for application to practice. A sample of 113 nurses practicing in 10 hospitals (randomly selected from the medium-sized hospitals in North Carolina) completed questionnaires that measured the nurses' awareness and use of the study findings. The results indicated much variation across the 14 studies. For example, from 34% to 94% of the nurses reported awareness of the various innovations. Coyle and Sokop used Brett's original scheme to categorize each study according to its stage of adoption: awareness (indicating knowledge of the innovation); persuasion (indicating the nurses' belief that nurses should use the innovation in practice); occasional use in practice; and regular use in practice. Only 1 of the 14 studies was at the regular-use stage of adoption. Six of the studies were in the persuasion stage, indicating that the nurses knew of the innovation and thought it *should* be incorporated into

		AWARE (%)	**PERSUADED (%)**	**USE SOMETIMES (%)**	**USE ALWAYS (%)**
STAGE	**NURSING INNOVATION**				
Awareness	Elimination of lactose from the formulas of tube-feeding diets for adult patients minimizes diarrhea, distention, flatulence, and fullness and reduces patient rejection of feedings (Horsley, Crane, & Haller, 1981)	38	36	13	19
Persuasion	Accurate monitoring of oral temperatures can be achieved on patients receiving oxygen therapy by using an electronic thermometer placed in the sublingual pocket (Lim-Levy, 1982)	68	55	35	29
Occasional use	A formally planned and structured preoperative education program preceding elective surgery results in improved patient outcomes (King & Tarsitano, 1982)	83	81	48	23
Regular use	A closed sterile system of urinary drainage is effective in maintaining the sterility of urine in patients who are catheterized for less than 2 weeks; continuity of the closed drainage system should be maintained during irrigations, sampling procedures, and patient transport (Horsley, Crane, Haller, & Bingle, 1981)	94	91	84	6

TABLE 26-1   Extent of Adoption of Four Nursing Practices*

*Based on findings reported in Coyle, L. A., & Sokop, A. G. (1990). Innovation adoption behavior among nurses. *Nursing Research, 39,* 176–180. The sample consisted of 113 practicing nurses.

nursing practice but were not basing their own nursing decisions on it. Table 26-1 describes 4 of the 14 nursing innovations, one for each of the four stages of adoption.

More recently, Rutledge, Greene, Mooney, Nail, and Ropka (1996) studied the extent to which oncology staff nurses adopted eight research-based practices. More than 1000 nurses were surveyed. The researchers found that awareness levels were high, with between 53% and 96% of the oncology nurses reporting awareness of the eight practices. Awareness and use were strongly linked: Almost 90% of aware nurses used seven of the practices at least some of the time.

The results of the recent studies are more encouraging than the studies by Ketefian and Kirchhoff because they suggest that, on average, practicing nurses are aware of many innovations based on research results, are persuaded that the innovations should be used, and are beginning to use them on occasion. Of course, it is possible that the respondents overstated their awareness and use of nursing innovations.

It is clear that a gap exists between knowledge production and knowledge utilization in nursing and in other disciplines. Some gap is inevitable and, given the imperfection of disciplined research as a means of knowing, even desirable. Nevertheless, it is clear that nurses are becoming enlightened with regard to the value of research by a growing body of research that is challenging traditional ways of practicing nursing.

Efforts To Improve Utilization

The need to reduce the gap between nursing research and nursing practice has been the topic of much discussion. In this section, we briefly describe a few of the formal projects that have been undertaken to achieve that goal.

THE WICHE PROJECT

One of the earliest research utilization projects was the Western Interstate Commission for Higher Education (WICHE) Regional Program for Nursing Research Development. The project, a 6-year effort funded by the Division of Nursing of the U.S. Department of Health, Education, and Welfare, had as its original goal investigating the feasibility of increasing nursing research activities through regional collaborative activities (Krueger, Nelson, & Wolanin, 1978). The three major project activities were (1) collaborative, nontargeted research (bringing together nurses from educational and practice settings to design studies based on mutually identified nursing problems); (2) collaborative, targeted research (multiple studies in different settings all designed to investigate a specific concept, quality of care); and (3) research utilization. The project team visualized research utilization as part of a five-phase resource linkage model. In this model, nurses were conceived as organizational change agents who could provide a link between research and practice. Through a support system (e.g., through workshops, conferences, and consultations), participant nurses were to utilize research results to solve problems identified as occurring in practice.

Nurses who participated in the WICHE project were given the opportunity to identify problems that needed research-based solutions and were then provided with opportunities to develop skills in reading and evaluating research for use in practice. They also developed detailed plans for introducing research innovations into their clinical practice settings. The final report indicated that the project was successful in increasing research utilization, but it also identified a stumbling block. The problem that posed the greatest difficulty was finding scientifically sound, reliable nursing studies with clearly identified implications for nursing care.

THE CURN PROJECT

The best-known nursing research utilization project is the Conduct and Utilization of Research in Nursing (CURN) Project, a 5-year development project awarded to the Michigan Nurses' Association by the Division of Nursing. The major objective of the CURN project was to increase the use of research findings in the daily practice of registered nurses by disseminating current research findings, facilitating organizational changes needed for the implementation of innovations, and encouraging the conduct of collaborative research that has relevance to nursing practice.

One of the activities of the CURN project was to stimulate the conduct of research in clinical settings. The project resulted in a set of nine volumes on various clinical problems. The titles of these volumes (e.g., *Pain, Preventing Decubitus Ulcers, Structured Preoperative Teaching,* and *Reducing Diarrhea in Tube-Fed Patients*) indicate that a wide range of clinical issues were studied.

The CURN project also focused on helping nurses to use research findings in their practice. The CURN project staff saw research utilization as primarily an organizational process (Horsley, Crane, & Bingle, 1978). According to their view, the commitment of organizations that employ practicing nurses to the research utilization process is essential for research to have any impact on nursing practice. They conceptualized the six phases of the research utilization process as follows (Horsley, Crane, Crabtree, & Wood, 1983):

1. Identification of practice problems that need solving and assessment of valid research bases to use in nursing practice
2. Evaluation of the relevance of the research-based knowledge as it applies to the identified clinical problem, the organization's values, current policies, and potential costs and benefits
3. Design of a nursing practice innovation that addresses the clinical problem but does not exceed the scientific limitations of the research base
4. Clinical trial and evaluation of the innovation in the practice setting
5. Decision making to adopt, revise, or reject the innovation
6. Development of strategies to extend the innovation to other appropriate settings

The CURN project team concluded that research utilization by practicing nurses is feasible, but only if the research is relevant to practice and if the results are broadly disseminated.

OTHER UTILIZATION PROJECTS

In the past decade, utilization projects have been undertaken by a growing number of hospitals and organizations, and descriptions of these projects are appearing with greater regularity in the nursing research literature. Only a few examples of broadly focused projects will be cited here to illustrate the types of approach that have been used to close the research–practice gap.

Bostrom and Wise (1994) described the efforts of one project implemented at a western hospital. The project, referred to as the Retrieval and Application of Research in Nursing (RARIN) project, was designed to facilitate the transfer of clinically relevant nursing information to nursing practice. A major component of the project involved training nurses to retrieve scientific information electronically.

A project in California focused on the building of organizational capacity as a tool for increasing research utilization (Rutledge & Donaldson, 1995). The Orange County Research Utilization in Nursing (OCRUN) project developed a regional network of 20 nursing service organizations and 6 academic institutions. During a 3-year period, nearly 400 nurses from those institutions participated in continuing education courses that focused on the development of research utilization competency. According to Rutledge and Donaldson, the project influenced nurse executives' perceptions of organizational readiness for change and ultimately influenced each participating organization's utilization processes and outcomes.

Dozens of more focused utilization projects are being implemented to address specific clinical issues. A few of these will be described in the Research Example section of this chapter.

BARRIERS TO UTILIZING NURSING RESEARCH

Typically, several years elapse between the time a researcher conceptualizes and designs a study and the time the results are reported in the research literature. Many more years may elapse between the time the results are reported and the time practicing nurses learn about the results and attempt to incorporate them into practice. Thus, it is not unusual for there to be an interim of a decade or so between the posing of a research problem and the implementation of a solution—if, in fact, there is *ever* an effort to implement. In the next section of this chapter, we discuss some strategies for bridging the gap between nursing research and nursing practice. First, however, we review some of the barriers to research utilization in nursing. These barriers can be broadly grouped into four categories relating to characteristics of the source of the barrier: (1) the research itself, (2) practicing nurses, (3) organizational settings, and (4) the nursing profession.

Research Characteristics

Studies reported in the nursing literature often do not warrant the incorporation of their findings into practice. Flaws in research design, sample selection, data collection instruments, or data analysis often raise questions about the soundness or generalizability of the study findings. Thus, a major impediment to research utilization by practicing nurses is that, for many problems, an extensive base of valid, reliable, and generalizable study results has not yet been developed.

As we have repeatedly stressed throughout this book, most studies have flaws of one type or another. The study may be flawed conceptually or methodologically, and the flaws may be minor or major. There are few, if any, perfect studies. If one were to wait for the perfect study before basing clinical decisions and interventions on research findings, however, one would have a very long wait indeed. It is precisely because of the limits of our research methods that replication becomes essential. When repeated testing of a hypothesis in different settings and with different types of sub-

jects yields similar results, then there can be greater confidence that the truth has been discovered. Isolated studies can almost never provide an adequate basis for making changes in nursing practice. Therefore, another constraint to research utilization is the dearth of reported replications of studies.

Nurses' Characteristics

Practicing nurses as individuals have characteristics that impede the incorporation of research findings into nursing care. Perhaps the most obvious is the educational preparation of nurses. Most practicing nurses—graduates of diploma or associate degree programs—have not received any formal instruction in research. They may therefore lack the skills to judge the merits of scientific projects. In a survey of some 600 nurses in England, 93% reported not being satisfied with their research skills (Pearcey, 1995). Furthermore, because research has played a limited role in the training of most nurses, they may not have developed positive attitudes toward research and may not be aware of the beneficial role it can play in the delivery of nursing care. Champion and Leach (1989) found that nurses' attitudes toward research were strong predictors of the utilization of research findings. Courses on research methods are now typically offered in baccalaureate nursing programs, but there is generally insufficient attention paid to research utilization. The ability to critique a research report is a necessary, but not sufficient, condition for effectively incorporating research results into daily decision making.

Another characteristic is one that is common to most humans. People are generally resistant to change. Change requires effort, retraining, and restructuring one's work habits. Change may also be perceived as threatening; for example, proposed changes may be perceived as potentially affecting one's job security. Thus, there may in some cases be opposition to introducing innovations in the practice setting. However, there is evidence from a recent survey of more than 1200 nurses that nurses value nursing research and want more time for research-related activities (Rizzuto, Bostrom, Suter, & Chenitz, 1994), so the time may be ripe for innovation.

Organizational Characteristics

Some of the impediments to research utilization, as the CURN project staff so astutely noted, stem from the organizations that train and employ practicing nurses. Organizations, perhaps to an even greater degree than individuals, resist change, unless there is a strong organizational perception that there is something fundamentally wrong with the status quo. In many settings, the organizational climate is simply not conducive to research utilization. To challenge tradition and accepted practices, a spirit of intellectual curiosity and openness must prevail.

In many practice settings, administrators have established protocols and procedures to reward expertise and competence in nursing practice. However, few practice settings have established a system to reward nurses for critiquing nursing studies, for utilizing research in practice, or for discussing research findings appropriate to clients. Thus, organizations have failed to motivate or reward nurses to seek ways to implement appropriate findings into their practice. Research review and utilization are often considered appropriate activities only when time is available, but available time is generally limited. In a national survey of nearly 1000 clinical nurses, one of the greatest reported barriers to research utilization was "insufficient time on the job to implement new ideas," which was reported as a moderate or great barrier by about 75% of the sample (Funk, Champagne, Wiese, & Tornquist, 1991).

Finally, organizations may be reluctant to expend the necessary resources for attempting utilization projects or for implementing changes to organizational policy. Resources may be required for the use of outside consultants, for staff release time, for administrative review, for evaluating the effects of an innovation, and so on. With the push toward cost containment in health care settings, resource constraints may therefore pose a barrier to research utilization—unless the utilization project has cost containment as an explicit goal.

Overall, in the national survey of perceived barriers, those stemming from the organizational setting were viewed by clinical nurses as posing the greatest obstacles to research utilization (Funk, Champagne, Wiese & Tornquist, 1991).

Characteristics of the Nursing Profession

Some of the impediments that contribute to the gap between research and practice are more global than those discussed previously and can be described as reflecting the state of the nursing profession or, even more broadly, the state of western society.

It has sometimes been difficult to encourage clinicians and researchers to interact and collaborate. They are generally in different settings, have many different professional concerns, interact with different networks of nurses, and operate according to different philosophical systems. Relatively few systematic attempts have been made to form collaborative arrangements, and to date, even fewer of these arrangements have been institutionalized as formal, permanent entities. Moreover, attempts to develop such collaboration will not necessarily be welcomed by either group. As Phillips (1986) observed, there is often a deep-seated lack of trust between nurse researchers and nurse clinicians.

A related issue is that communication between practitioners and researchers is problematic. Most practicing nurses do not read nursing research journals, nor do they usually attend professional conferences where research results are reported. Many nurses involved in the direct delivery of care are too overwhelmed by the jargon, the statistical symbols, and the wealth of quantitative information contained in research reports to understand fully such reports even when they do read them. Furthermore, nurse researchers may attend too infrequently to the needs of clinical nurses as identified in specialty journals. For research utilization to happen, there must be two-way communication between the practicing nurse and the nurse researcher. The recent emergence of two journals—*Applied Nursing Research* and *Clinical Nursing Research*—represents an important step in this direction.

Phillips (1986) also noted two other noteworthy barriers to bridging the research–practice gap. One is the shortage of appropriate role models. Phillips commented that, "even if a nurse wants to assume the role of nursing research consumer, there are few colleagues available to give support for the endeavor and fewer still available to emulate" (p. 8). The other barrier is the historical "baggage" that has defined nursing in such a way that practicing nurses may not typically perceive themselves as independent professionals capable of recommending changes based on nursing research results. If practicing nurses believe that their role is to await direction from the medical community, and if they believe they have no power to be self-directed, then they will have difficulty in initiating innovations based on nursing research results. In the previously mentioned national survey, the barrier perceived by the largest percentage of nurses was the nurse's feeling that he or she did not have "enough authority to change patient care procedures" (Funk, Champagne, Wiese, & Tornquist, 1991).

TIPS FOR IMPROVING RESEARCH UTILIZATION

Where does the responsibility for bridging the gap between research and practice lie? Should individual practicing nurses pursue appropriate nursing innovations? Should organizations and their administrative staff take the lead? Or should the direction come from researchers themselves? In our view, the entire nursing community must be involved in the process of putting research into practice. In this section, we discuss some research utilization strategies that various segments of the nursing community can adopt.

Strategies for Researchers

A great deal of the responsibility for research utilization rests in the hands of researchers. There is little point in doing research if the results do not get used, so it behooves researchers to take steps to ensure that utilization can occur. Some suggestions for strategies that researchers could implement to foster better adoption of their research results are as follows:

- *Do high-quality research.* A major impediment to utilizing nursing research results, as indicated in the previous section, is that there is often an inadequate basis for introducing innovations or for making changes. The quality of nursing studies has improved dramatically in the past two decades, but much progress remains to be made. The inadequacy of sampling plans remains one of the greatest weaknesses of nursing studies. If a study is based on an unrepresentative sample of 50 subjects, then utilization efforts based on the study findings are likely to be inappropriate.
- *Do relevant outcomes research.* In order for the nursing community to adopt innovations in nursing practice, there must be evaluations of the extent to which the innovations can achieve the desired outcomes. Researchers must develop a knowledge base about the cost-effectiveness and efficacy of interventions. They must design research that sheds light on the maximally beneficial "dosage" of the intervention; the client population that would most benefit from the intervention;

the context and circumstances under which the intervention can best be applied; and the intended and unintended effects of the intervention. In other words, researchers can address clinical problems in such a way that the utilization potential of the study is enhanced.

- *Replicate.* As noted earlier, utilization of research results can almost never be justified on the basis of a single isolated study, so researchers must make a real commitment to replicating studies. It is also important to publish the results of replications even if—in fact, especially if—the results are exactly the same as those obtained in an earlier investigation. The journal *Clinical Nursing Research* has explicitly noted its intent to publish the results of replication studies (Hayes, 1993).

- *Collaborate with practitioners.* Academic researchers will never succeed in having much of an impact on nursing practice unless they become better attuned to the needs of practicing nurses and the clients they serve, the problems that practicing nurses face in delivering nursing care, and the constraints that operate in practice settings. Practicing nurses will be more willing to change their behaviors and modes of delivering care if they perceive that researchers are addressing issues of concern and importance to them. Researchers should seek opportunities to exchange ideas for research problems with nurse clinicians. They also need to involve clinicians in the actual conduct of research and in the interpretation of study results. Indeed, it has repeatedly been found that nurses who are involved in research-related activities such as data collection develop more positive attitudes toward research and are more likely to use research findings in the clinical setting (e.g., Bostrom, 1991; Bostrom & Suter, 1993; Dufault et al., 1995).

- *Disseminate aggressively.* If a researcher fails to communicate the results of a completed study to other nurses, it is obvious that the results will never be utilized by practicing nurses. Even studies with a variety of methodologic shortcomings can make a contribution, if only to illuminate the researcher's conceptualization of a practice problem or to suggest how the research question might be better addressed in some subsequent study. It is the researcher's *responsibility* to find some means of communicating research results. Researchers should submit their manuscripts to at least two or three journals before abandoning hope of getting their reports published.

- *Disseminate broadly.* A researcher's responsibility for dissemination does not end at the point at which an article has been accepted for publication. Most nurses read only one or two professional journals, so a researcher who is truly committed to having his or her results known by the nursing community often publishes study results in several journals. It is unethical to submit *exactly* the same manuscript to two different journals, but a study generally yields more information than can be concisely reported in a single journal anyway. It is especially important from a utilization standpoint for researchers to report their results in specialty journals, which are more likely to be read by practicing nurses than the nursing research journals. Researchers should also take steps to disseminate study findings at conferences, colloquia, and workshops that are known to be attended by nurse clinicians. Collaboration with practicing nurses should prove useful in developing effective dissemination plans.

- *Communicate clearly.* It is not always possible to present the results of a research project in a way that is readily comprehensible to clinicians. However, researchers need to be encouraged to avoid unnecessary jargon whenever possible, to define any terms that are technically difficult, to construct tables carefully so that a nonresearcher can get a sense of the findings, and to compose the abstract of the report so that virtually any intelligent reader can understand the research problem, the general approach, and the most salient findings. A general aim should be to write research reports that are user-friendly.

- *Suggest clinical implications.* In the introduction to a research report, the researcher should explain the potential clinical significance of the study. In the discussion section, the researcher should suggest how the results of their research can be utilized by practicing nurses: How would a staff nurse currently working in the area apply the findings? Of course, the researcher should also be careful to discuss study limitations and to make some assessment of the generalizability of the study findings. If an implications section with suggestions for clinical practice became a standard feature of research reports, then the burden of utilization would be much lighter for the nurse clinician.

Strategies for Scholars and Educators

Some overlap exists between the categories of nurse researcher and nurse academician, but the overlap is imperfect because not all educators are researchers and not all researchers are in academia. Several of the following suggested strategies could, however, be undertaken by nonacademic researchers as well as by educators.

- *Incorporate research findings into the curriculum.* Research findings should be integrated throughout the curriculum. Whenever possible, faculty should document the efficacy of a specific procedure or technique by referring to a relevant study. When there is no relevant research, the instructor can note the absence of empirical evidence supporting the technique—this could help to stimulate the students' interest in research-based verification.

- *Encourage research and research utilization.* Either by acting as role models to students (e.g., by discussing their own research) or by clearly demonstrating positive attitudes toward research and its use in nursing, instructors can help to foster a spirit of inquiry and openness that is a precondition to effective utilization of research. Instructors of research methods can also encourage students to become better consumers of nursing research, to do their own research, or to develop a plan for a utilization project.

- *Prepare integrative reviews.* There is an urgent need for high-quality critical reviews of research on specific research topics. If a research question has been studied by several different researchers—in other words, if there have been several replications of a study—then the question may be ripe for a review that will summarize the state of knowledge. Such reviews can play an invaluable role for practicing nurses, who generally do not have the time to do extensive literature reviews and who may have some difficulty in critically evaluating individual studies. When an integrative review takes the form of a meta-analysis—which involves the use of statistical procedures to integrate the findings—the researcher should take pains to translate the results into clinical terms. Integrative reviews should ideally conclude with some strong statements about the implications of the body of research for nursing practice. As an example of a useful model, Beyea and Nicoll (1995) undertook a critical review of research on the administration of medications by intramuscular injection, with the aim of developing a clinical practice protocol.

- *Place demands on researchers.* Faculty (especially if they have done research themselves) are often asked to be anonymous reviewers of research proposals and reports. Funding sources that offer financial support for the conduct of nursing research generally rely on a panel of experts to help them review research proposals before awarding any grants. Peer reviewers of such proposals should demand that researchers demonstrate the proposed study's potential for practical utility. Moreover, peer reviewers can demand that the researchers include a specific plan for dissemination or utilization. Reviewers of journal articles of completed research should also criticize reports that have failed to include a discussion of the study's implications for practice.

Strategies for Practicing Nurses and Nursing Students

Practicing nurses cannot by themselves launch institution-wide utilization projects, but their behaviors and attitudes are nevertheless critical to the success of any efforts to base nursing interventions and nursing diagnoses on research findings. Furthermore, individual nurses can engage in and benefit from conceptual utilization. Therefore, every nurse has an important role to play in utilizing nursing research.

- *Read widely and critically.* Professionally accountable nurses continue their nursing education on an ongoing basis by keeping abreast of important developments in their field. All nurses should regularly read journals relating to their specialty, including the research reports in them. Research reports should be critically appraised, according to guidelines such as those suggested in Chapter 25. It is especially important for nurse clinicians to read critical reviews of research that integrate numerous studies on a problem. Brett's (1987) study confirms the importance of reading. Her findings revealed that nurses who spent more time each

week reading professional journals were more likely to adopt a research-based innovation than nurses who read infrequently.

- *Attend professional conferences.* Many nursing conferences include presentations of studies that have clinical relevance. It is often more rewarding to attend research presentations at a conference than to read a research report because the lag time between the conduct of a study and a conference presentation is generally less than the lag time for publication. Thus, conference attendees usually hear of an innovation much sooner than those who wait to read about it in a journal. Furthermore, those attending a conference get an opportunity to meet the researcher and to ask questions about practice implications. Brett's (1987) utilization study revealed a positive relationship between nurses' conference attendance and the degree to which they adopt research-based innovations. Some hospitals and other institutions offer stipends to defray the cost of attending such conferences.

- *Learn to expect evidence that a procedure is effective.* Every time nurses or nursing students are told about a standard nursing procedure, they have a right to ask: Why? Nurses need to develop expectations that the decisions they make in their clinical practice are based on sound rationales. It is not inappropriate for the nursing student or practitioner to challenge the principles and procedures that are currently in use, although tact is advisable so that defensiveness is not engendered by such challenges.

- *Seek environments that support research utilization.* Organizations differ in their openness to research utilization, so nurses interested in basing their practice on research have some control through their employment decisions. If organizations perceive that nurses are basing their employment decisions on such factors as the organizational climate regarding research, there will be some pressure to support research utilization.

- *Become involved in a journal club.* Many organizations that employ nurses sponsor journal clubs that meet regularly to review research articles that have potential relevance to practice. Generally, members take turns reviewing and critically appraising a study and presenting the critique to the club's members. If there is no such club in existence, it might be possible to work with the organization to initiate one (see, e.g., Tibbles & Sanford, 1994). Although the bulk of the responsibility for disseminating research results lies with the researcher, this is a responsibility that can be shared by practitioners.

- *Collaborate with a nurse researcher.* Collaboration, which we previously mentioned as a strategy for nurse researchers, is a two-way street. Practicing nurses who have identified a clinical problem in need of a solution and who lack methodologic skills for the conduct of a study should consider initiating a collaborative relationship with a local nurse researcher. Collaboration with a nurse researcher could also be a useful approach for formal, institutional utilization projects.

- *Pursue and participate in institutional utilization projects.* Sometimes, ideas for utilization projects come from staff nurses. Although large-scale utilization projects require organizational and administrative support, individual nurses or groups of nurses can propose such a project to the nursing department. For example, an idea for such a project may emerge in the context of a journal club. If the idea for a research utilization effort originates from within the administration, then individual nurses are still likely to play an important role in carrying out the project. Indeed, a utilization project can easily be undermined by reluctant or uncooperative staff. Although change is not always easy, it is in the interest of the profession to have practicing nurses who are open-minded about the possibility that a new technique or procedure can improve the quality of care that nurses provide.

- *Pursue appropriate personal utilization projects.* Not all findings from research studies are ones that require organizational commitment or policy directives. For example, a study might reveal that the health beliefs of an immigrant group are different from those of the predominant cultural group, and this may lead a nurse to ask several additional questions informally of clients of that immigrant group during assessment. If the nurse discovers that important and relevant information is gleaned from these additional questions, it may then be appropriate to recommend to the administration a more formal utilization project, which might involve changes to the standard assessment protocols. Of course, not all research findings are amenable to such informal personal utilization projects. If the results of a study or series of studies suggest an action or decision that is contrary to organizational policy or that has *any* potential risk for the clients, then nurses should not pursue such projects without supervisory approval. Some criteria for research utilization are discussed in the next section of this chapter.

Strategies for Administrators

According to several models of research utilization, the organizations that employ nurses play a fundamental role in supporting or undermining the nursing profession's efforts to develop a scientific base of practice. In the national survey, respondents viewed "enhancing administrative support and encouragement" as the single most effective means of facilitating research utilization (Funk, Champagne, Wiese, & Tornquist, 1991). Although the readers of this book are not likely to include a large audience of nursing or hospital administrators, the following suggested strategies are included primarily to alert practicing nurses to the kinds of issues facing these groups.

- *Foster a climate of intellectual curiosity.* If there is a great deal of administrative rigidity and opposition to change, then the staff's interest in research utilization is unlikely to become ignited. The administrator can take steps to encourage reading and critical thinking about the challenges facing practicing nurses. Open communication is an important ingredient in persuading staff nurses that their experiences and problems are important and that the administration is willing to consider innovative solutions.
- *Offer emotional or moral support.* If nurse administrators are unsupportive of research utilization, then there is little chance that any utilization efforts will get off the ground. Administrators need to make their support visible by informing staff and prospective staff on an individual basis, by establishing research utilization committees, by helping to develop research journal clubs, and so on. Administrators can perhaps offer the greatest degree of personal support by being a role model for the staff nurses. They can accomplish this, for example, by engaging in their own program of research, by actively participating themselves in the research journal clubs, and by playing a role in utilization projects.
- *Offer financial or resource support for utilization.* Utilization projects often require some resources, although resource demands may not be great. Resources may be required for release time for nurses engaged in utilization projects, for outside consultation, for supplies and computer time, for registration at conferences, and so on. If the administration expects nurses to engage in research utilization activities on their own time and at

their own expense, then the not-so-subtle message is that research utilization is unimportant to those running the organization.

- *Reward efforts for utilization.* When administrators evaluate nursing performance, they use a number of different criteria. Although research utilization should not be a primary criterion for evaluating a nurse's performance, its inclusion as one of several important criteria is likely to have a large impact on nurses' behaviors.

THE UTILIZATION PROCESS AND CRITERIA FOR UTILIZATION

A number of different models of research utilization have been developed during the past few decades. These models offer guidelines for designing and implementing a utilization project in a practice setting. One such model is the Stetler Model for Research Utilization (Stetler, 1994), which involves six phases of activities (preparation, validation, comparative evaluation, decision making, translation/application, and evaluation). Another model, the Iowa Model of Research in Practice (Titler et al., 1994), involves a series of activities with two critical decision points: (1) deciding whether there is a sufficient research base for utilization and (2) deciding whether the change is appropriate for adoption in practice. Some utilization projects have used as a framework Rogers' diffusion of innovation model, which describes a process involving five stages: knowledge, persuasion, decision, implementation, and confirmation (Rogers, 1995).

In this section, we discuss how a research utilization project can be planned and executed, using a model that we have adapted from several existing utilization models. Although the processes described here are ones that most likely will apply to an organization or a group of nurses working together, many of the steps in the processes are important ones for individual nurses to consider as they attempt to base their clinical decisions on scientific findings.

Approaches to Research Utilization

Nurses interested in utilizing research findings in their nursing practice generally set about the task in one of two ways. One approach to utilization, shown schematically as path A in Figure 26-1, begins with the identification of a clinical problem that needs solution (in the Iowa Model of Research in Practice, this corresponds to what is called **problem-focused triggers**). Such a problem identification may arise in the normal course of clinical practice or in the context of a quality assessment or quality improvement effort. This problem identification approach, which corresponds to the first step in the six-phase process described by the CURN project team, is likely to have considerable internal staff support if the selected problem is one that numerous nurses in the practice setting have encountered. This approach to utilization is likely to have much clinical relevance because a specific clinical situation generated the interest in resolving the problem in the first place.

Once a clinical problem has been identified, the next step is a search for relevant literature to determine whether nurse researchers have addressed the problem through disciplined research. If there is no research base related to the identified problem, then there are two choices for the utilization effort: (1) to abandon the original problem and select an alternative one; or (2) to consider initiating an original research project on the topic (i.e., to initiate steps to *create* a knowledge base). This decision is likely to depend on the research skills of the staff and on the availability of research consultants.

Next, the knowledge base must be assessed. If the knowledge base is sound (according to criteria to be described later), then the subsequent step is to conduct an **implementation assessment**. If, however, the existing knowledge base inspires little confidence that the research could effectively be utilized by nurses, then there remain the two previously suggested alternatives: (1) to "go back to the drawing board" and select a new problem or (2) to investigate the possibility of doing original research to improve the knowledge base.

The implementation assessment involves three primary aspects: (1) an assessment of the transferability of the research findings, (2) an analysis of the cost/benefit ratio, and (3) an evaluation of the feasibility of implementing the innovation. These criteria will be elaborated in the next section. If all the implementation criteria are met, the team can then proceed to design the protocols for the innovation and its clinical evaluation, test the innovation in the practice setting, evaluate its effectiveness and costs, and then decide whether the new practice should be institutionalized. A final optional step, but one that is highly advisable, is the dissemination of the results of the utilization project so that other practicing nurses can benefit. If the implementation analysis suggests that there might be problems in testing the innovation within that particular practice setting, then the team can either identify a new problem and begin the process anew or consider adopting a plan to improve the implementation potential (e.g., seeking external resources if cost considerations were the inhibiting factor).

The second major approach to conducting a utilization project, shown schematically as path B in Figure 26-1, has many of the same components as the first approach. The major difference, however, is the starting point. Here, the process starts with the research literature—corresponding to the **knowledge-focused triggers** identified in the Iowa model. This approach could occur if, for example, a utilization project emerged as a result of discussions within a journal club. In this approach, the team would proceed through most of the same steps as outlined previously, except that a preliminary assessment would need to be made of the clinical relevance of the re-

A. Problem Identification Approach

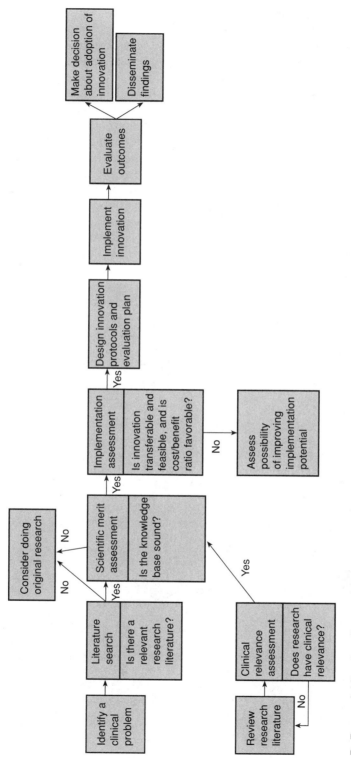

B. Research Literature Approach

Figure 26-1. A model for research utilization.

search findings. If it is determined that the research base is not clinically relevant, then the next step involves further reading and reviewing of the research literature.

Both these approaches involve several types of assessments, the results of which affect the appropriateness of proceeding with the utilization project. Criteria for making these assessments are presented next.

Utilization Criteria

As the model shown in Figure 26-1 suggests, there are three broad classes of criteria that are important in undertaking a utilization project: clinical relevance, scientific merit, and implementation potential. Each of these criteria is elaborated on here.

CLINICAL RELEVANCE

Of critical importance is whether the problem and its solution have a high degree of **clinical relevance**. The central issue here is whether a problem of significance to nurses will be solved by making some change or introducing a new intervention. There is little point in undertaking a utilization project if the nursing profession or the clients it serves cannot benefit from the effort. If, under the best of circumstances, there is little potential for solving a nursing problem or helping nurses to make important clinical decisions, then the project probably should not be undertaken.

The five questions relating to clinical relevance, shown in Box 26-1, can be applied to a research report or set of related reports and can generally be answered based on a reading of the introduction to the reports. According to Tanner (1987), from whom these questions were adapted, if the answer is yes to any one of the five questions, then the next step in the process can be pursued because the innovation has the potential for being useful in practice. If, however, the answers to all the questions are negative, then the prospect of clinical relevance is small, and there is probably little point in pursuing the problem area any further.

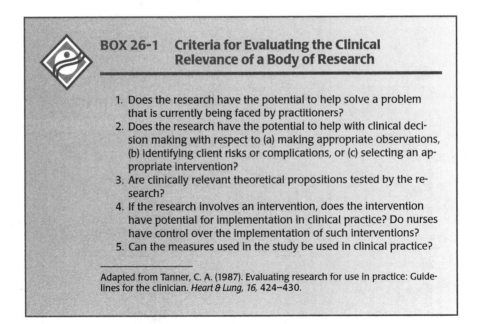

BOX 26-1   Criteria for Evaluating the Clinical Relevance of a Body of Research

1. Does the research have the potential to help solve a problem that is currently being faced by practitioners?
2. Does the research have the potential to help with clinical decision making with respect to (a) making appropriate observations, (b) identifying client risks or complications, or (c) selecting an appropriate intervention?
3. Are clinically relevant theoretical propositions tested by the research?
4. If the research involves an intervention, does the intervention have potential for implementation in clinical practice? Do nurses have control over the implementation of such interventions?
5. Can the measures used in the study be used in clinical practice?

Adapted from Tanner, C. A. (1987). Evaluating research for use in practice: Guidelines for the clinician. *Heart & Lung, 16,* 424–430.

SCIENTIFIC MERIT

We have discussed the criteria for **scientific merit** throughout this book and, in Chapter 25, we presented guidelines for assessing whether the findings and conclusions of a study are accurate, believable, and generalizable or transferable. When it comes to utilization, however, some additional concerns must be kept in mind. First and foremost is the issue of replication, the repeating of a study in a new setting, with a new sample of study participants. It is unwise to base an entire utilization project on a single study that has not been replicated, even if the study is extremely rigorous. Ideally, there would be several replications—each providing similar evidence of the effectiveness of the innovation being considered. At least one and ideally more of the studies should have been conducted in a clinical setting, with real clients.

Replications are seldom exact duplications of an earlier study; usually, a replication involves making some changes to some aspects of the research methods, such as the data collection instruments, the sampling plan, and so on. It is not essential that the replications be identical to provide a useful basis for pursuing a utilization project. Rather, it is more important that the *problem* being addressed is the same and that the innovations being tested are conceptually similar to each other. For example, several nurse researchers have investigated the use of therapeutic touch as a means of reducing stress and enhancing the psychological well-being of patients. Although these studies have all operationalized therapeutic touch in somewhat different ways and have examined somewhat different outcomes, it would be reasonable for a utilization project to consider the whole body of research on therapeutic touch.

IMPLEMENTATION POTENTIAL

Even when it has been determined that a problem has clinical significance and when there is a sound knowledge base relating to that clinical problem, it is not necessarily true that a utilization project can be planned and implemented. A number of other issues must be considered with regard to **implementation potential**, which we have grouped under three headings: the transferability of the knowledge, the feasibility of implementation, and the cost/benefit ratio of the innovation. Box 26-2 presents some assessment questions for these categories.

Transferability. The main issue in the transferability question is whether it makes good sense to attempt the selected innovation in the new practice setting. If there is some aspect of the practice setting that is fundamentally incongruent with the innovation—in terms of its philosophy, the type of clients it serves, its personnel, or its financial or administrative structure—then it makes little sense to try to transfer the innovation, even if a clinically significant innovation has been shown to be effective in various research contexts.

Feasibility. The feasibility questions address a number of practical concerns about the availability of resources, the availability of staff, the organizational climate, the need for and availability of external assistance, and the potential for clinical evaluation. An important issue here is whether nurses will have control over the innovation (often this means having the ability to manipulate the independent variable). When nurses do not have full control over the new procedure being introduced, it is important to recognize the interdependent nature of the utilization project and to proceed as early as possible to establish the necessary cooperative arrangements.

Cost/Benefit Ratio. A critical part of any decision to proceed with a utilization project is a careful assessment of the costs and benefits of the innovation. The **cost/benefit assessment** should encompass likely costs and benefits to various groups, including clients, staff, the or-

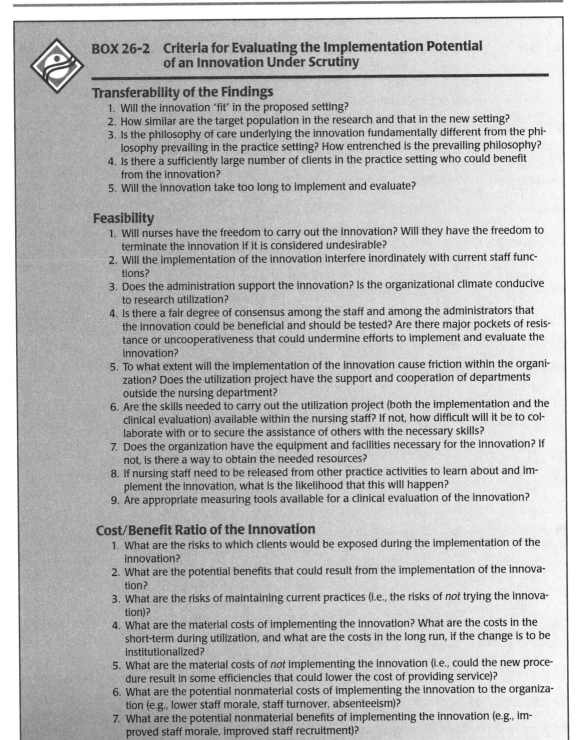

BOX 26-2   Criteria for Evaluating the Implementation Potential of an Innovation Under Scrutiny

Transferability of the Findings

1. Will the innovation "fit" in the proposed setting?
2. How similar are the target population in the research and that in the new setting?
3. Is the philosophy of care underlying the innovation fundamentally different from the philosophy prevailing in the practice setting? How entrenched is the prevailing philosophy?
4. Is there a sufficiently large number of clients in the practice setting who could benefit from the innovation?
5. Will the innovation take too long to implement and evaluate?

Feasibility

1. Will nurses have the freedom to carry out the innovation? Will they have the freedom to terminate the innovation if it is considered undesirable?
2. Will the implementation of the innovation interfere inordinately with current staff functions?
3. Does the administration support the innovation? Is the organizational climate conducive to research utilization?
4. Is there a fair degree of consensus among the staff and among the administrators that the innovation could be beneficial and should be tested? Are there major pockets of resistance or uncooperativeness that could undermine efforts to implement and evaluate the innovation?
5. To what extent will the implementation of the innovation cause friction within the organization? Does the utilization project have the support and cooperation of departments outside the nursing department?
6. Are the skills needed to carry out the utilization project (both the implementation and the clinical evaluation) available within the nursing staff? If not, how difficult will it be to collaborate with or to secure the assistance of others with the necessary skills?
7. Does the organization have the equipment and facilities necessary for the innovation? If not, is there a way to obtain the needed resources?
8. If nursing staff need to be released from other practice activities to learn about and implement the innovation, what is the likelihood that this will happen?
9. Are appropriate measuring tools available for a clinical evaluation of the innovation?

Cost/Benefit Ratio of the Innovation

1. What are the risks to which clients would be exposed during the implementation of the innovation?
2. What are the potential benefits that could result from the implementation of the innovation?
3. What are the risks of maintaining current practices (i.e., the risks of *not* trying the innovation)?
4. What are the material costs of implementing the innovation? What are the costs in the short-term during utilization, and what are the costs in the long run, if the change is to be institutionalized?
5. What are the material costs of *not* implementing the innovation (i.e., could the new procedure result in some efficiencies that could lower the cost of providing service)?
6. What are the potential nonmaterial costs of implementing the innovation to the organization (e.g., lower staff morale, staff turnover, absenteeism)?
7. What are the potential nonmaterial benefits of implementing the innovation (e.g., improved staff morale, improved staff recruitment)?

ganization as a whole, and even the nursing profession as a whole. Clearly, the most important factor is the client. If the degree of risk in introducing a new procedure is high, then the potential benefits must be great. Moreover, if there are risks to client well-being, it is essential that the knowledge base be sound. That is, an innovation that involves client risks should only be implemented when there is a solid body of evidence from several methodologically rigorous studies that the new practice is effective. A cost/benefit assessment should consider the reverse side of the coin as well: the costs and benefits of *not* implementing the innovation. It is sometimes easy to forget that the status quo bears its own risks and that failure to change—especially when such change is based on a firm knowledge base—is costly to clients, to organizations, and to the entire nursing community.

RESEARCH EXAMPLE

Many utilization projects are being undertaken by nurses in practice settings, and during the

1990s, many of these projects were described in the nursing literature. Table 26-2 provides examples of several research utilization projects. Another project, described in greater detail below, illustrates the potential of such projects to result in improved nursing care.

Kilpack, Boehm, Smith, and Mudge (1991) undertook a utilization project that focused on efforts to decrease patient falls in their hospital, the Dartmouth-Hitchcock Medical Center. The project began when the hospital's Nursing Quality Assurance Committee noted an increase in patient falls and established a study group to address the problem.

The group began by undertaking a thorough review of the literature to identify nursing interventions that have been documented as being effective in reducing patient falls. After the review, a fall prevention program was implemented in the two units that had especially high rates of inpatient falls. The special program was designed to prevent repeat falls among those who had a fall identified by an incident report.

During the 1-year study period, incident reports were screened, and for each patient who

TABLE 26-2 Examples of Research Utilization Projects		
INNOVATION	**RESULT OF UTILIZATION PROJECT**	**CITATION**
Use of saline flushes in lieu of heparinized flushes for adult patients	Change fully implemented on all units in three hospitals that previously used heparin locks	Shively, Riegal, Waterhouse, Burns, Templin, & Thomason, 1997
Alternatives to use of restraints	Reduced use of restraints for patients in two nursing homes and two extended care units	Stratmann, Vinson, Magee, & Hardin, 1997
Decision rules for choosing needles for peripheral intravenous therapy	Nursing procedure for needle choice decisions changed; 25% cost savings realized	Olson & Gomes, 1996
Skin care protocol	Protocol for the treatment of pressure ulcers successfully implemented in a large, long-term care facility	Specht, Bergquist, & Frantz, 1995

had experienced a fall, the staff nurse caring for the patient completed a form that listed the research-based interventions that previously had been identified in the literature review. The nurse was asked to select those interventions that he or she thought should be incorporated into the plan of care. With this information, the clinical nurse specialist developed a written plan of care using the nursing diagnosis of Potential for Injury. The staff nurse was asked to implement the plan, and adherence to the plan was monitored. Care plans were adjusted as needed when there was a recurrence of a fall.

The researchers gathered data on falls during the study period and documented their incidence and nature; they also documented the interventions that were utilized. They found that the patient fall rate on the two targeted units decreased (relative to the previous year), whereas the overall rate in the hospital increased. As a result of the project, six major clinical practice recommendations were made to the institution, and all six were implemented.

SUMMARY

In nursing, **research utilization** refers to the use of some aspect of a scientific investigation in a clinical application unrelated to the original research. Research utilization can best be characterized on a continuum, with direct utilization of some specific innovation (**instrumental utilization**) at one end and more diffuse situations in which users are influenced in their thinking about an issue based on some research (**conceptual utilization**) at the other end.

There is tremendous potential for research utilization at all points along this continuum throughout the nursing process. To date, however, there is little evidence that utilization has occurred—at least not with respect to instrumental utilization. It seems likely, though, that more diffuse forms of utilization have oc-

curred as nurses have increased their research productivity and their awareness of the need for research.

Several major utilization projects have been implemented, the most noteworthy being the WICHE and CURN projects. These utilization projects demonstrated that it is possible to increase research utilization, but they also shed light on some of the barriers to utilization. These barriers include such factors as an inadequate scientific base, nursing staff with little training in research and utilization, resistance to change among nurses and institutions that employ them, unfavorable organizational climates, resource constraints, limited collaboration among practitioners and researchers, poorly developed communication channels among these two groups, and the shortage of appropriate role models.

Responsibility for research utilization should be borne by the entire nursing community. Researchers, educators, members of peer review panels, practicing nurses, nursing students, and nurse administrators can adopt a number of strategies to improve the extent to which research findings form the basis for nursing practice.

A number of different models of research utilization have been developed, one of which was described in this chapter. In planning a major utilization project, practicing nurses can begin with the identification of an important clinical problem (**problem-focused triggers**) and then proceed to identify and critique the knowledge base and perform an assessment of the implementation potential of the innovation. Under favorable conditions, the nurses can then plan the innovation protocols, implement and evaluate the innovation, and make a rational decision regarding the adoption of the innovation based on the evaluation. Alternatively, nurses can begin with the knowledge base (**knowledge-focused triggers**) and then perform an evaluation of the clinical relevance of a research area before proceeding through the other steps of the utilization process. In either case, there are three major categories of **utilization criteria** that must be considered before proceeding with a utilization plan: **clinical relevance, scientific merit,** and **implementation potential.** The implementation potential category includes the dimensions of transferability of knowledge, feasibility of utilization in the particular setting, and the **cost/benefit ratio** of the innovation.

STUDY ACTIVITIES

Chapter 26 of the *Study Guide to Accompany Nursing Research: Principles and Methods,* 6th ed., offers various exercises and study suggestions for reinforcing the concepts taught in this chapter. Additionally, the following study questions can be addressed:

1. Find an article in a recent issue of a nursing research journal that does not discuss the implications of the study for nursing practice. Evaluate the study's relevance to nursing practice, and if appropriate, write one to two paragraphs summarizing the implications.

2. Consider your personal situation. What are the barriers that might inhibit your use of research findings? What steps might be taken to address those barriers?

SUGGESTED READINGS

Methodologic References

American Nurses' Association. (1991). *Standards of clinical nursing practice.* Kansas City, MO: ANA.

Barnard, K. E., & Hoehn, R. E. (1978). *Nursing child assessment satellite training: Final report.* Hyattsville, MD: Department of Health, Education, and Welfare, Division of Nursing.

Beyea, S. C., & Nicoll, L. H. (1995). Administration of medications via the intramuscular route: An integrative review of the literature and re-search-based protocol for the procedure. *Applied Nursing Research, 8,* 23–33.

Bostrom, J. (1991). Data collection as an educational process. *Journal of Continuing Education in Nursing, 22,* 248–253.

Bostrom, J., & Suter, W. N. (1993). Research utilization: Making the link to practice. *Journal of Nursing Staff Development, 9,* 28–34.

Bostrom, J., & Wise, L. (1994). Closing the gap between research and practice. *Journal of Nursing Administration, 24,* 22–27.

Brodish, M. S., Tranbarger, R. E., & Chamings, P. A. (1987). Clinical nursing research: A model for collaboration. *Journal of Nursing Administration, 17,* 6, 32.

Caplan, N., & Rich, R. F. (1975). *The use of social science knowledge in policy decisions at the national level.* Ann Arbor, MI: Institute for Social Research, University of Michigan.

Dufault, M. A., Bielecki, C., Collins, E., & Willey, C. (1995). Changing nursees' pain assessment practice: A collaborative research utilization approach. *Journal of Advanced Nursing, 21,* 634–45.

Funk, S. G., Champagne, M. T., Wiese, R. A., & Tornquist, E. M. (1991). Barriers to using research findings in practice: The clinician's perspective. *Applied Nursing Research, 4,* 90–95.

Funk, S. G., Tornquist, E. M., & Champagne, M. T. (1989a). A model for improving the dissemination of nursing research. *Western Journal of Nursing Research, 11,* 361–367.

Funk, S. G., Tornquist, E. M., & Champagne, M. T. (1989b). Application and evaluation of the dissemination model. *Western Journal of Nursing Research, 11,* 485–491.

Gennaro, S. (1994). Research utilization: An overview. *Journal of Obstetric, Gynecologic, and Neonatal Nursing, 23,* 313–319.

Green, S., & Houston, S. (1993). Promoting research activities: Institutional strategies. *Applied Nursing Research, 6,* 97–98.

Haller, D., Reynolds, M., & Horsley, J. (1979). Developing research-based innovation protocols: Process, criteria, and issues. *Research in Nursing & Health, 2,* 45–51.

Hayes, P. (1993). Replicative studies. *Clinical Nursing Research, 2,* 243–244.

Horsley, J. A., Crane, J., & Bingle, J. D. (1978). Research utilization as an organizational process. *Journal of Nursing Administration, 8,* 4–6.

Horsley, J., Crane, J., Crabtree, M., & Wood, D. (1983). *Using research to improve nursing practice: A guide.* New York: Grune & Stratton.

Jackel, M. (1989). Presenting research to nurses in clinical practice. *Applied Nursing Research, 2,* 191–193.

Janken, J. K., Rudisill, P., & Benfield, L. (1992). Product evaluation as a research utilization strategy. *Applied Nursing Research, 5,* 188–194.

Keefe, M. R., Pepper, G., & Stoner, M. (1988). Toward research-based nursing practice: The Denver collaborative research network. *Applied Nursing Research, 1,* 109–115.

Krueger, J. C., Nelson, A. H., & Wolanin, M. O. (1978). *Nursing research: Development, collaboration, and utilization.* Germantown, MD: Aspen Systems.

Lambert, C. E., & Lambert, V. A. (1988). Clinical nursing research: Its meaning to the practicing nurse. *Applied Nursing Research, 1,* 54–57.

Larson, E. (1989). Using the CURN project to teach research utilization in a baccalaureate program. *Western Journal of Nursing Research, 11,* 593–599.

Maurin, J. T. (1990). Research utilization in the social-political arena. *Applied Nursing Research, 3,* 48–51.

Pearcey, P. A. (1995). Achieving research-based nursing practice. *Journal of Advanced Nursing, 22,* 33–39.

Phillips, L. R. F. (1986). *A clinician's guide to the critique and utilization of nursing research.* Norwalk, CT: Appleton-Century-Crofts.

Reynolds, M. A., & Haller, K. B. (1986). Using research in practice: A case for replication in nursing. *Western Journal of Nursing Research, 8,* 113–116.

Rizzuto, C., Bostrom, J., Suter, W. N., & Chenitz, W. C. (1994). Predictors of nurses' involvement in research activities. *Western Journal of Nursing Research, 16,* 193–204.

Rogers, E. M. (1995). *Diffusion of innovations* (4th ed.). New York: Free Press.

Rutledge, D. N., & Donaldson, N. E. (1995). Building organization capacity to engage in research utilization. *Journal of Nursing Administration, 25,* 12–16.

Rutledge, D. N., Greene, P., Mooney, K., Nail, L. M., & Ropka, M. (1996). Use of research-based practices by oncology staff nurses. *Oncology Nursing Forum, 23,* 1235–1244.

Stetler, C. B. (1985). Research utilization: Defining the concept. *Image—The Journal of Nursing Scholarship, 17,* 40–44.

Stetler, C. B. (1994). Refinement of the Stetler/Marram model for application of research findings into practice. *Nursing Outlook, 42,* 15–25.

Tanner, C. A. (1987). Evaluating research for use in practice: Guidelines for the clinician. *Heart and Lung, 16,* 424–430.

Tibbles, L., & Sanford, R. (1994). The research journal club: A mechanism for research utilization. *Clinical Nurse Specialist, 8,* 23–26.

Titler, M. G., Kleiber, C., Steelman, V., Goode, C., Rakel, B., Barry-Walker, J. & Small, S. (1994). Infusing research into practice to promote quality care. *Nursing Research, 43,* 307–313.

Weiss, C. (1980). Knowledge creep and decision accretion. *Knowledge: Creation, Diffusion, Utilization, 1,* 381–404.

Substantive References

Brett, J. L. L. (1987). Use of nursing practice research findings. *Nursing Research, 36,* 344–349.

Brett, J. L. L. (1989). Organizational integrative mechanisms and adoption of innovations by nurses. *Nursing Research, 38,* 105–110.

Champion, V. L., & Leach, A. (1989). Variables related to research utilization in nursing. *Journal of Advanced Nursing, 14,* 705–710.

Coyle, L. A., & Sokop, A. G. (1990). Innovation adoption behavior among nurses. *Nursing Research, 39,* 176–180.

Horsley, J., Crane, J., & Haller, J. (1981). *Reducing diarrhea in tube-fed patients (CURN Project).* New York: Grune & Stratton.

Horsley, J., Crane, J., Haller, J., & Bingle, J. (1981). *Closed urinary drainage system (CURN Project).* New York: Grune & Stratton.

Ketefian, S. (1975). Application of selected nursing research findings into nursing practice. *Nursing Research, 24,* 89–92.

Kilpack, V., Boehm, J., Smith, N., & Mudge, B. (1991). Using research-based interventions to decrease patient falls. *Applied Nursing Research, 4,* 50–56.

King, I., & Tarsitano, E. (1982). The effect of structured and unstructured preoperative teaching: A replication. *Nursing Research, 31,* 324–329.

Kirchhoff, K. T. (1982). A diffusion survey of coronary precautions. *Nursing Research, 31,* 196–201.

Lim-Levy, F. (1982). The effect of oxygen inhalation on oral temperature. *Nursing Research, 31,* 150–152.

Longman, A. J., Verran, J. A., Ayoub, J., Neff, J., & Noyes, A. (1990). Research utilization: An evaluation and critique of research related to oral temperature measurement. *Applied Nursing Research, 3,* 14–19.

Nichols, G. A., & Verhonick, P. J. (1968). Placement times for oral temperatures: A nursing study replication. *Nursing Research, 17,* 159–161.

Olson, K. L., & Gomes, V. (1996). Intravenous therapy needle choices in ambulatory cancer patients. *Clinical Nursing Research, 5,* 453–461.

Shively, M., Riegel, B., Waterhouse, D., Burns, D., Templin, K., & Thomason, T. (1997). Testing a community level research utilization intervention. *Applied Nursing Research, 10,* 121–127.

Specht, J. P., Bergquist, S., & Frantz, R. A. (1995). Adoption of a research-based practice for treatment of pressure ulcers. *Nursing Clinics of North America, 30,* 555–563.

Stratmann, S., Vinson, M. H., Magee, R., & Hardin, S. B. (1997). The effects of research on clinical practice: The use of restraints. *Applied Nursing Research, 10,* 39–43.

CHAPTER **27**

Writing a Research Proposal

This chapter brings us, in a sense, full circle: back to the beginning of a research project. A **research proposal** is a written document specifying what the investigator proposes to study and therefore is written before the project has commenced. Proposals serve to communicate the research problem, its significance, and planned procedures for solving the problem to some interested party.

Proposals are written for various reasons. A student enrolled in a research class is often expected to submit a brief plan to the professor before data collection actually begins. Most universities require a formal proposal and a proposal hearing for students about to engage in research for a thesis or dissertation. Funding agencies that sponsor research almost always award funds competitively and use proposals as a basis for their funding decisions.

Proposals prepared for different reasons vary in the amount of detail expected but, like research reports, often have similar content. In the next section, we provide some general information regarding the content and preparation of research proposals. In a subsequent section, we offer more specific guidelines for the preparation of a proposal for the National Institutes of Health (NIH), the federal agency that sponsors a great number of nursing stud-

ies through its National Institute for Nursing Research.

OVERVIEW OF PROPOSAL PREPARATION

Reviewers of research proposals, whether they are faculty, funding sponsors, or peer reviewers, want a clear idea of what the researcher plans to do, how and when various tasks are to be accomplished, and whether the researcher is capable of successfully following the proposed plan of action. Proposals are generally evaluated on a number of criteria, including the importance of the research question, its theoretical relevance, the adequacy of the research methods, the availability of appropriate personnel and facilities, and, if money is being requested, the reasonableness of the budget. General guidelines for preparing research proposals follow.

Proposal Content

A researcher preparing a proposal will almost always be given a set of instructions that indicate the format to be followed. Funding agencies often supply an application kit that includes forms to be completed and a specified format for organizing the contents of the proposal. Despite the fact that formats and the amount of detail required may vary widely, there is considerable similarity in the type of information that is expected in research proposals. The major components normally included in research proposals are described in the following sections.

ABSTRACT

Proposals often begin with a brief synopsis of the proposed research. The abstract helps to establish a frame of reference for the reviewers as they begin to read the proposal. The abstract should be brief (usually about 200 to 300 words in length) and should state concisely the study objectives and methods to be used.

STATEMENT OF THE PROBLEM

The problem that the intended research will address is ordinarily identified early in the proposal. The problem should be stated in such a way that its importance is apparent to the reviewer. On the other hand, the researcher should not promise more than can be produced. A broad and complex problem is unlikely to be solvable or manageable.

SIGNIFICANCE OF THE PROBLEM

The proposal needs to describe clearly how the proposed research will make a contribution to knowledge. The proposal should indicate the expected generalizability of the research, its contribution to theory, its potential for improving nursing practice and patient care, and possible applications or consequences of the knowledge to be gained.

BACKGROUND OF THE PROBLEM

A section of the proposal is often devoted to an exposition of how the intended research

builds on what has already been done in an area. The background material should strengthen the author's arguments concerning the significance of the study, orient the reader to what is already known about the problem, and indicate how the proposed research will augment that knowledge; it should also serve as a demonstration of the researcher's command of current knowledge in a field.

OBJECTIVES

Specific, achievable objectives provide the reader with clear criteria against which the proposed research methods can be assessed. Objectives stated as research hypotheses or specific models to be tested are often preferred. Whenever the theoretical background of the study, existing knowledge, or the researcher's experience permits an explicit prediction of outcomes, these predictions should be included in the proposal. Avoid the use of null hypotheses, which create an amateurish impression. In exploratory or descriptive research, the formulation of hypotheses might not be feasible. Objectives, in such cases, may be most conveniently phrased as questions.

METHOD

The explanation of the research method should be thorough enough that a reader will have no question about how the research objectives will be addressed. A thorough method section includes a description of the sampling plan, research design, instrumentation, specific procedures, and analytic strategies, together with a discussion of the rationale for the methods, potential methodologic problems, and intended strategies for handling such problems.

THE WORK PLAN

Researchers often describe in the proposal their plan for managing the flow of work on a research project. The researchers indicate in the **work plan** the sequence of tasks to be performed, the anticipated length of time required for their completion, and the personnel required for their accomplishment. The work plan indicates to the reader how realistic and thorough the researcher has been in designing the study.

PERSONNEL

In proposals addressed to funding agencies, the qualifications of key project personnel should be described. The research competencies of the project director and other team members are typically given major consideration in evaluating a proposal.

FACILITIES

The proposal should document the extent to which special facilities required by the project will be available. Access to physiologic instrumentation, libraries, data processing equipment, computers, special documents or records, and subjects should be described to reassure sponsors or advisers that the project will be able to proceed as planned. The willingness of the institution with which the researcher is affiliated to allocate space, equipment, services, or data should also be indicated.

BUDGET

The budget translates the project activities into monetary terms. It is a statement of how much money will be required to accomplish the various tasks. A well-conceived work plan greatly facilitates the preparation of the budget. If there are inordinate difficulties in detailing financial needs, there may be reason to suspect that the work plan is insufficiently developed.

General Tips on Proposal Preparation

Although it would be impossible to tell readers exactly what steps to follow to produce a suc-

cessful proposal, we can offer some advice that might help to minimize the anxiety and frustration that often accompany the preparation of a proposal. Many of the tips we provide are especially relevant for researchers who are preparing a proposal for the purpose of securing funding for a research project.

1. **Review a successful proposal.** Although there is no substitute for actually doing one's own proposal as a learning experience, beginning proposal writers can often profit considerably by actually seeing the real thing. The information in this chapter is useful in providing some guidelines, but reviewing an actual successful proposal can do more to acquaint the novice with how all the pieces fit together than all the textbooks in the world.

   Chances are some of your colleagues or advisors have written a proposal that has been accepted (either by a funding sponsor or by a dissertation committee), and many people are glad to share their successful efforts with others. Also, proposals funded by the federal government are generally in the public domain. That means that you can ask to see a copy of proposals that have obtained federal funding by writing to the sponsoring agency.

   In recognition of the need of beginning researchers to become familiar with successful proposals, several journals (including *The Western Journal of Nursing Research* and *Research in Nursing & Health*) have published proposals in their entirety (with the exception of administrative information such as budgets), together with the critique of the proposal prepared by a panel of expert reviewers. For example, the first such published proposal was a grant application funded by the Division of Nursing entitled, "Couvade: Patterns, Predictors, and Nursing Management" (Clinton, 1985). A more recent example is a proposal for a study of comprehensive discharge planning for the elderly (Naylor, 1990). Another journal, *Grants Magazine,* also publishes successful proposals.

2. **Pay attention to reviewers' criteria.** In most instances in which research funding is at stake, the funding agency will provide the researcher with information about the criteria that reviewers use in making funding decisions. In some cases, the criteria will simply consist of a list of questions that the reviewers must address in making a global assessment of the proposal's quality. In other cases, however, the agency will be able to specify exactly how many points will be assigned to different aspects of the proposal on the basis of specified criteria. As an example, the National Institute of Child Health and Human Development funded some research projects relating to fertility regulation using the following evaluation criteria:

   a. *Conceptualization of the problem.* Ability of the researcher to conceptualize the problem, including the operationalizing and quantifying of measures, and the development of a theoretical or conceptual framework (0 to 30 points)

   b. *Project staff qualifications and availability.*

      Adequacy of the relevant training and experience of the proposed staff (0 to 15 points)

      Appropriateness of allocation of personnel and time to accomplish objectives of the project (0 to 10 points)

   c. *Data sources and analysis.* Demonstration of capability for identifying and obtaining access to pertinent and relevant sources of data and adequacy of plans for data analysis (0 to 20 points)

   d. *Review and analysis of literature.* Adequacy of the review and analysis of the literature in terms of scope and depth and extent to which research needs are delineated in theoretical, methodologic, and analytic areas (0 to 15 points)

   e. *Facilities and equipment.* Adequacy of computer facilities and other equipment that would be needed in the performance of the research (0 to 10 points)

      In this example, a maximum of 100 points was awarded for each competing proposal. The proposals with the highest scores would ordinarily be most likely to obtain funding. Therefore, the researcher should pay particular attention to those aspects of the proposal that contribute most to an overall high score. In this example, it would have made little sense to put 85% of the proposal development effort into the literature review section, when a maximum of 15 points could be given for this part of the proposal.

      Different agencies establish different criteria for different types of research projects. The wise researcher will learn what those criteria are and pay careful attention to them in the development of the proposal.

3. **Be judicious in putting together a research team.** For projects that are funded, reviewers often give considerable weight to the qualifications of the people who will conduct the research. In the example cited earlier, a full 25 of the 100 points were based on the expertise of the research personnel and their time allocations.

      The person who is in the lead role on the project—often referred to as the principal investigator (PI)—should carefully scrutinize the qualifications of the research team. It is not enough to have a team of competent people; it is necessary to have the right mix of competence. A project team of three brilliant theorists without statistical skills in a project that proposes sophisticated multivariate techniques may have difficulty convincing reviewers that the project would be successful. Gaps and weaknesses can often be compensated for by the judicious use of consultants.

Another shortcoming of many project teams is that they often look as though there are too many managers. It is generally unwise to load up a project staff with five or more top-level professionals who are only able to contribute 5% to 10% of their time to the project. Such projects often run into management difficulties because no one person is ever really in control of the flow of work. Although collaborative efforts are to be commended, you should be able to *justify* the inclusion of every staff person and to identify the unique contribution that each will make to the successful completion of the project.

4. **Justify and document your decisions.** Unsuccessful proposals often fail because they do not provide the reviewer with confidence that adequate thought and consideration have been given to a rationale for decisions. Almost every aspect of the proposal involves a decision—the problem selected, the population studied, the size of the sample, the data collection procedures to be used, the comparison group to be used, the extraneous variables to be controlled, the analytic procedures to be used, the personnel who will work on the project, and so on. These decisions should be made carefully, keeping in mind the costs and benefits of an alternative decision. When you are satisfied that you have made the right decision, you should be ready to defend your decision by sharing the rationale with the reviewers. In general, insufficient detail is more detrimental to the proposal than an overabundance of detail, although page constraints may make full detail impossible.

5. **Arrange for a critique of the proposal.** Before formal submission of a proposal, a draft should be reviewed by at least one other person, preferably someone with relevant methodologic and substantive strengths in the proposed area of research. (Ideally, if the proposal is being submitted for funding, then the reviewer will be someone who is knowledgeable about the funding source.) If a consultant has been proposed because of specialized expertise that you believe will strengthen the study, then it would be advantageous to have that consultant participate in the proposal development by reviewing the draft and making recommendations for its improvement.

GRANT APPLICATIONS TO THE NATIONAL INSTITUTES OF HEALTH

The National Institutes of Health (NIH) funds a considerable number of nursing research studies through the National Institute of Nursing Research (NINR) and through other institutes and agencies within NIH. Applications for grant funding through NIH are made by completing Public Health Service Grant Application Form PHS 398 (revised, May 1995), which is available through the research offices of most universities and hospitals. Copies of the application kit can also be obtained by writing to the following address:

Extramural Outreach and Information Resources
National Institutes of Health
6701 Rockledge Drive, Room 6207
Bethesda, MD 20892–7910
Tel.: 301–435–0714
Fax: 301–480–0525
e-mail: grantsinfo@nih.gov
website: www.nih.gov/grants/forms

New grant applications are generally processed in three cycles annually. The schedule for

TABLE 27-1   Schedule for Processing General National Institutes of Health Grant Applications

RECEIPT DATES	INITIAL (PEER) REVIEW DATES	NATIONAL ADVISORY COUNCIL REVIEW DATES	EARLIEST POSSIBLE START DATES
February 1	June/July	September/October	December 1
June 1	October/November	January/February	April 1
October 1	February/March	May/June	July 1

submission and review of new grant applications is shown in Table 27–1. Proposals (grant applications) may be submitted on the proper forms at any time during the year. However, proposals received after one receipt date will be held for another cycle. For example, if a proposal is received by NIH on February 2, it will be considered with the proposals received by June 1, not February 1.

Types of NIH Grants

The NIH awards different types of grants, and each has its own objectives and review criteria. Five types of grants that represent the bulk of awards are discussed next, but other types are also available.

The basic grant program—and the primary funding mechanism for independent research—is the **Research Project Grant** (R01). The objective of the R01 grant is to support discrete, specific research projects in areas reflecting the interests and competencies of a PI. As of February 1998, the five explicitly stated review criteria are as follows:

1. *Significance.* How will scientific knowledge be advanced? What effect will the study have on concepts or methods in the field? Is the problem being addressed an important one?
2. *Approach.* Are the conceptual framework, research design, methods, and analyses adequately developed and appropriate for the study objectives? Are

potential problem areas identified with consideration given to possible solutions?
3. *Innovation.* Does the proposed project use original and innovative concepts, approaches, or methods? Does the project challenge existing paradigms or develop new methods or technologies?
4. *Investigator.* Are the investigator and other members of the research team appropriately trained and qualified to carry out the project?
5. *Environment.* Does the research environment in which the research will be conducted contribute to the probability of the project's success? Is there evidence of institutional support?

In addition to these five explicit criteria, other factors are relevant in evaluating R01 proposals, including the reasonableness of the proposed budget, the adequacy of the proposed means for protecting human subjects or research animals, and the appropriateness of the sampling plan in terms of the inclusion of women and minorities as participants in the study.

There are also a limited number of **Small Grants** (R03) that provide funding for small-scale studies, pilot work, or feasibility studies in specific areas that are announced annually by NIH institutes. These grants award up to $35,000 of project funds (nonrenewable) for a project period of up to 2 years.

A special program (R15) has been established for researchers working in educational institutions that have not been major participants in NIH programs. These are the **Academic Research Enhancement Awards (AREA)**, the objective of which is to stimulate research in institutions that provide baccalaureate training for many individuals who go on to do health-related research. AREA grants enable qualified researchers to obtain support for small-scale research projects. The review criteria for AREA grants are basically the same as for R01 grants.

Another special program has been established for new investigators. The **First Independent Research Support and Transition**, or **FIRST (R29)**, program is designed to provide an initial period of support for newly independent researcher scientists. These grants are intended to provide an opportunity for new scientists to demonstrate creativity and productivity and to assist them in making the transition to other NIH grants. FIRST awards are made for a period of 5 years, and the total direct costs must not exceed $350,000. The review criteria are essentially the same as those for R01 grants, but less emphasis is placed on the investigator's experience than on his or her potential for productive research. Letters of reference must accompany the proposal and are carefully evaluated.

Finally, a relatively new type of grant program is referred to as the **Mentored Research Scientist Development Award** (K01). These grants provide sponsored research experience for doctorally prepared researchers who need a mentored research experience with an expert sponsor. The awards provide an opportunity for individuals to gain expertise in new research areas or in areas that would demonstrably enhance their research careers.

If you have an idea for a study and are not sure which type of grant program is best suited to your project—or you are not sure whether the project is one in which NINR or another institute within NIH might be interested—it is advisable to contact NINR directly. NINR's Division of Extramural Affairs has staff who can provide feedback about whether your proposed project will fit within the program interests of NINR. The telephone number is 301–594–6906; information about NINR's ongoing areas of research interests and specific areas of current opportunity are available on the Internet (www.nih.gov/ninr).

Preparing a Grant Application for NIH

As indicated earlier, proposals to NIH must be submitted according to procedures described in the Public Health Service application kit. Each kit specifies exactly how the grant application should be prepared and what forms are to be used for supplying critical pieces of information. It is important to follow these instructions precisely. In the sections that follow, we describe the various components of an application and provide some tips that should be helpful in completing certain sections.*

FRONT MATTER

The **front matter** of the grant application consists of various forms that help in the processing of the application or that provide administrative information about the conduct of the research. Proposal writers often fail to give this section the attention it merits because all the intellectual work is presented in the research plan section. However, we urge researchers to pay as much attention to detail in this first section as in the second. Each form included in Section 1 is briefly described to acquaint the reader with its contents.

- *Face page.* On the face page form, the researcher provides the title of the application (not to exceed 56 spaces), the name and institutional affiliation of the PI, the costs for the initial budget period and for the entire proposed period of support, the

---

*The application kit for NIH grants changes periodically. Therefore, the instructions in a current version of Form PHS 398 should be carefully reviewed and followed in preparing a grant application rather than relying exclusively on information in this chapter.

proposed time period of the project, and other administrative information.

- *Abstract of research plan.* Page 2 is a form that asks for a half-page abstract or description of the proposed study, the designation of the performance sites, and a listing of the key professional personnel who would work on the study. The abstract *must* fit into the space allocated.
- *Table of contents.* Page 3 indicates on what pages various sections and subsections of the proposal are to be found.
- *Budget.* Pages 4 and 5 consist of budgetary forms. Page 4 asks for an itemization of all costs that would be incurred by the project during the first 12 months. Page 5 asks for a summary of the budget for the entire project period. For R01 grants, support can be requested for up to 5 years, but most projects are completed in 3 years or less. Beginning at the bottom of page 5 (and continuing for as many pages as necessary), the researcher must provide a narrative justification of all budgeted items. New researchers often make the mistake of submitting a budget justification that is insufficiently detailed. Remember that the reviewers need to be able to tell whether the budget is reasonable, and part of your job is to convince them that you would use funding judiciously. Normally, two or three single-spaced pages are needed to justify budgetary items.

Figure 27–1 presents a hypothetical page 4 (detail of first-year expenditures), and Figure 27–2 presents a hypothetical page 5 for a study that would require 2 years of support. The bottom of Figure 27–2 presents the first few paragraphs of a budget justification, showing the level of detail that is ordinarily considered appropriate. For most projects, personnel costs (wages and fringe benefits) represent the bulk of the requested funds, and personnel costs are generally represented as a percentage of a person's time (e.g., 20 hours

per week would be designated as a 50% level of effort on the proposed project). Other costs include the cost for consultants, project-specific equipment, supplies, travel costs, patient care costs, costs associated with a subcontract or consortium arrangements, and other expenses. The final category might include such items as laboratory fees, subject stipends, transcriptions, computer time, and data entry expenses. Note that the NIH budget forms should indicate **direct costs** (specific project-related costs) only. **Indirect costs** (institutional **overhead**) are not shown on the budget forms. Beginning researchers are likely to need the assistance of a research administrator or an experienced, funded researcher in developing their first budget.

- *Biographic sketches.* Forms are provided to summarize salient aspects of the education and experience of key project personnel. The PI and any other proposed staff who are considered important contributors to the project's success must have their biographic sketches included. A maximum of two pages is permitted for each person.
- *Other support.* Key personnel must identify any sources of support they are now receiving or sources of support that they have pending on the form of other planned or submitted proposals. This form is designed to help reviewers determine whether important staff may be overcommitted and therefore potentially unable to devote a sufficient amount of time to the proposed project.
- *Resources.* On this form, the author must designate the availability of needed facilities and equipment in the following categories: laboratory, clinical, animal, computer, office, and other.

RESEARCH PLAN SECTION

The main section of the NIH grant application is reserved for the investigator's research plan.

DD							

Principal Investigator/Program Director *(Last, first, middle):* <u>Singleton, Sheila F.</u>

DETAILED BUDGET FOR INITIAL BUDGET PERIOD **DIRECT COSTS ONLY**				**FROM** 12/1/99	**THROUGH** 11/30/2000		

| PERSONNEL *(Applicant organization only)* | | TYPE APPT. *(months)* | % EFFORT ON PROJ. | INST. BASE SALARY | DOLLAR AMOUNT REQUESTED *(omit cents)* | | |
NAME	ROLE ON PROJECT				SALARY REQUESTED	FRINGE BENEFITS	TOTALS
Sheila Singleton	Principal Investigator	12	25%	$80,000	$20,000	6,000	26,000
Carol Joyce	Co-Invest.	12	25%	40,000	10,000	3,000	13,000
Diane Dodd	Interviewer	9	100%	30,000	22,500	6,750	29,250
To Be Hired	Res. Asst.	12	20%	15,000	3,000	900	3,900
To Be Hired	Secretary	12	40%	20,000	8,000	2,400	10,400
SUBTOTALS ⟶					63,500	19,050	82,550

CONSULTANT COSTS
Lou Cohen, Statistical consultant   5 days @ $400/day
<u>Nancy Butcher, Programming consultant   20 days @ $250/day</u>   7,000
EQUIPMENT *(Itemize)*

Laptop Computer   2,000

SUPPLIES *(Itemize by category)*
Office supplies $75/month × 12
Photocopying $50/month × 12
Postage/Courier $50/month × 12
Subject stipends   200 @ $15
Telephone $1,000   6,100

TRAVEL 1 professional conference ($1,000); interviewer travel ($750)   1,750

| PATIENT CARE COSTS | INPATIENT | |
| | OUTPATIENT | |

ALTERATIONS AND RENOVATIONS *(Itemize by category)*

OTHER EXPENSES *(Itemize by category)*

SUBTOTAL DIRECT COSTS FOR INITIAL BUDGET PERIOD		$	99,400
CONSORTIUM/CONTRACTUAL COSTS	DIRECT COSTS		
	INDIRECT COSTS		
TOTAL DIRECT COSTS FOR INITIAL BUDGET PERIOD *(Item 7a, Face Page)* ⟶		$	99,400

PHS 398 (Rev. 5/95)   *(Form Page 4)* Page _____   DD
Number pages consecutively at the bottom throughout the application. Do <u>not</u> use suffixes such as 3a, 3b..

Figure 27-1. Example of a first-year budget for an NIH grant.

EE _____   Principal Investigator/Program Director *(Last, first, middle):* _____Singleton, Sheila F._____

BUDGET FOR ENTIRE PROPOSED PERIOD OF SUPPORT
DIRECT COSTS ONLY

BUDGET CATEGORY TOTALS		INITIAL BUDGET PERIOD *(from Form Page 4)*	ADDITIONAL YEARS OF SUPPORT REQUESTED			
			2nd	3rd	4th	5th
PERSONNEL: *Salary and fringe benefits* Applicant organization only		82,550	90,800			
CONSULTANT COSTS		7,000	9,000			
EQUIPMENT		2,000	0			
SUPPLIES		6,100	5,000			
TRAVEL		1,750	2,000			
PATIENT CARE COSTS	INPATIENT	0	0			
	OUTPATIENT	0	0			
ALTERATIONS AND RENOVATIONS		0	0			
OTHER EXPENSES		0	1,000			
SUBTOTAL DIRECT COSTS		99,400	107,800			
CONSORTIUM/ CONTRACTUAL COSTS	DIRECT					
	INDIRECT					
TOTAL DIRECT COSTS		99,400	107,800			

TOTAL DIRECT COSTS FOR ENTIRE PROPOSED PERIOD OF SUPPORT *(Item 8a, Face Page)* → | $ 207,200

JUSTIFICATION. Follow the budget justification instructions exactly. Use continuation pages as needed.

Personnel

Dr. Singleton, the PI, will be responsible for overall project management, instrument development, data quality control, data analysis, and report preparation. She is budgeted for 25% effort in the first 18 months of the project. In the final 6 months, Dr. Singleton will devote 50% of her time to the project to perform the data analyses and prepare the final report.

Dr. Joyce, the Co-PI, will devote 25% of her time to the project throughout the 2-year period. She will participate in the instrumentation, training of the interviewer, development of a coding scheme, analysis of the data, and report preparation.

The interviewer, Diane Dodd, will begin project work in Month 4. She will work 15 months at 100% effort and will be responsible for the collection of data. A research assistant (RA) will be hired to assist with such tasks as library research, instrument pretests, and data coding. The RA will work at 20% effort in both years of the project. A secretary will be hired at 40% effort to perform secretarial and clerical functions.

A 5% salary increase has been budgeted for all personnel in Year 2.

Consultants

Dr. Lou Cohen, a prominent statistician with expertise in LISREL, will provide consultation with regard to the statistical analysis of the data. Dr. Cohen is budgeted for 5 days in Year 1 of the project and for 10 days in Year 2.

Figure 27-2.   Example of an overall summary budget for an NIH grant.

This section consists of nine parts (though not all nine are relevant to every application). Parts a through d of the research plan, combined, must not exceed 25 single-spaced pages, including any figures, charts, or tables. If the proposal does not adhere to this page restriction, then the application will be returned without review. Within the overall 25-page limitation, the text can be distributed among Parts a through d in any manner the researcher considers appropriate, although guidelines are suggested.

a. *Specific aims*. The researcher must provide a succinct summary of the research problem and the specific objectives to be undertaken during the course of the project, including any hypotheses to be tested. The application guidelines suggest that Part a be restricted to a single page.

b. *Background and significance*. In Part b, the researcher must convince the review panel that the proposed study idea is sound and has important clinical or theoretical relevance. In this section of the research plan, the researcher provides the context for the conduct of the study, usually through a brief analysis of existing knowledge on the topic and through a discussion of a conceptual framework. Within this context, the investigator must demonstrate the significance of, and need for, the proposed new project. Beginning researchers often have an especially difficult time with this section because of the recommendation to restrict this section to two to three pages. This is often a challenging task, especially if you have a firm grasp on the broad range of literature relating to your topic. However, we again urge researchers not to be tempted to exceed the three-page guideline. Space should be conserved for a full elaboration of the proposed research methods.

c. *Preliminary studies*. This section is reserved for a description of the project team's previous studies that are relevant to the new proposed investigation. Many novice researchers mistakenly believe that this section is designed for a literature review. If you make this mistake, it will indicate that you are a novice and unable to follow instructions. This section (although it is optional for new applications and is only required for continuation proposals) provides an opportunity to persuade the reviewers that you have the skills and background needed to do the research. Because the biographic sketch included in the front matter is limited to only two pages, the Preliminary Studies section provides a forum for the description of any relevant work you and other key staff have either completed or are in the process of doing. If the only relevant research you have completed is your dissertation, here is an opportunity to describe that research in full. If you have completed relevant research that has led to publications, you should reference them in this section and include copies of them as appendices. Other items that might be described in this section include previous uses of an instrument or an experimental procedure that will be used in the new study, relevant clinical or teaching experience, membership on task forces or in organizations that have provided you with a perspective on the research problem, or the results of a pilot study that involved the same research problem. The point is that this section allows you to demonstrate that the proposed work grew out of some ongoing commitment to, interest in, or experience with the topic. For new applications, no more than six to eight pages should be devoted to Part c, and fewer pages are often sufficient.

d. *Research design and methods*. It is in Part d that you must describe the methods you will use to conduct the study. This section should be succinct but with sufficient detail to persuade reviewers that you have a sound rationale for your methodologic decisions. Although there are no specific page limitations associated with this section of the application, keep in mind that you have up to 25 pages in total for Parts a through d combined.

The number of subsections in the methods section varies from one application to another. Each subsection should be labeled clearly to facilitate the review process. As is true in organizing any written material, it is often useful to begin with an outline. Here is an outline of the sections used in a successful grant application for a nonexperimental study of parenting behavior and family environments among low-income teenage mothers:

• Overview of the Research Design
• Sampling Considerations
• Research Variables and Measuring Instruments
• Data Collection Procedures
• Data Analysis
• Research Products
• Project Schedule

If there is an experimental intervention, that intervention should be described in full. Protocols for the implementation of the intervention also need to be discussed. If there is to be a control group, clearly identify how the control group will be selected. If the design involves a comparison group rather than a randomly assigned control group, then you will need to discuss your rationale for the selection of the specified group, any shortcomings in using this group, and why this group is preferable to some alternative. For example, if you were to study the psychological consequences of an abortion in an effort to determine the need for follow-up interventions, there are at least four alternative comparison groups: (1) same-aged, never-pregnant women; (2) same-aged women who had a miscarriage; (3) same-aged women who were still pregnant and had not decided how to resolve the pregnancy; or (4) same-aged women who had delivered a baby. Each group might be expected to introduce different types of selection biases, so your rationale for selecting one over the other would be a critical reflection of your conceptualization of the problem and your methodologic sophistication.

In quantitative studies, the design section should also indicate how the research situation will be structured to control for extraneous variables. The proposal should specify what variables might represent contaminating sources of influence; which variables will be controlled (and how); why other variables will not be controlled; and what the probable impact of the uncontrolled variables on the study outcome will be. Krathwohl (1988) observed that "probably nobody knows better than the researcher the multiple sources of contamination which might affect the study. Convincingly indicate the nature and basis of the particular compromise which is being proposed and the reasons for accepting it" (p. 31).

A number of things should be included in a section on sampling. The reviewer normally expects to find a description of the population, the proposed sampling design, and the number of study participants to be included in the study. The section should include both a description of the sampling plan and a justification for its use. If you cannot use random sampling, explain the constraints (e.g., the costs of implementing such a design) and—in a quantitative study—discuss steps you would take to make the sample as representative as possible and to document any biases. Increasingly, review panels expect to see a power analysis that justifies the adequacy of the specified sample size in quantitative projects. It is also advisable to document your access to the specified subject pool. For instance, if the proposal indicates that patients and personnel from Park Memorial Hospital will participate in the study, then you should include a letter of cooperation from an administrator of the hospital with the application. The reviewers need to have confidence that the proposed study, if funded, would actually be done as planned. One further issue relating to the sample is that NIH policy requires that women and members of minority groups be included in all NIH-supported projects involving humans, unless a clear and compelling justification for their exclusion can be established. Guidelines for the inclusion of women and minorities should be reviewed before developing a sampling plan; the guidelines can be found on the NIH website (www.nih.gov) in the *NIH Guide for Grants and Contracts*, Volume 23, March 11, 1994. NIH is also developing new policies regarding the inclusion of children in research projects; a preliminary statement on this policy was issued in the *NIH Guide*, Volume 26, January 31, 1997, but further policy statements are forthcoming and should be reviewed.

Normally, a subsection of the grant application is devoted to data collection and instrumentation. The use of particular measuring instruments should be justified as appropriate for the purposes of the study. It is inadequate to select a well-known measure without explicitly demonstrating its relevance and valued qualities. For established measures, the proposal should describe reported evidence of the measure's reliability and validity. If a new instrument is to be developed, then the anticipated procedures for its development *and* evaluation

should be described. If possible, sample items or the entire instrument should be included in an appendix. In qualitative studies, the data collection section should describe the procedures that will be implemented to enhance and assess the trustworthiness of the data.

A subsection should be devoted to the specific procedures that will be used to collect the research data. This subsection should include such information as where and when the data will be collected, how subjects will be recruited, how research personnel such as interviewers or observers will be trained, whether study participants will be paid a stipend for their time, what quality-control procedures will be implemented to ensure the integrity of the data, and how the security of the data will be maintained. If the study is longitudinal, then it is also important to describe the schedule for waves of data collection (and a rationale for the schedule) as well as information on how the problem of attrition will be managed.

The grant application should include, in as much detail as possible, the plan for the analysis of data. This is typically one of the weakest sections of proposals. Some applications say little more than, "Trust me—I'll figure out what to do with the data once I have collected them." You may not be able to tell in advance every analytic strategy you will try, but you should be able to work through the general procedures you will use in testing the hypotheses or answering the research questions.

Although the grant application kit does not specifically request a project schedule or work plan, it is often useful to include one (unless the page limitation makes it impossible to do so). A work plan helps reviewers assess how realistic you have been in planning the project, and it should help you to develop an estimate of needed resources (i.e., your budget). Flow charts and other diagrams are often useful for highlighting the sequencing and interrelationships of project activities. One of the simplest and most effective types of charts is called a **Gantt chart,** named after its inventor, Henry Gantt. Figure 27–3 presents a Gantt chart for the 30-month study on teenage parents. Other, more sophisticated charting techniques, such as the **Program Evaluation Review Technique (PERT)** and the **Critical Path Method,** are sometimes used for complex projects. These are briefly described by Krathwohl (1988).

Preparing a research proposal for a qualitative study is particularly challenging because the investigator typically does not know in advance exactly how the study will proceed. That is, the research design, sampling plan, and even data collection methods often evolve in the field as the researcher develops and refines his or her understanding of the phenomenon under study. However, it is important to explain in the proposal some basic strategies and to indicate how decisions are likely to get made—for example, how will the investigator make a decision about when to stop sampling? A research proposal for a qualitative study should devote considerable space to a description of how data quality will be assessed and how emerging conceptualizations will be validated.

e. *Human subjects.* If the research involves data collected from humans, then this section must describe the procedures that will be used to protect their rights

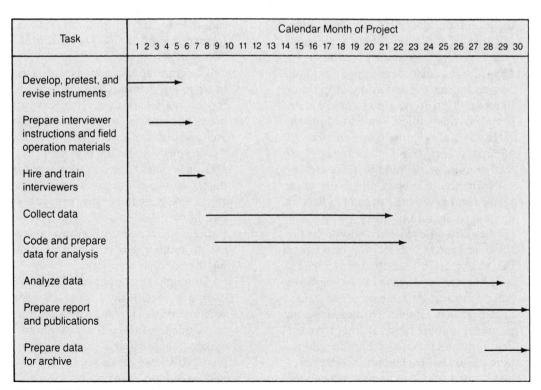

Figure 27-3.   Example of a Gantt chart.

and to minimize the risks that they will take. The application kit specifies six questions that need to be addressed (an example is presented in Appendix A). This section of the proposal often serves as the cornerstone of the document submitted to the Institutional Review Board of your institution before funding (you should check with your office of research administration for Institutional Review Board requirements).

f. *Vertebrate animals.* If your proposed research involves the use of vertebrate animals, then this section must contain a justification of their use and a description of the procedures used to safeguard their welfare.

g. *Literature cited.* This subsection of the Research Plan consists of a list of references used in the text of the grant application. Any reference style is acceptable. This section is restricted to six pages.

h. *Consortium or contractual arrangements.* If the proposed project will involve the collaboration of two or more different institutions (e.g., if a separate organization will be used to perform laboratory analyses, under a subcontract agreement), then details about the nature of the arrangements must be described in this section.

i. *Consultants.* If you plan to include consultants to help with specific tasks on the proposed project, you must include a letter from each consultant, confirming his or her willingness to serve on the project. Letters are also needed from collaborators on the project, if they are affiliated with an institution different from your own.

APPENDIX

The concluding section of the grant application is reserved for appended materials. These materials may include actual instruments to be used in the project, detailed calculations on sample size estimates, scoring or coding instructions for instruments, proposed letters of consent, letters of cooperation from institutions that will provide access to subjects, complex statistical models, and other supplementary materials in support of the application. The researcher can also submit copies of up to 10 published papers or papers accepted for publication (but *not* papers submitted for publication but not yet accepted). The appended materials are not made available to the entire review panel, so essential information should not be relegated to the appendix.

The Review Process

Grant applications submitted to NIH are received by the NIH Center for Scientific Review (CSR), where they are reviewed for completeness and relevance to the overall mission of NIH. Acceptable applications are assigned to an appropriate Institute or Center. Figure 27–4 presents the NIH Institutes and Centers, as of March 1998. Most applications by nurse researchers are assigned to NINR, unless the content of the proposal is better suited to another Institute. NIH encourages applicants to enclose a cover letter with their applications suggesting an assignment to a specific Institute and outlining how the research is congruent with the mission of that Institute.

As the schedule in Table 27–1 indicates, NIH uses a sequential, dual review system for making decisions about its grant applications. The first level involves a panel of peer reviewers (not employed by NIH), who evaluate the grant application for its scientific merit. These review panels are called **scientific review groups** (SRGs) or, more commonly, **study sections**. Each panel consists of about 15 to 20 researchers with backgrounds appropriate to the specific study section for which they have been selected. Appointments to the review panels are generally for 4-year terms and are staggered so that about one fourth of each panel is new each year. The second level of review is by a National Advisory Council, which includes

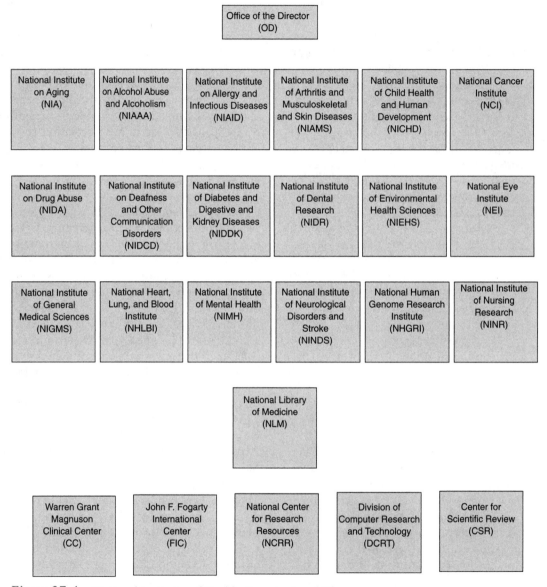

Figure 27-4.   National Institutes of Health Organizational Chart

both scientific and lay representatives. The National Advisory Council considers not only the scientific merit of an application but also the relevance of the proposed study to the programs and priorities of the Center or Institute to which the application has been submitted as well as budgetary considerations.

NIH has recently instituted a triage system for the first level of review, referred to as a **streamlined review procedure**. Study section members are sent applications and asked to evaluate whether the applications are in the upper half of lower half in terms of their quality and likelihood for funding. Normally, each application is formally reviewed and critiqued by at least two assigned reviewers. If two reviewers agree that an application is not in the upper half, that application will be designated "NC" (not considered) and will not be discussed at the study section meeting nor assigned a score.

Applications in the upper half are discussed in full at the study section meeting and privately assigned a priority score that reflects each reviewer's opinion of the merit of the application.* The ratings range from 1.0 (the best possible score) to 5.0 (the least favorable score), in increments of 0.1. Before the streamlined review procedures were instituted, priority scores typically ran the full range from 1.0 to 5.0. However, the full range is no longer routinely used because the only applications assigned a score are those previously designated as being in the upper half. Thus, the priority scores tend to be in the 1.0 to 2.5 range. However, reviewers are free to "vote their conscience" and may therefore provide any priority score they believe to be appropriate.

The individual ratings from different panel members are then combined, averaged, and multiplied by 100 to yield scores that (technically) range from 100 to 500, with 100 being the best possible score. Among all scored applications, only those with the lowest priority scores actually obtain funding. Cutoff scores for funding vary from agency to agency and year to year. It is often necessary to obtain a rating of 200 or lower to become funded. Within NIH overall, fewer than 20% of all grant applications are actually funded; within NINR, about one out of every four applications is funded.

Applications for clinical research, defined as human biomedical and behavioral studies of the etiology, epidemiology, prevention (and preventive strategies), diagnosis, or treatment of diseases, disorders, or conditions, are also evaluated based on whether the proposed project appropriately includes women and minorities in the study population. The study section codes each scored application "acceptable" or "unacceptable" in terms of gender and minority representation. Special guidelines for what is acceptable are applied to clinical trials.

Each grant applicant, regardless of the decision of the study section, is sent a summary of the peer review panel's evaluation. These **pink sheets** (so called because they are printed on pink paper) summarize the reviewers' comments in seven areas: (1) an overall description of the project; (2) a critique of the strengths and weaknesses of the proposal, based on the five criteria described under R01 grants; (3) an overall evaluation of the project; (4) an evaluation of gender and minority representation; (5) a review of procedures relating to human subjects and animal welfare; (6) an assessment of the reasonableness of the budget; and (7) a discussion of other considerations, with emphasis on the protection of the rights of human subjects or the welfare of animal subjects. The applicant is also advised of the application's average priority score and percentile rank.

Unless an unfunded proposal is criticized in some fundamental way (e.g., the problem area

---

*Occasionally, a review panel will vote to defer an application. **Deferrals** are relatively rare and usually involve an application that the review panel considers meritorious but missing some crucial information that would permit the panel to make a final determination.

was not judged to be significant, or the basic design was considered inappropriate), it is often worthwhile to resubmit an application, making revisions that reflect the concerns of the peer review panel. Unfunded proposals that receive encouraging priority scores (in the 200 to 250 range) are especially likely to fare well in a resubmission. When a proposal is resubmitted, the next review panel members are usually given a copy of the original application and the pink sheet so that they can evaluate the degree to which the original criticisms have been addressed.

FUNDING FOR RESEARCH PROPOSALS

Funding for research projects is becoming more and more difficult to obtain. The problem lies not only in research cutbacks and inflation but also in the extremely keen and growing competition among researchers. As increasing numbers of nurses become prepared to carry out significant research, so too will applications for research funds increase. Successful proposal writers need to have good research and proposal-writing skills, and they must also know how and from whom funding is available. The combined set of skills and knowledge is sometimes referred to as **grantsmanship**.

Federal Funding

The federal government is the largest contributor to the support of research activities. The two major types of federal disbursements are grants and contracts. **Grants** are awarded for proposals in which the research idea is developed by the investigator. The researcher who identifies an important research problem can seek federal funds through a grant program of one or more agencies of the government.

There are three basic mechanisms for the funding of federal grants. One mechanism is for agencies and institutes to issue broad objectives relating to an overall mission. For example, as discussed in Chapter 1, NINR identified five areas of special interest for 1995 through 1999 (e.g., "behavioral factors related to immunocompetence"). A second mechanism is for an agency to issue **program announcements** periodically, which describe new, continuing, or expanded program interests. For example, in 1997, NINR issued program announcements titled "Self-Care Behavior and Aging," "Managing the Symptoms of Cognitive Impairment," and "Understanding and Improving Antiretroviral Regimen Adherence." The program announcements identify various specific objectives within a topic area and invite grant applications that address the objectives. Researchers apply for funding from this general grants program through the process described in the preceding section. Program announcements are publicized by various government agencies on the Internet. Also, *The Catalogue of Federal Domestic Assistance* publishes information about all federal programs that provide any kind of aid. Information from this publication can be accessed through the Internet (www.gsa.gov/fdac).

The second grant-funding mechanism offers federal agencies a means of identifying a more specific topic area in which they are especially interested in receiving applications by a **Request for Applications (RFA)**. As an example, NINR issued an RFA titled "Sex and Gender-related Differences in Pain and Analgesic Response" in 1997. Unlike a program announcement, an RFA usually specifies a deadline for the receipt of proposals. General guidelines and goals for the competition are also specified, but the researcher has considerable liberty to develop the specific research problem. Notices of such grant competitions are announced on the Internet on the websites specific to each funding agency and are also published in *The Federal Register*, which is a daily publication of the Government Printing Office (www.access.gpo.gov/su_docs).

The second type of government funding (and this may occur at both the federal and state level) is in the form of **contracts.** An agency that identifies the need for a specific study issues a **Request for Proposals (RFP),** which details the *exact* work that the government wants done and the specific problem to be addressed. Proposals in response to RFPs describe the methods the researcher would use in addressing the research problem, the project staff and facilities, and the cost of doing the study in the proposed way. Contracts are usually awarded to only one of the competitors. The contract method of securing research support severely constrains the kinds of work in which investigators can engage—the researcher responding to an RFP generally has no latitude in developing the research objectives. For this reason, most nurse researchers probably will want to compete for grants rather than contracts. Nevertheless, many interesting RFPs have been issued by NIH and other agencies. For example, one recent NIH RFP called for proposals for a study of "Ethnic Differences in Life Style, Psychological Factors, and Medical Care During Pregnancy."

A summary of every federal RFP is printed in the *Commerce Business Daily,* which is published every government workday; information can be accessed on the Internet (cbdnet. gpo.gov). Also, NIH publishes a weekly bulletin called the *NIH Guide for Grants and Contracts;* the contents of the bulletin are available on the Internet through the NIH website. This bulletin announces new NIH initiatives, including RFAs and RFPs issued by NIH. An example of a portion of an RFA for NINR, listed in the January 7, 1994 issue of the *NIH Guide,* is presented in Figure 27–5.

Private Funds

Health care research is supported by a number of philanthropic foundations, professional organizations, and corporations. Many investigators prefer private funding to government support because there is often less "red tape." Private organizations are typically less rigid in their proposal regulations, reporting requirements, clearance of instruments, and monitoring of progress. Not surprisingly, private organizations are besieged with proposed research projects.

Information about philanthropic foundations that support research is available through the Foundation Center (Internet address: fdncenter.org). The Foundation Center offers a wide variety of resources on foundation funding and how to secure it. Some on-line assistance is available at the Center's website (e.g., you can do a preliminary search of foundations by subject area or geographic location), but the most comprehensive resource for identifying funding opportunities is the Center's *The Foundation Directory.* This volume, which is updated regularly, lists nearly 8000 foundations whose annual grants are at least $200,000, and *The Foundation Directory, Part 2* lists foundations that have annual grant programs from $50,000 to $200,000. (The Foundation Center's database is also available on CD-ROM.) These directories list the purposes and activities of the foundations and information for contacting them. A growing number of foundations now have their own websites.

Professional associations, such as the American Nurses' Foundation, Sigma Theta Tau, the American Association of University Women, and the Social Science Research Council, offer funds for conducting research. Health organizations, such as the American Heart Association and the American Cancer Society, also support research activities.

Finally, funds for research are sometimes donated by private corporations, particularly those dealing with health care products. The Foundation Center publishes a directory called *Corporate Foundation Profiles* and also provides links through its website to a number of corporate philanthropic programs. Additional

SYMPTOM MANAGEMENT: ACUTE PAIN

RFA AVAILABLE: NR-94-003
National Institute of Nursing Research

Letter of Intent Receipt Date: March 15, 1994
Application Receipt Data: April 21, 1994

THIS IS A NOTICE OF AVAILABILITY OF A REQUEST FOR APPLICATIONS (RFA); IT IS ONLY AN ABSTRACT OF THE RFA. POTENTIAL APPLICANTS MUST REQUEST THE COMPLETE RFA, WHICH CONTAINS ESSENTIAL INFORMATION FOR THE PREPARATION OF AN APPLICATION, FROM THE CONTACT LISTED IN "INQUIRIES," BELOW. FAILURE TO FOLLOW THE INSTRUCTION IN THE COMPLETE RFA MAY RESULT IN AN INCOMPLETE APPLICATION, WHICH WILL BE RETURNED TO THE APPLICANT WITHOUT REVIEW.

PURPOSE

The focus of this RFA is on interventions to improve the assessment, management, and prevention of acute pain. Studies that address the multidimensional nature of pain, which includes a range of physiological, sensory, affective, behavioral, cognitive, and sociocultural factors, are encouraged in order to provide a scientific basis for clinical practice.

ELIGIBILITY REQUIREMENTS

Applications may be submitted by domestic and foreign for-profit and non-profit organizations, public and private, such as universities, colleges, hospitals, laboratories, units of state and local governments, and eligible agencies of the Federal Government. Applications from minority individuals and women are encouraged.

MECHANISM OF SUPPORT

This RFA will use the National Institutes of Health (NIH) individual research project grant (R01)...The total project period for applications submitted in response to the present RFA may not exceed three years. The anticipated award date is September 30, 1994. Because the nature and scope of the research proposed in response to this RFA may vary, it is anticipated that the size of an award will vary also, but will generally be in the range of $150,000 to $180,000 direct costs. This RFA is a one-time solicitation.

FUNDS AVAILABLE

Approximately $1,200,000 in total costs for the first year will be committed to fund applications submitted in response to this RFA. It is anticipated that four to six applications will be funded.

**This is an excerpt from an RFA that appeared in the NIH Guide for Grants and Contracts, Vol. 23, No. 1, January 7, 1994, pp. 36-38.*

Figure 27-5. Example of a request for application.

information concerning the requirements and interests of corporations should be obtained either from the organization directly or from personnel in research administration offices of universities, hospitals, or other agencies with which you are affiliated.

 ## CONCLUSION

Proposals represent the means for opening communication between researchers and parties interested in the conduct of research. Those parties may be funding agencies, faculty advisers, or institutional officers, depending on the circumstances. An accepted proposal is a two-way contract: Those accepting the proposal are effectively saying, "We are willing to offer our (emotional or financial) support, as long as the investigation proceeds as proposed," and those writing the proposal are saying, "If you will offer support, then I will conduct the project as proposed." Therefore, the proposal offers some assurance that neither party will be disappointed.

Beginning proposal writers sometimes forget that, in essence, they are selling a product: themselves and their ideas. It is not inappropriate, therefore, to do a little marketing. If the researcher does not sound convinced that the proposed study is important and will be executed with skill, then the reviewers will not be convinced either. The proposal should be written in a positive, confident tone. Instead of saying, "The study will *try* to . . . ," it is better to indicate more positively that the study *will* achieve some goals. Similarly, it is more optimistic to specify what the investigator *will* do, rather than what he or she *would* do, if approved. There is no need to brag or promise what cannot be accomplished. Rather, it is a question of putting the actual project accomplishments and significance in a positive light.

As another aspect of marketing, the proposal should be as physically attractive as possible. A neat and pleasing appearance invites the re-

viewer to read a proposal and suggests that care has been devoted to its preparation. Flashy and expensive binders, figures, and so forth are unnecessary, but the physical presentation should not leave a bad impression on readers.

Grantsmanship, like research skills, is both a skill and an art. The skill can be acquired through further reading, by attending a course on grantsmanship, or by working with a mentor. We also hope that we have been helpful in communicating some of what goes into the skill part, and we offer all readers our best wishes in cultivating the art of doing and writing about research and acquiring support to pursue it.

SUMMARY

A **research proposal** is a written document specifying what a researcher intends to study and is written with the intent of obtaining approval and support—often financial support. The major components of a research proposal include the following: an abstract, statement of the problem, significance of the problem, background, objectives, methods, work plan, personnel, facilities, and a budget.

A major source of funding for nurse researchers is the National Institutes of Health (NIH), within which is housed the National Institute of Nursing Research (NINR). Nurses can apply for a variety of grants from NIH, the most common being the **Research Project Grant** (R01 grant), **Small Grant** (R03), **FIRST Grant** (R29), or **AREA Grant** (R15). Grant applications to NIH, which are submitted on special forms and which must follow strict formatting guidelines, are reviewed three times a year in a dual review process. The first phase involves a review by a peer **study section** that evaluates each proposal's scientific merit, and the second phase is a review by a National Advisory Council. In NIH's new **streamlined review procedure**, the study section assigns **priority scores** only to applications judged to be in the top half of proposals based on their quality. A score of 100 represents the most meritorious ranking, and a score of 500 is the lowest possible score. A detailed critique of the proposal, together with information on the priority score and percentile ranking, is sent back to the researcher in the form of a **pink sheet**.

The federal government is the largest source of research funds for health researchers. In addition to regular grants programs, agencies of the federal government announce special funding programs in the form of **program announcements** and **Requests for Applications** (**RFAs**) for **grants** and **Requests for Proposals** (**RFPs**) for **contracts**. Other sources of funding include foundations, professional associations, and private corporations. The set of skills associated with learning about funding opportunities and developing proposals that can be funded is sometimes referred to as **grantsmanship**.

STUDY ACTIVITIES

Chapter 27 of the *Study Guide to Accompany Nursing Research: Principles and Methods, 6th ed.*, offers various exercises and study suggestions for reinforcing the concepts taught in this chapter. Additionally, the following study questions can be addressed:

1. Suppose that you were planning to study the self-care behaviors of aging patients with AIDS.
   a. Outline the methods you would recommend adopting.
   b. Develop a work plan.
   c. Prepare a hypothetical budget.
2. Suppose that you were interested in studying separation anxiety in hospitalized children. Using the references cited in this chapter, identify potential funding sources for your project.

SUGGESTED READINGS

Bauer, D. G., & the American Association of Colleges of Nursing (1988). *The complete grants source book for nursing and health*. New York: Macmillan.

Brooten, D., Munro, B. H., Roncoli, M., Arnold, L., Brown, L., York, R., Hollingsworth, A., Cohen, S., & Rubin, M. (1989). Developing a program grant for use in model testing. *Nursing and Health Care, 10*, 315–318.

Brown, L. P., Meier, P., Spatz, D. L., Spitzer, A., Finkler, S. A., Jacobsen, B. S., & Zukowsky, K. (1997). Resubmission of a grant application. *Nursing Research, 46*, 119–122.

Clinton, J. (1985). Couvade: Patterns, predictors, and nursing management: A research proposal submitted to the Division of Nursing. *Western Journal of Nursing Research, 7*, 221–248.

Cohen, M. Z., Knafl, K., & Dzurec, L. C. (1993). Grant writing for qualitative research. *Image—The Journal of Nursing Scholarship, 25*, 151–156.

Foundation Center Staff. (1996). *National guide to foundation funding in health*. New York: The Foundation Center.

Foundation Center Staff. (1997). *The foundation directory* (17th ed.). New York: The Foundation Center.

Frels, L. (1992). Sources and means of acquiring grant support for selected projects. *AANA Journal, 60*, 362–364.

Fuller, E. O., Hasselmeyer, E. G., Hunter, J. C., Abdellah, F. G., & Hinshaw, A. S. (1991). Summary statements of the NIH nursing research grant applications. *Nursing Research, 40*, 346–351.

Kim, M. J. (1993). The current generation of research proposals: Reviewers' viewpoints. *Nursing Research, 42*, 118–119.

Krathwohl, D. R. (1988). *How to prepare a research proposal* (3rd ed.). Syracuse, NY: Syracuse University Bookstore.

Lindquist, R. D., Tracy, M. F., & Treat-Jacobson, D. (1995). Peer review of nursing research proposals. *American Journal of Critical Care, 4*, 59–65.

McCormick, K. S., Cohen, E., Reed, M., Sparks, S., & Wasem, C. Funding nursing informatics activities: Internet access to announcements of government funding. *Computers in Nursing, 14,* 315–322.

Naylor, M. D. (1990). An example of a research grant application: Comprehensive discharge planning for the elderly. *Research in Nursing & Health, 13,* 327–347.

Sandelowski, M., Davis, D., & Harris, B. (1989). Artful design: Writing the proposal for research in the naturalist paradigm. *Research in Nursing & Health, 12,* 77–84.

Tornquist, E. M., & Funk, S. G. (1990). How to write a research grant proposal. *Image—The Journal of Nursing Scholarship, 22,* 44–51.

GLOSSARY

abstract A brief description of a completed or proposed study; in research journals, usually located at the beginning of the journal article.

accessible population The population of people available for a particular study; often a nonrandom subset of the target population.

accidental sampling Selection of the most readily available persons (or units) as participants in a study; also known as *convenience sampling*.

acquiescence response set A bias in self-report instruments, especially in social psychological scales, created when study participants characteristically agree with statements ("yea-say") independent of their content.

adjusted means The mean group values for the dependent variable, after removing the effects of covariates through regression procedures.

after-only design An experimental design in which data are collected from subjects only after the experimental intervention has been introduced.

alpha (α) (1) In tests of statistical significance, the level designating the probability of committing a Type I error; (2) in estimates of internal consistency, a reliability coefficient, as in Cronbach's alpha.

analysis A process of organizing and synthesizing data in such a way that research questions can be answered and hypotheses tested.

analysis of covariance (ANCOVA) A statistical procedure used to test mean differences among groups on a dependent variable, while controlling for one or more extraneous variables (covariates).

analysis of variance (ANOVA) A statistical procedure for testing mean differences among three or more groups by comparing the variability between groups with the variability within groups.

analytic induction A method of analyzing qualitative data that involves an iterative approach to testing research hypotheses.

anonymity Protection of participants in a study such that even the researcher cannot link individuals with the information provided.

applications The tasks that computers can be used to perform (e.g., word processing, database management, statistical analysis).

applied research Research that concentrates on finding a solution to an immediate practical problem.

ASCII format A set of standardized codes used in computers to represent keyboard characters; a file saved in ASCII (an acronym for American Standard Code for Information Interchange) is stripped of proprietary codes specific to the software that created the original file.

assumptions Basic principles that are accepted as being true on the basis of logic or reason, without proof or verification.

asymmetric distribution A distribution of data values that is skewed, that is, has two halves that are not mirror images of each other.

attribute variables Preexisting characteristics of the study participants, which the researcher simply observes or measures.

attrition The loss of participants during the course of a study, which can introduce bias by changing the composition of the sample initially drawn—particularly if more participants are lost from one group than another; attrition can thereby be a threat to the internal validity of a study.

audit trail The systematic collection and documentation of material that allows an independent auditor in an inquiry audit of qualitative data to draw conclusions about the data.

axial coding The second-level of coding in a grounded theory study, involving the process of categorizing, recategorizing, and condensing all first-level codes by connecting a category and its subcategories.

baseline measure A measure of the dependent variable before the introduction of an experimental intervention.

basic research Research designed to extend the base of knowledge in a discipline for the sake of knowledge production or theory construction, rather than for solving an immediate problem.

before–after design An experimental design in which data are collected from research subjects both before and after the introduction of the experimental intervention.

behavioral objective An intended outcome of a program or intervention, stated in terms of the behavior of the individuals at whom the program is aimed.

beneficence A fundamental ethical principle that seeks to prevent harm and exploitation of, and to maximize benefits for, study participants.

beta (β) (1) In multiple regression, the standardized coefficients indicating the relative weights of the independent variables in the regression equation; (2) in statistical testing, the probability of a Type II error.

between-subjects design A research design in which separate groups of people are being compared (e.g., smokers and nonsmokers).

bias Any influence that produces a distortion in the results of a study.

bimodal distribution A distribution of data values with two peaks (high frequencies).

bivariate statistics Statistics derived from the analysis of two variables simultaneously for the purpose of assessing the empirical relationship between them.

"blind" review The review of a manuscript or proposal such that neither the author nor the reviewer is identified to the other party.

borrowed theory A theory borrowed from another discipline or field to guide nursing practice or research.

bracketing In phenomenologic inquiries, the process of identifying and holding in abeyance any preconceived beliefs and opinions one has about the phenomena under study.

bricolage The tendency in qualitative research to derive a complex array of data from a variety of sources, using a variety of methods.

byte A single character, such as a number, letter, or specialized symbol, in a computer's memory.

canonical analysis A statistical procedure for examining the relationship between two or more independent variables *and* two or more dependent variables.

case-control study A research design, typically found in retrospective ex post facto research, that involves the comparison of a "case" (i.e., a person with the condition under scrutiny, such as lung cancer) and a matched control (a similar person without the condition).

case study A research method that involves a thorough, in-depth analysis of an individual, group, institution, or other social unit.

categorical variable A variable with discrete values rather than values incrementally placed along a continuum (e.g., a person's marital status).

category system In observational studies, the prespecified plan for organizing and recording the behaviors and events under observation.

causal modeling The development and statistical testing of an explanatory model of hypothesized causal relationships among phenomena.

causal relationship A relationship between two variables such that the presence or absence of one variable (the "cause") determines the presence or absence, or value, of the other (the "effect").

cell (1) The intersection of a row and column in a table with two or more dimensions; (2) in an experimental design, a cell is the representation of an experimental condition in a schematic diagram.

census A survey covering an entire population.

central processing unit (CPU) The portion of a computer, comprising the control unit and arithmetic/logic unit, where all decisions and calculations are performed.

central tendency A statistical index of the "typicalness" of a set of scores that comes from the center of the distribution of scores; the three most common indices of central tendency are the mode, the median, and the mean.

chi-square test A nonparametric test of statistical significance used to assess whether a relationship exists between two nominal-level variables; symbolized as χ^2.

clinical relevance The degree to which a study addresses a problem of significance to the practice of nursing; a major criterion for research utilization.

clinical research Research designed to generate knowledge to guide nursing practice.

clinical trial An experiment involving a test of the effectiveness of a clinical treatment, generally involving a large and heterogeneous sample of subjects.

closed-ended question A question that offers respondents a set of mutually exclusive and jointly exhaustive alternative replies, from which the one that most closely approximates the "right" answer must be chosen.

cluster analysis A multivariate statistical procedure used to cluster people or things based on patterns of association.

cluster randomization The random assignment of intact groups of subjects—rather than individual subjects—to treatment conditions.

cluster sampling A form of sampling in which large groupings ("clusters") are selected first (e.g., nursing schools), with successive subsampling of smaller units (e.g., nursing students).

code of ethics The fundamental ethical principles that are established by a discipline or institution to guide researchers' conduct in research with human (or animal) subjects.

codebook A record that documents the researcher's categorization and coding decisions.

coding The process of transforming raw data into standardized form for data processing and analysis; in quantitative research, the process of attaching numbers to categories; in qualitative research, the process of identifying recurring words, themes, or concepts within the data.

coefficient alpha (Cronbach's alpha) A reliability index that estimates the internal consistency or homogeneity of a measure composed of several items or subparts.

coercion In a research context, the explicit or implicit use of threats (or excessive rewards) to get people to agree to participate in a study.

cognitive questioning A method sometimes used during the pretest phase of instrument development in which respondents are asked to think aloud about the meaning of a question and what comes to mind when they hear a question.

cohort study A kind of trend study that focuses on a specific subpopulation (which is often an age-related subgroup) from which different samples are selected at different points in time (e.g., the cohort of nursing students who graduated between 1970 and 1974).

comparison group A group of subjects whose scores on a dependent variable are used as a basis for evaluating the scores of the group of primary interest (e.g., nonsmokers as a comparison group for smokers); term used in lieu of *control group* when the investigation does not involve a true experimental design.

computer An electronic device that performs simple operations with extreme accuracy and speed.

computer program A set of instructions to a computer.

concealment A tactic involving the unobtrusive collection of research data without the participants' knowledge or consent, used as a means of obtaining an accurate view of naturalistic behavior when the known presence of an observer would distort the behavior of interest.

concept   An abstraction based on observations of certain behaviors or characteristics (e.g., stress, pain).

conceptual model   Interrelated concepts or abstractions that are assembled together in some rational scheme by virtue of their relevance to a common theme; sometimes referred to as *conceptual framework*.

conceptual utilization   The use of research findings in a general, conceptual way to broaden one's thinking about an issue, although the knowledge is not put to any specific, documentable use.

concurrent validity   The degree to which scores on an instrument are correlated with some external criterion, measured at the same time.

confidence interval   The range of values within which a population parameter is estimated to lie.

confidence level   The estimated probability that a population parameter lies within a given confidence interval.

confidentiality   Protection of participants in a study such that their individual identities will not be linked to the information they provide and will never be publicly divulged.

confirmability   A criterion for evaluating data quality with qualitative data, referring to the objectivity or neutrality of the data.

consent form   A written agreement signed by a study participant and a researcher concerning the terms and conditions of a study participant's voluntary participation in a study.

consistency check   A procedure performed in cleaning a set of data to ensure that the data are internally consistent.

constant comparison   A procedure often used in a grounded theory analysis wherein newly collected data are compared in an ongoing fashion with data obtained earlier, to refine theoretically relevant categories.

construct   An abstraction or concept that is deliberately invented (constructed) by researchers for a scientific purpose (e.g., health locus of control).

construct validity   The degree to which an instrument measures the construct under investigation.

consumer   An individual who reads, reviews, and critiques research findings and who attempts to use and apply the findings in practice.

contact information   Information obtained from study participants in longitudinal studies that facilitates their relocation at a future date.

contamination   The inadvertent, undesirable influence of one experimental treatment condition on another treatment condition.

content analysis   The process of organizing and integrating narrative, qualitative information according to emerging themes and concepts; classically, a procedure for analyzing written or verbal communications in a systematic and objective fashion, typically with the goal of quantitatively measuring variables.

content validity   The degree to which the items in an instrument adequately represent the universe of content.

contingency table   A two-dimensional table that permits cross-tabulation of the frequencies of two categorical variables.

continuous variable   A variable that can take on an infinite range of values along a specified continuum (e.g., height).

control   The process of holding constant possible influences on the dependent variable under investigation.

control group   Subjects in an experiment who do not receive the experimental treatment and whose performance provides a baseline against which the effects of the treatment can be measured (see also *comparison group*).

convenience sampling   Selection of the most readily available persons (or units) as participants in a study; also known as *accidental sampling*.

convergent validity   An approach to construct validation that involves assessing the degree to which two methods of measuring a construct are similar (i.e., converge).

core category In a grounded theory study, the central phenomenon that is used to integrate all categories of data.

correlation A tendency for variation in one variable to be related to variation in another variable.

correlation coefficient An index that summarizes the degree of relationship between two variables. Correlation coefficients typically range from +1.00 (for a perfect positive relationship) through 0.0 (for no relationship) to −1.00 (for a perfect negative relationship).

correlation matrix A two-dimensional display showing the correlation coefficients between all combinations of variables of interest.

correlational research Research that explores the interrelationships among variables of interest without any active intervention on the part of the researcher.

cost/benefit analysis An evaluation of the financial costs of a program or intervention relative to the financial gains attributable to it.

cost–benefit assessment The assessment of relative costs and benefits, to individuals, organizations, and society, of implementing an innovation.

counterbalancing The process of systematically varying the order of presentation of stimuli or treatments to control for ordering effects, as in counterbalancing the order of treatments in a repeated-measures design.

covariate A variable that is statistically controlled (held constant) in analysis of covariance. The covariate is typically an extraneous, confounding influence on the dependent variable or a preintervention measure of the dependent variable.

covert data collection The collection of information in a study without the participant's knowledge.

Cramér's V An index describing the magnitude of relationship between nominal-level data, used when the contingency table to which it is applied is larger than 2×2.

credibility A criterion for evaluating the data quality of qualitative data, referring to confidence in the truth of the data.

criterion variable The criterion against which the effect of an independent variable is tested; sometimes used instead of *dependent variable*.

criterion-related validity The degree to which scores on an instrument are correlated with some external criterion.

critical case sampling A sampling approach used by qualitative researchers that involves the purposeful selection of cases that are especially important or illustrative.

critical incident technique A method of obtaining data from study participants by in-depth exploration of specific incidents and behaviors related to the matter under investigation.

critical region The area in the sampling distribution representing values that are "improbable" if the null hypothesis is true.

critique An objective, critical, and balanced appraisal of a research report's various dimensions (e.g., conceptual, methodologic, ethical).

Cronbach's alpha A widely-used reliability index that estimates the internal consistency or homogeneity of a measure composed of several subparts; also referred to as *coefficient alpha*.

crossover design See *repeated-measures design*.

cross-sectional study A study based on observations of different age or developmental groups at a single point in time for the purpose of inferring trends over time.

cross-tabulation A determination of the number of cases occurring when two variables are considered simultaneously (e.g., gender—male/ female—cross-tabulated with smoking status—smoker/nonsmoker). The results are typically presented in a table with rows and columns divided according to the values of the variables.

data The pieces of information obtained in the course of a study (singular is *datum*).

data analysis The systematic organization and synthesis of research data, and the testing of research hypotheses using those data.

data cleaning The preparation of data for analysis by performing checks to ensure that the data are consistent and correct.

data collection The gathering of information needed to address a research problem.

data entry The process of entering data onto an input medium for computer analysis.

data saturation See *saturation*.

data transformation A step often undertaken before the analysis of research data, to put the data in a form that can be analyzed meaningfully (e.g., recoding of values).

debriefing Communication with study participants, generally after their participation has been completed, regarding various aspects of the study.

deception The deliberate withholding of information, or the provision of false information, to research participants, usually to reduce potential biases.

deductive reasoning The process of developing specific predictions from general principles (see also *inductive reasoning*).

degrees of freedom (*df*) A concept used in conjunction with statistical tests, referring to the number of sample values that are free to vary (e.g., with a given sample mean, all but one value would be free to vary); degrees of freedom is often $N - 1$, but different formulas are relevant for different tests.

Delphi technique A method of obtaining judgments from a panel of experts. The experts are questioned individually, and a summary of the judgments is circulated to the entire panel. The experts are questioned again, with further iterations introduced as needed until there is some consensus.

demonstration A program or intervention that is being tested, often on a large scale, to determine its effectiveness and the desirability of changing policies or procedures.

dependability A criterion for evaluating data quality in qualitative data, referring to the stability of data over time and over conditions.

dependent variable The outcome variable of interest; the variable that is hypothesized to depend on or be caused by another variable, the *independent variable*.

descriptive research Research studies that have as their main objective the accurate portrayal of the characteristics of persons, situations, or groups and/or the frequency with which certain phenomena occur.

descriptive statistics Statistics that are used to describe and summarize data (e.g., mean, standard deviation).

descriptive theory A broad characterization that thoroughly accounts for a single phenomenon.

determinism The belief that phenomena are not haphazard or random, but rather have antecedent causes; an assumption in the positivist paradigm.

deviation score A score computed by subtracting an individual score value from the mean of the distribution of scores.

dichotomous variable A variable having only two values or categories (e.g., gender).

direct costs Specific project-related costs incurred in the course of a study (e.g., for personnel working on the study, supplies, travel, and so on).

directional hypothesis A hypothesis that makes a specific prediction about the direction and nature of the relationship between two variables.

discrete variable A variable that has a finite number of values between two points.

discriminant function analysis A statistical procedure used to predict group membership or status on a categorical (nominal-level) variable on the basis of two or more independent variables.

discriminant validity An approach to construct validation that involves assessing the degree to which a single method of measuring two constructs yields different results (i.e., discriminates the two).

disproportionate sample A sample that results when the researcher samples differing proportions of study participants from different strata in the population to ensure adequate representation from strata that are comparatively smaller.

double-blind experiment An experiment in which neither the subjects nor those who administer the treatment know who is in the experimental or control group.

dummy variables Dichotomous variables created for use in many multivariate statistical analyses, typically using codes of 0 and 1 (e.g., female = 1, male = 0).

effect size A statistical expression of the magnitude of the relationship between two variables, or the magnitude of the difference between two groups, with regard to some attribute of interest.

eigenvalue In factor analysis, the value equal to the sum of the squared weights for each factor.

electronic database Bibliographic files that can be accessed by computer for the purpose of conducting a literature review.

element The most basic unit of a population, from which a sample will be drawn; in nursing research, the element is typically humans.

eligibility criteria The criteria used by a researcher to designate the specific attributes of the target population, and by which participants are selected for participation in a study.

emergent design A design that unfolds in the course of a qualitative study as the researcher makes ongoing design decisions reflecting what has already been learned.

emic perspective A term used by ethnographers to refer to the way members of a culture view their world; the "insider's view."

empirical evidence Evidence that is rooted in objective reality and that is gathered through the collection of data using one's senses; used as the basis for generating knowledge.

endogenous variable In path analysis, a variable whose variation is determined by other variables within the model.

equivalence The degree of similarity between alternate forms of a measuring instrument.

error of measurement The deviation between true scores and obtained scores of a measured characteristic.

eta squared A statistic calculated, in ANOVA, to indicate the proportion of variance in the dependent variable explained by the independent variables, analogous to R in multiple regression.

ethics A system of moral values that is concerned with the degree to which research procedures adhere to professional, legal, and social obligations to the study participants.

ethnography A branch of human inquiry, associated with the field of anthropology, that focuses on the culture of a group of people, with an effort to understand the world view of those under study.

ethnomethodology A branch of human inquiry, associated with sociology, that focuses on the way in which people make sense of their everyday activities and come to behave in socially acceptable ways.

ethnonursing research The study of human cultures, with a focus on a group's beliefs and practices relating to nursing care and related health behaviors.

etic perspective A term used by ethnographers to refer to the "outsider's" view of the experiences of a cultural group.

evaluation research Research that investigates how well a program, practice, or policy is working.

event sampling In observational studies, a sampling plan that involves the selection of integral behaviors or events.

ex post facto research Research conducted after the variations in the independent variable have occurred in the natural course of events; a form of nonexperimental research in which causal explanations are inferred "after the fact."

exogenous variable In path analysis, a variable whose determinants lie outside the model.

experiment A research study in which the investigator controls (manipulates) the independent variable and randomly assigns subjects to different conditions.

experimental group   The subjects who receive the experimental treatment or intervention.

experimental intervention   (experimental treatment) See *intervention; treatment.*

exploratory research   A study designed to explore the dimensions of a phenomenon or to develop or refine hypotheses about the relationships between phenomena.

external criticism   In historical research, the systematic evaluation of the authenticity and genuineness of data.

external storage device   A device external to a computer for storing computer files and programs (e.g., a floppy disk).

external validity   The degree to which the results of a study can be generalized to settings or samples other than the ones studied.

extraneous variable   A variable that confounds the relationship between the independent and dependent variables and that needs to be controlled either in the research design or through statistical procedures.

extreme case sampling   A sampling approach used by qualitative researchers that involves the purposeful selection of the most extreme or unusual cases.

extreme response set   A bias in self-report instruments, especially in social psychological scales, created when participants express their opinions in terms of extreme response alternatives (e.g., "strongly agree") independent of the question's content.

F-ratio   The statistic obtained in several statistical tests (e.g., ANOVA) in which variation attributable to different sources (e.g., between groups and within groups) is compared.

face validity   The extent to which a measuring instrument looks as though it is measuring what it purports to measure.

factor analysis   A statistical procedure for reducing a large set of variables into a smaller set of variables with common characteristics or underlying dimensions.

factorial design   An experimental design in which two or more independent variables are simultaneously manipulated; this design permits a separate analysis of the main effects of the independent variables, plus the interaction effects of those variables.

field notes   The notes taken by researchers describing the unstructured observations they have made in the field, and their interpretation of those observations.

field research   Research in which the data are collected "in the field" from individuals in their normal roles, with the aim of understanding the practices, behaviors, and beliefs of individuals or groups as they normally function in real life.

file   A collection of information that can be accessed by a computer by reference to a specific name

findings   The results of the analyses of the research data; in quantitative studies, the results of the hypothesis tests.

Fisher's exact test   A statistical procedure used to test the significance of the difference in proportions, used when the sample size is small or cells in the contingency table have no observations.

fixed-alternative question   A question that offers respondents a set of prespecified responses, from which the respondent must choose the alternative that most closely approximates the correct response.

focus group interview   An interview with a group of individuals assembled to answer questions on a given topic.

focused interview   A loosely structured interview in which the interviewer guides the respondent through a set of questions using a topic guide.

follow-up study   A study undertaken to determine the outcomes of individuals who have a specified condition or who have received a specified treatment.

formative evaluation   An ongoing assessment of a product or program as it is being developed, designed to optimize the ultimate quality of that product or program.

framework   The conceptual underpinnings of a study; often referred to as a *theoretical* *framework* in studies based on a theory, or as a *conceptual framework* in studies that have roots in a specific conceptual model.

frequency distribution A systematic array of numeric values from the lowest to the highest, together with a count of the number of times each value was obtained.

frequency polygon Graphic display of a frequency distribution, in which dots connected by a straight line indicate the number of times a score value occurs in a set of data.

Friedman test A nonparametric analogue of ANOVA, used when the researcher is working with paired groups or a repeated-measures situation.

full disclosure The communication of complete information to potential research participants regarding the nature of the study, the person's right to refuse participation, and the likely risks and benefits that would be incurred.

functional relationship A relationship or association between two variables wherein it cannot be assumed that one variable caused the other; however, it can be said that the variable *X* changes values as a function of changes in variable *Y*.

gaining entrée The process of gaining access to study participants in qualitative field studies through the cooperation of key actors in the selected community or site.

Gantt chart A chart depicting the scheduling of activities (tasks) in a research study and highlighting the sequencing and interrelationships among activities.

generalizability The degree to which the research procedures justify the inference that the findings represent something beyond the specific observations on which they are based; in particular, the inference that the findings can be generalized from the sample to the entire population.

grand theory A broad theory aimed at describing large segments of the physical, social, or behavioral world; also referred to as a *macro-theory.*

grand tour question A broad question asked in an unstructured interview to gain a general overview of a phenomenon, on the basis of which more focused questions are subsequently asked.

grant A financial award made to a researcher or team of researchers for the conduct of a proposed project.

grantsmanship The combined set of skills and knowledge needed to secure financial support for one's research ideas.

graphic rating scale A scale in which respondents are asked to rate something (e.g., a concept, issue, institution) along an ordered bipolar continuum (e.g., "excellent" to "very poor").

grounded theory An approach to collecting and analyzing qualitative data with the aim of developing theories and theoretical propositions grounded in real-world observations.

hardware The physical electronic equipment that makes up a computer.

Hawthorne effect The effect on the dependent variable resulting from subjects' awareness that they are participants under study.

hermeneutics A qualitative research tradition, closely related to phenomenology, that uses the lived experiences of humans as a tool for better understanding the social, cultural, political, and/or historical context in which those experiences occurred.

heterogeneity The degree to which objects are dissimilar (i.e., characterized by high variability) with respect to some attribute.

histogram A graphic presentation of frequency distribution data.

historical research Systematic studies designed to establish facts and relationships concerning past events.

history threat A threat to the internal validity of a study; refers to the occurrence of events external to the intervention but concurrent with it, which can affect the dependent variable of interest.

homogeneity (1) In terms of the reliability of an instrument, the degree to which the subparts are internally consistent (i.e., are measuring the same critical attribute). (2) More generally, the degree to which objects are similar (i.e., characterized by low variability).

homegeneous sampling A sampling approach used by qualitative researchers that involves the deliberate selection of cases with limited variation.

hypothesis A statement of predicted relationships between variables.

impact analysis An evaluation of the effects of a program or intervention on outcomes of interest, net of other factors influencing those outcomes.

implementation analysis An evaluation that describes the process by which a program or intervention was implemented in practice.

implementation potential The extent to which an innovation is amenable to implementation in a new setting, an assessment of which is usually made in a research utilization project; includes the criteria of transferability, feasibility, and the cost/benefit ratio of the innovation.

independent variable The variable that is believed to cause or influence the dependent variable; in experimental research, the manipulated (treatment) variable.

indirect costs The institutional costs that are included in a research budget, over and above the specific (direct) costs of conducting the study; also referred to as *overhead*.

inductive reasoning The process of reasoning from specific observations to more general rules (see also *deductive reasoning*).

inferential statistics Statistics that permit inferences on whether relationships observed in a sample are likely to occur in a larger population of concern.

informant A term used to refer to those individuals who provide information to researchers about a phenomenon under study, often used in qualitative studies.

informed consent An ethical principle that requires researchers to obtain the voluntary participation of subjects, after informing them of possible risks and benefits.

input devices Those parts of a computer system that allow data and commands to be entered into the computer (e.g., a keyboard or terminal).

inquiry audit An independent scrutiny of qualitative data and relevant supporting documents by an external reviewer, a method used to determine the dependability and confirmability of qualitative data.

Institutional Review Board (IRB) A group of individuals from an institution who convene to review proposed and ongoing studies with respect to ethical considerations.

instrument The written device that a researcher uses to collect data (e.g., questionnaires, tests, observation schedules, etc.).

instrumental utilization Clearly identifiable attempts to base some specific action or intervention on the results of research findings.

instrumentation threat The threat to the internal validity of the study that can arise if the researcher changes the measuring instrument between two points of data collection.

intensity sampling A sampling approach used by qualitative researchers that involves the purposeful selection of intense (but not extreme) cases.

interaction effect The effect of two or more independent variables acting in combination (interactively) on a dependent variable rather than as unconnected factors.

intercoder reliability The degree to which two coders, operating independently, assign the same codes to variables.

internal consistency The degree to which the subparts of an instrument are all measuring the same attribute or dimension, as a measure of the instrument's reliability.

internal criticism In historical research, an evaluation of the worth of the historical evidence.

internal validity The degree to which it can be inferred that the experimental treatment (independent variable), rather than uncontrolled, extraneous factors, is responsible for observed effects.

Internet The electronic "highway" that interconnects thousands of computer networks around the world over telephone lines.

interrater (interobserver) reliability The degree to which two raters or observers, operating independently, assign the same ratings or values for an attribute being measured or observed.

interval estimation A statistical estimation approach in which the researcher establishes a range of values that are likely, within a given level of confidence, to contain the true population parameter.

interval measure A level of measurement in which an attribute of a variable is rank-ordered on a scale that has equal distances between points on that scale (e.g., Fahrenheit degrees).

intervention In experimental research, the experimental treatment or manipulation.

interview A method of data collection in which one person (an interviewer) asks questions of another person (a respondent); interviews are conducted either face-to-face or by telephone.

interview schedule The formal instrument, used in structured self-report studies, that specifies the wording of all questions to be asked of respondents.

inverse relationship A negative correlation between two variables; i.e., a relationship characterized by the tendency of high values on one variable to be associated with low values on the second variable.

isomorphism In measurement, the correspondence between the measures an instrument yields and reality.

item A single question on a test or questionnaire, or a single statement on an attitude or other scale (e.g., a final examination might consist of 100 items).

journal club A group that meets regularly (often in clinical settings) to discuss and critique research reports appearing in research journals, sometimes with the goal of assessing the utilization potential of the findings.

judgmental sampling A type of nonprobability sampling method in which the researcher selects participants for the study on the basis of personal judgment about which ones will be most representative or productive, also referred to as *purposive sampling*.

Kendall's tau A correlation coefficient used to indicate the magnitude of a relationship between ordinal-level data.

key informant A person well-versed in the phenomenon of research interest and who is willing to share the information and insight with the researcher; key informants are often used in needs assessments.

known-groups technique A technique for estimating the construct validity of an instrument through an analysis of the degree to which the instrument separates groups that are predicted to differ on the basis of known characteristics or a theory.

Kruskal-Wallis test A nonparametric test used to test the difference between three or more independent groups, based on ranked scores.

Kuder-Richardson (KR-20) formula A method of calculating an internal consistency reliability coefficient for a scaled set of items when the items are dichotomous.

latent variable An unmeasured variable that represents an underlying, abstract construct (usually in the context of a LISREL analysis).

law A theory that has accrued such persuasive empirical support that it is accepted as truth (e.g., Boyle's law of gases).

least-squares estimation A commonly used method of statistical estimation in which the solution minimizes the sums of squares of error terms; sometimes referred to as *ordinary least squares* (OLS).

level of measurement A system of classifying measurements according to the nature of the measurement and the type of mathematic operations to which they are amenable; the four levels are nominal, ordinal, interval, and ratio.

level of significance The risk of making a Type I error, established by the researcher before the statistical analysis (e.g., the .05 level).

life history A narrative self-report about a person's life experiences regarding some theme of interest to the researcher.

life table analysis A statistical procedure used when the dependent variable represents a time interval between an initial event (e.g., onset of a disease) and an end event (e.g., death); also referred to as *survival analysis*.

Likert scale A composite measure of attitudes that involves summation of scores on a set of items (statements) to which respondents are asked to indicate their degree of agreement or disagreement.

LISREL The widely used acronym for *linear structural relation analysis*, typically used for testing causal models.

listwise deletion A method of dealing with missing values in a data set that involves the elimination of cases with missing data.

literature review A critical summary of research on a topic of interest, often prepared to put a research problem in context or as the basis for an implementation project.

log In participant observation studies, the observer's daily record of events and conversations that took place.

logical positivism The philosophy underlying the traditional scientific approach; see also *positivist paradigm*.

logistic regression A multivariate regression procedure that analyzes relationships between multiple independent variables and categorical dependent variables; also referred to as *logit analysis*.

longitudinal study A study designed to collect data at more than one point in time, in contrast to a cross-sectional study.

macro-theory A broad theory aimed at describing large segments of the physical, social, or behavioral world; also referred to as a *grand theory*.

main effects In a study with multiple independent variables, the effects of a single independent variable on the dependent variable.

mainframe A large, multiuser computer system.

manifest variable An observed, measured variable that serves as an indicator of an underlying construct (i.e., a latent variable).

manipulation An intervention or treatment introduced by the researcher in an experimental or quasi-experimental study; the researcher manipulates the independent variable to assess its impact on the dependent variable.

manipulation check In experimental studies, a test to determine whether the manipulation was implemented as intended.

Mann-Whitney *U* test A nonparametric statistic used to test the difference between two independent groups, based on ranked scores.

MANOVA See *multivariate analysis of variance*.

matching The pairing of subjects in one group with those in another group based on their similarity on one or more dimensions, done to enhance the overall comparability of groups.

maturation threat A threat to the internal validity of a study that results when changes to the outcome measure (dependent variable) result from the passage of time.

maximum likelihood estimation An estimation approach (sometimes used in lieu of the least squares approach) in which the estimators are ones that estimate the parameters most likely to have generated the observed measurements.

maximum variation sampling A sampling approach used by qualitative researchers that involves the purposeful selection of cases with a wide range of variation.

McNemar test A statistical test for comparing differences in proportions, when the values are derived from paired (nonindependent) groups.

mean A descriptive statistic that is a measure of central tendency, computed by summing all scores and dividing by the number of subjects.

measurement The assignment of numbers to objects according to specified rules to characterize quantities of some attribute.

measurement model In LISREL, the model that stipulates the hypothesized relationships among the manifest and latent variables.

median A descriptive statistic that is a measure of central tendency, representing the exact middle score or value in a distribution of scores; the median is the value above and below which 50% of the scores lie.

median test A nonparametric statistical test that involves the comparison of median values of two independent groups to determine if the groups derive from populations with different medians.

mediating variable A variable that mediates or acts like a "go-between" in a chain linking two other variables (e.g., coping skills may be said to mediate the relationship between stressful events and anxiety).

member check A method of validating the credibility of qualitative data through debriefings and discussions with informants.

meta-analysis A technique for quantitatively combining and thus integrating the results of multiple studies on a given topic.

methodologic notes In observational field studies, the notes kept by the researcher regarding the methods used in collecting the data.

methodologic research Research designed to develop or refine procedures for obtaining, organizing, or analyzing data.

methods (research) The steps, procedures, and strategies for gathering and analyzing the data in a research investigation.

microcomputer See *personal computer.*

middle-range theory A theory that focuses on only a piece of reality or human experience, involving a selected number of concepts (e.g., theories of stress).

minimal risk Anticipated risks that are no greater than those ordinarily encountered in daily life or during the performance of routine tests or procedures.

missing values Values missing from a data set for some study participants, due, for example, to refusals, researcher error, or skip patterns.

modality A characteristic of a frequency distribution describing the number of peaks, that is, values with high frequencies.

mode A descriptive statistic that is a measure of central tendency; the score or value that occurs most frequently in a distribution of scores.

model A symbolic representation of concepts or variables and interrelationships among them.

molar approach A way of making observations about behaviors that entails studying large units of behavior and treating them as a whole.

molecular approach A way of making observations about behavior that uses small and highly specific behaviors as the unit of observation.

mortality threat A threat to the internal validity of a study, referring to the differential loss of participants (attrition) from different groups.

multimethod research Generally, research in which multiple approaches are used to address the research problem; often used to designate research in which both qualitative and quantitative data are collected and analyzed.

multimodal distribution A distribution of values with more than one peak (high frequency).

multiple classification analysis A variant of multiple regression and ANCOVA that yields group means on the dependent variable adjusted for the effects of covariates.

multiple comparison procedures Statistical tests, normally applied after an ANOVA indicates statistically significant group differences, that compare different pairs of groups; also referred to as *post hoc tests.*

multiple correlation coefficient An index that summarizes the degree of relationship between two or more independent variables and a dependent variable; symbolized as *R.*

multiple regression analysis A statistical procedure for understanding the simultaneous effects of two or more independent (predictor) variables on a dependent variable.

multistage sampling A sampling strategy that proceeds through a set of stages from larger to smaller sampling units (e.g., from states, to nursing schools, to faculty members).

multitrait–multimethod matrix approach A method of establishing the construct validity of an instrument that involves the use of multiple measures for a set of subjects; the target instrument is valid to the extent that there is a strong relationship between it and other measures purporting to measure the same attribute (convergence) and a weak relationship between it and other measures purporting to measure a different attribute (discriminability).

multivariate analysis of variance (MANOVA) A statistical procedure used to test the significance of differences between the means of two or more groups on two or more dependent variables, considered simultaneously.

multivariate statistics Statistical procedures designed to analyze the relationships among three or more variables; commonly used multivariate statistics include multiple regression, analysis of covariance, and factor analysis.

N Often used to designate the total number of study participants (e.g., "the total N was 500").

n Often used to designate the number of participants in a subgroup or in a cell of a study (e.g., "each of the four groups had an *n* of 125, for a total N of 500").

naturalistic paradigm An alternative paradigm to the traditional positivist paradigm that holds that there are multiple interpretations of reality, and that the goal of research is to understand how individuals construct reality within their context; often associated with qualitative research.

naturalistic setting A setting for the collection of research data that is natural to those being studied (e.g., homes, places of work, and so on).

needs assessment A study in which a researcher collects data for estimating the needs of a group, community, or organization; usually used as a guide to policy planning and resource allocation.

negative case analysis A method of refining a hypothesis or theory in a qualitative study that involves the inclusion of cases that appear to disconfirm earlier hypotheses.

negative relationship A relationship between two variables in which there is a tendency for higher values on one variable to be associated with lower values on the other (e.g., as temperature increases, people's productivity may decrease); also referred to as an *inverse relationship*.

negative results Research results that fail to support the researcher's hypotheses.

negatively skewed distribution An asymmetric distribution of data values such that a disproportionately high number of cases have high values—that is, fall at the upper end of the distribution; when displayed graphically, the tail points to the left.

network sampling The sampling of participants based on referrals from others already in the sample, sometimes referred to as *snowball sampling*.

nominal measure The lowest level of measurement that involves the assignment of characteristics into categories (e.g., males, category 1; females, category 2).

nondirectional hypothesis A research hypothesis that does not stipulate in advance the direction and nature of the relationship between variables.

nonequivalent control group design A quasi-experimental design involving a comparison group that was not developed on the basis of random assignment, but from whom preintervention data are obtained to assess the initial equivalence of the groups.

nonexperimental research Studies in which the researcher collects data without introducing any treatment or changes.

nonparametric statistics A general class of inferential statistics that does not involve rigorous assumptions about the distribution of the critical variables; most often used when the data are measured on the nominal or ordinal scales.

nonprobability sampling The selection of participants or sampling units from a population using nonrandom procedures; examples include convenience, judgmental, and quota sampling.

nonrecursive model A causal model that hypothesizes reciprocal effects wherein a variable can be both the cause of and an effect of another variable.

nonresponse bias A bias that can result when a nonrandom subset of people invited to participate in a study fail to participate.

nonsignificant result The result of a statistical test indicating that group differences or a relationship between variables could have occurred as a result of chance, at a given level of significance, sometimes abbreviated as *NS* in research journals.

normal distribution A theoretical distribution that is bell-shaped and symmetrical; also referred to as a *normal curve.*

norms Test-performance standards, based on the collection of test score information from a large, representative sample.

null hypothesis The hypothesis that states there is no relationship between the variables under study; used primarily in connection with tests of statistical significance as the hypothesis to be rejected.

objectivity The extent to which two independent researchers would arrive at similar judgments or conclusions (i.e., judgments not biased by personal values or beliefs); considered a desirable attribute within the positivist paradigm.

observational notes In field studies, the observer's descriptions about observed events and conversations.

observational research Studies in which the data are collected by observing and recording behaviors or activities of interest.

obtained (observed) score The actual score or numeric value assigned to a person on a measure.

one-tailed test A test of statistical significance in which only values at one extreme (tail) of a distribution are considered in determining significance; used when the researcher has predicted the direction of a relationship (see *directional hypothesis*).

open-ended question A question in an interview or questionnaire that does not restrict the respondents' answers to preestablished alternatives.

open coding The first level of coding in a grounded theory study, referring to the basic descriptive coding of the content of narrative materials.

operating system The software that controls the overall operation of a computer system; examples for IBM-type personal computers include MS/DOS and Windows 95.

operational definition The definition of a concept or variable in terms of the operations or procedures by which it is to be measured.

operationalization The process of translating research concepts into measurable phenomena.

ordinal measure A level of measurement that yields rank orders of a variable along some dimension.

outcome analysis An evaluation of what transpires with respect to outcomes of interest after implementing a program or intervention, without use of an experimental design to assess net effects; see also *impact analysis.*

outcome variable A term sometimes used to refer to the dependent variable in experimental research; that is, the measure that captures the outcome of the experimental intervention.

outcomes research Research designed to document the effectiveness of health care services and the end results of patient care.

outliers Values that lie outside the normal range of values for other cases in a data set.

output devices Those parts of a computer system that communicate information back to the computer user (e.g., a printer).

p value In statistical testing, the probability that the obtained results are due to chance alone; the probability of committing a Type I error.

pair matching See *matching.*

pairwise deletion A method of dealing with missing values in a data set that involves the deletion of cases with missing data on a selective basis (i.e., deletion of a case only when one variable is paired with another variable that has missing data).

panel study A type of longitudinal study in which data are collected from the same people at two or more points in time.

paradigm A way of looking at natural phenomena that encompasses a set of philosophical assumptions and that guides one's approach to inquiry.

parameter A characteristic of a population (e.g., the mean age of all U.S. citizens).

parametric statistics A class of inferential statistics that involves (a) assumptions about the distribution of the variables, (b) the estimation of a parameter, and (c) the use of interval or ratio measures.

participant See *study participant.*

participant observation A method of collecting data through the observation of a group or organization in which the researcher participates as a member.

path analysis A regression-based procedure for testing causal models, typically using nonexperimental data.

Pearson's r The most widely used correlation coefficient, designating the magnitude of relationship between two variables measured on at least an interval scale; also referred to as the *product-moment correlation.*

peer reviewer A person who reviews and critiques a research report or proposal, who himself or herself is a researcher (usually working on similar types of research problems as those under review), and who makes a recommendation about publishing or funding the research.

perfect correlation A correlation between two variables such that the values of one variable permit perfect prediction of the values of the other; designated as 1.00 or −1.00.

personal computer (PC) A small computer used by individual users; also referred to as a microcomputer.

personal notes In field studies, written comments about the observer's own feelings during the research process.

personal interview A face-to-face interview between an interviewer and a respondent.

phenomenon The abstract entity or concept under investigation in a study, most often used by qualitative researchers in lieu of the term "variable."

phenomenology A qualitative research tradition, with roots in philosophy and psychology, that focuses on the lived experience of humans.

phi coefficient A statistical index describing the magnitude of relationship between two dichotomous variables.

pilot study A small-scale version, or trial run, done in preparation for a major study.

pink sheet For grant applications submitted to the National Institutes of Health, the evaluation form containing the comments and priority score of the peer review panel.

point estimation A statistical estimation procedure in which the researcher uses information from a sample to estimate the single value (statistic) that best represents the value of the population parameter.

population The entire set of individuals (or objects) having some common characteristics (e.g., all RNs in the state of California); sometimes referred to as *universe.*

positive relationship A relationship between two variables in which there is a tendency for high values on one variable to be associated with high values on the other (e.g., as physical activity increases, pulse rate also increases).

positive results Research results that are consistent with the researcher's hypotheses.

positively skewed distribution An asymmetric distribution of values such that a disproportionately high number of cases have low values, that is, fall at the lower end of the distribution; when displayed graphically, the tail points to the right.

positivist paradigm The traditional paradigm underlying the scientific approach, which assumes that there is a fixed, orderly reality that can be objectively studied; often associated with quantitative research.

post hoc test A test for comparing all possible pairs of groups following a significant test of overall group differences (e.g., in an ANOVA).

posttest The collection of data after the introduction of an experimental intervention.

posttest-only design An experimental design in which data are collected from subjects only after the experimental intervention has been introduced; also referred to as an *after-only design.*

power In research design, the ability of a design to detect existing relationships among variables.

power analysis A procedure for estimating either the likelihood of committing a Type II error or sample size requirements.

prediction The use of empirical evidence to make forecasts about how variables of interest will behave in a new setting and with different individuals.

predictive validity The degree to which an instrument can predict some criterion observed at a future time.

preexperimental design A research design that does not include mechanisms to compensate for the absence of either randomization or a control group.

pretest (1) The collection of data before the experimental intervention; sometimes referred to as *baseline data;* (2) the trial administration of a newly developed instrument to identify flaws or assess time requirements.

pretest–posttest design An experimental design in which data are collected from research subjects both before and after the introduction of the experimental intervention; also referred to as a *before–after design.*

primary source First-hand reports of facts, findings, or events; in terms of research, the primary source is the original research report as prepared by the investigator who conducted the study.

principal investigator (PI) The person who is the lead researcher and who will have primary responsibility for overseeing the project.

probability sampling The selection of participants or sampling units from a population using random procedures; examples include simple random sampling, cluster sampling, and systematic sampling.

probing Eliciting more useful or detailed information from a respondent in an interview than was volunteered in the first reply.

problem statement The statement of the research problem, often phrased in the form of a research question.

process analysis An evaluation focusing on the process by which a program or intervention gets implemented and used in practice.

process consent In a qualitative study, an ongoing, transactional process of negotiating consent with study participants, allowing them to play a collaborative role in the decision making regarding their continued participation.

product–moment correlation coefficient (r) The most widely used correlation coefficient, designating the magnitude of relationship between two variables measured on at least an interval scale; also referred to as *Pearson's r.*

program See *computer program.*

projective techniques Methods for measuring psychological attributes (values, attitudes, personality) by providing respondents with unstructured stimuli to which to respond.

prolonged engagement In qualitative research, the investment of sufficient time in the collection of data to have an in-depth understanding of the group under study; a mechanism for achieving data credibility.

proportional hazards model A model applied in multivariate analyses in which independent variables are used to predict the risk (hazard) of experiencing an event at a given point in time.

proportionate sample A sample that results when the researcher samples from different strata of the population in direct proportion to their representation in the population.

proposal A document specifying what the researcher proposes to study; a proposal communicates the research problem, its significance, planned procedures for solving the problem, and, when funding is sought, how much the study will cost.

prospective study A study that begins with an examination of presumed causes (e.g., cigarette smoking) and then goes forward in time to observe presumed effects (e.g., lung cancer).

psychometric evaluation An assessment of the quality of an instrument, based primarily on evidence of its reliability and validity.

psychometrics The theory underlying principles of measurement and the application of the theory in the development of measuring tools.

purposive (purposeful) sampling A type of nonprobability sampling method in which the researcher selects participants for the study on the basis of personal judgment about which ones will be most representative or productive; also referred to as *judgmental sampling*.

Q-by-Q The detailed question-by-question instructions that inform interviewers about the intent of questions in an interview schedule and the type of information that should be obtained from respondents.

Q sort A data collection method in which the participant sorts statements into a number of piles (usually 9 or 11) according to some bipolar dimension (e.g., most like me/least like me; most useful/least useful).

qualitative analysis The organization and interpretation of nonnumeric data for the purpose of discovering important underlying dimensions and patterns of relationships.

qualitative data Information collected in narrative (nonnumeric) form, such as the transcript of an unstructured interview.

qualitative research The investigation of phenomena, typically in an in-depth and holistic fashion, through the collection of rich narrative materials using a flexible research design.

quantitative analysis The manipulation of numeric data through statistical procedures for the purpose of describing phenomena or assessing the magnitude and reliability of relationships among them.

quantitative data Information collected in a quantified (numeric) form.

quantitative research The investigation of phenomena that lend themselves to precise measurement and quantification, often involving a rigorous and controlled design.

quasi-experiment A study in which subjects are not randomly assigned to treatment conditions, but the researcher does manipulate the independent variable and exercises certain controls to enhance the internal validity of the results.

quasi-statistics An "accounting" system used to assess the validity of conclusions derived from qualitative analysis.

questionnaire A method of gathering self-report information from respondents through self-administration of questions in a paper-and-pencil format; also referred to as a self-administered questionnaire or SAQ.

quota sampling The nonrandom selection of participants in which the researcher prespecifies characteristics of the sample to increase its representativeness.

r The symbol typically used to designate a bivariate correlation coefficient, summarizing the magnitude and direction of a relationship between two variables.

R The symbol used to designate the multiple correlation coefficient, indicating the magnitude (but not direction) of the relationship between the dependent variable and multiple independent variables, taken together.

R^2 The squared multiple correlation coefficient, indicating the proportion of variance in the dependent variable accounted for or explained by a group of independent variables.

random assignment The assignment of subjects to treatment conditions in a random manner (i.e., in a manner determined by chance alone); also known as *randomization*.

random number table A table displaying hundreds of digits (from 0 to 9) set up in such a way that each number is equally likely to follow any other; used in randomization and random sampling.

random sampling The selection of a sample such that each member of a population has an equal probability of being included.

randomization The assignment of subjects to treatment conditions in a random manner (i.e., in a manner determined by chance alone); also known as *random assignment*.

range A measure of variability, consisting of the difference between the highest and lowest values in a distribution of scores.

ratio measure A level of measurement in which there are equal distances between score units and which has a true meaningful zero point (e.g., weight).

reactivity A measurement distortion arising from the study participant's awareness of being observed, or, more generally, from the effect of the measurement procedure itself.

readability The ease with which research materials (e.g., a questionnaire) can be read by people with varying reading skills, often empirically determined through readability formulas.

rectangular matrix A matrix of data (variables by subjects) that contains no missing values for any of the variables.

recursive model A path model in which the causal flow is unidirectional, without any feedback loops; opposite of a nonrecursive model.

refereed journal A journal that makes decisions about the acceptance of manuscripts on the basis of recommendations from peer reviewers.

regression A statistical procedure for predicting values of a dependent variable based on the values of one or more independent variables.

relationship A bond or a connection between two or more variables.

reliability The degree of consistency or dependability with which an instrument measures the attribute it is designed to measure.

reliability coefficient A quantitative index, usually ranging in value from .00 to 1.00, that provides an estimate of how reliable an instrument is; computed through such procedures as Cronbach's alpha technique, the split-half technique, test–retest approach, and interrater approaches.

repeated-measures design An experimental design in which one group of subjects is ex-

posed to more than one condition or treatment in random order; sometimes referred to as a *crossover design*.

replication The deliberate repetition of research procedures in a second investigation for the purpose of determining if earlier results can be repeated.

representative sample A sample whose characteristics are highly similar to those of the population from which it is drawn.

research Systematic inquiry that uses orderly, disciplined methods to answer questions or solve problems.

research control See *control*.

research design The overall plan for addressing a research question, including specifications for enhancing the integrity of the study.

research problem A situation involving an enigmatic, perplexing, or conflictful condition that can be investigated through disciplined inquiry.

research proposal See *proposal*.

research question A statement of the specific query the researcher wants to answer to address a research problem.

research report A document that summarizes the main features of a study, including the research question, the methods used to address it, the findings, and the interpretation and implications of the findings.

research utilization The use of some aspect of a scientific investigation in an application unrelated to the original research.

residuals In multiple regression, the error term or unexplained variance.

respondent In a self-report study, the research participant who responds to questions posed by the researcher.

response rate The rate of participation in a study, calculated by dividing the number of persons participating by the number of persons sampled.

response-set bias The measurement error introduced by the tendency of some individuals to respond to items in characteristic ways (e.g., always agreeing), independently of the item's content.

results The answers to research questions, obtained through an analysis of the collected data; in a quantitative study, the information obtained through statistical tests.

retrospective study A study that begins with the manifestation of the dependent variable in the present (e.g., lung cancer) and then links this effect to some presumed cause occurring in the past (e.g., cigarette smoking).

right justification A convention used in data entry, when a fixed format mode is used, such that values are placed as far to the right as possible within a designated field (e.g., the value 1 in a two-column field would be entered 01).

risk/benefit ratio The relative costs and benefits, to an individual subject and to society at large, of participation in a study; also, the relative costs and benefits of implementing an innovation.

rival hypothesis An alternative explanation, competing with the researcher's hypothesis, for understanding the results of a study.

sample A subset of a population selected to participate in a research study.

sampling The process of selecting a portion of the population to represent the entire population.

sampling bias Distortions that arise when a sample is not representative of the population from which it was drawn.

√ **sampling distribution** A theoretical distribution of a statistic, using the values of the statistic computed from an infinite number of samples as the data points in the distribution.

√ **sampling error** The fluctuation of the value of a statistic from one sample to another drawn from the same population.

sampling frame A list of all the elements in the population, from which the sample is drawn.

SAQ See *questionnaire*.

saturation The process of collecting data in a grounded theory study to the point at which a sense of closure is attained because new data yield only redundant information.

scale A composite measure of an attribute, involving the combination of several items that have a logical and empirical relationship to each other, resulting in the assignment of a score to place people on a continuum with respect to the attribute.

scatter plot A graphic representation of the relationship between two variables.

scientific approach A set of orderly, systematic, controlled procedures for acquiring dependable, empirical—and typically quantitative—information; the methodologic approach associated with the positivist paradigm.

scientific merit The degree to which a study is methodologically and conceptually sound; a major criterion for research utilization.

screening instrument The instrument used to determine whether potential subjects for a study meet all the eligibility criteria.

secondary analysis A form of research in which the data collected by one researcher are reanalyzed by another investigator to answer new research questions.

secondary source Second-hand accounts of events or facts; in a research context, a description of a study or studies prepared by someone other than the original researcher.

selective coding The third level of coding in a grounded theory study that involves the process of selecting the core category, systematically integrating relationships between the core category and other categories, and validating those relationships.

selection threat (self-selection) A threat to the internal validity of the study resulting from pre-existing differences between the groups under study; the differences affect the dependent variable in ways extraneous to the effect of the independent variable.

self-determination A person's ability to decide voluntarily whether to participate in a study.

self-report Any procedure for collecting data that involves a direct report of information by the person who is being studied (e.g., by interview or questionnaire).

semantic differential A technique used to measure attitudes that asks respondents to rate a concept of interest on a series of bipolar rating scales.

sensitivity   In measurement, the ability of the measuring tool to make fine discriminations between objects, with differing amounts of the attribute being measured.

setting   The physical location and conditions in which data collection takes place in a study.

significance level   The probability that an observed relationship could be caused by chance (i.e., as a result of sampling error); significance at the .05 level indicates the probability that a relationship of the observed magnitude would be found by chance only 5 times out of 100.

sign system   In structured observational research, a system for listing the behaviors of interest to the researchers, in situations in which the observation focuses on specific behaviors that may or may not be manifested by the study participants.

sign test   A nonparametric test for comparing two paired groups based on the relative ranking of values between the pairs.

simple random sampling   The most basic type of probability sampling, wherein a sampling frame is created by enumerating all members of a population of interest, and then selecting a sample from the sampling frame through completely random procedures.

skewed distribution   The asymmetric distribution of a set of data values around a central point.

snowball sampling   The selection of participants by means of nominations or referrals from earlier participants; also referred to as *network sampling.*

social desirability response set   A bias in self-report instruments created when participants have a tendency to misrepresent their opinions in the direction of answers consistent with prevailing social norms.

software   The instructions for performing operations made to a computer and the documentation for those instructions.

Solomon four-group design   An experimental design that uses a before–after design for one

pair of experimental and control groups and an after-only design for a second pair.

Spearman-Brown prophecy formula   An equation for making corrections to a reliability estimate that was calculated by the split-half method.

Spearman's rank-order correlation (Spearman's rho)   A correlation coefficient indicating the magnitude of a relationship between variables measured on the ordinal scale.

split-half technique   A method for estimating the internal consistency reliability of an instrument by correlating scores on half of the measure with scores on the other half.

standard deviation   The most frequently used statistic for measuring the degree of variability in a set of scores.

standard error   The standard deviation of a sampling distribution, such as the sampling distribution of means.

standard scores   Scores expressed in terms of standard deviations from the mean, with raw scores transformed to have a mean of zero and a standard deviation of one; sometimes referred to as *z* scores.

statement of purpose   A broad declarative statement of the overall goals of a research project.

statistic   An estimate of a parameter, calculated from sample data.

statistical analysis   The organization and analysis of quantitative data using statistical procedures, including both descriptive and inferential statistics.

statistical inference   The process of inferring attributes about the population based on information from a sample, using laws of probability.

statistical significance   A term indicating that the results obtained in an analysis of sample data are unlikely to have been caused by chance, at some specified level of probability.

statistical test   An analytic procedure that allows a researcher to determine the probability that obtained results from a sample reflect true population parameters.

stipend   A monetary payment to individuals participating in a study to serve as an incentive for participation and/or to compensate for time and expenses.

strata Subdivisions of the population according to some characteristic (e.g., males and females); singular is *stratum*.

stratified random sampling The random selection of study participants from two or more strata of the population independently.

structured data collection An approach to collecting information from participants, either through self-report or observations, wherein the researcher determines in advance the categories of interest.

study section Within the National Institutes of Health, a group of peer reviewers that evaluates grant applications in the first phase of the review process.

study participant An individual who participates and provides information in a research investigation.

subgroup effects The differential effect of the independent variable on the dependent variable for various subsets of the sample.

subject An individual who participates and provides data in a study; term used primarily in quantitative research.

summated rating scale See *Likert scale*.

survey research Nonexperimental research that focuses on obtaining information regarding the activities, beliefs, preferences, and attitudes of people through direct questioning of a sample of respondents.

survival analysis A statistical procedure used when the dependent variable represents a time interval between an initial event (e.g., onset of a disease) and an end event (e.g., death); also referred to as *life table analysis*.

symmetric distribution A distribution of values that has two halves that are mirror images of each other; a distribution that is not skewed.

systematic sampling The selection of study participants such that every kth (e.g., every 10th) person (or element) in a sampling frame or list is chosen.

table of random numbers See *random number table*.

table shells A table without any numeric values, prepared in advance of data analysis as a guide to the analyses to be performed.

target population The entire population in which the researcher is interested and to which he or she would like to generalize the results of a study.

test statistic A statistic used to test for the statistical significance of relationships between variables; the sampling distributions of test statistics are known for circumstances in which the null hypothesis is true; examples include chi-square, F-ratio, t-test, and Pearson's r.

test–retest reliability Assessment of the stability of an instrument by correlating the scores obtained on repeated administrations.

testing threat A threat to the internal validity of a study that occurs when the administration of a pretest or baseline measure of a dependent variable results in changes on the variable, apart from any effect of the independent variable.

theme A recurring regularity emerging from an analysis of qualitative data.

theoretical notes In field studies, notes detailing the researcher's interpretations of observed behavior.

theoretical sampling In qualitative studies, the selection of sample members based on emerging findings as the study progresses, to ensure adequate representation of important themes.

theory An abstract generalization that presents a systematic explanation about the relationships among phenomena.

thick description A rich and thorough description of the research context in a qualitative study.

time sampling In observational research, the selection of time periods during which observations will take place.

time series design A quasi-experimental design that involves the collection of information over an extended period of time, with multiple data collection points both before and after the introduction of a treatment.

topic guide   A list of broad question areas to be covered in a semi-structured interview or focus group interview.

transferability   (1) A criterion for evaluating the quality of qualitative data, referring to the extent to which the findings from the data can be transferred to other settings or groups—analogous to generalizability; (2) also, a criterion used in an implementation assessment of a utilization project.

treatment   The experimental intervention under study; the condition being manipulated.

treatment group   The group receiving the intervention being tested; the experimental group.

trend study   A form of longitudinal study in which different samples from a population are studied over time with respect to some phenomenon (e.g., annual Gallup polls on abortion attitudes).

triangulation   The use of multiple methods or perspectives to collect and interpret data about some phenomenon, to converge on an accurate representation of reality.

true score   A hypothetical score that would be obtained if a measure were infallible; the portion of the observed score not due to random error or measurement bias.

trustworthiness   A term used in the evaluation of qualitative data, assessed using the criteria of credibility, transferability, dependability, and confirmability.

t-test   A parametric statistical test used for analyzing the difference between two means.

Type I error   An error created by rejecting the null hypothesis when it is true (i.e., the researcher concludes that a relationship exists when in fact it does not).

Type II error   An error created by accepting the null hypothesis when it is false (i.e., the researcher concludes that *no* relationship exists when in fact it does).

unimodal distribution   A distribution of values with one peak (high frequency).

unit of analysis   The basic unit or focus of a researcher's analysis; in nursing research, the unit of analysis is typically the individual study participant.

univariate descriptive study   A study that gathers information on the occurrence, frequency of occurrence, or average value of the variables of interest, one variable at a time, without focusing on interrelationships among variables.

univariate statistics   Statistical procedures for analyzing a single variable for purposes of description.

unstructured interview   An oral self-report in which the researcher asks a respondent questions without having a predetermined plan regarding the specific content or flow of information to be gathered.

unstructured observation   The collection of descriptive information through direct observation, whereby the observer is guided by some general research questions but does not follow a prespecified plan for observing, enumerating, or recording the information.

utilization   See *research utilization.*

utilization criteria   The criteria that are brought to bear in considering whether an innovation is amenable to utilization in a practice setting; includes the criteria of clinical relevance, scientific merit, and implementation potential.

validity   The degree to which an instrument measures what it is intended to measure.

validity coefficient   A quantitative index, usually ranging in value from .00 to 1.00, that provides an estimate of how valid an instrument is; usually computed in conjunction with the criterion-related approach to validating an instrument.

variability   The degree to which values on a set of scores are widely different or dispersed.

variable   An attribute of a person or object that varies, that is, takes on different values (e.g., body temperature, age, heart rate).

variance   A measure of variability or dispersion, equal to the standard deviation squared.

vignette   A brief description of an event, person, or situation to which respondents are asked to react and to describe their reactions.

visual analogue scale   A scaling procedure used to measure a variety of clinical symptoms (e.g., pain, fatigue) by having people indicate on a straight line the intensity of the attribute being measured.

vulnerable subjects   Special groups of people whose rights in research studies need special protection because of their inability to provide meaningful informed consent or because their circumstances place them at higher-than-average-risk of adverse effects; examples include young children, the mentally retarded, and unconscious patients.

weighting   A correction procedure used to arrive at population values when a disproportionate sampling design has been used.

Wilcoxon signed ranks test   A nonparametric statistical test for comparing two paired groups, based on the relative ranking of values between the pairs.

wild code   A coded value that is not legitimate within the coding scheme for that data set.

Wilk's lambda (λ)   An index used in discriminant function analysis to indicate the proportion of variance in the dependent variable *un*accounted for by predictors; $\lambda = 1 - R^2$.

windows   A mechanism for dividing a computer's display screen into rectangles for viewing two or more applications or parts of a single application at the same time.

within-subjects design   A research design in which a single group of subjects is compared under different conditions or at different points in time (e.g., before and after surgery).

z score   A standard score, expressed in terms of standard deviations from the mean.

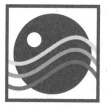

APPENDIX **A**

Human Subject Protocol*

(1) Describe the characteristics of the subject population, such as their anticipated number, age ranges, sex, ethnic background, and health status. Identify the criteria for inclusion or exclusion. Explain the rationale for the use of special classes of subjects, such as fetuses, pregnant women, children, institutionalized mentally disabled, prisoners, or others who are likely to be vulnerable.

1. Characteristics of the population. The sample for the proposed research will consist of approximately 300 women aged 18–22 who first became pregnant before their eighteenth birthday and who subsequently delivered a child. The women were interviewed initially in 1980–1981 as part of an evaluation of the special program for teenage mothers—Project Redirection. At the time of the initial interview, the women were residing in 6 communities: Phoenix, San Antonio, Fresno, Riverside (CA), Harlem and Bedford-Stuyvesant (NY).

---

*Grant applications under the Public Health Service (see Chapter 27) must include a section on the protection of human subjects, which must address six specific questions. This appendix contains the actual responses to those six questions for a funded study of parenting among low-income teenage mothers. Such a protocol often serves as the focal point of an evaluation by an Institutional Review Board.

The initial eligibility criteria for the Project Redirection study are indicated below:
*   either pregnant or a parent;
*   living in a household that met certain poverty guidelines;
*   17 years old or younger; and
*   without a high school diploma or GED certificate.

The sample size for the proposed study is based on the teens in the six sites who completed three rounds of interviews thus far:

• Phoenix, AZ	81
• San Antonio, TX	86
• Harlem, NY	38
• Bedford-Stuyvesant, NY	54
• Riverside, CA	32
• Fresno, CA	38
TOTAL	329

(2) Identify the sources of research material obtained from individually identifiable living human subjects in the form of specimens, records, or data. Indicate whether the material or data will be obtained specifically for research purposes or whether use will be made of existing specimens, records, or data.

2. Sources of Data. Three rounds of interviews have already been completed with the research sample, and information from

these earlier interviews will be used in the present study. Additionally, data will be gathered in a fourth round of in-home interviews, to be collected in 1986–1987 if the proposed research is funded. Data will be gathered by a combined interview/observation approach, using a specially constructed interview schedule and several standardized instruments.

(3) Describe plans for the recruitment of subjects and the consent procedures to be followed, including the circumstances under which consent will be sought and obtained, who will seek it, the nature of the information to be provided to prospective subjects and the method of documenting consent.

3.   Recruitment and Consent. Subjects have already been recruited for this study—i.e., they were participants in three earlier rounds of interviewing as part of another research project. For the present study, letters will be mailed to respondents at their most recently known address and they will be asked to verify their current address and telephone number (if available). For respondents for whom there is no return postcard, tracking procedures to ascertain the respondents' present address will be undertaken.

For those respondents who are located through these procedures, an interviewer will contact them and explain the general nature and purpose of the research, the confidential nature of the interviews, the time commitments, and the stipend ($25) that would be paid to them in compensation for their time. The respondents will also be told that their children should be present at the time of the interview, so that appropriate observations can be made. Upon consent to be included in this wave of the research, an interview will be scheduled. At the time of the interview, the interviewers, who will receive extensive train-

ing for this project, will repeat the description of the research prior to commencing. The respondent will be told that her participation is voluntary; that no information she gives will be divulged to anyone other than research staff; that her participation will have no effect on any services that she might be receiving; that she can stop the interview at any time; and that she can decline to answer individual questions if she so chooses. This information will be included in a Consent Form, which each respondent will be requested to sign prior to the interview.

(4) Describe any potential risks—physical, psychological, social, legal, or other—and assess their likelihood and seriousness. Where appropriate, describe alternative treatments and procedures that might be advantageous to the subjects.

4.   Risks. There is relatively minor risk, in interviewing these young women about their family life, that the interview will be stressful to them. Furthermore, our procedures are designed to minimize any discomfort on the respondents' parts. We will use female interviewers who will be trained not only with respect to the research instruments but also with regard to the stresses of parenthood in disadvantaged populations. In the event of any signs of distress during the interview, interviewers will be instructed to refrain from further questioning, proceeding only if the respondent desires. Our experience in dealing with this sample leads us to believe, however, that the women are more likely to find a conversation with an objective but sympathetic listener therapeutic rather than stressful.

(5) Describe the procedures for protecting against or minimizing any potential risks, including risks to confidentiality, and assess their likely effectiveness. Where ap-

propriate, discuss provisions for insuring necessary medical or professional intervention in the event of adverse effects to the subjects. Also, where appropriate, describe the provisions for monitoring the data collected to insure the safety of subjects.

5. Confidentiality. Measures to protect the confidentiality of the respondents will be instituted throughout the course of this project. Data security procedures to protect the identity of individuals will be implemented during interviewer training, data collection, data analysis, and after completion of the project. Respondents will be fully informed as to these confidentiality procedures at the outset of the interview.

The issue of confidentiality and data security will be stressed during the training of data collectors. The need for confidentiality and the specific policies and procedures related to this issue will be explained to all interviewers. Thereafter, the interviewers will be required to sign a confidentiality statement prior to conducting interviews.

All identifying information will be removed from the interview schedule upon receipt from the field staff. Names, addresses, telephone numbers and any other identifying information will be recorded *only* on a cover sheet of the interview. The interview form itself, which will be kept in a locked file, will bear only a numeric identification code. The cover sheet will be removed from completed interviews and kept in a separate locked file. Access to this file will be restricted to key project personnel.

(6) Discuss why the risks to subjects are reasonable in relation to the anticipated benefits to subjects and in relation to the importance of the knowledge that may reasonably be expected to result.

6. Anticipated Benefits. In theory, no direct benefits to the respondents are anticipated. However, as mentioned above, we have found that respondents often enjoy the interview experience. Nevertheless, the primary benefit expected from the project is indirect. The study is expected to generate knowledge that will be useful in the formulation of social policy and in the design and delivery of appropriate services for young disadvantaged mothers and their children. Since we believe that the risks to subjects are negligible, we believe that the benefits provide justification for the conduct of this research.

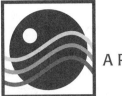

A P P E N D I X **B**

Statistical Tables

TABLE B-1. Distribution of *t* Probability

	LEVEL OF SIGNIFICANCE FOR ONE-TAILED TEST					
	.10	*.05*	*.025*	*.01*	*.005*	*.0005*
			Level of Significance for Two-Tailed Test			
DF	*.20*	*.10*	*.05*	*.02*	*.01*	*.001*
1	3.078	6.314	12.706	31.821	63.657	636.619
2	1.886	2.920	4.303	6.965	9.925	31.598
3	1.638	2.353	3.182	4.541	5.841	12.941
4	1.533	2.132	2.776	3.747	4.604	8.610
5	1.476	2.015	2.571	3.376	4.032	6.859
6	1.440	1.953	2.447	3.143	3.707	5.959
7	1.415	1.895	2.365	2.998	3.449	5.405
8	1.397	1.860	2.306	2.896	3.355	5.041
9	1.383	1.833	2.262	2.821	3.250	4.781
10	1.372	1.812	2.228	2.765	3.169	4.587
11	1.363	1.796	2.201	2.718	3.106	4.437
12	1.356	1.782	2.179	2.681	3.055	4.318
13	1.350	1.771	2.160	2.650	3.012	4.221
14	1.345	1.761	2.145	2.624	2.977	4.140
15	1.341	1.753	2.131	2.602	2.947	4.073
16	1.337	1.746	2.120	2.583	2.921	4.015
17	1.333	1.740	2.110	2.567	2.898	3.965
18	1.330	1.734	2.101	2.552	2.878	3.922
19	1.328	1.729	2.093	2.539	2.861	3.883
20	1.325	1.725	2.086	2.528	2.845	3.850
21	1.323	1.721	2.080	2.518	2.831	3.819
22	1.321	1.717	2.074	2.508	2.819	3.792
23	1.319	1.714	2.069	2.500	2.807	3.767
24	1.318	1.711	2.064	2.492	2.797	3.745
25	1.316	1.708	2.060	2.485	2.787	3.725
26	1.315	1.706	2.056	2.479	2.779	3.707
27	1.314	1.703	2.052	2.473	2.771	3.690
28	1.313	1.701	2.048	2.467	2.763	3.674
29	1.311	1.699	2.045	2.462	2.756	3.659
30	1.310	1.697	2.042	2.457	2.750	3.646
40	1.303	1.684	2.021	2.423	2.704	3.551
60	1.296	1.671	2.000	2.390	2.660	3.460
120	1.289	1.658	1.980	2.358	2.617	3.373
∞	1.282	1.645	1.960	2.326	2.576	3.291

TABLE B-2. Significant Values of *F*
$\alpha = .05$ (Two-Tailed) $\alpha = .025$ (one-tailed)

$\frac{df_B}{df_w}$	1	2	3	4	5	6	8	12	24	∞
1	161.4	199.5	215.7	224.6	230.2	234.0	238.9	243.9	249.0	254.3
2	18.51	19.00	19.16	19.25	19.30	19.33	19.37	19.41	19.45	19.50
3	10.13	9.55	9.28	9.12	9.01	8.94	8.84	8.74	8.64	8.53
4	7.71	6.94	6.59	6.39	6.26	6.16	6.04	5.91	5.77	5.63
5	6.61	5.79	5.41	5.19	5.05	4.95	4.82	4.68	4.53	4.36
6	5.99	5.14	4.76	4.53	4.39	4.28	4.15	4.00	3.84	3.67
7	5.59	4.74	4.35	4.12	3.97	3.87	3.73	3.57	3.41	3.23
8	5.32	4.46	4.07	3.84	3.69	3.58	3.44	3.28	3.12	2.93
9	5.12	4.26	3.86	3.63	3.48	3.37	3.23	3.07	2.90	2.71
10	4.96	4.10	3.71	3.48	3.33	3.22	3.07	2.91	2.74	2.54
11	4.84	3.98	3.59	3.36	3.20	3.09	2.95	2.79	2.61	2.40
12	4.75	3.88	3.49	3.26	3.11	3.00	2.85	2.69	2.50	2.30
13	4.67	3.80	3.41	3.18	3.02	2.92	2.77	2.60	2.42	2.21
14	4.60	3.74	3.34	3.11	2.96	2.85	2.70	2.53	2.35	2.13
15	4.54	3.68	3.29	3.06	2.90	2.79	2.64	2.48	2.29	2.07
16	4.49	3.63	3.24	3.01	2.85	2.74	2.59	2.42	2.24	2.01
17	4.45	3.59	3.20	2.96	2.81	2.70	2.55	2.38	2.19	1.96
18	4.41	3.55	3.16	2.93	2.77	2.66	2.51	2.34	2.15	1.92
19	4.38	3.52	3.13	2.90	2.74	2.63	2.48	2.31	2.11	1.88
20	4.35	3.49	3.10	2.87	2.71	2.60	2.45	2.28	2.08	1.84
21	4.32	3.47	3.07	2.84	2.68	2.57	2.42	2.25	2.05	1.81
22	4.30	3.44	3.05	2.82	2.66	2.55	2.40	2.23	2.03	1.78
23	4.28	3.42	3.03	2.80	2.64	2.53	2.38	2.20	2.00	1.76
24	4.26	3.40	3.01	2.78	2.62	2.51	2.36	2.18	1.98	1.73
25	4.24	3.38	2.99	2.76	2.60	2.49	2.34	2.16	1.96	1.71
26	4.22	3.37	2.98	2.74	2.59	2.47	2.32	2.15	1.95	1.69
27	4.21	3.35	2.96	2.73	2.57	2.46	2.30	2.13	1.93	1.67
28	4.20	3.34	2.95	2.71	2.56	2.44	2.29	2.12	1.91	1.65
29	4.18	3.33	2.93	2.70	2.54	2.43	2.28	2.10	1.90	1.64
30	4.17	3.32	2.92	2.69	2.53	2.42	2.27	2.09	1.89	1.62
40	4.08	3.23	2.84	2.61	2.45	2.34	2.18	2.00	1.79	1.51
60	4.00	3.15	2.76	2.52	2.37	2.25	2.10	1.92	1.70	1.39
120	3.92	3.07	2.68	2.45	2.29	2.17	2.02	1.83	1.61	1.25
∞	3.84	2.99	2.60	2.37	2.21	2.09	1.94	1.75	1.52	1.00

(continued)

TABLE B-2.   Significant Values of F
$\alpha = .01$ (Two-Tailed) (Continued) $\alpha = .005$ (one-tailed)

df_B df_W	1	2	3	4	5	6	8	12	24	∞
1	4052	4999	5403	5625	5764	5859	5981	6106	6234	6366
2	98.49	99.00	99.17	99.25	99.30	99.33	99.36	99.42	99.46	99.50
3	34.12	30.81	29.46	28.71	28.24	27.91	27.49	27.05	26.60	26.12
4	21.20	18.00	16.69	15.98	15.52	15.21	14.80	14.37	13.93	13.46
5	16.26	13.27	12.06	11.39	10.97	10.67	10.29	9.89	9.47	9.02
6	13.74	10.92	9.78	9.15	8.75	8.47	8.10	7.72	7.31	6.88
7	12.25	9.55	8.45	7.85	7.46	7.19	6.84	6.47	6.07	5.65
8	11.26	8.65	7.59	7.01	6.63	6.37	6.03	5.67	5.28	4.86
9	10.56	8.02	6.99	6.42	6.06	5.80	5.47	5.11	4.73	4.31
10	10.04	7.56	6.55	5.99	5.64	5.39	5.06	4.71	4.33	3.91
11	9.65	7.20	6.22	5.67	5.32	5.07	4.74	4.40	4.02	3.60
12	9.33	6.93	5.95	5.41	5.06	4.82	4.50	4.16	3.78	3.36
13	9.07	6.70	5.74	5.20	4.86	4.62	4.30	3.96	3.59	3.16
14	8.86	6.51	5.56	5.03	4.69	4.46	4.14	3.80	3.43	3.00
15	8.68	6.36	5.42	4.89	4.56	4.32	4.00	3.67	3.29	2.87
16	8.53	6.23	5.29	4.77	4.44	4.20	3.89	3.55	3.18	2.75
17	8.40	6.11	5.18	4.67	4.34	4.10	3.78	3.45	3.08	2.65
18	8.28	6.01	5.09	4.58	4.29	4.01	3.71	3.37	3.00	2.57
19	8.18	5.93	5.01	4.50	4.17	3.94	3.63	3.30	2.92	2.49
20	8.10	5.85	4.94	4.43	4.10	3.87	3.56	3.23	2.86	2.42
21	8.02	5.78	4.87	4.37	4.04	3.81	3.51	3.17	2.80	2.36
22	7.94	5.72	4.82	4.31	3.99	3.76	3.45	3.12	2.75	2.31
23	7.88	5.66	4.76	4.26	3.94	3.71	3.41	3.07	2.70	2.26
24	7.82	5.61	4.72	4.22	3.90	3.67	3.36	3.03	2.66	2.21
25	7.77	5.57	4.68	4.18	3.86	3.63	3.32	2.99	2.62	2.17
26	7.72	5.53	4.64	4.14	3.82	3.59	3.29	2.96	2.58	2.13
27	7.68	5.49	4.60	4.11	3.78	3.56	3.26	2.93	2.55	2.10
28	7.64	5.45	4.57	4.07	3.75	3.53	3.23	2.90	2.52	2.06
29	7.60	5.42	4.54	4.04	3.73	3.50	3.20	2.87	2.49	2.03
30	7.56	5.39	4.51	4.02	3.70	3.47	3.17	2.84	2.47	2.01
40	7.31	5.18	4.31	3.83	3.51	3.29	2.998	2.66	2.29	1.80
60	7.08	4.98	4.13	3.65	3.34	3.12	2.82	2.50	2.12	1.60
120	6.85	4.79	3.95	3.48	3.17	2.96	2.66	2.34	1.95	1.38
∞	6.64	4.60	3.78	3.32	3.02	2.80	2.51	2.18	1.79	1.00

(continued)

TABLE B-2. Significant Values of *F*

α = .001 (Two-Tailed) (Continued)   α = .0005 (one-tailed)

df_B / df_w	1	2	3	4	5	6	8	12	24	∞
1	405284	500000	540379	562500	576405	585937	598144	610667	623497	636619
2	998.5	999.0	999.2	999.2	999.3	999.3	999.4	999.4	999.5	999.5
3	167.5	148.5	141.1	137.1	134.6	132.8	130.6	128.3	125.9	123.5
4	74.14	61.25	56.18	53.44	51.71	50.53	49.00	47.41	45.77	44.05
5	47.04	36.61	33.20	31.09	29.75	28.84	27.64	26.42	25.14	23.78
6	35.51	27.00	23.70	21.90	20.81	20.03	19.03	17.99	16.89	15.75
7	29.22	21.69	18.77	17.19	16.21	15.52	14.63	13.71	12.73	11.69
8	25.42	18.49	15.83	14.39	13.49	12.86	17.04	11.19	10.30	9.34
9	22.86	16.39	13.90	12.56	11.71	11.13	10.37	9.57	8.72	7.81
10	21.04	14.91	12.55	11.28	10.48	9.92	9.20	8.45	7.64	6.76
11	19.69	13.81	11.56	10.35	9.58	9.05	8.35	7.63	6.85	6.00
12	18.64	12.97	10.80	9.63	8.89	8.38	7.71	7.00	6.25	5.42
13	17.81	12.31	10.21	9.07	8.35	7.86	7.21	6.52	5.78	4.97
14	17.14	11.78	9.73	8.62	7.92	7.43	6.80	6.13	5.41	4.60
15	16.59	11.34	9.34	8.25	7.57	7.09	6.47	5.81	5.10	4.31
16	16.12	10.97	9.00	7.94	7.27	6.81	6.19	5.55	4.85	4.06
17	15.72	10.66	8.73	7.68	7.02	6.56	5.96	5.32	4.63	3.85
18	15.38	10.39	8.49	7.46	6.81	6.35	5.76	5.13	4.45	3.67
19	15.08	10.16	8.28	7.26	6.61	6.18	5.59	4.97	4.29	3.52
20	14.82	9.95	8.10	7.10	6.46	6.02	5.44	4.82	4.15	3.38
21	14.59	9.77	7.94	6.95	6.32	5.88	5.31	4.70	4.03	3.26
22	14.38	9.61	7.80	6.81	6.19	5.76	5.19	4.58	3.92	3.15
23	14.19	9.47	7.67	6.69	6.08	5.65	5.09	4.48	3.82	3.05
24	14.03	9.34	7.55	6.59	5.98	5.55	4.99	4.39	3.74	2.97
25	13.88	9.22	7.45	6.49	5.88	5.46	4.91	4.31	3.66	2.89
26	13.74	9.12	7.36	6.41	5.80	5.38	4.83	4.24	3.59	2.82
27	13.61	9.02	7.27	6.33	5.73	5.31	4.76	4.17	3.52	2.75
28	13.50	8.93	7.19	6.25	5.66	5.24	4.69	4.11	3.46	2.70
29	13.39	8.85	7.12	6.19	5.59	5.18	4.64	4.05	3.41	2.64
30	13.29	8.77	7.05	6.12	5.53	5.12	4.58	4.00	3.36	2.59
40	12.61	8.25	6.60	5.70	5.13	4.73	4.21	3.64	3.01	2.23
60	11.97	7.76	6.17	5.31	4.76	4.37	3.87	3.31	2.69	1.90
120	11.38	7.31	5.79	4.95	4.42	4.04	3.55	3.02	2.40	1.56
∞	10.83	6.91	5.42	4.62	4.10	3.74	3.27	2.74	2.13	1.00

TABLE B-3.   Distribution of χ^2 Probability

DF	LEVEL OF SIGNIFICANCE				
	.10	.05	.02	.01	.001
1	2.71	3.84	5.41	6.63	10.83
2	4.61	5.99	7.82	9.21	13.82
3	6.25	7.82	9.84	11.34	16.27
4	7.78	9.49	11.67	13.28	18.46
5	9.24	11.07	13.39	15.09	20.52
6	10.64	12.59	15.03	16.81	22.46
7	12.02	14.07	16.62	18.48	24.32
8	13.36	15.51	18.17	20.09	26.12
9	14.68	16.92	19.68	21.67	27.88
10	15.99	18.31	21.16	23.21	29.59
11	17.28	19.68	22.62	24.72	31.26
12	18.55	21.03	24.05	26.22	32.91
13	19.81	22.36	25.47	27.69	34.53
14	21.06	23.68	26.87	29.14	36.12
15	22.31	25.00	28.26	30.58	37.70
16	23.54	26.30	29.63	32.00	39.25
17	24.77	27.59	31.00	33.41	40.79
18	25.99	28.87	32.35	34.81	42.31
19	27.20	30.14	33.69	36.19	43.82
20	28.41	31.41	35.02	37.57	45.32
21	29.62	32.67	36.34	38.93	46.80
22	30.81	33.92	37.66	40.29	48.27
23	32.01	35.17	38.97	41.64	49.73
24	33.20	36.42	40.27	42.98	51.18
25	34.38	37.65	41.57	44.31	52.62
26	35.56	38.89	42.86	45.64	54.05
27	36.74	40.11	44.14	46.96	55.48
28	37.92	41.34	45.42	48.28	56.89
29	39.09	42.56	46.69	49.59	58.30
30	40.26	43.77	47.96	50.89	59.70

TABLE B-4. Significant Values of the Correlation Coefficient

	LEVEL OF SIGNIFICANCE FOR ONE-TAILED TEST				
	.05	*.025*	*.01*	*.005*	*.0005*
	Level of Significance for Two-Tailed Test				
df	*.1*	*.05*	*.02*	*.01*	*.001*
1	.98769	.99692	.999507	.999877	.9999988
2	.90000	.95000	.98000	.990000	.99900
3	.8054	.8783	.93433	.95873	.99116
4	.7293	.8114	.8822	.91720	.97406
5	.6694	.7545	.8329	.8745	.95074
6	.6215	.7067	.7887	.8343	.92493
7	.5822	.6664	.7498	.7977	.8982
8	.5494	.6319	.7155	.7646	.8721
9	.5214	.6021	.6851	.7348	.8471
10	.4973	.5760	.6581	.7079	.8233
11	.4762	.5529	.6339	.6835	.8010
12	.4575	.5324	.6120	.6614	.7800
13	.4409	.5139	.5923	.5411	.7603
14	.4259	.4973	.5742	.6226	.7420
15	.4124	.4821	.5577	.6055	.7246
16	.4000	.4683	.5425	.5897	.7084
17	.3887	.4555	.5285	.5751	.6932
18	.3783	.4438	.5155	.5614	.5687
19	.3687	.4329	.5034	.5487	.6652
20	.3598	.4227	.4921	.5368	.6524
25	.3233	.3809	.4451	.5869	.5974
30	.2960	.3494	.4093	.4487	.5541
35	.2746	.3246	.3810	.4182	.5189
40	.2573	.3044	.3578	.3932	.4896
45	.2428	.2875	.3384	.3721	.4648
50	.2306	.2732	.3218	.3541	.4433
60	.2108	.2500	.2948	.3248	.4078
70	.1954	.2319	.2737	.3017	.3799
80	.1829	.2172	.2565	.2830	.3568
90	.1726	.2050	.2422	.2673	.3375
100	.1638	.1946	.2301	.2540	.3211

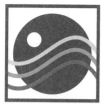

SUBJECT INDEX

Page numbers in bold type indicate glossary entries.

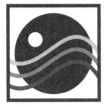

NAME INDEX

A

Abbott, R. D., 235
Acton, G.J., 71
Adler, L. M., 364
Ahijevych, K., 443
Ailinger, R. L., 113, 302
Ainsworth-Vaughan, N., 252
Aish, A. E., 113
Ajzen, I., 116, 117
Alcott, L. M., 249
Alcozer, F. R., 302
Aldrich, M. S., 159
Alexander, D. J., 378
Algase, D. L., 375
Allan, J. D., 302, 612
Allen, M., 123
Allison, P. D., 533
Alpert-Gillis, L. J., 235
Amsel, R., 166, 344
Anastasi, A., 401
Anderson, B., 113
Anderson, D.C., 16
Anderson, G., 609
Anderson, G.C., 31
Anderson, K. H., 115
Andrews, C.M., 44
Andrews, H. A., 112
Angelini, P. J., 166
Armstrong, M. L., 443
Armstrong, S., 203, 204
Armstrong-Persily, C., 270
Arnaud, S. S., 379
Artinian, B.M., 72
Ashcroft, T., 60
Ashley, N. D. 424
Astrom, G., 242
Atkinson, 246
Austin, J. K., 608
Auvil-Novak, S. E., 121

B

Bach, C. A., 617
Baggs, J. G., 302
Baier, M., 115
Baigis-Smith, J., 204
Bailey, D., 375
Baker, H. M., 252

Ballantyne, A., 355
Banasik, J. L., 386
Bandura, A., 123
Bargagliotti, L. A., 259
Barham, L.N., 100
Barkman, A., 568
Barroso, J., 159
Bartlett, D.B., 376
Barton, J. A., 582
Bassford, T. L., 612
Bearinger, L. H., 165
Beaton, R. D., 345, 539
Beattie, E., 375
Beck, C., 203, 364
Becker, H. S., 582
Becker, M., 116
Becker, M. A., 491
Becker, P. T., 375
Beech, B., 208
Beel-Bates, C. A., 375
Belknap, D.C., 16, 185
Benner, P., 121, 332
Bennett, S. J., 424
Benoliel, J. Q., 608
Bensley, L., 261
Berelson, B., 209
Berg, J., 158, 539
Bergquist, S., 665
Berk, R. A., 204
Berkey, N., 116
Berman, R. L., 612
Bernardo, M. L., 114
Bernhard, L. A., 464
Bernstein, I. H., 415
Berry, R. A., 502
Besch, C. L., 209
Betz, M. L., 204
Betz, N. E., 401
Beyea, S. C., 656
Bingle, J. D., 646, 649, 651
Bishop, B. A., 235
Blalock, H. M., 529
Blane, C., 364
Blieley, A., 355
Blixen, C. E., 210
Blum, R. W., 165
Bodensteiner, A., 616
Boehm, J., 665
Bond, E. F., 389

Bookbinder, M., 192
Borum, J., 199
Bos, H., 267
Bostrom, J., 204, 651, 653, 655
Bostrom-Ezrati, J., 540
Bott, M., 272
Bott, M. J., 609
Bottorff, J. L., 110, 252
Boumans, N. P. G., 301
Bourbonnais, F. F., 113
Bournaki, M. C., 114, 377
Bowen, J. M., 390
Bowlby, J., 123
Bowman, J. M., 116
Boyette, B. G., 158
Boyle, R., 111
Bradley, C., 636
Bradley, C. B., 199
Brandt, K.A., 44
Brecht, M. L., 443, 539
Brengelmann, G. L., 389
Brett, J. L. L., 648, 657
Brewer, J., 259, 263
Bridge, R. G., 400
Bright, M. A., 587
Brink, P. J., 251
Britt, J., 502
Brittin, M., 185
Brodsky, M.S., 101
Brooks, E. M., 113
Brooks, J. A., 344
Brown, E.L., 5
Brown, J. K., 206, 390
Brown, J. S., 290
Brown, L. D., 502
Brown, S. T., 116
Bryan, J. L., 364
Buchanan, L. M., 344
Buchko, B. L., 235
Buchwald, D. S., 390
Buckwalter, K. C., 377
Budin, W.C., 71
Buhle, E. L., 597
Bull, M.J., 18
Burgener, S. C., 326, 375
Burke, S.O., 91
Burns, D., 665
Burns, K.J., 60
Burr, R., 344